Bratton's Family Medicine

BOARD REVIEW

Editor-in-Chief
Robert A. Baldor, MD, FAAFP

EDITION

5

Bratton's Family Medicine

BOARD REVIEW

Editor-in-Chief

Robert A. Baldor, MD, FAAFP
Professor and Vice-Chair, Educational Affairs
Department of Family Medicine and Community Health
University of Massachusetts Medical School/UMass Memorial HealthCare
Worcester, Massachusetts

Section Editors

Margarita C. Castro-Zarraga, MD
Assistant Professor and Residency
  Advocate for Underserved
  Populations
UMass/Fitchburg Family Medicine
  Residency
University of Massachusetts Medical
  School/UMass Memorial HealthCare
Worcester, Massachusetts

Anita Kostecki, MD
Assistant Professor and Director for
  FM Maternal & Newborn Inpatient
  Services
Department of Family Medicine &
  Community Health
University of Massachusetts Medical
  School
Worcester, Massachusetts

Christine Runyan, PhD, ABPP
Clinical Associate Professor and Director
  Behavioral Science
UMass/Worcester Family Medicine Residency
University of Massachusetts Medical School/
  UMass Memorial HealthCare
Worcester, Massachusetts

Felix B. Chang, MD, DABMA
Assistant Professor and Director Inpatient Medicine
UMass/Fitchburg Family Medicine
  Residency
University of Massachusetts Medical
  School/UMass Memorial HealthCare
Worcester, Massachusetts

Frank J. Domino, MD
Professor and Predoctoral Director
Department of Family Medicine &
  Community Health
University of Massachusetts
  Medical School/UMass Memorial
  HealthCare
Worcester, Massachusetts

5

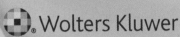
. Wolters Kluwer
Health

Philadelphia • Baltimore • New York • London
Buenos Aires • Hong Kong • Sydney • Tokyo

Executive Editor: Rebecca Gaertner
Senior Product Development Editor: Kristina Oberle
Production Project Manager: Alicia Jackson
Senior Manufacturing Manager: Beth Welsh
Marketing Manager: Stephanie Manzo
Design Coordinator: Joan Wendt
Production Service: S4Carlisle Publishing Services

© 2014 Wolters Kluwer Health
Two Commerce Square
2001 Market Street
Philadelphia, PA 19103 USA
LWW.com

3rd edition, © 2011 by Lippincott Williams & Wilkins, a Wolters Kluwer Business
2nd edition, © 2002 by Lippincott Williams & Wilkins
1st edition, © 1998 by Lippincott Williams & Wilkins

Printed in China

Library of Congress Cataloging-in-Publication Data

Bratton's family medicine board review / editor, Robert A. Baldor ; section editors, Margarita C. Castro-Zarraga, Anita Kostecki, Christine Runyan, Felix B. Chang, Frank J. Domino. — Fifth edition.
    p. ; cm.
Family medicine board review
Includes bibliographical references and index.
ISBN 978-1-4511-9078-6
I. Baldor, Robert A., editor of compilation.   II. Title: Family medicine board review.
[DNLM: 1. Family Practice—Examination Questions. WB 18.2]
RC58
610.76—dc23

2013051127

Care has been taken to confirm the accuracy of the information presented and to describe generally accepted practices. However, the authors, editors, and publisher are not responsible for errors or omissions or for any consequences from application of the information in this book and make no warranty, expressed or implied, with respect to the currency, completeness, or accuracy of the contents of the publication. Application of the information in a particular situation remains the professional responsibility of the practitioner.

The authors, editors, and publisher have exerted every effort to ensure that drug selection and dosage set forth in this text are in accordance with current recommendations and practice at the time of publication. However, in view of ongoing research, changes in government regulations, and the constant flow of information relating to drug therapy and drug reactions, the reader is urged to check the package insert for each drug for any change in indications and dosage and for added warnings and precautions. This is particularly important when the recommended agent is a new or infrequently employed drug.

Some drugs and medical devices presented in the publication have Food and Drug Administration (FDA) clearance for limited use in restricted research settings. It is the responsibility of the health care provider to ascertain the FDA status of each drug or device planned for use in their clinical practice.

To purchase additional copies of this book, call our customer service department at (800) 638-3030 or fax orders to (301) 223-2320. International customers should call (301) 223-2300.

Visit Lippincott Williams & Wilkins on the Internet: at LWW.com. Lippincott Williams & Wilkins customer service representatives are available from 8:30 am to 6 pm, EST.

10 9 8 7 6 5 4 3 2 1

Dedication

I'd like to dedicate this 5th edition to Robert L. Bratton, MD, the initial author who conceptualized and developed this board review text. This book has been an incredibly helpful tool for residents and practicing physicians to use while preparing for their ABFM board certification examinations. In taking over as the editor of this book, I have tried to match Dr. Bratton's standard in providing realistic questions along with insightful answers to help the readers further their education as they prepare for the board exams.

I'd also like to recognize my fellow section editors (Drs. Frank Domino, Tina Runyan, Anita Kostecki, Felix Chang, and Margarita Castro-Zarraga), all key members of the University of Massachusetts family medicine residency faculty, who have committed their professional careers to educating the next generation of family physicians. I applaud their interest in constantly improving the quality of medical education and sincerely thank them for their efforts in helping me update this 5th edition.

Finally, this dedication would not be complete without my acknowledgment of the incredible support provided to me by my amazing wife and devoted partner Rebecca. I could not have completed this task without her understanding and tolerance for the many hours spent working on this book; she is truly deserving of my gratitude and heartfelt thanks!

Robert A. Baldor, MD

Contributing Authors

Mohammad Alhabbal, MD, FHM
Assistant Professor
Department of Family Medicine & Community Health
University of Massachusetts Medical School/UMassMemorial
    HealthCare
Worcester, Massachusetts

Philip Bolduc, MD
Assistant Professor
Department of Family Medicine & Community Health
University of Massachusetts Medical School
Worcester, Massachusetts

Cassandra Dorvil, DO, MBS
UMass/Fitchburg Family Medicine Residency
University of Massachusetts Medical School/UMassMemorial
    HealthCare
Worcester, Massachusetts

Rebecca G. Kinney, MD
Partnership Health Center
Clinical Instructor
Family Medicine Residency of Western Montana
University of Washington, School of Medicine
Missoula, Montana

Rocio Nordfeldt, MD
Assistant Professor
UMass/Fitchburg Family Medicine Residency
University of Massachusetts Medical School/UMassMemorial
    HealthCare
Worcester, Massachusetts

Jennifer Smith, MD
UMass/Fitchburg Family Medicine Residency
University of Massachusetts Medical School/UMassMemorial
    HealthCare
Worcester, Massachusetts

J. Herbert Stevenson, MD
Associate Professor and Director of Sports Medicine
Director of the Sports Medicine Fellowship Program
Department of Family Medicine & Community Health
Department of Orthopedics & Rehabilitation
University of Massachusetts Medical School/UMassMemorial
    HealthCare
Worcester, Massachusetts

Jeff Wang, MD, MPH
UMass/Fitchburg Family Medicine Residency
University of Massachusetts Medical School/UMassMemorial
    HealthCare
Worcester, Massachusetts

Edmund Zaccaria, MD
Assistant Professor
Department of Family Medicine & Community Health
University of Massachusetts Medical School/UMassMemorial
    HealthCare
Worcester, Massachusetts

Preface

Bratton's Family Medicine Board Review, fifth edition, is a directed review of important topics that typically appear on American Board of Family Medicine (ABFM) in-training, board certification, and recertification examinations. This material is not intended to be a comprehensive review but, instead, should direct the examinee to areas of weakness that may need further review.

Family medicine is a broad field, and to provide a complete, comprehensive review of all topics that may be covered is impractical. Courses are available that attempt to provide this type of review; however, this book is more abbreviated and focuses on topics that are commonly found on board examinations.

Adequate preparation for any test is the key to success and rewarding results. Given this, we all know the importance of practice tests and the benefits of testing our knowledge base before the actual examination. This review book is structured for the examinee with an established foundation of knowledge within the field of family medicine. Its primary purpose is to identify areas of weakness that can be improved upon, and to that end, each answer has a suggested "Additional Reading" to assist the reader in further study on identified topics of weakness as they prepare for the board examination.

This edition updates the existing content, with revised information to reflect changes that have occurred in the medical field since the last edition. The ABFM restructures the examination on a yearly basis, so it is important to visit its Website, *www.theabfm.org*, to get updates on the structure of each examination. I hope that you will find this book enlightening and, most of all, beneficial in your studies for the ABFM examinations. If you have any suggestions to help improve this material, please contact me with your suggestions at robert.baldor@umassmed.edu. Our goal is to help you prepare for and, then, pass your board examination!

The ABFM Board Certification Process

Introduction

To be certified as a diplomat of the American Board of Family Medicine requires completion of an accredited family medicine residency, obtaining a full, unrestricted medical license and passing a certification examination. Below outlines the requirements for taking the ABFM certification examinations depending on whether you are still in training, seeking initial certification, or maintaining ABFM certification.

Residency *In-Training* Examination

The "in-training examination" is for current family medicine residents enrolled in an accredited training program. Individual registration is not required as the registration is handled by the residency office. The Residency Director should have all the necessary details. The test is administered annually to each resident during the 3 years of residency training. All residents receive the same test. However, there are no pass or fail ratings; instead the results are scored and grading is based on the level of training. The examination is given in the fall, and most residency programs make any necessary arrangements to relieve residents of clinical responsibilities for the examination day. The purpose of the "in-training exam" is to assess resident's knowledge base as they progress through training and to objectively evaluate the residency education program. Scores are reported to each resident with a comparison of the results with those of the respective peers in training. The in-training exam scores are also reported to the residency director, so that he or she may track individual resident's educational development and look for areas of weakness across the residency training program.

The Initial Board Certification Examination

To obtain board certification, not only must candidates successfully complete the initial board certification examination, but their Program Director must also verify that the resident has successfully met all of the ACGME program requirements and the candidate must hold a current valid, full, and unrestricted license to practice medicine in the United States or Canada.

The residency program can assist in the process of initial certification; however, recertification is the responsibility of each physician. The examination is held in testing centers throughout the country on various dates twice a year (usually each fall and spring). As stated by the ABFM, "The American Board of Family Medicine Certification and Recertification Examinations are tests of cognitive knowledge and problem-solving abilities relevant to Family Medicine. Appropriate subject areas of the following disciplines are included: Internal Medicine, Surgery, Obstetrics, Community Medicine, Pediatrics, Psychiatry and Behavioral Sciences, Geriatrics and Gynecology. Elements of the examinations include but are not limited to, diagnosis, management, and prevention of illness."

The Maintain of Certification (MC-FP) Process

Following the initial board certification as a family medicine specialist, the diplomat must participate in the "Maintain of Certification" (MC-FP) process in order to maintain their certification status. This process has been required of all specialties (not just for family medicine) by the American Board of Medical Specialties (ABMS) in order to continuously assess the competence of physicians and their knowledge base and skill sets. The MC-FP process emphasizes the importance of ongoing participation in assessment activities between recertification examinations, rather than just relying on a periodic recertification examination every several years. The MC-FP is a requirement that encourages clinical excellence and benefits both physicians and their patients. The MC-FP assessment process consists of four parts:

Part I. Professionalism (current, valid license)
Part II. Self-assessment and lifelong learning (SAM educational modules and CME requirements)
Part III. Cognitive expertise (the recertification examination)
Part IV. Performance in practice (PPM practice quality-improvement exercises)

The current guidelines for the MC-FP program require that each certified diplomat successfully complete a series of these requirements in three separate (3-year) stages.

The Part II requirement refers to the successful completion of (almost annual) Self-Assessment Modules (SAMs). These modules include a 60-question cognitive exam and an interactive simulated patient care exercise that includes an assessment of the diagnosis and management plan for the patient scenario. These modules are completed online by the individual physician, although group learning sessions are often available (such as at the American Academy of Family Physician [AAFP] Annual Scientific Assembly). The ABFP runs the examination process, not the AAFP. SAM topics have included the following:

- Asthma
- Care of the elderly
- Coronary artery disease
- Depression
- Diabetes
- Childhood illness
- Health behavior
- Heart failure
- Hypertension

- Maternity care
- Pain management
- Well child care

A SAM module can take from 2 to 8 hours to complete. CME credits are awarded for successfully completing each SAM module. The American Board of Family Medicine (ABFM) Website (https://www.theabfm.org/MC-FP/index.aspx) has the complete details about the SAM modules.

The Part IV requirement refers to completion of Performances in Practice Modules (PPMs). The ABFM offers Web-based, quality-improvement modules that generally correspond to the SAMs. To complete these modules, a physician assesses the care of their patients using evidence-based quality indicators. Data from 10 patients are entered into the ABFM Website, and feedback is provided for several quality indicators. The physician chooses an indicator and designs a quality-improvement plan, submits the plan, and implements the plan in practice. After a period of time (at least a week), the physician again assesses the care provided to 10 patients in the chosen health area and enters the data into the ABFM Website. The physician is then able to compare their pre- and postintervention performance and compare the results to those of their peers. Alternative methods of meeting the Part IV requirement are available for those physicians who do not currently have a continuity practice (e.g., urgent care practice, administration). CME credits are awarded for successfully completing each PPM.

The Recertification Examination

The recertification examination is held annually in testing centers throughout the country on various dates twice a year (usually each fall and spring). Registration for the board recertification examination is done by contacting the American Board of Family Medicine (ABFM), and a formal application (www.theabfm.org/cert/index.aspx) must be submitted. However, before sitting for the recertification examination, family physicians must have completed the Maintenance of Certification (MC-FP) process as outlined above. Applicants must have successfully completed Parts I (the applicant holds a current, valid, full, and unrestricted license to practice medicine in the United States or Canada), Part II (completed the required number of SAMs and provide evidence that they have met the required continuing medical education [CME] hours), and Part IV (completion of the PPM practice quality-improvement exercises). Successfully passing the recertification examination is required to complete Part III.

Summary

Once you have inquired about the certification/recertification examination (as noted above), you will receive registration information from the ABFM, including selection of your preferred testing site location. Prometric is the computer-based testing vendor that the ABFM has used to administer the exam with approximately 345 locations in the United States and Canada and 140 international locations. It is important to register early to ensure that you get your first choice of location. The exam is offered in the spring and fall, but typically the fall examination has limited seating and is primarily for those physicians who were unable to take the spring examination and for off-cycle residents who did not complete training in time to take the spring examination. Additionally, candidates who are unsuccessful on the spring administration can apply to retake the examination in the fall. There is no limit to the number of times a candidate may take the examination, provided qualifications are met with each reapplication.

Before the test, you will receive additional material that includes your assigned testing site and a registration number. Make sure you bring the information including your registration number and photo identification along with an additional form of identification to the test site on the day of the test. Failure to do this may prevent you from taking the test, or it may delay you in the on-site registration process. This is not required for in-training residency examinations.

More information is available by contacting the ABFM office or accessing their Website:

The American Board of Family Medicine, Inc.
1648 McGrathiana Parkway Suite 550
Lexington, KY 40511-1247
Phone: 859-269-5626 or 888-995-5700
Fax: 859-335-7501 or 859-335-7509
Email: help@theabfm.org

Preparing for the Exam

Introduction

Just when we thought that the standardized tests we had to pass in high school, college, and medical school were behind us, the American Board of Family Medicine (ABFM) requires an in-training examination (in some cases referred to as the *in-service examination*) yearly during residency training and we must pass a board examination at the end of that residency training in order to receive board certification. Additionally, ABFM diplomats must also pass a recertification examination every 10 years to maintain their board certification. For many, the board examination process is a stressful time. In addition to using this book to review your family medicine knowledge, it is always helpful to review some basic test-taking strategies. The following are some general guidelines for preparing for your examination.

Examination Formats

The *in-training examination* consists of 240 multiple-choice questions and uses a content outline that is identical to the blueprint for the ABFM certification examination. The examination includes 4 to 8 pictorial items, which may be radiographs, EKGs, pictures of dermatologic conditions, or other images. The entire computer-based test is single-best-answer multiple-choice questions, with each question having four or five answers to choose from. The study questions and answers that are provided in this book will help you to study covered topics in a similar format. There is no penalty for guessing, so if you reach the end of the test and are short of time, make sure you have answered all the questions.

The *initial certification* and *recertification* examinations are full-day computer-based exams that contain multiple-choice (one best answer) questions. There are five sections with scheduled (optional) breaks in between each section. Additionally, all candidates should be prepared to choose two 'module topics' that they will select during the exam application process. The 'module topic' areas include ambulatory family medicine, child and adolescent care, geriatrics, women's health, maternity care, emergent/urgent care, hospital medicine, and sports medicine.

The first 2-hour section of the exam consists of 120 multiple choice questions. The next 2 sections are 45 minute each, and the content is based on your selected module topics. There are 15-minute breaks between each section and a longer break over the lunch hour. The afternoon consists of two 80-multiple-choice-question sections, each about 90 minutes long with a 15-minute break in between.

The ABFM Website can be accessed at www.theabfm.org and is an excellent resource for more detailed information.

The Exam Day

The certification and recertification examinations are given at specific computer-based testing centers across the United States and may require a significant amount of traveling to reach the location. Insure that you have identified the site and are familiar with the surrounding traffic patterns and parking locations. On arrival, you are photographed and fingerprinted for access to and from the testing site. You must have two forms of identification (one with photo) when you check in.

Adequate sleep is imperative as you prepare for any test, and this test is no exception. It is a good idea to arrange your call schedule to allow plenty of sleep the week before the test so that you arrive well rested. On the morning of the test, eat a light breakfast and consider bringing a lunch for the board and recertification examinations (not necessary for the in-training examination, because you are usually through with the test at around 1:00 pm). Pack your own lunch and find a quiet place to enjoy your meal and relax during the scheduled lunch break. Bring along aspirin, ibuprofen, or acetaminophen if a headache should occur during the test. Cough drops and allergy medication (nonsedating) should be remembered. Remember that calculators or watches are not allowed, and beeping electronic devices or cellular phones should be left at home. Earplugs may help mute unwanted noises that distract you.

The examinations require you to sit for extended periods of time. Bring a lightweight jacket or sweater in case it gets cold and loose-fitting clothing with comfortable shoes. Also, don't forget your glasses. You are *not* allowed to take any additional materials, into the testing room for the certification/recertification examination. Personal items are to be left in a secure locker provided by the testing site. The testing site does offer hard candy or mints and you are given a small white erasable board with a magic marker for making notes or doing calculations.

Make sure you use the bathroom before entering the testing room; having to leave requires you to raise your hand and the proctor must log you out from your computer and allow you to leave the room and then fingerprint you when you return; needless to say, this can waste a lot of valuable test-taking time. While in the examination room, you are seated at a small, isolated cubicle with fellow test-takers (who might even be high school students taking their SATs!) at your left and right. A proctor is seated behind a glass enclosure and observes all who are taking the test. Additionally, you are monitored by video cameras during the examination.

Test-Taking Skills

Anxiety is a natural response when faced with a test situation. The important thing is to not let anxiety affect your performance deleteriously. Relaxation techniques, such as stretching or deep breathing exercises can be used. However, a little anxiety can be good for you and may improve your performance.

Answer the easiest questions first. Start with the first question of each section and answer all the questions you can with reasonable certainty. If there is a difficult question, skip over it and return when you have finished the section. The computerized examination format allows you to flag questions that you are unsure about, so that you can return to them later.

Check your pace and be mindful of the time. On the computer, you should see the time in a small box at the bottom of the screen. Pay attention to these reminders and adjust your pace as necessary. A good rule of thumb is to plan for a minute per question. Don't spend an excessive amount of time on any one question, which could put you at risk for not being able to answer easy questions at the end of the test because you ran out of time.

A strategy that can be helpful when taking examinations is to read the answers first. If you don't have a good understanding of the test question, you can't answer it correctly based on your knowledge. Reading the answers can activate your knowledge about the question, and when you then read the question, the 'activated knowledge' impacts on your understanding of the question.

A common test-taking error is failing to read ALL of the question and/or ALL of the choices before actually marking your response. General skimming of the question can lead to premature closure and result in a wrong answer. Self-assessment is important as you may not even realize that you tend to skim the question or fail to read all the choices. Be mindful of making such errors when you answer the questions in this book and mark any such errors on your "Study Grid."

Being "lured by a distractor" is another common error. One strategy to address this is to read the actual question to be answered first, before reading through the background information/vignette. For example, there may be a sentence or two leading up to the question, "What is the best treatment?" If you read the question first you become aware that the question is about treatment, so that you begin to think about treatment decisions as you read the question, rather than being distracted by other information presented in the question. Avoid reading extra meaning into the questions. The ABFM does not structure questions to try to outsmart the test-taker. Questions are designed to be fair and not have hidden agendas. Therefore, take questions literally and do not imply hidden meanings.

As you read questions, try to identify "keywords." Typical keywords to look for include the specific symptoms that are present, the duration of the symptoms, and current treatments. Be mindful of other keywords that are sometimes ignored such as age and diagnoses other than those related to chief complaint. Other "nonmedical" terms (e.g., season, social issues, and miscellaneous adjectives) can also be important to consider.

Guess if you do not know the answer, but use what you know (partial knowledge) to narrow down the choices and resist: being lured by an unknown distracter; choosing on the basis of "technical words" that must be right; or using "tricks" rather than actual knowledge (i.e., two are same, one of those must be right). Consider similarities and differences between answers—use these to either serve as a memory trigger to help recall the forgotten information or to make a guess by choosing the outlier. However, this is a last ditch effort because there may be more similarities and differences between options other than that which discriminates the correct answer.

You are penalized only for an incorrect or unanswered question; therefore, all questions should be answered even if they require a guess. Also, it is important to remember that if the answer uses absolute terminology, such as always, never, all, or none, it usually is a false response. Very little in the world of medicine is absolute.

If time allows, review your work. Sometimes you will want to consider changing a previously answered question. If this is based on being cued from another question, a clerical error, or realizing the question was misread, you have a good chance of changing to the correct answer. However, if this is just based on a "reconsideration of the original answer," you have a 50:50 chance of being correct, as this is usually just changing one guess to another. So only change an answer if you realized that you misread the question, or you have new knowledge through spontaneous recall, or another question gave you content information or jogged your memory, or you noticed you made a clerical error.

Using This Book

Although most who sit for the ABFM examinations pass, that should not be taken for granted. A poor score could result in not becoming board certified or losing board certification status. This book is meant as a study guide to help you identify areas of weakness. Although highlighting topics previously covered by ABFM tests, it is not an exhaustive review of all information and not meant to be used as reference to support medical practice. Hence, the answers are not formally referenced, rather followed by an "Additional Reading" suggestion to help you learn more about the topic.

Adopt a structured study program that is started 6 to 8 weeks before the examination. Use this book as a study review tool for 2 hours nightly during the week (reserving the weekends for family, friends, and rest). Answer 20 questions and then take a break. Use the "Study Grid" found in this book as a way of tracking your progress. Each question is marked with one of the broad ABFM knowledge categories—every time you get a question wrong, place a mark in the category so that you can identify your areas of weakness. During the week before the test, focus on key areas of weakness, addressing those categories that are addressed more frequently in the exam. For example, if you are having trouble with the cardiovascular or respiratory categories, that is a concern because typically each of these areas are covered by a significant portion (10% to 12%) of exam questions versus 1% to 2% for other areas such as for hematology questions. Additionally be mindful of any test-taking errors that you are consistently making and be mindful of those as a way of enhancing your performance.

Contents

The Conscious Uncoupling book

↓ reactivity

———— ○ ————

Care of the Adult Patient

QUESTIONS

Each of the following questions or incomplete statements is followed by four or five suggested answers or completions. Select the ONE BEST ANSWER in each case.

1. All of the following can be helpful in preventing recurrent diverticulitis except
A) Increased dietary fiber
B) Exercise
C) Smoking cessation
D) Avoiding nuts, corn, or popcorn
E) Mesalamine and *Lactobacillus casei*

Answer and Discussion

The answer is D. Interventions to prevent recurrences of diverticulitis include increased intake of dietary fiber, exercise, and, in persons with a body mass index (BMI) of 30 kg per m^2 or higher, weight loss. Counseling for smoking cessation is recommended because smoking is associated with an increased incidence of complicated diverticulitis and less favorable outcomes (e.g., surgery at a younger age, higher risk of recurrence). Evidence from a prospective cohort study of 47,228 men in the United States found no evidence that avoiding nuts, corn, or popcorn decreases the risk of diverticulosis or diverticular complications, such as diverticulitis. A small prospective study found that mesalamine and *Lactobacillus casei* are effective in preventing recurrence. A meta-analysis of four randomized controlled trials with 1,660 patients who had experienced at least one episode of diverticulitis found that rifaximin (Xifaxan) plus fiber provided 1 year of complete relief and fewer complications compared with fiber alone.

> Additional Reading: Diagnosis and management of acute diverticulitis. *Am Fam Physician.* 2013; 87(9):612–620.

> Category: Gastroenterology system

2. Which one of the following represents an optimal screening strategy for colorectal cancer?
A) Colonoscopy every 5 years
B) Computed tomographic (CT) colonography every 10 years
C) High-sensitivity fecal occult blood test (FOBT) every 2 years
D) Sigmoidoscopy every 5 years with high-sensitivity FOBT every 3 years
E) Sigmoidoscopy every 5 years

Answer and Discussion

The answer is D. The U.S. Preventive Services Task Force (USPSTF) recommends screening for colorectal cancer in adults 50 to 75 years of age using colonoscopy, sigmoidoscopy, or high-sensitivity FOBT. Studies show that the optimal intervals for these tests are colonoscopy every 10 years; high-sensitivity FOBT annually; and sigmoidoscopy every 5 years combined with high-sensitivity FOBT every 3 years. Sigmoidoscopy every 5 years without high-sensitivity FOBT is significantly less effective in detecting colorectal cancer than are other screening tests. The USPSTF concluded that there is insufficient evidence to determine the net benefit of CT colonography and fecal DNA testing.

> Additional Reading: Screening for colorectal cancer. *Am Fam Physician.* 2010; 81(8):1017–1018.

> Category: Gastroenterology system

3. Which of the following *p* values reflects the best chance that the findings are not the result of chance?
A) *p* value < 0.5
B) *p* value < 0.1
C) *p* value < 0.05
D) *p* value < 0.01
E) *p* value = 1

Answer and Discussion

The answer is B. The *p* value is defined as the measured probability of a finding occurring (i.e., rejecting the null hypothesis) by chance alone, given that the null hypothesis is actually true. By convention, a *p* value < 0.05 is often considered significant. ("There is less than a 5% probability that the finding [null hypothesis rejected] was due to chance alone.")

> Additional Reading: Terms used in evidence-based medicine. *Am Fam Physician.* From: http://www.aafp.org/journals/afp/authors/ebm-toolkit/glossary.html.

> Category: Patient/Population-based care

4. Which of the following statements is true regarding influenza?

A) Treatment with antivirals should be initiated within 48 hours of the onset of symptoms.

B) Anitiviral agents reduce the duration of fever by 1 week.

C) Amantadine is effective for both influenza types A and B.

D) Prophylactic therapy is the single most important measure to prevent influenza outbreaks.

E) Amantadine is the only agent approved for prophylaxis.

Answer and Discussion

The answer is A. Influenza causes significant morbidity and mortality and is responsible for considerable medical expenditures especially in the elderly. Vaccination is the single most important public health measure to prevent this illness. Amantadine (Symmetrel) and rimantadine (Flumadine) are older antiviral agents (M2 inhibitors). Oseltamivir (Tamiflu) and zanamivir (Relenza) are chemically related antiviral medications known as neuraminidase inhibitors that have activity against both influenza A and B viruses. Both are also approved for prophylaxis. For antiviral agents to be effective, they must be initiated within 48 hours of the onset of influenza symptoms. Antiviral agents reduce the duration of fever and illness by 1 day and also reduce the severity of some symptoms. For optimal use of antiviral agents, patients with influenza symptoms must present early, and family physicians must accurately and rapidly diagnose the illness.

> **Additional Reading:** Influenza antiviral medications. Centers for disease control and prevention. From: http://www.cdc.gov/flu/professionals/antivirals/summary-clinicians.htm. Accessed 8/22/2013.

> **Category:** Respiratory system

5. Primary insomnia is usually associated with

A) Sleep apnea

B) Restless legs syndrome (RLS)

C) Periodic limb movements

D) Circadian rhythm sleep disorders

E) None of the above

Answer and Discussion

The answer is E. Insomnia is defined as inadequate or poor-quality sleep characterized by one or more of the following: difficulty falling asleep, difficulty maintaining sleep, waking up too early in the morning, or sleep that is not refreshing. Insomnia also involves daytime consequences such as fatigue, difficulty concentrating, and irritability. Periods of insomnia lasting between 1 night and a few weeks are defined as acute insomnia. Chronic insomnia refers to sleep difficulty occurring at least 3 nights per week for 1 month or more. Insomnia may be associated with specific sleep disorders, including RLS, periodic limb movement disorder, sleep apnea, and circadian rhythm sleep disorders.

RLS is characterized by unpleasant sensations in the legs or feet that are temporarily relieved by movement. Symptoms are worse in the evening, especially when a person is lying down and remaining still. The sensations cause difficulty falling asleep and are often accompanied by periodic limb movements. Periodic limb movement disorder is characterized by bilateral repeated and rhythmic, small-amplitude jerking or twitching movements in the lower extremities and, less frequently, in the arms. These movements occur every 20 to 90 seconds and can lead to awakenings, which are usually not noticed by the patient. Often the patient reports that sleep is not refreshing. In many cases, the bed partner is more likely to report the movement problem.

Obstructive sleep apnea is most commonly associated with snoring, daytime sleepiness, and obesity but occasionally presents with insomnia. Circadian rhythm sleep disorders including sleep-work insomnia are characterized by an inability to sleep because of a disturbance between the circadian sleep rhythm and the desired or required sleep schedule.

Primary insomnia occurs in the absence of the previously mentioned conditions. When the insomnia persists beyond 1 or 2 nights or becomes predictable, treatment should be considered. Pharmacologic treatment is usually effective, especially short-acting hypnotics. Sleep hygiene measures may also be useful. Chronic insomnia may be more difficult to treat. Because chronic insomnia is often multifactorial in etiology, a patient may need multiple treatment modalities, including medication (antidepressants, antihistamines, melatonin) and behavioral therapy. If an underlying medical or psychiatric condition is identified, this condition should be treated first. ✂

> **Additional Reading:** Primary insomnia in older persons. *Am Fam Physician.* 2013; 87(4):280–281.

> **Category:** Neurology

6. A 65-year-old man presents to your office and reports urinary incontinence. Examination reveals an enlarged prostate. You suspect overflow incontinence. Which of the following measurements of postvoid residual (PVR) volumes would represent the threshold for a normal amount?

A) 50 mL

B) 100 mL

C) 200 mL

D) 500 mL

E) 1,000 mL

Answer and Discussion

The answer is A. Urge incontinence results from bladder contractions that exceed the ability of the brain to prevent them. Causes include inflammation or irritation within the bladder, resulting from calculi, malignancy, infection, or atrophic vaginitis-urethritis. Other central causes include stroke, Parkinson's disease or dementia, drugs such as hypnotics or narcotics, or metabolic disorders such as hypoxemia and encephalopathy. Additionally, urge incontinence can occur when ambulation is impaired, making it difficult for patients to get to the bathroom in time. This condition is referred to as "functional incontinence."

Stress incontinence is caused by a malfunction of the urethral sphincter that causes urine to leak from the bladder when intra-abdominal pressure increases, such as during coughing or sneezing. Causes for stress incontinence include pelvic prolapse, urethral hypermobility, or displacement of the urethra and bladder neck from their normal anatomic alignment. Stress incontinence can also occur as a result of intrinsic sphincter deficiency, in which the sphincter is weak because of a congenital condition or denervation resulting from α-adrenergic blocking drugs, surgical trauma, or radiation damage. Overflow bladder incontinence occurs as a result of urine retention with bladder distention. Urine collects in the bladder until maximum bladder capacity is reached. It then leaks as a result of "overflow," usually manifesting as dribbling. Increased intra-abdominal pressure may also cause loss of urine, so that overflow incontinence sometimes mimics stress incontinence.

Overflow incontinence can be caused by medications that relax the bladder detrusor muscle (e.g., anticholinergic agents, calcium-channel blockers [CCBs]). It can also be caused by denervation of the detrusor resulting from a neurologic abnormality that affects bladder innervation (e.g., diabetic neuropathy) or because of damage to bladder innervation (e.g., tumors, radiation, surgery). Additionally, overflow incontinence can be caused by obstructed urinary outflow resulting from prostate enlargement, fecal impaction, urethral stricture, or urethral constriction related to α-adrenergic agonist medications.

The workup should include a urinalysis, which can identify acute urinary tract infection (UTI) and diabetes-induced glycosuria, both of which can cause or aggravate urge incontinence. These conditions are reversible with treatment. If appropriate, a urine culture should also be obtained. The basic evaluation of urinary incontinence should also include measurement of PVR urine volume to detect urinary retention (i.e., overflow bladder). PVR volume measurement can detect retention caused by potentially reversible factors (e.g., anticholinergic or other drugs, fecal impaction). Urinary retention not obviously resulting from a transient cause generally requires further evaluation, including cystometry, to determine why the bladder does not empty properly. The PVR urine volume can be measured by one of two methods. The first and most common method is "in and out" urethral catheterization after the patient has urinated to empty the bladder. The quantity of urine obtained is measured. PVR volume can also be measured with pelvic ultrasonography. Ultrasonography is a useful alternative to catheterization, especially for measuring the PVR volume in men with suspected prostate obstruction, because catheterizing these patients may cause urinary infection or obstruction. Normally, <50 mL of residual urine is present after voiding. Volumes of >200 mL are abnormal. Intermediate volumes (50 to 200 mL) are considered equivocal, and the test should be repeated. Other tests include office cystometry and office stress testing. Office cystometry consists of aliquots of sterile saline that are infused into the bladder via a catheter with an open syringe attached to the catheter. Contractions are detected by monitoring the fluid level that appears in the syringe after several aliquots of water have been instilled. A rise and fall in the fluid level indicates pressure changes (i.e., contractions) within the bladder. Severe feelings of urgency or bladder contractions at <300 mL of bladder volume constitute a presumptive diagnosis of urge incontinence. For the diagnosis of urge incontinence, simple cystometry can be used. In this test, the patient lies supine on the examination table with a full bladder and coughs forcefully. The physician places a gauze pad in front of the perineum. If urine leaks onto the gauze pad during coughing, a presumptive diagnosis of stress incontinence is made. The physician then places his or her fingers on either side of the patient's urethra and elevates the structure. The patient is then asked to cough. In patients with stress incontinence, urethral elevation prevents further urine leakage. If no incontinence is noted in the supine position, the maneuvers should be repeated with the patient standing. If no incontinence occurs in either position, the patient probably does not have stress incontinence.

Additional Reading: Diagnosis of urinary incontinence. *Am Fam Physician.* 2013; 87(8):543–550.

Category: Nephrologic system

7. Which of the following is considered a risk factor for retinal detachment?
A) Glaucoma
B) Diabetic retinopathy
C) Hyphema
D) Myopia

Answer and Discussion
The answer is D. Retinal detachment is a preventable cause of vision loss. It is relatively common after the age of 60. There are three types of retinal detachments: exudative, tractional, and rhegmatogenous. The most common type is rhegmatogenous, which results from retinal breaks caused by vitreoretinal traction. Exudative (or serous) retinal detachment results from the accumulation of serous and/or hemorrhagic fluid in the subretinal space because of hydrostatic factors (e.g., severe acute hypertension), or inflammation (e.g., sarcoid uveitis), or neoplastic effusions. Exudative retinal detachment generally resolves with adequate treatment of the underlying disease, and restoration of normal vision is often excellent. Tractional retinal detachment occurs via centripetal mechanical forces on the retina, usually mediated by fibrotic tissue resulting from previous hemorrhage, injury, surgery, infection, or inflammation. Risk factors for retinal detachment include advancing age, previous cataract surgery, myopia, and trauma. Other eye conditions including hyphema, glaucoma, and diabetic retinopathy are not considered risk factors for retinal detachment. Patients typically present with symptoms such as light flashes, floaters, peripheral visual field loss, and blurred vision. Retinal tears may occur without symptoms, but often photopsia (light flashes) is noted. Photopsia results from vitreoretinal traction. When the retina tears, blood and retinal pigment epithelium cells may enter the vitreous cavity and are perceived as "floaters." Immediate intervention can prevent retinal detachment. Patients with the acute onset of flashes or floaters should be referred to an ophthalmologist.

Additional Reading: Evaluation and management of suspected retinal detachment. *Am Fam Physician.* 2004;69:1691–1698.

Category: Special sensory

8. Which of the following medications is considered the treatment of choice for *Bordetella pertussis* infection?
A) Penicillin
B) Ciprofloxacin
C) Azithromycin
D) Tetracycline
E) Cefuroxime

Answer and Discussion
The answer is C. Recent epidemiologic studies have shown that the incidence and prevalence of *Bordetella pertussis* infection in adults are much greater than previously reported. In studies of adults with chronic cough, 20% to 25% were found to have serologic evidence of recent *B. pertussis* infection. However, pertussis is rarely considered in adults because the signs and symptoms are nonspecific. Apart from a prolonged cough, there are no specific symptoms suggestive of pertussis in older individuals who have been immunized. With this in mind, pertussis should be considered in the differential diagnosis of persistent cough in previously immunized children and adults. Administration of erythromycin or other macrolide (azithromycin or clarithromycin) may be a consideration in patients presenting with persistent cough. Prophylaxis of exposed persons before culture or serologic results are available would be another consideration. Early treatment with a macrolide should limit the spread of infection to persons whose immunity has waned or in unimmunized children. The acellular vaccine may allow booster immunization, which can be a method of preventing *B. pertussis* infection after immunity from the pertussis vaccination has waned.

Additional Reading: Prevention and treatment of pertussis. *Med Lett Drugs Ther.* 2012;54(1399):73–74.

Category: Respiratory system

9. Mrs Jones, a 52-year-old teacher, presents with a sudden onset of dyspnea. Which one of the following makes a pulmonary embolus more likely?

A) Fever >38.0°C (100.4°F)
B) Chest pain
C) Orthopnea
D) Wheezes
E) Rhonchi

Answer and Discussion

The answer is B. Chest pain is common in patients with pulmonary embolism (PE). When evaluating a patient for possible PE, the presence of orthopnea suggests heart failure, fever suggests an infectious process, wheezing suggests asthma or chronic obstructive pulmonary disease (COPD), and rhonchi suggest heart failure, interstitial lung disease, or infection. These generalizations are supported by a 2008 study designed to improve the diagnosis of PE on the basis of the history, physical examination, EKG, and chest radiograph.

> **Additional Reading:** Diagnosis of deep venous thrombosis and pulmonary embolism. *Am Fam Physician.* 2012;86(10):913–919

> **Category:** Cardiovascular system

10. A 23-year-old auto mechanic is brought to the emergency department with slurred speech, confusion, and ataxia. He appears intoxicated and has a history of binge drinking, but denies recent alcohol intake and no odor of alcohol is noted on his breath. Abnormalities on the metabolic profile include a carbon dioxide content of 10 mmol per L (N 20 to 30). His blood alcohol level is <10 mg per dL (0.01%). A urinalysis shows calcium oxalate crystals and a red blood cell (RBC) count of 10 to 20 per hpf. Woods lamp examination of the urine shows fluorescence. His arterial pH is 7.25. Which one of the following would be the most appropriate at this point?

A) Immediate hemodialysis
B) Gastric lavage
C) Administration of activated charcoal
D) Fomepizole (Antizol)

Answer and Discussion

The answer is D. Ethylene glycol poisoning should be suspected in patients with metabolic acidosis of unknown cause and subsequent renal failure, as rapid diagnosis and treatment will limit the toxicity and decrease both morbidity and mortality. This diagnosis should be considered in a patient who appears intoxicated but does not have an odor of alcohol, and has anion gap acidosis, hypocalcemia, urinary crystals, and nontoxic blood alcohol levels. Ethylene glycol is found in products such as engine coolant, de-icing solution, and carpet and fabric cleaners. Ingestion of 100 mL of ethylene glycol by an adult can result in toxicity.

Until recently, ethylene glycol poisoning was treated with sodium bicarbonate, ethanol, and hemodialysis. Treatment with fomepizole (Antizol) has this specific indication, however, and should be initiated immediately when ethylene glycol poisoning is suspected. If ethylene glycol poisoning is treated early, hemodialysis may be avoided, but once severe acidosis and renal failure have occurred hemodialysis is necessary. Ethylene glycol is rapidly absorbed, and use of ipecac or gastric lavage is therefore not effective. Large amounts of activated charcoal will only bind to relatively small amounts of ethylene glycol, and the therapeutic window for accomplishing this is less than 1 hour.

> **Additional Reading:** Methanol and ethylene glycol poisoning. In: Basow DS, ed. *UpToDate.* Waltham, MA: UpToDate; 2013.

> **Category:** Nonspecific system

11. The Health Insurance Portability and Accountability Act (HIPAA) standards ensure that

A) Patients have control and access to their medical records
B) Insurance companies have unlimited access to health information
C) Physicians can protect themselves from liability
D) Attorneys have unrestricted access to health care records

Answer and Discussion

The answer is A. HIPAA is three sets of standards developed by the Department of Health and Human Services in 1996: (1) Transactions and Code Sets, (2) Privacy, and (3) Security. The goals of the standards are to simplify the administration of health insurance claims and lower costs, give patients more control and access to their medical information, and protect individually identifiable medical information from real or potential threats of disclosure or loss. Privacy and security are closely related. *Privacy* is the patient's right over the use and disclosure of his or her own personal health information. Privacy includes the right to determine when, how, and to what extent personal information is shared with others. The HIPAA privacy rules grant new rights to patients to gain access to and control the use and disclosure of their personal health information. *Security* is the specific measures a health care provider must take to protect personal health information from unauthorized breaches of privacy, as in situations where information is stolen or sent to the wrong person in error. Security also includes measures taken to ensure against the loss of personal health information, as in situations where a patient's records are lost or destroyed by accident. The HIPAA privacy rules require general security measures be put in place, and the proposed security rules follow a detailed and comprehensive set of activities to guard against unauthorized disclosure of personal health information stored or transmitted electronically or on paper.

> **Additional Reading:** HIPAA again: confronting the updated privacy and security rules. *Fam Pract Manag.* 2013; 20(3):18–22.

> **Category:** Patient/Population-based care

12. You are asked to perform a preoperative evaluation on a 55-year-old white woman with type 2 diabetes mellitus prior to elective femoral–anterior tibial artery bypass surgery. She is unable to climb a flight of stairs or do heavy work around the house. She denies exertional chest pain and is otherwise healthy. Based on current guidelines, which one of the following diagnostic studies would be appropriate prior to surgery because the results could alter the management of this patient?

A) Pulmonary function studies
B) Coronary angiography
C) Carotid angiography
D) A dipyridamole-thallium scan
E) A hemoglobin A1c level

Answer and Discussion

The answer is D. A preoperative evaluation prior to noncardiac surgery requires an assessment of the perioperative cardiovascular risk of the procedure involved, the functional status of the patient, and clinical factors that can increase the risk, such as diabetes mellitus, stroke, renal insufficiency, compensated or prior heart failure, mild angina, or previous myocardial infarction (MI). This patient is not undergoing emergency surgery, nor does she have an active cardiac condition; however, she is undergoing a high-risk procedure (>5% risk of perioperative MI) with vascular surgery. As she cannot climb a flight of stairs or do heavy housework, her functional status is <4 METs, and she should be considered for further evaluation. The patient's diabetes is an additional clinical risk factor.

With vascular surgery being planned, appropriate recommendations include proceeding with the surgery with heart rate control, or performing noninvasive testing if it will change the management of the patient. Coronary angiography is indicated if the noninvasive testing is abnormal. Pulmonary function studies are most useful in patients with underlying lung disease or those undergoing pulmonary resection. Hemoglobin A1c is a measure of long-term diabetic control and is not particularly useful perioperatively. Carotid angiography is not indicated in asymptomatic patients being considered for lower-extremity vascular procedures.

Additional Reading: Perioperative cardiac risk reduction. *Am Fam Physician*. 2012;85(3):239–246.

Category: Cardiovascular system

13. Which of the following tumor markers is correct for the condition?
A) CA (cancer antigen) 27.29 for metastatic cervical cancer
B) CA (cancer antigen) 125 for hepatic carcinoma
C) AFP (α-fetoprotein) for ovarian carcinoma
D) CA (cancer antigen) 19–9 for pancreatic cancer
E) β-hCG (beta unit of human chorionic gonadotropin) for ovarian cancer

Answer and Discussion

The answer is D. Recognized tumor markers are most appropriate for monitoring response to therapy and detecting early recurrence. Cancer antigen (CA) 27.29 is most often used to follow response to therapy in patients with metastatic breast cancer. CA 27.29 is highly associated with breast cancer, although levels are elevated in several other malignancies (colon, gastric, hepatic, lung, pancreatic, ovarian, and prostate cancers). CA 27.29 also can be found in patients with benign disorders of the breast, liver, and kidney and in patients with ovarian cysts. CA 27.29 levels higher than 100 units per mL are rare in benign conditions.

Carcinoembryonic antigen (CEA) is used to detect relapse of colorectal cancer. CEA elevations also occur with other malignancies. Nonmalignant conditions associated with elevated CEA levels include cigarette smoking, peptic ulcer disease, inflammatory bowel disease, pancreatitis, hypothyroidism, biliary obstruction, and cirrhosis. Levels exceeding 10 ng per mL are rarely due to benign disease. Fewer than 25% of patients with disease confined to the colon have an elevated CEA level. Therefore, CEA is not useful in screening for colorectal cancer or in the diagnostic evaluation of an undiagnosed illness. A CEA level should be utilized only after malignancy has been diagnosed.

CA 19–9 may be helpful in diagnosing pancreatic abnormalities. Levels >1,000 units per mL are correlated with pancreatic cancer. Benign conditions such as cirrhosis, cholestasis, cholangitis, and pancreatitis can also result in CA 19–9 elevations, although values are usually <1,000 units per mL.

CA 125 is useful for evaluating pelvic masses in postmenopausal women, monitoring response to therapy in women with ovarian cancer, and detecting recurrence of ovarian carcinoma. Postmenopausal women with asymptomatic palpable pelvic masses and CA 125 levels >65 units per mL likely have ovarian cancer. Because premenopausal women have more benign causes of elevated CA 125 levels, testing for the marker is less useful in this population.

α-Fetoprotein (AFP) is a marker for hepatocellular carcinoma. It is used to screen highly selected populations and to assess hepatic masses in patients at particular risk for developing hepatic malignancy.

Testing for the β-subunit of human chorionic gonadotropin (β-hCG) is an integral part of the diagnosis and management of gestational trophoblastic disease. Combined AFP and β-hCG testing is an essential adjunct in the evaluation and treatment of nonseminomatous germ cell tumors and in monitoring the response to therapy. AFP and β-hCG are useful in evaluating potential origins of poorly differentiated metastatic cancer.

Prostate-specific antigen (PSA) is used to screen for prostate cancer and detects recurrence of the malignancy.

Additional Reading: Serum tumor markers. *Am Fam Physician*. 2003;68:1075–1082.

Category: Nonspecific system

14. Which one of the following is the greatest risk factor for abdominal aortic aneurysm (AAA)?
A) Cigarette smoking
B) Diabetes mellitus
C) Hypertension
D) African American race
E) Female gender

Answer and Discussion

The answer is A. Cigarette smokers are five times more likely than nonsmokers to develop an AAA. The risk is associated with the number of years the patient has smoked and declines with cessation. Diabetes mellitus is protective, decreasing the risk of AAA by half. Women tend to develop AAA in their sixties, 10 years later than men. Whites are at greater risk than African Americans. Hypertension is less of a risk factor than cigarette smoking.

Additional Reading: The U.S. Preventive Services Task Force (USPSTF) recommendations on screening for abdominal aortic aneurysm. From: http://www.uspreventiveservicestaskforce.org/uspstf/uspsaneu.htm

Category: Cardiovascular system

15. A 23-year-old otherwise healthy white woman presents complaining of dizziness. She was fine until about a week ago when she developed a case of diarrhea, which other members of her family have also had. Since that time she has been lightheaded when standing, feels her heart race, and gets headaches or blurred vision if she does not sit or lie down. She has not passed out but has been unable to work. She has not taken any medications. On exam, no abnormalities are detected except for her heart rate, which increases from 72 beats per minute when she is sitting to 112 beats per minute when she stands. Her blood pressure remains unchanged with positional changes. Routine laboratory tests and an EKG are normal. What is the most likely cause of this patient's condition?
A) Myocarditis
B) A seizure disorder
C) Postural orthostatic tachycardia syndrome (POTS)
D) Systemic lupus erythematosus (SLE)
E) Somatization disorder

Answer and Discussion

The answer is C. POTS is manifested by a rise in heart rate >30 beats per minute or by a heart rate >120 beats per minute within 10 minutes of being in the upright position. Symptoms usually include position-dependent headaches, abdominal pain, light-headedness, palpitations, sweating, and nausea. Most patients will not actually pass out, but some will if they are unable to lie down quickly enough. This condition is most prevalent in white women between the ages of 15 and 50 years. Often these patients are hardworking, athletic, and otherwise in good health. There is a high clinical correlation between POTS and chronic fatigue syndrome. Although no single etiology for POTS has been found, the condition is thought to have a genetic predisposition, is often incited after a prolonged viral illness, and has a component of deconditioning. The recommended initial management is encouraging adequate fluid and salt intake, followed by the initiation of regular aerobic exercise combined with lower-extremity strength training, and then the use of β-blockers.

Additional Reading: Dizziness: a diagnostic approach. *Am Fam Physician*. 2010;82(4):361–368, 369; and Postural orthostatic tachycardia syndrome: a clinical review. *Pediatr Neurol*. 2010;42(2):77–85.

Category: Cardiovascular system

16. Of the following conditions, which is related to the development of osteoporosis in men?
A) Prolactinoma
B) Hypogonadism
C) Prostate cancer
D) Renal stones
E) Inguinal hernia

Answer and Discussion

The answer is **B**. Men, like women, are at risk of developing osteoporosis that may lead to increased risk of fractures. Hypogonadism is an independent risk factor for osteoporosis. Dual-energy x-ray absorptiometry should be performed in men who are at increased risk of osteoporosis and who are candidates for drug therapy. Initial labs in men with osteoporosis should include a complete blood count, liver function testing, thyroid-stimulating hormone (TSH) level, serum testosterone, creatinine, calcium, and 25-OH vitamin D levels. Twenty-four-hour urine calcium and creatinine levels to identify hypercalciuria is indicated in men with osteoporosis that occurs before the age of 60 years or if initial diagnostic methods fail to determine a cause of low bone mass.

Bisphosphonates decrease the risk of vertebral fracture in men with osteoporosis. Teriparatide (Forteo) decreases the risk of vertebral fractures and can be used for treatment of severe osteoporosis. Men should have an adequate intake of calcium (1,200 mg daily) along with vitamin D (800 IU daily) to prevent osteoporosis.

Additional Reading: Osteoporosis in men. *Am Fam Physician*. 2010;82(5):503–508.

Category: Endocrine system

17. In patients treated with disulfiram (Antabuse) for alcohol abuse, which test is necessary for monitoring during treatment?
A) Alkaline phosphatase
B) Amylase
C) Creatinine
D) Alanine aminotransferase (ALT)
E) Ammonia level

Answer and Discussion

The answer is **D**. In the United States, disulfiram, acamprosate (Campral), and naltrexone (Revia) are approved for the treatment of alcohol dependence. Although disulfiram is reported to be effective as an aversive drug, placebo-controlled clinical trials have been inconclusive. Disulfiram inhibits the metabolism of anticoagulant drugs, phenytoin, and isoniazid. It should be used cautiously in patients with liver disease and is contraindicated during pregnancy and in patients with ischemic heart disease. Disulfiram can cause hepatitis, and therefore monitoring of liver function studies is essential. Acamprosate is a newer agent that works by its effect on the GABA system. Side effects include diarrhea, insomnia, anxiety, depression, pruritus, and dizziness. The third drug approved for use in the treatment of alcohol dependence is the opioid antagonist naltrexone. Naltrexone is believed to reduce consumption of alcohol and increase abstinence by reducing the craving for alcohol. The rate of relapse is highest within the first 90 days of abstinence, and it is during this time that

naltrexone may be beneficial. Daily dosages may range from 25 to 100 mg. Side effects include nausea, headache, anxiety, and sedation. Naltrexone can be hepatotoxic at higher dosages and should be used with caution in patients with chronic liver disease. Selective serotonin reuptake inhibitors (SSRIs), including fluoxetine and sertraline, have been found to decrease alcohol intake in heavy drinkers without a history of depression. However, in some trials SSRIs were found to be no more effective than a placebo. Any drug therapy should be combined with psychotherapy or group therapy to help address the social and psychologic aspects of alcohol dependence.

Additional Reading: Management of alcohol withdrawal syndrome. *Am Fam Physician*. 2010;82(4):344–347.

Category: Psychogenic

> **Disulfiram can cause hepatitis, and therefore monitoring of liver function studies is essential.**

18. The test of choice for the diagnosis of ureteral obstruction secondary to renal lithiasis is
A) Noncontrast helical computed tomography (CT)
B) Ultrasound
C) Intravenous pyelogram
D) Magnetic resonance imaging (MRI)
E) Plain radiographs

Answer and Discussion

The answer is **A**. The most common cause of the sudden onset of flank pain in adults is acute urolithiasis. Identification of a stone in the ureter with resultant partial or complete ureteral obstruction confirms the suspected diagnosis. Noncontrast helical CT has the advantages of avoiding contrast exposure, identifying radiolucent calculi, evaluating nearby structures and requires a shorter time for examination. As a result, helical CT is a better test for assessing acute urolithiasis. Abdominal ultrasound has a high specificity in evaluating stones, but its sensitivity is lower than helical CT. Plain films are used to follow patients with known radiopaque (i.e., calcium) stones.

Additional Reading: Guidelines on urolithiasis. *European association of urology (EAU)*. 2008; 128 p.

Category: Nephrologic

19. Which of the following infections is least likely in a patient with COPD?
A) Streptococcus pneumoniae
B) Haemophilus influenzae
C) Moraxella catarrhalis
D) Mycoplasma pneumoniae

Answer and Discussion

The answer is **D**. COPD is a disease process involving progressive chronic airflow obstruction because of chronic bronchitis, emphysema, or both. Chronic bronchitis is defined clinically as excessive cough and sputum production on most days for at least 3 months during at least 2 consecutive years. Emphysema is characterized by chronic dyspnea resulting from the destruction of lung tissue and the enlargement of air spaces. Asthma, which features airflow obstruction, airway inflammation, and increased airway responsiveness to various stimuli, may be distinguished from COPD by reversibility of pulmonary function deficits. Acute exacerbations of COPD are treated with oxygen (in hypoxemic patients), inhaled β2 agonists, inhaled anticholinergics, antibiotics, and systemic corticosteroids. Theophylline may be considered in patients who do not respond to other bronchodilators.

Antibiotic therapy is directed at the most common pathogens, including *Streptococcus pneumoniae*, *Haemophilus influenzae*, and *Moraxella catarrhalis*. Mild-to-moderate exacerbations of COPD are usually treated with broad-spectrum antibiotics such as doxycycline, trimethoprim-sulfamethoxazole, and amoxicillin-clavulanate potassium. Treatment with extended-spectrum penicillins, fluoroquinolones, third-generation cephalosporins, or aminoglycosides may be considered in patients with severe exacerbations. The management of chronic stable COPD includes smoking cessation and oxygen therapy. Inhaled β2 agonists, inhaled anticholinergics, and systemic corticosteroids are also used in patients with chronic stable disease. Inhaled corticosteroids decrease airway reactivity and can reduce the use of health care services for management of respiratory symptoms. Avoiding acute exacerbations helps to reduce long-term complications. Long-term oxygen therapy, regular monitoring of pulmonary function, and referral for pulmonary rehabilitation are often utilized and can improve the quality of life and reduce hospitalizations. Influenza and pneumococcal vaccines should be administered. Selected patients who do not respond to standard therapies may benefit from lung-reduction surgery.

Additional Reading: ACP updates guideline on diagnosis and management of stable COPD. *Am Fam Physician*. 2012;85(2): 204–205.

Category: Respiratory system

20. Because of safety concerns, which one of the following asthma medications should be used only as additive therapy and not as monotherapy?
A) Inhaled corticosteroids
B) Leukotriene-receptor antagonists
C) Short-acting β-agonists
D) Long-acting β-agonists
E) Mast-cell stabilizers

Answer and Discussion

The answer is D. Because of the risk of asthma exacerbation or asthma-related death, the Food and Drug Administration (FDA) has added a warning against the use of long-acting β-agonists as monotherapy. Inhaled corticosteroids, leukotriene-receptor antagonists, short-acting β-agonists, and mast-cell stabilizers are approved and accepted for both monotherapy and combination therapy in the management of asthma.

Additional Reading: Drugs for asthma and COPD. *Treat Guidel Med Lett*. 2013;132:75.

Category: Respiratory system

21. A 65-year-old with a history of chronic atrial fibrillation is being monitored while on warfarin therapy. The nurse calls to inform you the patient's international normalized ratio (INR) is measured at 7. He has no active signs of bleeding, but is at increased risk of bleeding. Appropriate management at this time includes which of the following:
A) Stop warfarin, observe, and repeat INR in 3 days.
B) Stop warfarin and observe; repeat INR in 24 hours.
C) Stop warfarin, give vitamin K, and repeat INR in 24 hours.
D) Stop warfarin, give vitamin K and fresh-frozen plasma with daily INRs.

Answer and Discussion

The answer is C. Warfarin inhibits the formation of clotting factors II, VII, IX, and X. The drug is highly protein-bound to albumin. Because of this inverse relationship between the levels of albumin and free warfarin, acutely ill patients with poor nutritional states and postoperative patients may need lower dosages of warfarin. The INR is the patient's prothrombin time divided by the mean of the normal prothrombin time, with this ratio raised to the international sensitivity index. After starting warfarin therapy, a steady-state response is not typically achieved for approximately 2 weeks. A dosage of 4 to 5 mg per day is typical, although the required dosage may be variable (as low as 0.5 mg or as high as 50 mg per day). Elderly patients should start at a lower dosage. Checking the INR approximately 24 hours after the first dose can help determine the second dose. If there has been little or no rise in the INR (which is to be expected), a 5-mg dose on the second day should be safe. If an INR is not available on the day after the first dose, it can be obtained on days 2, 3, or 4. If the initial INR (on days 1 through 4) is high, the patient is likely sensitive to warfarin's effects; therefore, a lower dose should be given. Patients who are restarting warfarin therapy after a time off the drug can safely begin with their previous maintenance dose. Guidelines recommend that the INR be checked at least four times during the first week of therapy. This frequency could then be gradually decreased on the basis of the stability of the INR. Because the risk of bleeding is greatest in the first 6 to 12 weeks of treatment, checking the INR weekly is appropriate. The maximum time between tests should be no more than 4 to 6 weeks. If a patient's INR has been stable and then fluctuates by more than 0.2 below or 0.4 above the goal INR, the patient should be evaluated for the cause of the change. Associated causes include laboratory error, noncompliance, drug interactions with warfarin, dietary interactions, or a change in the patient's health. If no reversible cause is found, a change in dosage may be made, with a repeat INR within 2 weeks. Close follow-up with repeated testing is needed because the patients who have the most variation in results are most likely to develop bleeding or thromboembolism. In asymptomatic patients whose INR is elevated, temporary discontinuation of the drug is often used, but administration of vitamin K shortens the time to return to the target INR. There is indirect evidence that use of vitamin K is associated with a lower incidence of hemorrhage. Oral vitamin K is effective and may have fewer risks than the parenterally administered form. When a patient's INR is between 5 and 9, the recommendations include temporary discontinuation of warfarin therapy. If the patient is at risk for hemorrhage (e.g., is taking nonsteroidal anti-inflammatory drugs [NSAIDs]), low-dose oral vitamin K (1.0 to 2.5 mg) also should be given. However, the lowest dose available in tablet form is 5 mg, and often only 1 or 2 mg is needed. The parenteral form can be given orally and mixed in a flavored drink if needed. If the patient cannot be treated orally, 0.5 to 1 mg of intravenous vitamin K should be administered. For INRs of 9 or higher, vitamin K also should be given at a higher dose (2.5 mg intravenously or 5 mg orally). A repeat INR should be obtained within 24 hours. Additional vitamin K may be needed, depending on the result of the repeat INR. If the INR is elevated and the patient is bleeding, fresh-frozen plasma or a concentrate of clotting factors should be administered. A repeat INR should be obtained shortly after the fresh-frozen plasma is given. Additional fresh-frozen plasma may be needed because of its short duration of action. A large dose of vitamin K (10 mg) should also be given. Additional vitamin K may be necessary because the half-life of warfarin is longer than the half-life of vitamin K. Daily INR measurements should be instituted.

Additional Reading: A systematic approach to managing warfarin doses. *Fam Pract Manag.* 2005;12(5):77–83.

Category: Cardiovascular system

22. A 60-year-old man presents to your office inquiring about prostate cancer screening. Choose the correct statement:
A) PSA is the gold standard test for prostate cancer screening.
B) PSA should be checked annually starting at 50 years of age to screen for prostate cancer.
C) PSA can produce false-positive results, which can be associated with negative psychological effects.
D) Men who have false-positive test are less likely to have additional testing.
E) The USPSTF recommends PSA testing to screen for prostate cancer at age 60.

Answer and Discussion

The answer is C. Convincing evidence demonstrates that the PSA test often produces false-positive results; approximately 80 percent of positive PSA test results are false-positive when cutoffs between 2.5 and 4.0 ng per mL (2.5 and 4.0 µg per L) are used. There is adequate evidence that false-positive PSA test results are associated with negative psychological effects, including persistent worry about prostate cancer. Men who have a false-positive test result are more likely to have additional testing, including one or more biopsies, in the following year than those who have a negative test result.

There is also convincing evidence that a substantial percentage of men who have asymptomatic cancer detected by PSA screening have a tumor that either will not progress or will progress so slowly that it would have remained asymptomatic for the man's lifetime.

Although the precise, long-term effect of PSA screening on prostate cancer–specific mortality remains uncertain, existing studies adequately demonstrate that the reduction in prostate cancer mortality after 10 to 14 years is, at most, very small, even for men in what seems to be the optimal age range of 55 to 69 years. There is no apparent reduction in all-cause mortality. In contrast, the harms associated with the diagnosis and treatment of screen-detected cancer are common, occur early, often persist, and include a small but real risk of premature death.

Additional Reading: U.S. Preventive Services Task Force. Screening for prostate cancer: Recommendation statement. *Am Fam Physician.* 2013;87(4):267–273.

Category: Reproductive system

23. Type II renal tubular acidosis (RTA) is associated with
A) The proximal tubules having decreased ability to absorb bicarbonate
B) Urine pH that is normal when plasma bicarbonate levels are normal
C) Chronic metabolic alkalosis
D) Plasma bicarbonate levels that are easily restored with supplementation
E) Hyperkalemia

Answer and Discussion

The answer is A. Type I (distal) RTA is a disorder that affects adults and is considered a familial disorder in children. Sporadic cases may be primary (especially in women) or secondary (e.g., to an autoimmune disease such as Sjögren's syndrome; medications including amphotericin B or lithium therapy; kidney transplantation; nephrocalcinosis; renal medullary sponge kidney; chronic

renal obstruction). Familial cases may be autosomal dominant and are often associated with hypercalciuria. In type I RTA, the urine pH is never <5.5.

Type II (proximal) RTA is associated with several inherited diseases (e.g., Fanconi's syndrome, fructose intolerance, Wilson's disease, Lowe's syndrome), multiple myeloma, vitamin D deficiency, and chronic hypocalcemia with secondary hyperparathyroidism. It may occur after renal transplant, exposure to heavy metals, and after treatment with certain medications, including acetazolamide, sulfonamides, tetracycline, and streptozocin.

In type II RTA, the ability of the proximal tubules to reabsorb HCO_3^- is decreased, so that urine pH is >7 at normal levels of plasma HCO_3^-, but may be <5.5 at low levels of plasma HCO_3^-. Type III RTA is a combination of types I and II and is seldom seen.

Type IV RTA is a condition associated with mild renal insufficiency in adults with diabetes mellitus, human immunodeficiency virus (HIV) nephropathy, or interstitial renal damage (SLE, obstructive uropathy, sickle cell disease). It may also be produced by drugs that interfere with the renin–aldosterone system (e.g., NSAIDs, angiotensin-converting enzyme [ACE] inhibitors, potassium-sparing diuretics, trimethoprim). Aldosterone deficiency or unresponsiveness of the distal tubule to aldosterone results in type IV RTA. This reduces potassium excretion, causing hyperkalemia, which reduces ammonia production and acid excretion by the kidney. Urine pH is usually normal.

Types I and II RTA are associated with chronic metabolic acidosis, mild volume loss, and hypokalemia. Hypokalemia may lead to muscle weakness, hyporeflexia, and paralysis. Type I RTA has decreased citrate excretion in the urine, increased mobilization of bone calcium, and hypercalciuria, which results in osteopenia, bone pain, and kidney stones or nephrocalcinosis. Renal parenchymal damage and chronic renal failure may develop. Type IV RTA is usually asymptomatic with only mild acidosis, but cardiac arrhythmias or paralysis may develop if hyperkalemia is extreme. Sodium bicarbonate relieves symptoms and prevents or stabilizes renal failure and bone disease. In adults with type I RTA, sodium bicarbonate eliminates acidosis and reduces the occurrence of kidney stones. In type II RTA, the plasma HCO_3^- cannot be restored to the normal range. HCO_3^- replacement should exceed the acid load of the diet. Additional HCO_3^- replacement increases potassium bicarbonate losses in the urine. Citric acid/sodium citrate (Bicitra) or potassium citrate/citric acid (Polycitra-K) can be substituted for sodium bicarbonate and may be better tolerated. Potassium supplements may be required in patients who become hypokalemic when given sodium bicarbonate, but are not recommended in patients with normal or high serum potassium levels. In type IV RTA, the hyperkalemia is treated with fluid administration and potassium-depleting diuretics. A few patients may need mineralocorticoid replacement therapy.

Additional Reading: Overview of renal tubular acidosis. In: Basow DS, ed. *UpToDate.* Waltham, MA: UpToDate; 2013.

Category: Nephrologic

24. Which of the following is considered a first-line medication in the treatment of hypertension?
A) Chlorthalidone
B) Lisinopril
C) Clonidine
D) Losartan
E) Amlodipine

Answer and Discussion

The answer is A. A 2009 Cochrane review was undertaken to compare the effects of thiazide diuretics, β-blockers, ACE inhibitors, and CCBs with placebo. Thiazide diuretics (e.g., chlorthalidone, hydrochlorothiazide) lowered mortality and morbidity from stroke, heart attack, and heart failure more than β-blockers. ACE inhibitors (e.g., lisinopril) and CCBs (e.g., amlodipine) reduced mortality and morbidity as much as thiazide diuretics, but the evidence is less robust. Because the use of thiazide diuretics is supported by a strong body of evidence and no other class of antihypertensive medications has been shown to be better at improving outcomes, they are the first-line drugs for most patients with hypertension.

Doxazosin is an α-blocker and is not indicated for first-line treatment. Losartan is an angiotensin-receptor blocker (ARB), which should be reserved for patients who cannot tolerate ACE inhibitors. Unfortunately, there are no high-quality randomized controlled trials (RCTs) to fully evaluate the effects of ARBs or α-blockers and current evidence does not support using β-blockers as first-line therapy for hypertension.

Diuretics remain the preferred first-step drug and an important part of any multidrug regimen for the treatment of hypertension. ACE inhibitors and CCBs appear to be as effective as thiazide diuretics, but the evidence is not as strong.

Additional Reading: First-line treatment for hypertension. *Am Fam Physician.* 2010;81(11):1333–1335.

Category: Cardiovascular system

> **Low-dose thiazides reduce all morbidity and mortality outcomes.**

25. Which of the following drugs offers protection from osteoporosis?
A) Hydrochlorothiazide
B) Metoprolol
C) Enalapril
D) Verapamil
E) Losartan

Answer and Discussion

The answer is A. In healthy elderly adults, low-dose hydrochlorothiazide preserves bone mineral density at the hip and spine. Hydrochlorothiazide produces small positive benefits on cortical bone density that are sustained for at least the first 4 years of treatment. They provide a further option in the prevention of postmenopausal bone loss, especially for women with hypertension or a history of kidney stones. None of the other listed medications provides this protection.

Additional Reading: The effect of treatment with a thiazide diuretic for 4 years on bone density in normal postmenopausal women. *Osteoporo Int.* 2007;18(4):479–486.

Category: Endocrine system

26. An ankle-brachial index of _____ is considered normal.
A) 0.95
B) 0.75
C) 0.50
D) 0.25
E) 0.15

Answer and Discussion

The answer is A. Symptoms of claudication include pain, ache, cramp, or tired feeling that occurs on walking. They are most common in the calf but may occur in the foot, thigh, hip, or buttocks. The condition is worsened by walking rapidly or uphill and usually relieved in 1 to 5 minutes by rest (sitting is not necessary); the patient can walk the same distance again before pain recurs. Disease progression is indicated by a reduction in the distance that the patient can walk without symptoms. Eventually, ischemic pain may occur at rest, beginning in the most distal parts of a limb as a severe, unrelenting pain aggravated by elevation and often interfering with sleep. If intermittent claudication is the only symptom, the extremity may appear normal, but the pulses are reduced or absent. The level of arterial occlusion and the location of intermittent claudication closely correlate (e.g., aortoiliac disease frequently causes claudication in the buttocks, hips, and calves, and the femoral pulses are reduced or absent). In men, impotence is common and depends on the location and extent of occlusion. In femoropopliteal disease, claudication is typically in the calf, and all pulses below the femoral are absent. In patients with small vessel disease (e.g., thromboangiitis obliterans, diabetes mellitus), femoropopliteal pulses may be present, but foot pulses are absent. Pallor of the involved foot after 1 to 2 minutes of elevation, followed by redness on dependency, helps confirm arterial insufficiency. Normal venous filling time with dependency after elevation is 15 seconds. If symptoms of claudication occur with good distal pulses, spinal stenosis should be considered. A severely ischemic foot is painful, cold, and often numb. In chronic cases, the skin may be dry and scaly, with poor nail and hair growth. As ischemia worsens, ulceration may appear (typically on the toes or heel, occasionally on the leg), especially after local trauma. Edema is usually not present unless the patient has kept the leg in a dependent position for pain relief. More extensive blockage may compromise tissue viability, leading to necrosis or gangrene. Ischemia with redness, pain, and swelling of the foot on dependency may mimic cellulitis or venous insufficiency. Although arterial occlusion in the extremities can usually be diagnosed clinically, noninvasive tests confirm the diagnosis and are useful in follow-up. Invasive tests can document the location and extent of disease if angioplasty, local fibrinolytic therapy, or surgical bypass is contemplated. Doppler ultrasonography is most widely used. Arterial stenosis and occlusion can be detected using a velocity detector (Doppler probe). A colored signal shows the direction of flow (color Doppler). The simplest method for estimating blood flow to the lower extremities is to compare systolic BP at the level of the ankle with brachial systolic pressure (ankle-brachial indices). During this procedure, a blood pressure cuff is applied to the ankle, inflated above brachial systolic pressure, and deflated slowly. Ankle systolic blood pressure can be obtained accurately with a Doppler probe placed over the dorsalis pedis or posterior tibial arteries. This blood pressure at rest normally is ≥90% of the brachial systolic pressure; with mild arterial insufficiency, it is 70% to 90%; with moderate insufficiency, 50% to 70%; and with severe insufficiency, <50%.

Additional Reading: Critical review of the ankle brachial index. *Curr Cardiol Rev.* 2008;4(2):101–106.

Category: Cardiovascular system

27. A secondary cause of RLS is
A) Vitamin B_{12} deficiency
B) Heavy metal intoxication
C) Alcohol abuse
D) Iron deficiency
E) Bismuth overdose

Answer and Discussion

The answer is D. RLS is a neurologic movement disorder that is often associated with a sleep disturbance. Patients with RLS have an irresistible urge to move their legs, which is usually secondary to uncomfortable sensations that are worse during periods of inactivity and often interfere with sleep. It is estimated that between 2% and 15% of the population may experience symptoms of RLS. Primary RLS may have a genetic origin. The diagnosis of RLS is based primarily on the patient's history. Pharmacologic treatment of RLS includes dopaminergic agents, opioids, benzodiazepines, and anticonvulsants.

Secondary causes of RLS include iron deficiency, neurologic lesions, pregnancy, and uremia. Patients with iron deficiency may receive symptom relief by taking supplemental iron. A ferritin level of less than 50 ng per mL may cause or exacerbate RLS. Although levels above 10 to 20 ng per mL are reported as normal, supplemental iron may improve symptoms in individuals with levels less than 50 ng per mL. Iron is not beneficial in individuals with ferritin above this level. RLS also may occur secondarily to the use of certain medications.

Additional Reading: Restless legs syndrome. *Am Fam Physician.* 2008;78(2):235–240.

Category: Neurologic

28. In appropriate patients, thrombolytic therapy can be given up to __hours after onset of stroke symptoms.
A) 1 hour
B) 2 hours
C) 3 hours
D) 24 hours
E) 36 hours

Answer and Discussion

The answer is C. Transient ischemic attack (TIA) is considered a significant warning sign of impending stroke. It is crucial to recognize these events to prevent permanent disability or death in affected individuals. The 90-day risk of stroke after a TIA has been estimated to be approximately 10%, with one-half of strokes occurring within the first 2 days of the attack. The 90-day stroke risk is even higher when a TIA results from internal carotid artery disease. Most patients reporting symptoms of TIA should be referred to an emergency department for further evaluation. Patients who arrive at the emergency department within 180 minutes of symptom onset should undergo evaluation to determine if they are candidates for thrombolytic therapy. Initial testing should include complete blood count with platelet count, prothrombin time, international normalized ratio, partial thromboplastin time, and electrolyte and glucose levels. CT scanning of the head should be performed immediately to ensure that there is no evidence of brain hemorrhage or mass. Risk factors for stroke should be evaluated in patients who have had a TIA. Blood pressure, lipid levels, and diabetes mellitus should be controlled. If indicated, smoking cessation and weight loss are also important. ACE inhibitor therapy may help prevent stroke. Aspirin is the treatment of choice for stroke prevention in patients who do not require anticoagulation. Clopidogrel (Plavix) is an alternative therapy in patients who do not tolerate aspirin. Atrial fibrillation, a known cardioembolic source (confirmed thrombus), or a highly suspected cardioembolic source (e.g., recent large MI, dilated cardiomyopathy, mechanical valve, rheumatic mitral valve stenosis) is an indication for anticoagulation with warfarin therapy.

Additional Reading: Transient ischemic attacks: Part I. Diagnosis and evaluation. *Am Fam Physician.* 2004;69:1665–1674, 1679–1680.

Transient ischemic attacks: Part II. Treatment. *Am Fam Physician.* 2004;69:1681–1688.

Category: Neurologic

29. Of the following, which is *least* likely to be seen in strep throat?
A) Fever
B) Malaise
C) Tonsilar exudates
D) Palatine petechiae
E) Rhinorrhea

Answer and Discussion

The answer is E. Sore throat is one of the most common reasons for visits to family physicians. Although most patients with sore throat have an infectious cause (pharyngitis), <20% have a clear indication for antibiotic therapy (i.e., group A β-hemolytic streptococcal infection). Viral pharyngitis is the most common cause of sore throat. Infectious mononucleosis (IM) is most common in patients 15 to 30 years of age. Patients typically present with fever, sore throat, and malaise. On examination, there is pharyngeal redness with exudates. Posterior cervical lymphadenopathy is common in patients with IM, and its absence makes the diagnosis much less likely. Hepatosplenomegaly also may be present. If these patients are treated with amoxicillin or ampicillin, 90% develop a classic maculopapular rash. Patients with bacterial pharyngitis generally do not have rhinorrhea, cough, or conjunctivitis. Children younger than 15 are more likely to have strep throat. Symptoms of strep throat may include pharyngeal erythema and swelling, tonsillar exudate, edematous uvula, palatine petechiae, and anterior cervical lymphadenopathy. Untreated, strep pharyngitis lasts 7 to 10 days. Patients with untreated streptococcal pharyngitis are infectious during the acute phase of the illness and for 1 additional week. Antibiotic therapy shortens the infectious period to 24 hours, reduces the duration of symptoms by about 1 day, and prevents most complications. The incidence of complications with strep infection, such as rheumatic fever and peritonsillar abscess, is low. Peritonsillar abscess occurs in <1% of patients treated with antibiotics. Patients with peritonsillar abscess typically have a toxic appearance and may present with a muffled voice, fluctuant peritonsillar mass, and asymmetric deviation.

Additional Reading: Pharyngitis. *Am Fam Physician.* 2004;69:1465–1470.

Category: Respiratory system

30. Angioneurotic edema is associated with the use of
A) ACE inhibitors
B) β-Blockers
C) Loop diuretics
D) α-Receptor blockers
E) CCBs

Answer and Discussion

The answer is A. Angioneurotic edema, which occurs in 0.1% to 0.2% of patients, usually develops within the first week of therapy but can occur at any time. This life-threatening adverse effect also occurs with angiotensin II-receptor blockers, but to a lesser extent. Any patient with a history of angioneurotic edema, whether related to an ACE inhibitor, ARBs, or another cause, should not be given an ACE inhibitor. Other contraindications include pregnancy, renal artery stenosis, and previous allergy to ACE inhibitors.

Additional Reading: Drugs for Hypertension. *Treat Guidel Med Lett.* 2012;10(113):1–10.

Category: Cardiovascular system

31. Genital warts
A) Rarely resolve spontaneously
B) Are treated on the basis of cost, convenience, and adverse affects
C) Do not remain in tissue after treatment
D) Are treated with an alternative method if a single treatment fails to eradicate the wart

Answer and Discussion

The answer is B. Untreated visible genital warts may resolve spontaneously, remain the same, or increase in size. The primary treatment goal is removal of symptomatic warts. Some evidence suggests that treatment may also reduce the persistence of human papillomavirus (HPV) DNA in genital tissue and therefore may reduce the incidence of cervical cancer. The choice of therapy is based on the number, size, site, and morphology of lesions, as well as patient preference, treatment cost, convenience, adverse effects, and physician experience. Assuming that the diagnosis is certain, switching to a new treatment modality is appropriate if there is no response after three treatment cycles. Routine follow-up at 2 to 3 months is advised to monitor response to therapy and evaluate for recurrence. Treatment methods can be chemical or ablative.

Additional Reading: Management of genital warts. *Am Fam Physician.* 2004;70:2335–2342, 2345–2346.

Category: Integumentary

32. In which of the following cases is comprehensive evaluation necessary when a patient is affected by a deep venous thrombosis (DVT)?
A) 45-year-old man with an idiopathic DVT
B) 65-year-old with a recent transatlantic flight and DVT of left thigh
C) 55-year-old who develops a calf DVT after a 4-hour car ride
D) 75-year-old with a history of non–small cell cancer of lung with left leg DVT
E) 72-year-old with a right thigh DVT and no history of travel

Answer and Discussion

The answer is A. Treatment goals for DVT include stopping clot propagation and preventing the recurrence of thrombus, the occurrence of PE, and the development of pulmonary hypertension, which can be a complication of multiple recurrent pulmonary emboli. About 30% of patients with DVT or PE have a thrombophilia. A comprehensive evaluation is suggested in patients younger than 50 years with an idiopathic episode of DVT, patients with recurrent thrombosis, and patients with a family history of thromboembolism. Intravenous administration of unfractionated heparin followed by oral administration of warfarin remains the mainstay of treatment for DVT. Subcutaneous low-molecular-weight (LMW) heparin is at least as effective as unfractionated heparin given in a continuous intravenous route. LMW heparin is the agent of choice for treating DVT in pregnant women and patients with cancer. On the basis of validated protocols, warfarin can be started at a dosage of 5 or 10 mg per day. The intensity and duration of warfarin therapy depends on the individual patient, but treatment of at least 3 months usually is required. Some patients with thrombophilias require lifetime anticoagulation. Treatment for PE is similar to that for DVT. Because of the risk of respiratory failure and hemodynamic instability, in-hospital management is advised. Unfractionated heparin is commonly used, although LMW heparin is safe and effective. Thrombolysis is used in patients with massive PE. Subcutaneous heparin, LMW heparin, and warfarin have been approved for use in surgical prophylaxis. Elastic compression stockings are useful in patients at lowest risk for thromboembolism. Intermittent pneumatic leg compression is a useful adjunct to anticoagulation and an alternative when anticoagulation is contraindicated.

Additional Reading: Diagnosis of deep venous thrombosis and pulmonary embolism. *Am Fam Physician.* 2012;86(10):913–919

Category: Cardiovascular system

33. Which of the following statements is correct concerning hepatitis C virus (HCV)?
A) There is no risk to infants if the mother is affected.
B) There is no risk associated with sexual intercourse with an individual with hepatitis C.
C) Cesarean section should be performed on mothers who test positive for hepatitis C to prevent transmission to the newborn.
D) Hepatitis C can be spread by contaminated water supplies.
E) Hepatitis C does not appear to be transmitted in breast milk.

Answer and Discussion

The answer is E. In an effort to reduce the risk of transmission to others, HCV-positive patients should be advised not to donate blood, organs, tissue, or semen; not to share toothbrushes, dental appliances, razors, or other personal care articles that might have blood on them; and to cover cuts and sores on the skin to keep from spreading infectious blood or secretions. HCV-positive patients with one long-term, steady sex partner do not need to change their sexual practices. They should, however, discuss the risk (which is low but not absent) with their partner. If they want to lower the small chance of spreading HCV to their partner, they may decide to use barrier precautions such as latex condoms. HCV-positive women do not need to avoid pregnancy or breast-feeding. Potential, expectant, and new parents should be advised that about 5 of every 100 infants born to HCV-infected women become infected. This infection occurs at the time of birth, and no treatment has been shown to prevent the transmission. There is no evidence that the method of delivery is related to transmission; therefore, the need for cesarean section versus vaginal delivery should not be determined on the basis of HCV-infection status. Limited data on breast-feeding indicate that it does not transmit HCV, although it may be prudent for HCV-positive mothers to abstain from breast-feeding if their nipples are cracked or bleeding. Infants born to HCV-positive women should be tested for HCV infection and, if positive, evaluated for the presence or development of chronic liver disease. HCV is not spread by sneezing, hugging, coughing, food or water, sharing eating utensils or drinking glasses, or casual contact. Persons should not be excluded from work, school, play, child care, or other settings on the basis of HCV-infection status. HCV-positive persons should be evaluated to assess for biochemical evidence of chronic liver disease. These patients should be assessed for severity of disease and possible treatment according to current practice guidelines in consultation with, or by referral to, a specialist knowledgeable in this field.

Additional Reading: Hepatitis C: diagnosis and treatment. *Am Fam Physician.* 2010;81(11):1351–1357.

Category: Gastroenterology system

> ⦿ HCV-positive women do not need to avoid pregnancy or breast-feeding.

34. Which of the following classes of drugs can be used safely with NSAIDs without needing to closely monitor the patient's renal function, potassium levels, and/or blood pressure?
A) ACE inhibitors
B) CCBs
C) Diuretics
D) β-Blockers

Answer and Discussion

The answer is B. Combined use of NSAIDs and hypertensive medication (i.e., diuretics, β-blockers, α-blockers, and ACE inhibitors) may decrease the effectiveness of antihypertensive medication and cause serious complications. Thus, when using the two in combination, renal function, potassium levels, and blood pressure should be monitored. CCBs and central α-agonists can usually be used without these concerns.

> **Additional Reading:** Mechanisms and treatment of resistant hypertension. *J Clin Hypertens (Greenwich)*. 2008;10(3):239–244.

> **Category:** Cardiovascular system

35. Which of the following statements about sunscreens and sun exposure is true?
A) The most dangerous rays are the ultraviolet A (UVA) type.
B) Sunscreens with a skin protection factor of 10 are adequate protection.
C) Patients allergic to thiazide diuretics may react adversely to *para*-aminobenzoic acid (PABA).
D) Steroids should be avoided in patients with sunburns because of their immunosuppressant properties.
E) Repeated use of sunscreens can increase the risk of sun poisoning.

Answer and Discussion

The answer is C. Sun-produced UV light is divided into two types of rays: UVA (320 to 400 nm) and UVB (280 to 320 nm). The dangerous rays are in the UVB range. Sunscreens of at least skin protection factor 15 (and preferably SPF-30) should be used when persons are exposed to the sun. *Para*-aminobenzoic acid, which is used in many sunscreens, is very effective at preventing sunburns. Unfortunately, patients with sensitivities to thiazides, benzocaine, or sulfonamides may react adversely to *para*-aminobenzoic acid. In most cases, sunburn is prevented with simple precautions. Sunburn (usually a first-degree burn) appears within the first 24 hours and can be very painful. Sunburn is treated with cold-water compresses. In severe cases, sunburns can be treated with steroids.

> **Additional Reading:** Sunscreens revisited. *Med Lett Drugs Ther*. 2011;53(1359):17–18.

> **Category:** Integumentary

36. Which of the following tests is recommended to be used to screen when celiac sprue is suspected?
A) Shilling's test
B) Antigliadin IgA and IgG antibodies
C) IgA tissue transglutaminase antibodies (tTG)
D) Withdrawal of lactose from the diet to monitor for improvement of symptoms
E) Scotch tape test

Answer and Discussion

The answer is C. Celiac sprue is an inherited disorder that is characterized by an intolerance to gluten, a cereal-type protein found in wheat, rye, oats, and barley. Symptoms in infancy include colic, failure to thrive, and, in severe cases, iron-deficiency anemia with the development of edema. In adults, symptoms include abdominal bloating and discomfort, with diarrhea, anemia, weight loss, arthralgias, and edema. Steatorrhea is usually present. Laboratory findings usually include iron-deficiency anemia (in children), folate-deficiency anemia (in adults), low protein levels, and electrolyte abnormalities and coagulation studies may be abnormal.

Celiac disease can be difficult to diagnose and may be confused with irritable bowel syndrome, inflammatory bowel disease, diverticulitis, intestinal infections, iron-deficiency anemia caused by menstrual blood loss, and chronic fatigue syndrome. IgA tissue transglutaminase antibodies (tTG) and IgA endomysial antibodies (EMA) are appropriate first-line serologic tests to rule in celiac disease. The tTG test uses a less costly enzyme-linked immunosorbent assay (ELISA); therefore, it is the recommended single serologic test for celiac disease screening in the primary care setting. However, a minority of patients with celiac disease have IgA deficiency. Therefore, if the serum IgA tTG result is negative but clinical suspicion for the disease is high, a serum total IgA level may be considered. Antigliadin IgA and IgG antibodies are elevated in >90% of patients; however, they are nonspecific and no longer recommended to test for celiac disease. A positive IgA tTG result should prompt small bowel biopsy to confirm the diagnosis. A jejunum biopsy would show a flat mucosa with a loss of intestinal villi. Before being tested, one should continue to eat a diet that includes foods with gluten, such as breads and pastas. If a person stops eating foods with gluten before being tested, the results may be negative for celiac disease even if the disease is present.

The Schilling test is used to diagnose pernicipous aneamia in patients with vitamin B_{12} deficiency, and the Scotch tape test is used in the diagnosis of pin worms. Withdrawal of lactose from the diet to monitor for improvement of symptoms can be utilized when assessing patients for lactose deficiency.

Treatment involves dietary counseling to avoid gluten-containing foods and supplementary vitamins. In severe cases, corticosteroids are used to induce a refractory stage.

> **Additional Reading:** Celiac disease. *Am Fam Physician*. 2007; 76(12):1795–1802.

> **Category:** Gastroenterology system

37. Pain associated with the distal second metatarsal head is most likely a result of
A) Morton's neuroma
B) Jones fracture
C) Gout
D) Metatarsalgia

Answer and Discussion

The answer is D. Metatarsalgia is characterized by pain and sometimes swelling associated with the second (and, less commonly, the third) metatarsal head. The pain is secondary to a synovitis that affects the joint. Patients with hammertoes are at an increased risk because of stress placed at the head of the metatarsals. In most cases, radiographs are normal; however, more severe cases may show subluxation or dislocation of the metacarpal joint. NSAIDs, hot soaks, and metatarsal pads may help; however, if subluxation or dislocation is present, surgery may be necessary. Morton's neuroma usually presents with a feeling as if the patient is standing on a pebble in their shoe, with a burning sensation in the ball of your foot that may radiate into the toes. A Jones fracture is a fairly common fracture of the fifth metatarsal, and gout typically involves pain and inflammation at the first metatarsophalangeal joint, although other toes can be involved.

Additional Reading: Busconi BD, Stevenson JH. Approach to the athlete with metatarsalgia. *Sports Medicine Consult: A Problem-Based Approach to Sports Medicine for the Primary Care Physician.* Philadelphia, PA: Lippincott, Williams & Wilkins; 2009

Category: Musculoskeletal system

38. Desensitization immunotherapy may be used in the treatment of
A) Chronic urticaria
B) Hymenoptera allergies
C) Atopic dermatitis
D) Milk allergy
E) None of the above

Answer and Discussion

The answer is B. Desensitization immunotherapy is used in the treatment of severe allergic rhinitis and beesting (hymenoptera) allergies. The patient is given gradually increasing concentrations of the allergen over an increasing period. Typically, there is a decrease in the mast-cell response with a decrease in histamine production when the patient is exposed to the allergen. In addition, IgE levels decrease. In most cases, the injections are continued year-round and may be spaced out as the desired response occurs. Injections should always be given in the presence of a physician, and appropriate equipment must be available to treat potential anaphylaxis. Patients must be observed for at least 30 minutes after administration of the injections. Desensitization immunotherapy is not appropriate for the treatment of chronic urticaria, milk allergies, or atopic dermatitis.

Additional Reading: Allergen immunotherapy. *Am Fam Physician.* 2004;70(4):689–696.

Category: Nonspecific system

39. A 21-year-old man is brought to the emergency room after suffering a seizure. He is tachycardic and hypertensive and has a temperature of 38.6°C. Physical examination shows that the patient is in a postictal state and has a nasal septum perforation. Electrocardiogram (ECG) findings suggest acute MI. Friends of the patient report recent cocaine use. Which of the following drugs is indicated?
A) Elumazenil
B) Diazepam
C) Dexfenfluramine
D) Propranolol
E) Phenytoin

Answer and Discussion

The answer is B. Cocaine is a strong narcotic stimulant that is often abused. Its mechanism of action involves the increased release of norepinephrine and the blockage of its reuptake. Effects of cocaine begin within 3 to 5 minutes (within 8 to 10 seconds with smoking "crack" cocaine), and peak effects occur at 10 to 20 minutes. The effects rarely last more than 1 hour. Cocaine toxicity is characterized by seizures; hyperpyrexia; tachycardia; mental status changes, including paranoid behavior; hypertension; cerebrovascular accidents; MIs; and rhabdomyolysis. Nasal septum perforation may also occur.

In most cases, treatment involves the use of diazepam for aggitation, hypertension, and tachycardia. Nitroprusside or CCBs can be used for hypertensive crisis. β-Blockers should be avoided given the risk of coronary vasoconstriction and paradoxical hypertension. Other complications, such as cerebrovascular accidents, rhabdomyolysis, and MIs, should be managed in a conventional manner. Fortunately, cocaine has a short half-life and symptoms are usually self-limited. Individuals who use cocaine may become rapidly addicted.

Additional Reading: Cocaine overdose. *Epocrates online.* From: https://online.epocrates.com/

Category: Psychogenic

40. Goodpasture's syndrome is associated with
A) Osteoporosis and renal lithiasis
B) Pathologic fractures and thyroiditis
C) Hepatitis and recurrent cystitis
D) Pulmonary hemorrhage and glomerulonephritis
E) Pica and angioedema

Answer and Discussion

The answer is D. Goodpasture's syndrome is a condition manifested by pulmonary hemorrhages and progressive glomerulonephritis. Circulating basement membrane antibodies are responsible for the renal and pulmonary abnormalities. Patients with Goodpasture's syndrome are typically young males (5 to 40 years; male:female ratio of 6:1); however, there is a bimodal peak at approximately 60 years of age. Men and women are equally affected at older ages. Symptoms include severe hemoptysis, shortness of breath, and renal failure. Laboratory findings include iron-deficiency anemia, hematuria, proteinuria, cellular and granular casts in the urine, and circulating antiglomerular antibodies. Chest radiographs show progressive, bilateral, fluffy infiltrates that may migrate and are asymmetrical. Renal biopsy may be necessary to make the diagnosis. Treatment involves high-dose steroids, immunosuppression, and plasmapheresis, which may help preserve renal function. If significant injury to the kidneys occurs, then dialysis or transplant may be necessary. Untreated, Goodpasture's syndrome can be fatal.

Additional Reading: Pathogenesis and diagnosis of anti-GBM antibody (goodpasture's) disease. In: Basow DS, ed. *UpToDate.* Waltham, MA: UpToDate; 2013.

Category: Nephrologic system

> Goodpasture's syndrome is a condition manifested by pulmonary hemorrhages and progressive glomerulonephritis. Circulating basement membrane antibodies are responsible for the renal and pulmonary abnormalities.

41. Black cohosh has been advocated to treat
A) Muscle and joint pain
B) The common cold
C) Depression
D) Menopausal symptoms
E) Osteoporosis

Answer and Discussion

The answer is D. The herb black cohosh, or *Actaea racemosa* (formerly named *Cimicifuga racemosa*), is native to North America. The roots and rhizomes of this herb are widely used in the treatment of menopausal symptoms and menstrual dysfunction. Although the clinical trials on black cohosh are of insufficient quality to support definitive statements, this herbal medicine may be effective in the short-term treatment of menopausal symptoms. The mechanism of action is unclear, and early reports of an estrogenic effect have not been proved in recent studies. Although black cohosh may be useful in treating some menopausal symptoms, there is currently no evidence regarding any protective effect of black cohosh against the development of osteoporosis. Adverse effects are extremely uncommon, and there are no known significant adverse drug interactions.

Additional Reading: Black cohosh. *Am Fam Physician*. 2003; 68:114–116.

Category: Nonspecific system

42. A 32-year-old man with a history of Wolff–Parkinson–White syndrome (WPW) presents to the emergency department with his "heart racing again." He is alert and in no acute distress. His blood pressure is 130/70 mm Hg, pulse rate 220 beats per minute, and oxygen saturation 96%. An EKG reveals a regular, wide-complex tachycardia. He appears stable and his EKG is consistent with WPW. You decide to use pharmacologic conversion for his initial treatment; which one of the following would be the treatment of choice?
A) Verapamil (Calan)
B) Adenosine (Adenocard)
C) Procainamide
D) Digoxin

Answer and Discussion

The answer is C. Adenosine, digoxin, and calcium-channel antagonists act by blocking conduction through the atrioventricular (AV) node, which may increase the ventricular rate paradoxically, initiating ventricular fibrillation. These agents should be avoided in Wolff-Parkinson-White syndrome. Procainamide is usually the treatment of choice in these situations, although amiodarone may also be used.

> **Additional Reading:** Evaluation and initial treatment of supraventricular tachycardia. *N Engl J Med*. 2012;367:1438–1448.

Category: Cardiovascular system

43. A recognized complication of sleep apnea is
A) Hyperlipidemia
B) Diabetes mellitus
C) RLS
D) Migraines
E) Congestive heart failure (CHF)

Answer and Discussion

The answer is E. Obstructive sleep apnea occurs most often in moderately or severely obese persons. Men are affected more often than women (4% of men and 2% of women in middle age). Upper airway narrowing leads to obstruction during sleep. In severely obese persons, a combination of hypoxemia and hypercapnia may induce central apnea as well. By definition, apneic periods last at least 10 seconds (some for 2 minutes). Repeated nocturnal obstruction may cause recurring cycles of sleep, obstructive choking, and arousal with gasping for air. Daytime drowsiness usually results from the repeated cycles. Similar but less-pronounced cycles occur in nonobese persons, possibly secondary to developmental or congenital abnormalities of the upper airway. Complications of sleep apnea include cardiac abnormalities (e.g., sinus arrhythmias, extreme bradycardia, atrial flutter, ventricular tachycardia, heart failure), hypertension, excessive daytime sleepiness, morning headache, and slowed mentation. The mortality rate from stroke and MIs is significantly higher in persons with obstructive sleep apnea than in the general population.

> **Additional Reading:** Sleep apnea, obstructive. In: Domino F, ed. *The 5-Minute Clinical Consult*. Philadelphia, PA: Lippincott Williams and Wilkins; 2014.

Category: Neurologic

44. Which of the following medications is effective for RLS?
A) Levodopa/carbidopa
B) Diltiazem
C) Phenytoin
D) Haloperidol
E) Vitamin B$_6$

Answer and Discussion

The answer is A. RLS is a relatively common problem seen by family physicians. The condition is characterized by repeated movements and paresthesias of the lower extremities (occasionally the arms). Patients may describe a tingling irritation or a drawing or crawling sensation that prevents the onset of sleep or may disturb sleep. The symptoms are often relieved by movement. Laboratory and neurologic tests are normal. Associated conditions include iron deficiency, diabetes, uremia, pregnancy, rheumatoid arthritis, vitamin B$_{12}$ deficiency, and polyneuropathy. Treatment includes the use of ropinirole (Requip), pramipexole (Mirapex), pergolide (Permax), levodopa/carbidopa (Sinemet), gabapentin (Neurontin), carbamazepine (Carbatrol), and other antiepileptics, opiates, and benzodiazepines.

> **Additional Reading:** Restless legs syndrome. *Am Fam Physician*. 2008;78(2):235–240.

Category: Neurologic

45. Which of the following forms of hepatitis does NOT have a chronic state?
A) Hepatitis A
B) Hepatitis B
C) Hepatitis C
D) Hepatitis D

Answer and Discussion

The answer is A. Hepatitis is an inflammation of the liver that is characterized by nausea, anorexia, fever, right-upper abdominal discomfort, jaundice, and marked elevation of liver function tests. The condition is usually classified into the following types:

- *Hepatitis A*. Also known as infectious hepatitis, the causative agent is an RNA virus. The disease is common and often presents subclinically. It is estimated that as much as 75% of the U.S. population has positive antibodies to hepatitis A. The onset of clinical symptoms is usually acute, and children and young adults are usually affected. The transmission is via a fecal–oral route and has been linked to the consumption of contaminated shellfish (e.g., raw oysters). The course of the disease is usually mild, and the prognosis is usually excellent. There is neither an associated chronic state nor a carrier state. The diagnosis is made by the detection of elevated levels of IgM antibodies, which indicate active disease, and IgG antibodies, which indicate previous disease. Most cases require no special treatment other than supportive care, and symptoms usually resolve after several weeks. The disease can be prevented by administering Ig to those who are in close contact with those affected. Immunization, especially for travelers, is recommended to specifically prevent hepatitis A.

- *Hepatitis B*. This DNA viral disease is more severe than hepatitis A and causes more complications. It affects as much as 10% of the U.S. population. The infective Dane particle consists of a viral core and outer surface coat. The disease often develops insidiously and can affect persons of all ages. It is transmitted parenterally (through infected blood transfusions or infected needles used by intravenous drug abusers) and through sexual contact (especially in sexually active young adults and homosexuals). The symptoms are often severe and can be devastating to elderly patients or those who are debilitated. Approximately 10% of cases become chronic; up to 30% of affected patients become carriers of the virus after they are infected. The detection of the hepatitis B surface antigen (formerly known as the Australian antigen) supports the diagnosis of acute illness, and values become positive between 1 and 7 weeks before the symptoms become evident. The hepatitis B antibody appears weeks to months after the development of the clinical symptoms. The presence of a hepatitis B surface antibody indicates previous disease and represents immunity. Those who have received hepatitis B vaccination also have positive titers if they are immune. An anticore antibody (IgM) usually develops at the onset of the illness, and the IgG anticore antibody (which develops shortly after IgM appears) can be used as a marker for the disease during the "window period," which occurs when the hepatitis B surface antigen disappears and before the hepatitis B surface antibodies appear. The hepatitis B e antigen is found in those who are hepatitis B surface antigen–positive; its presence is associated with greater infectivity and a greater chance of progression to the chronic state. The delta agent (hepatitis D) is a separate virus that may coexist with hepatitis B; it is usually associated with a more severe case of hepatitis B and in cases of chronic hepatitis B in which there is reactivation of the virus. Prophylaxis of hepatitis B can be achieved with hepatitis B vaccine given at 1 month and 6 months after the initial injection, for a total of three injections. Persons exposed to hepatitis B (e.g., by needle stick) should also receive hepatitis B Ig at the time of exposure.

- *Hepatitis C.* This disease (also known as *non-A, non-B hepatitis,* or *posttransfusion hepatitis*) accounts for as many as 40% of the cases of hepatitis in the United States. It is the main indication for liver transplant in the United States when cirrhosis is present. The disease is transmitted by infected blood and is commonly seen in intravenous drug abusers and those who had blood transfusions infected with the virus. The disease is usually insidious in its presentation, and the severity is variable. As many as 50% of these patients may develop chronic disease, which may eventually lead to cirrhosis. The diagnosis is made by serologic means, and pegylated α-interferon and ribavirin have been used for treatment.
- *Hepatitis E.* The transmission is similar to the hepatitis A virus. The disease is found in India and Southeast Asia, Africa, and Mexico. Cases in the United States are usually related to travel to these endemic areas. Hepatitis E virus is associated with a high fatality in pregnant women.

Additional Reading: Hepatitis A. *Am Fam Physician.* 2012;86(11): 1027–1034

Category: Gastroenterology system

46. Which of the following factors is included in the criteria for administering streptokinase with MI?
A) Cardiogenic chest pain lasting at least 6 hours
B) ECG changes of at least 1 to 2 mm of ST elevation in two adjacent precordial leads
C) Streptokinase should not be administered 6 hours after the onset of chest pain
D) Q waves noted in the lateral precordial leads

Answer and Discussion

The answer is B. Streptokinase is a thrombolytic agent administered during MI. The majority of patients with an acute ST elevation myocardial infarction (STEMI) have a complete occlusion of a coronary artery due to thrombus. Thus, thrombolytic therapy has been important treatment option. However, primary percutaneous coronary intervention (PCI) is the preferred appraoch for reperfusion for most patients with STEMI as there are better outcomes (lower mortality and less recurrent ischemia) with fewer complications such as intracranial hemorrhage that occurs with thrombolytic use. However, such treatment remains an important reperfusion strategy in locations with limited availability of timely PCI.

Streptokinase is associated with a 1% to 2% rate of allergic reactions consisting of skin rashes and fever and ypotension occurs in another 10%. Because of the development of antibodies, patients previously treated with streptokinase should be given recombinant tissue plasminogen activator (alteplase) or reteplase plasminogen activator. The criteria for consideration of thrombolytics include chest pain (consistent with cardiogenic pain) for at least 30 minutes' duration and ECG changes that show at least 1 to 2 mm of ST elevation in two adjacent precordial leads. Medication should be given within 12 hours for maximal benefit. Although extremely variable depending on the source, the following is a list of absolute contraindications to thrombolytics:

- History of intracranial hemorrhage
- Other strokes or cerebrovascular events within 1 year
- Known intracranial neoplasm
- Unclear mental status
- Active gastrointestinal (GI) bleeding
- Aortic dissection
- Acute pericarditis

Relative contraindications include:

- Recent surgery (within 3 weeks)
- Prolonged (>10 minutes) cardiopulmonary resuscitation
- Recent vascular puncture in a noncompressible region (<2 weeks)

Prior stroke (nonhemorrhagic)

- Uncontrolled hypertension defined as systolic blood pressure (SBP) > 180 mm Hg or diastolic blood pressure (DBP) > 110 mm Hg

Major surgery (3 months or less)

- Pregnancy
- Bleeding diasthesis
- Active peptic ulcer disease

Minor hemorrhage, menstruation, and diabetic retinopathy are not contraindications to fibrinolytic therapy.

Additional Reading: Fibrinolytic therapy in acute ST elevation myocardial infarction: initiation of therapy. In: Basow DS, ed. *UpToDate.* Waltham, MA: UpToDate; 2013.

Category: Cardiovascular system

47. A 48-year-old alcoholic stops drinking 2 days before presenting to his physician. He is diaphoretic, nauseated, tachycardic, anxious, and hypertensive. The most appropriate management is to
A) Prescribe diazepam and refer the patient to a drug treatment program
B) Hospitalize the patient, administer diazepam, and closely observe his condition
C) Administer disulfiram and diazepam and follow up with the patient in 1 week
D) Reassure the patient, compliment his decision to stop drinking, and explain the symptoms that are to be expected
E) Refer the patient to psychiatry

Answer and Discussion

The answer is B. Symptoms of alcohol withdrawal usually occur 6 to 48 hours after the last alcoholic drink. These symptoms include sweating, anxiety, tremor, weakness, gastrointestinal (GI) discomfort, hypertension, tachycardia, fever, and hyperreflexia. Other symptoms include hallucinations and, in severe cases, delirium tremens that are characterized by disorientation with hallucinations, drenching sweats, severe tremors, and electrolyte disturbances that can lead to seizures. Treatment involves hospitalization and close observation. Antianxiety medications, including chlordiazepoxide, lorazepam, diazepam, midazolam, and oxazepam, are used for treatment and are slowly tapered to prevent withdrawal-related symptoms. Oral multivitamin supplementation with thiamine, folate, and pyridoxine is also recommended. Disulfiram is not used for alcohol withdrawal but can be used in the treatment of alcoholism to help discourage further drinking.

> **Additional Reading:** Management of alcohol withdrawal syndrome. *Am Fam Physician*. 2010;82(4):344–347.

Category: Psychogenic

48. Which of the following statements about Burner's syndrome is true?
A) The mechanism of injury involves acute hyperextension of the shoulder while the neck and head are forced in the same direction.
B) Symptoms include temporary weakness, pain, paresthesias, and decreased sensation of the distal extremity.
C) The injury involves traction forces on the spinal cord's dorsal columns.
D) Most cases cause permanent neurologic deficits.
E) The condition is associated with overuse injury of the knees.

Answer and Discussion

The answer is B. Burner's syndrome is seen mostly in football players and results from a tackling or blocking injury. The injury occurs when the contact shoulder is depressed and the head and neck are forced in the opposite direction of contact. The traction-type forces placed on the brachial plexus lead to variable symptoms of weakness, pain, paresthesias, limited motion, and decreased sensation of the affected extremity. Diminished reflexes may also be seen. The condition should be treated with caution, and cervical disc or bony injury should be ruled out. In most cases, the symptoms last only a few minutes; however, the athlete should not return to play until a complete evaluation can be performed and the symptoms resolve.

> **Additional Reading:** Busconi BD, Stevenson JH. Approach to the athlete with burners/stingers (Transient brachial plexopathy). *Sports Medicine Consult: A Problem-Based Approach to Sports Medicine for the Primary Care Physician.* Philadelphia, PA: Lippincott, Williams & Wilkins; 2009.

Category: Musculoskeletal system

> 🔔 **Burner's syndrome occurs when the contact shoulder is depressed and the head and neck are forced in the opposite direction of contact. The traction-type forces placed on the brachial plexus lead to variable symptoms of weakness, pain, paresthesias, limited motion, and decreased sensation of the affected extremity.**

49. Which of the following indicates a therapeutic effect for β-blockers?
A) Pupillary constriction
B) Drug level within the acceptable range
C) Heart rate between 60 and 70 bpm
D) Generalized fatigue
E) Peripheral cyanosis

Answer and Discussion

The answer is C. β-Blockers (e.g., propranolol, metoprolol, labetalol, nadolol) are used in the treatment of hypertension. They are considered a negative inotrope and chronotrope. In most cases, they are best suited for young patients who have a hyperdynamic cardiac status. β-Blockers should be used cautiously in patients with the following:

- Asthma and COPD, because nonselective β-blockers can induce bronchoconstriction
- Diabetes, because β-blockers can blunt the response of hypoglycemia
- History of CHF, because β-blockers can decrease cardiac output (however, recent evidence supports ardioselective β-blocker use in CHF with systolic dysfunction)
- Bradycardia or heart block

Other side effects include fatigue, impotence, impaired glucose tolerance, and rebound tachycardia and hypertension (if the drug is abruptly discontinued). β-Blockers are also used for migraine prophylaxis and to treat performance anxiety and tachycardia. Newer evidence supports that β-blockers are not deleterious for patients with depression as once thought. Finally, β-blockers are also used after MI to improve survival; they reduce myocardial oxygen demand by decreasing heart rate and contractility. Additionally, they should be given prior to surgery in those at risk for cardiac events. A therapeutic dose is determined by a recorded heart rate of 60 to 70 bpm.

> **Additional Reading:** Drugs for hypertension. *Treat Guidel Med Lett.* 2012;10(113):1–10.

Category: Cardiovascular system

50. A 54-year-old woman presents to your office with complaints of frequent sweating episodes, palpitations, nervousness, and sensitivity to heat with increased appetite and weight loss. The most likely diagnosis is
A) Hypothyroidism
B) Menopause
C) Addison's disease
D) Hyperthyroidism
E) Cushing's disease

Answer and Discussion

The answer is D. The manifestations of hyperthyroidism are numerous and include the following: goiter; widened pulse pressure; tachycardia; warm, moist skin; tremor; atrial fibrillation; nervousness; frequent diaphoresis; sensitivity to heat; palpitations; exophthalmos; pretibial myxedema; increased appetite with weight loss; diarrhea; and insomnia. The hallmark findings of Graves' disease include the triad of goiter, exophthalmos, and pretibial myxedema. Anemia, present with hypothyroidism, is not seen with hyperthyroidism. While menopausal symptoms would include hot flashes and night sweats, mood changes are also often seen, but slowed metabolism and weight gain are more likely than weight lost and there would be accompanying irregular periods.

Addison's disease is characterized by a gradual onset of fatigability, weakness, anorexia, nausea and vomiting, weight loss, skin and mucous membrane pigmentation, hypotension, and in some cases hypoglycemia depending on the duration and degree of adrenal insufficiency. The manifestations vary from mild chronic fatigue to life-threatening shock associated with acute destruction of the glands. Asthenia is the major presenting symptom.

Cushing's disease is not associated with sweats and palpatations—weight gain, especially truncal obesity and "moon facies" are common. While depression and irritability can be seen, so can menstrual irregularities.

Additional Reading: Overview of the clinical manifestations of hyperthyroidism in adults. In: Basow DS, ed. *UpToDate.* Waltham, MA: UpToDate; 2013.

Category: Endocrine system

51. Which of the following statements about altitude sickness is true?
A) Most people are affected at altitudes between 5,000 and 7,500 ft.
B) Dehydration is rarely an associated condition.
C) The most common symptom is headache.
D) Hydrochlorothiazide is used for prophylaxis.
E) A high carbohydrate diet can help prevent symptoms.

Answer and Discussion

The answer is C. As altitude increases, the partial pressure of oxygen decreases. Approximately 20% of people experience symptoms ascending to more than 8,000 ft in less than 1 day, and 80% show some symptoms at altitudes higher than 12,700 ft. Symptoms include headache (most common), impaired concentration, nausea, vomiting, fatigue, dyspnea and hyperventilation, palpitations, and insomnia. Any type of physical exertion usually aggravates the symptoms, and excessive hyperventilation leads to dehydration. In severe cases, pulmonary and cerebral edema can occur. The most common manifestation is acute mountain sickness, heralded by malaise and headache.

Risk factors include young age, residence at a low altitude, rapid ascent, strenuous physical exertion, and a previous history of altitude illness. However, activity restriction is not necessary for those with coronary artery disease (CAD) who are traveling to high altitudes. Acetazolamide (a carbonic anhydrase inhibitor) helps prevent respiratory alkalosis, which contributes to the symptoms. It is an effective prophylactic treatment started one day before ascent and continued until the patient acclimatizes to their final altitude. Dexamethasone is an effective alternative treatment for those with contraindictions to acetazolamide (which includes a sulfa allergy).

Treatment involves hydration and usually only symptomatic measures are necessary.

Additional Reading: Altitude illness: risk factors, prevention, presentation, and treatment. *Am Fam Physician.* 2010;82(9): 1103–1110.

Category: Respiratory system

52. Anemia that is seen in patients with chronic renal disease is usually caused by insufficient
A) Iron stores
B) Vitamin B_{12}
C) Renin levels
D) Erythropoietin levels
E) Folate stores

Answer and Discussion

The answer is D. Serum recombinant erythropoietin is used to treat refractory anemia in patients with chronic renal disease. The synthetic drug replaces erythropoietin that is normally produced by the kidneys. Although expensive, the drug is indicated if the patient has significant anemia that is not caused by other factors. The major side effect is hypertension, which must be monitored at regular intervals. Other side effects include polycythemia, with the possible development of thromboembolism, stroke, and MI. The drug does not appear to accelerate the preexisting renal disease. Close monitoring of serum hemoglobin is necessary with the use of erythropoietin. Iron supplementation must be given to achieve an adequate erythropoietin response.

Additional Reading: Peginesatide (Omontys) for anemia in chronic kidney disease. *Med Lett Drugs Ther.* 2012;54(1392): 45–46.

Category: Hematologic system

53. Which of the following statements is true of Lyme disease?
A) The disease is transmitted by the bite of a common wood tick.
B) The second stage may be characterized by fever, malaise, a stiff neck, back pain, and erythema chronicum migrans.
C) The first stage may involve carditis with atrioventricular (AV) block or pericarditis, peripheral neuropathies, and meningitis.
D) Treatment may be accomplished with doxycycline or amoxicillin.
E) It is predominant in the South Central and Western regions of the United States.

Answer and Discussion

The answer is D. Caused by the spirochete *Borrelia burgdorferi*, Lyme disease is transmitted by the bite of the deer tick (*Ixodes dammini*). Although reported in most states, it appears to be predominant in the Great Lakes area and the Western and Northeastern United States. The symptoms occur in three stages:

First stage. This stage usually begins with malaise, fever, headache, stiff neck, and back pain. Generalized lymphadenopathy with splenomegaly occurs, and a large annular erythematous lesion forms at the bite site and shows central clearing (erythema chronicum migrans). Multiple lesions may occur and affect other areas of the body. The lesions are warm but not often painful. As many as 25% may not exhibit skin manifestations. These symptoms usually appear within a few days to up to 1 month after the tick bite.

Second stage. This is the disseminated stage. Complications include carditis with AV block, palpitations, dyspnea, chest pain, and syncope. Pericarditis may also occur. Neurologic manifestations, including peripheral neuropathies and meningitis, are sometimes present. Large-joint arthritis is also common.

Chronic phase. After the second stage, a chronic phase may result. This phase is predominantly characterized with intermittent attacks of oligoarthritis lasting weeks to months. Other symptoms include subtle neurologic abnormalities (e.g., memory problems, mood or sleep disorders). Diagnosis is usually made by the clinical presentation; however, an ELISA followed by Western blot for positive results can help in the diagnosis but is somewhat unreliable.

Treatments for early disease include doxycycline, amoxicillin, and cefuroxime axetil. A single dose of doxycycline has been shown to reduce the likelihood of Lyme disease after a deer tick bite. A moderately effective recombinant vaccine for the prevention of Lyme disease has been removed from the market.

Additional Reading: Lyme disease. In: Domino F, ed. *The 5-Minute Clinical Consult.* Philadelphia, PA: Lippincott Williams and Wilkins; 2014.

Category: Nonspecific system

54. Which of the following conditions would disqualify a patient from passing a Department of Transportation (DOT) examination?
A) Diabetic taking insulin
B) Blood pressure reading of 158/94 mm Hg
C) Vision 20/40 in both eyes
D) Use of a hearing aid
E) Field of vision measured at 70 degrees in each eye

Answer and Discussion

The answer is A. Many physicians perform DOT physical examinations. The following are disqualifying conditions: A diabetic patient taking insulin cannot be certified for interstate driving. However, a driver who has diabetes controlled by oral medications and diet may be qualified if the disease is well controlled and the driver is under medical supervision. If diabetes is untreated or uncontrolled, certification should not be given.

From a cardiac standpoint, any condition known to be accompanied by sudden and unexpected syncope, collapse, or CHF is disqualifying. Conditions such as MI, angina, and cardiac dysrhythmias should, in most cases, be evaluated by a cardiologist before certification is issued. Holter monitors and exercise stress tests may be needed when a driver has multiple risk factors. Tachycardia or bradycardia should be investigated to rule out underlying cardiac disease. Asymptomatic dysrhythmia with no underlying disease process should not be disqualifying.

With regards to blood pressure, if the blood pressure is 159/99 mm Hg or lower, a full 1-year certification is appropriate. If the blood pressure is >160–179/100–109, temporary certification may be granted for 3 months to allow time for the driver to be evaluated and treated. If the initial pressure is 180/110 mm Hg or higher, the driver should not be certified. Once the driver's blood pressure is under control, certification can be issued for no more than 1 year at a time. Several readings should be taken over several days to rule out "white coat" hypertension. Significant target organ damage and additional risk factors increase the risk of sudden collapse and should be disqualifying.

Vision must be at least 20/40 in each eye with or without correction. Certification can be given once vision has been corrected, but not until. The driver should be advised to have his or her eyes evaluated, obtain corrective lenses, and then return for certification. Field of vision must be at least 70 degrees in each eye. Color vision must allow recognition of standard traffic signals (i.e., red, green, and amber).

The driver should pass a whispered voice test at 5 ft in at least one ear. A hearing aid may be worn for the test. If the test result is questionable, an audiogram is recommended. The better ear must not have an average hearing loss of more than 40 dB at 500, 1,000, and 2,000 Hz (to obtain an average, add the three decibel losses together and divide by 3).

Additional Reading: Commercial driver's license examination. In: Basow DS, ed. *UpToDate.* Waltham, MA: UpToDate; 2013.

Category: Patient/Population-based care

55. A 45-year-old woman presents to your office with petechiae noted on the lower extremities. A platelet count is obtained and noted to be 10,000. Which of the following conditions would not be associated with her thrombocytopenia?
A) Epistaxis
B) Hemarthrosis
C) Vaginal bleeding
D) Mucosal bleeding in the mouth
E) Ecchymosis at the site of minor trauma

Answer and Discussion

The answer is B. Thrombocytopenia is caused by decreased platelet production, splenic sequestration of platelets, increased platelet destruction or use, or dilution of platelets. Severe thrombocytopenia results in a characteristic pattern of bleeding: multiple petechiae in the skin, often most evident on the lower legs; scattered small ecchymoses at sites of minor trauma; mucosal bleeding (epistaxis, bleeding in the GI and genitourinary [GU] tracts, vaginal bleeding); and excessive bleeding following surgical procedures. Heavy GI bleeding and bleeding into the central nervous system (CNS) may be life threatening. Thrombocytopenia does not cause massive bleeding into tissues (e.g., deep visceral hematomas, hemarthroses), which is characteristic of bleeding secondary to coagulation disorders such as hemophilia. Medications associated with thrombocytopenia include heparin (up to 5%, even with very low doses), quinidine, quinine, sulfa preparations, oral antidiabetic drugs, gold salts, and rifampin.

Additional Reading: Thrombocytopenia. *Am Fam Physician.* 2012;85(6):612–622.

Category: Hematologic system

56. Iron-deficiency anemia is associated with
A) Hyperchromic, macrocytic features
B) Elevated serum iron levels
C) Increased total iron-binding capacity (TIBC)
D) Increased ferritin levels
E) Normal bone marrow biopsy results

Answer and Discussion

The answer is C. Iron-deficiency anemia produces a hypochromic, microcytic anemia. Causes include excessive menstruation, GI blood loss, inadequate iron consumption, malabsorption, pregnancy, or excessive growth in the absence of adequate iron consumption during infancy. Symptoms may include generalized weakness and fatigue, facial pallor, glossitis, cheilosis, and angular stomatitis. In chronic, severe cases patients may have pica (e.g., craving for dirt, paint), pagophagia (craving for ice), or dysphagia associated with a postcricoid esophageal web. Physical examination may show skin pallor, dry brittle nails, and tachycardia with perhaps a flow murmur. Laboratory tests show a depressed Hb with microcytic, hypochromic features; low serum iron concentration; low ferritin; and increased transferrin (TIBC). Bone marrow aspiration shows diminished iron stores with small, pale RBCs. Only when the hematocrit falls below 31% to 32% do the RBC indices become microcytic. Treatment is the administration of iron replacement for 6 to 12 months until iron stores are replenished. The addition of ascorbic acid enhances iron absorption without increasing gastric distress.

Additional Reading: Iron deficiency anemia: evaluation and management. *Am Fam Physician.* 2013;87(2):98–104.

Category: Hematologic system

57. Which of the following is not indicated in the emergent treatment of thyroid storm?
A) Propylthiouracil
B) Supersaturated potassium iodine
C) Propranolol
D) Aspirin
E) Acetaminophen

Answer and Discussion

The answer is D. Thyroid storm is a life-threatening condition seen in patients with hyperthyroidism. The condition is usually precipitated by stress, illness, or manipulation of the thyroid during surgery. Signs and symptoms include diaphoresis, tachycardia, palpitations, weight loss, diarrhea, fever, mental status changes, weakness, and shock. Treatment should be provided immediately and includes propylthiouracil, supersaturated potassium iodine, and propranolol. Other measures involve fluid replacement and control of fever with acetaminophen and cooling blankets. Avoid aspirin because it may increase T_3 and T_4 by reducing protein binding. Steroids may also be given to help prevent the conversion of T_3 and T_4 peripherally. The definitive therapy after control of the thyroid storm involves ablation of the thyroid gland with iodine-131 or surgery. After treatment, many patients become hypothyroid and may require replacement therapy.

Additional Reading: Overview of the clinical manifestations of hyperthyroidism in adults. In: Basow DS, ed. *UpToDate.* Waltham, MA: UpToDate; 2013.

Category: Endocrine system

58. Which of the following ECG findings is associated with sudden cardiac death?
A) Prolonged QT interval
B) First-degree AV block
C) Sinus arrhythmia
D) Right bundle branch block
E) Premature ventricular contractions

Answer and Discussion

The answer is A. A prolonged QT interval is a common entity associated with sudden arrhythmia death syndrome. Arrhythmias may be induced in normal hearts by medications; electrolyte abnormalities (e.g., hypokalemia, hypomagnesemia); myocarditis; and endocrine, CNS, or nutritional disorders. These arrhythmias are associated with prolongation of the QT interval. A group of inherited gene mutations has been identified associated with cardiac ion channels that cause long QT syndrome and carry an increased risk for sudden death. Some of the highest rates of inherited long QT syndrome occur in Southeast Asian and Pacific Rim countries. The average age of persons who die of long QT syndrome is 32 years; men are more commonly affected. In addition to a prolonged QT interval, which occurs in some but not all persons with long QT syndrome, another characteristic electrocardiographic abnormality is the so-called Brugada sign (an upward deflection of the terminal portion of the QRS complex). Most cardiac events are precipitated by vigorous exercise or emotional stress, but they also can occur during sleep. Torsades de pointes and ventricular fibrillation are the usual fatal arrhythmias. Long QT syndrome should be suspected in patients with recurrent syncope during exertion and those with family histories of sudden, unexpected death. Not all persons with long QT syndrome have warning symptoms or identifiable electrocardiographic abnormalities, and they may present with sudden death. β-Blockers, potassium supplements, and implantable defibrillators have been used for treatment of long QT syndrome. Identifying the specific gene mutation in a given patient with long QT syndrome can help guide prophylactic therapy.

Additional Reading: Sudden arrhythmia death syndrome: importance of the long QT syndrome. *Am Fam Physician.* 2003;68:483–488.

Category: Cardiovascular system

> Long QT syndrome should be suspected in patients with recurrent syncope during exertion and those with family histories of sudden, unexpected death.

59. A 21-year-old is brought to your clinic in status epilepticus. What drug should be administered initially?
A) Lorazepam
B) Phenytoin
C) Phenobarbital
D) Pentobarbital
E) Fosphenytoin

Answer and Discussion

The answer is A. Lorazepam should be administered intravenously and approximately 1 minute allowed to assess its effect. Diazepam or midazolam may be substituted if lorazepam is not available. If seizures continue at this point, additional doses of lorazepam should be infused and a second intravenous catheter placed in order to begin a concomitant phenytoin (or fosphenytoin) loading infusion. Even if seizures terminate after the initial lorazepam dose, therapy with phenytoin or fosphenytoin is generally indicated to prevent the recurrence of seizures.

Additional Reading: Status epilepticus in adults. In: Basow DS, ed. *UpToDate.* Waltham, MA: UpToDate; 2013.

Category: Neurologic

60. Which of the following statements about hyperglycemic hyperosmolar nonketotic coma is true?
A) It is usually associated with type I adult-onset diabetes mellitus.
B) It is associated with fluid overload.
C) Associated laboratory findings include elevated serum lactate.
D) Treatment involves intravenous administration of glucose.
E) Treatment involves fluid administration.

Answer and Discussion

The answer is E. Hyperosmolar nonketotic coma secondary to hyperglycemia usually occurs in patients with type II adult-onset diabetes mellitus. The condition occurs when serum glucose is elevated, leading to osmotic diuresis and the development of dehydration without ketosis. In most cases, the condition affects elderly, mildly obese patients who fail to keep adequate fluid intake to make up for the osmotic diuresis. Complications include mental status changes with the development of coma, acute renal failure, thrombosis, shock, and lactic acidosis. Diagnosis depends on the detection of plasma glucose >600 mg per dL, serum lactate >5 mmol, and a serum osmolality >320 mOsmol per kg. Sodium and potassium levels are usually normal; however, blood urea nitrogen (BUN) and creatinine are markedly elevated. Treatment consists of fluid replacement (usually approximately 10 L) with potassium supplementation and the cautious administration of insulin. Triggering conditions such as infection, MI, or stroke should be ruled out. Unfortunately, the mortality rate for hyperglycemic hyperosmolar nonketotic coma approaches 50% if not treated immediately.

> **Additional Reading:** Clinical features and diagnosis of diabetic ketoacidosis and hyperosmolar hyperglycemic state in adults. In: Basow DS, ed. *UpToDate*. Waltham, MA: UpToDate; 2013.

Category: Endocrine system

61. Which of the following statements about giardiasis is true?
A) Transmission occurs through fecal–oral contamination.
B) Chlorination of drinking water kills the cyst.
C) Diagnosis can be achieved by peripheral blood smears.
D) The cyst form is responsible for symptoms.
E) Asymptomatic carriers do not require treatment.

Answer and Discussion

The answer is A. *Giardia lamblia* is the causative agent in parasitic giardiasis. Most cases are asymptomatic. However, these patients pass infective cysts and must be treated. Symptoms occur 1 to 3 weeks after infection and include foul-smelling watery diarrhea, flatulence, abdominal cramps and distention, and anorexia. Outbreaks in day schools, nursing homes, and institutions for the mentally retarded are common. Transmission is through a fecal–oral route. The infective form is the cyst, and trophozoites are responsible for the symptoms. Cysts are transmitted in contaminated food or water. *Giardia* cysts are resistant to chlorination; therefore, filtration is used to clear cysts from drinking water supplies. *Giardia* is sensitive to heat, thus bringing water to a boil is effective before consumption. Diagnosis is accomplished by detecting cysts or the parasite in the stool (usually three samples) or in duodenal contents (by using endoscopy, the swallowed-string test, or Enterotest). Treatment includes metronidazole and furazolidone. The medication is available in suspension, making it useful for children. Close contacts should also be tested, especially when recurrent infections are found. Although *Giardia* is most commonly associated with beavers, there is evidence of sporadic transmission between infected dogs and people.

> **Additional Reading:** Parasites—Giardia. Centers for Disease Control and Prevention; 2013. From: http://www.cdc.gov/parasites/giardia/

Category: Gastroenterology system

62. A 32-year-old sportsman who recently attended a wild-game feed banquet consumed summer sausage made from bear meat. He complains of abdominal discomfort, diarrhea, and muscle tenderness. The most likely diagnosis is
A) Trichinosis
B) Salmonellosis
C) Giardiasis
D) Ascariasis
E) Shigellosis

Answer and Discussion

The answer is A. Trichinosis is a parasitic infection caused by the roundworm *Trichinella spiralis*. The condition results from eating inadequately prepared or raw pork, bear, or walrus meat that contains the encysted larva. Many cases are linked to the consumption of contaminated summer sausage. Many patients are asymptomatic; however, some may exhibit diarrhea, abdominal discomfort, and a low-grade fever. Ocular symptoms may also occur with edema of the eyelids, photophobia, and retinal or subconjunctival hemorrhages. Muscle soreness and urticaria may also be associated with the parasitic infection. Laboratory studies show an increasing eosinophilia with a leukocytosis. Diagnosis can be made by muscle biopsy showing the larva or cysts, serologic tests, or ELISA tests. Treatment is accomplished with thiabendazole with variable response. For severe cases, corticosteroids may be indicated. Complications include myocarditis, meningitis, and pneumonitis. The prognosis is usually good. Most cases can be avoided by thoroughly cooking pork before consumption.

> **Additional Reading:** Parasites—Trichinellosis (also known as Trichinosis). Centers for Disease Control and Prevention; 2013. From: http://www.cdc.gov/parasites/trichinellosis/

Category: Gastroenterology system

63. A 24-year-old long-distance runner has been training for a track meet. He reports localized pain, especially at night, and mild swelling over his proximal left tibia that has not responded to anti-inflammatory agents or ice therapy. Radiographs of the area are normal. The most likely diagnosis is
A) Stress fracture
B) Shin splints
C) Osteoid osteoma
D) Gastrocnemius tear
E) Iliotibial band (ITB) syndrome

Answer and Discussion

The answer is A. Stress fractures usually involve the tibia (commonly in the proximal two-thirds of the bone) and fibula (usually 5 to 7 cm above the lateral malleolus) after prolonged and repeated use. Stress fractures account for up to 10% of all sports injuries. Long-distance runners or athletes who are inadequately conditioned are frequently affected. Symptoms include pain over the lower leg in the affected area; the pain usually improves with rest but recurs with repeated activity. Localized erythema and swelling may occur over the fracture site. Night pain is a common feature, which should alert the clinician to the possibility of a stress fracture. Radiographs are normal in many cases; however, technetium bone scans can be used to demonstrate the fracture. Bone scans are the most cost-effective means to diagnose stress fractures. The MRI is also very sensitive but is more expensive. Treatment of stress fractures includes rest from exercise or competition for 6 to 8 weeks. Those who experience pain with ambulation or cannot adhere to limited activity for 6 to 8 weeks should be in a walking cast or boot for 4 to 6 weeks. When patients resume their activity, they should begin slowly and gradually work back to their normal routines. If pain should recur, nonunion of the fracture should be suspected and the athlete should be referred to an orthopaedist. The athlete may return to competition after 14 days without pain and no pain with gradual return to activity.

> **Additional Reading:** Busconi BD, Stevenson JH. Approach to the athlete with a tibial stress fracture. *Sports Medicine Consult: A Problem-Based Approach to Sports Medicine for the Primary Care*

Physician. Philadelphia, PA: Lippincott, Williams & Wilkins; 2009.

Category: Musculoskeletal system

64. Which of the following statements about familial periodic paralysis is true?
A) It is an autosomal-recessive transmitted disorder.
B) It involves disturbances of potassium regulation.
C) It is associated with permanent muscle weakness.
D) It is aggravated by administration of acetazolamide.
E) It most commonly affects the elderly.

Answer and Discussion

The answer is B. Familial periodic paralysis is an autosomal-dominant transmitted disorder that is characterized by episodes of paralysis, loss of deep tendon reflexes, and failure of the muscles to respond to electrical stimulation. Onset is usually early in life; episodic weakness beginning after age 25 is almost never due to periodic paralysis. There is no alteration in mental status—patients remain alert during attacks. Muscle strength is normal between attacks. There are two basic types:

1. *Hypokalemic.* Attacks usually begin in adolescence. Symptoms occur the day after vigorous exercise. The symptoms are usually mild and may affect particular muscle groups (proximal muscles) or involve all extremities at once. Oropharyngeal and respiratory muscles are unaffected. The weakness usually lasts 24 to 48 hours. Meals high in carbohydrates and sodium may precipitate the attacks.

2. *Hyperkalemic.* Attacks usually occur earlier in childhood. They are shorter in duration, more frequent, and less severe. Attacks are usually associated with myotonia. Most patients are actually normokalemic during the attacks; however, the administration of potassium can precipitate the attack—thus the name.

Diagnosis is made by the history, and serum potassium levels should be drawn during the attacks to determine the specific type of paralysis. Provocative testing with glucose and insulin can be used (in hypokalemic forms) with caution in those who have infrequent attacks. The treatment of choice for both types is acetazolamide. Potassium chloride may help abort hypokalemic attacks; calcium gluconate and furosemide may help abort hyperkalemic attacks.

Additional Reading: Evaluation of the patient with muscle weakness. *Am Fam Physician*. 2005;71(7):1327–1336.

Category: Neurologic

65. Crohn's disease is associated with which of the following?
A) Inflammation limited to the superficial layer of the bowel wall
B) The affinity to involve the rectosigmoid junction
C) Decreased risk of colon cancer
D) Continuous mucosal areas of ulceration that affect the anus
E) Fistula formation

Answer and Discussion

The answer is E. Crohn's disease is characterized by a transmural inflammation of the GI tract. It may affect any part of the GI tract but is usually associated with the terminal ileum, the colon, or both. On colonoscopy, areas of ulceration and submucosal thickening give the bowel a cobblestone appearance, with some skipped areas of normal bowel. In addition to the transmural inflammation, there are granulomas, abscesses, fissures, and fistula formation. Symptoms include fever, weight loss, abdominal pain (usually the right-lower quadrant), diarrhea (rarely with associated blood), and growth retardation in children. In children, Crohn's disease is more common than ulcerative colitis. Complications include intestinal obstruction; toxic megacolon, which is usually more common in ulcerative colitis; malabsorption, particularly associated with fat-soluble vitamins and especially vitamin B_{12}; intestinal perforation; fistula formation; and development of gall and kidney stones. There is also an increased risk—five times the average—for bowel cancer. Other areas may be affected, including the following:

- Joints: arthritis, ankylosing spondylitis
- Skin: erythema nodosum, aphthous ulcers, pyoderma gangrenosum
- Eyes: episcleritis, iritis, uveitis
- Liver: fatty liver, pericholangitis

The diagnosis is usually made with colonoscopy or flexible sigmoidoscopy with biopsy or with x-ray contrast studies (usually avoided in acute stages because of the risk of developing toxic megacolon with barium). Treatment involves the use of oral corticosteroids or steroid enemas, ciprofloxacin, metronidazole, antidiarrheal agents, and sulfasalazine (Azulfidine), olsalazine (Dipentum), or mesalamine (Asacol, Pentasa, Rowasa), all three of which contain 5-aminosalicylic acid. Infliximab is a drug that has been approved for the treatment of Crohn's disease. The drug is a potent antibody to tumor necrosis factor that is elevated in patients with Crohn's disease and can help close fistulas in up to 60% of patients. In severe cases, total parenteral nutrition may be necessary with surgery to remove the ulcerated bowel. Adalimumab is also used.

Additional Reading: Diagnosis and management of Crohn's disease. *Am Fam Physician*. 2011;84(12):1365–1375.

Category: Gastroenterology system

66. A 68-year-old patient is seen for a general examination. Current recommendations for immunizations include
A) Tetanus booster every 5 years
B) Influenza vaccination yearly
C) Pneumococcal vaccination yearly
D) Hepatitis booster every 5 years
E) Meningococcal vaccination

Answer and Discussion

The answer is B. Adult immunizations should include tetanus immunization every 10 years and influenza vaccination yearly beginning at age 50. Pneumococcal immunization should be given at age 65. Those at high risk receiving pneumococcal vaccination before age 65 and after 5 years may require boosters. Vaccination can be started earlier in patients at high risk for disease (e.g., patients who are immunocompromised, those with chronic lung disease or diabetes). Patients who do not have functional spleens should receive pneumococcal, meningococcal, and influenza immunization.

Additional Reading: Advisory committee on immunization practices (ACIP): recommended immunization schedule for adults aged 19 years and older—United States. *MMWR*. 2013;62(01):9–19.

Category: Patient/Population-based care

67. The treatment of choice for leishmaniasis is
A) Mebendazole
B) Quinine
C) Doxycycline
D) Ciprofloxacin
E) Antimonial compound

Answer and Discussion

The answer is E. The condition *leishmaniasis* refers to various clinical syndromes caused by a protozoa species. Leishmaniasis is endemic in many of the tropics, the subtropics, and southern Europe. It is typically a vector-borne disease, with rodents and canids as common reservoir hosts and humans as incidental hosts. In humans, visceral, cutaneous, and mucosal leishmaniasis results from infection of macrophages throughout the reticuloendothelial system, in the skin, and in the nasal and oropharyngeal mucosa. *Leishmania* parasites are transmitted by the bite of female sandflies. The transmission of *Leishmania* species typically is localized because of the limited area that sandflies inhabit. Typically these insects remain within a few hundred yards of their breeding ground. They are found in dark, moist places in areas ranging from deserts to rain forests. Many reside in debris or rubble near structures. The primary lesion at the site of an infected sandfly bite is small and usually not noticed. Parasites travel from the skin through the bloodstream to the lymph nodes, spleen, liver, and bone marrow. Clinical signs develop gradually after 2 weeks up to 1 year later. The typical syndrome consists of fevers, hepatosplenomegaly, pancytopenia, and polyclonal hypergammaglobulinemia with reversed albumin/globulin ratio. In up to 10% of patients, twice-daily temperature spikes occur. Death can occur within 1 to 2 years in a majority of untreated symptomatic patients. A subclinical form with vague minor symptoms resolves spontaneously in a majority of patients and can progress to full-blown visceral leishmaniasis in one-third of cases. Those infected are resistant to further attacks unless they are immunocompromised. One to 2 years after apparent cure, some patients develop nodular cutaneous lesions full of parasites, which can last for years and is often treated as folliculitis.

Treatment consists of a regimen of antimonial compounds. Pentavalent antimonial (SbV) compounds—the mainstays for treating leishmaniasis since the 1940s—are not licensed for U.S. commercial use. However, the SbV compound sodium stibogluconate (Pentostam®) is available to U.S.-licensed physicians through the Center for Disease Control and Prevention (CDC) Drug Service under an IND (Investigational New Drug) protocol approved by the FDA and by CDC's Institutional Review Board (IRB). Toxicity including myalgia, arthralgia, fatigue, elevated liver function tests, pancreatitis, and electrocardiographic abnormalities are more common as the length of treatment progresses but usually does not limit treatment and is reversible. No medications have been approved by FDA for treatment of cutaneous or mucosal leishmaniasis, although liposomal amphotericin B (AmBisome®) is FDA-approved for treatment of visceral leishmaniasis. Alternatives include amphotericin B and pentamidine. Many other agents have been recommended as alternatives or adjuncts to antimonial compounds often on the basis of suboptimal data.

Additional Reading: Parasites—leishmaniasis. Center for Disease Control and Prevention; 2013. From: www.cdc.gov/parasites/leishmaniasis/health_professionals/index.html#tx

Category: Nonspecific system

> Treatment of leishmaniasis consists of a regimen of antimonial compounds, which are available through the CDC via the IND (Investigational New Drug) protocol.

68. Which of the following statements is true regarding glaucoma?
A) Intraocular pressure is diagnostic for glaucoma.
B) Glaucoma suspects have normal intraocular pressure.
C) Measurement of intraocular pressures by primary care physicians to screen for glaucoma is not recommended.
D) Prostaglandin eye drops are contraindicated in the treatment of glaucoma.
E) Laser treatment is the treatment of choice once glaucoma is identified.

Answer and Discussion

The answer is C. Glaucoma is the second most common cause of legal blindness in the United States. Open-angle glaucoma is a condition that involves progressive optic neuropathy characterized by enlarging optic disc cupping and visual field loss. Most patients are asymptomatic. Patients at increased risk for open-angle glaucoma include African Americans above 40 years of age, whites older than 65 years, a personal history of diabetes or severe myopia, and persons with a family history of glaucoma. Elevated intraocular pressure is a risk factor for open-angle glaucoma, but it is not diagnostic. Some patients with glaucoma have normal intraocular pressure (i.e., normal-pressure glaucoma), and many patients with elevated intraocular pressure do not have glaucoma (i.e., glaucoma suspects). Screening patients for glaucoma by the primary physician is not recommended. Formal visual field testing (perimetry) by vision care is the mainstay of glaucoma diagnosis and management. Nonspecific β-blocker or prostaglandin analog eye drops are generally the first-line treatment to reduce intraocular pressure. Laser treatment and surgery are usually reserved for patients in whom medical treatment has failed. Without treatment, open-angle glaucoma can result in irreversible vision loss.

Additional Reading: Open-angle glaucoma: epidemiology, clinical presentation, and diagnosis. In: Basow DS, ed. *UpToDate*. Waltham, MA: UpToDate; 2013.

Category: Special sensory

69. Which of the following statements about acetaminophen overdose is correct?
A) Symptoms include extremity pain with physical findings of peripheral neuropathy.
B) Toxic effects rarely occur with ingestion of greater than 140 to 150 mg per kg of acetaminophen.
C) Elevations in liver tests peak 3 to 4 hours after ingestion.
D) Blood levels obtained 4 hours after ingestion determine treatment.
E) Treatment involves the use of deferoxamine.

Answer and Discussion

The answer is D. Acetaminophen overdose is not uncommon. Most cases involve children younger than 6 years. Toxic effects occur when the doses exceed 140 to 150 mg per kg or a total dose of 7.5 g. The drug primarily affects the liver 24 to 72 hours after ingestion by depleting glutathione stores and causing hepatocellular necrosis. Symptoms include nausea, vomiting, and right-upper quadrant abdominal pain. Acetaminophen levels should be checked 4 hours after ingestion and plotted on the Rumack–Matthew nomogram. Peak aspartate aminotransferase, alanine aminotransferase (ALT), bilirubin, and prothrombin time (PT) values are seen 3 to 4 days after ingestion. Treatment, including emesis induced by syrup of ipecac, gastric lavage, and administration of activated charcoal, should be initiated as soon as possible. A 4-hour acetaminophen level greater than 150 µg per mL requires administration of the antidote acetylcysteine (Mucomyst). For maximal therapeutic effect, *N*-acetylcysteine should be administered within 8 hours of acetaminophen ingestion.

> **Additional Reading:** Pharmaceutical drug overdose. *Treat Guidel Med Lett.* 2006; 4(49):61–66.

> **Category:** Nonspecific system

70. Which of the following statements about chronic fatigue syndrome is true?
A) Antibiotics may be beneficial.
B) Antidepressants may be beneficial.
C) The disease is most likely linked to the Epstein–Barr virus (EBV).
D) Symptoms rarely improve.
E) Bed rest is usually beneficial.

Answer and Discussion

The answer is B. Chronic fatigue syndrome is a poorly understood constellation of symptoms that includes generalized fatigue, sore throat, tender lymphadenopathy, headaches, and generalized myalgias. The disease does not appear to be associated with chronic infections of EBV or Lyme disease. It does appear to be associated with underlying psychiatric disorders, such as somatization disorder, depression, and anxiety. Chronic fatigue syndrome has no pathognomic features and remains a constellation of symptoms and a diagnosis of exclusion. Patients with this constellation of symptoms should receive supportive therapy and be encouraged to gradually increase their exercise program within their limits and participate in their usual activities. Alternative medicines and vitamins are popular with many chronic fatigue syndrome patients but generally are not very helpful. The use of antibiotics or antiviral agents is contraindicated. In some cases, patients may respond to antidepressant medications. Given enough time, most patients improve.

> **Additional Reading:** Chronic fatigue syndrome: diagnosis and treatment. *Am Fam Physician.* 2012;86(8):741–746.

> **Category:** Nonspecific system

71. Chronic gingivitis as a result of chronic plaque buildup can initially lead to
A) Periodontitis
B) Dental caries
C) Glossitis
D) Oropharyngeal cancer
E) Oropharyngeal candidiasis

Answer and Discussion

The answer is A. Periodontitis is the most common cause of tooth loss. It occurs when chronic gingivitis (a result of bacterial plaque buildup) leads to loss of supporting bone around the tooth root. Symptoms include deepening of the gingival pockets between the teeth with the accumulation of calculus deposits. The gums soon lose their attachment to the tooth, and bone loss occurs. Bacteria accumulate in the gingival pockets and can lead to progression of the disease. Later in the course of the disease, the gums recede and eventually tooth loss occurs. Treatment involves dental referral and, in severe cases, surgery. Regular dental visits twice yearly and proper brushing and flossing techniques help prevent plaque buildup.

> **Additional Reading:** Common dental infections in the primary care setting. *Am Fam Physician.* 2008;77(6):797–802.

> **Category:** Nonspecific system

72. Which of the following medications is contraindicated in pregnancy?
A) Lisinopril
B) Penicillin
C) Acetaminophen
D) α Methyldopa

Answer and Discussion

The answer is A. Women of childbearing age should be warned to notify their physicians as soon as possible if they become pregnant during ACE-inhibitor therapy. ACE inhibitors are not considered teratogenic if they are discontinued during the first trimester (class C), but they are considered teratogenic in the second and third trimesters (class D).

> **Additional Reading:** Angiotensin converting enzyme inhibitors and receptor blockers in pregnancy. In: Basow DS, ed. *UpToDate.* Waltham, MA: UpToDate; 2013.

> **Category:** Reproductive system

73. A 48-year-old woman presents to your office complaining of blurred vision and pain associated with the right eye. The patient also reports seeing halos around light sources as well as nausea, abdominal pain, and vomiting. Physical examination shows her right eye is red and the pupil is dilated. The most likely diagnosis is
A) Angle-closure glaucoma
B) Graves' disease
C) Digoxin toxicity
D) Hyphema
E) Atropine poisoning

Answer and Discussion

The answer is A. Glaucoma is classified into two types: open-angle and angle-closure.

- *Open-angle type* (90% of cases) results when the rate of aqueous fluid outflow is decreased and the ocular pressure is consistently increased, giving rise to optic atrophy with loss of vision. The disease usually is bilateral, affects African Americans more commonly than whites, and appears to have genetic predisposition. Examination may show optic disc cupping and an increase in intraocular pressure (normal: 10 to 21 mm Hg). The diagnosis should not be based on one reading. Treatment involves the use of intraocular β-blockers, such as timolol and pilocarpine. Surgical therapy may be necessary for patients whose conditions do not respond appropriately to medical treatment.

- *Angle-closure glaucoma* is less common, often more acute in onset, and is associated with a narrow anterior chamber and pupillary dilation that obstructs the normal flow of aqueous fluid. The condition constitutes an ophthalmologic emergency and is associated with stress, dark rooms, and pupillary dilation by medication used to perform eye examinations. Most patients experience pain and blurred vision with halos around lights. They may also present with abdominal pain and vomiting. Physical examination shows an eye that is red with the pupil dilated and unresponsive to light. Untreated, the condition can lead to blindness in 2 to 5 days. Treatment involves medication (miotics and carbonic anhydrase inhibitors) and laser peripheral iridectomy.

Patients older than 65 years should be screened for glaucoma every 1 to 2 years, or every year if there is a strong family history for glaucoma. African American individuals should be screened at an earlier age (40 years). The report of the United States Preventive Services Task Force does not recommend the routine performance of tonometry by primary care physicians. Instead, primary care physicians are encouraged to refer to an eye specialist for screening.

Additional Reading: Angle-closure glaucoma. In: Basow DS, ed. *UpToDate*. Waltham, MA: UpToDate; 2013.

Category: Special sensory

74. The ligament most commonly injured with an ankle sprain is the
A) Anterior talofibular ligament
B) Fibulocalcaneal ligament
C) Posterior talofibular ligament
D) Deltoid ligament

Answer and Discussion

The answer is A. Ankle sprains are graded according to the following criteria:

- *Grade 1:* Mild sprain with no evidence of ligamentous tear; associated with mild pain and swelling
- *Grade 2:* Moderate sprain with evidence of partial tear of ligaments; associated with moderate swelling, ecchymosis, and difficulty ambulating
- *Grade 3:* Severe sprain with evidence of a complete tear of the ligament; associated with significant swelling, ecchymosis, ankle instability, and the inability to walk

The ligaments involved include the anterior talofibular (which is the most commonly affected), the fibulocalcaneal, and the posterior talofibular ligament. A positive drawer sign (movement of the talus forward) indicates rupture of the anterior talofibular ligament. Treatment for grades 1, 2, and 3 sprains involves rest, ice, compression, elevation (RICE), use of air casts, and NSAIDs followed by early mobilization and physical therapy, which emphasizes strengthening and proprioceptive training. Sprains not responding to conservative care over 4 to 6 weeks or with atypical symptoms require specialty referral. High-ankle sprains are much less common and involve injury to the syndesmosis. Mechanism is from dorsi-flexion external rotation. Recovery time is increased with these injuries and requires initial non–weight-bearing for 1 to 3 weeks followed by graduated weight-bearing and PT.

Additional Reading: Busconi BD, Stevenson JH. Approach to the athlete with an ankle sprain. *Sports Medicine Consult: A Problem-Based Approach to Sports Medicine for the Primary Care Physician.* Philadelphia, PA: Lippincott, Williams & Wilkins; 2009.

Category: Musculoskeletal system

75. Of the following, the medication of choice for refractive hiccups is
A) Chlorpromazine
B) Acetazolamide
C) Gabapentin
D) Chloral hydrate
E) Clonidine

Answer and Discussion

The answer is A. Hiccups are sudden, repeated, involuntary contractions of the diaphragm followed by abrupt closure of the glottis. They result from stimulation of the efferent and afferent nerves that innervate the diaphragm. Causes include excitement, alcohol consumption, and gastric distention caused by overeating. Low CO_2 levels tend to accentuate hiccups, and high levels tend to prevent them. Advocated symptomatic treatment includes breathing

into a paper bag, rapidly drinking a glass of water, swallowing dry bread, holding one's breath, or consuming crushed ice. In addition, gastric decompression may provide relief. For refractive hiccups, chlorpromazine may be given orally or intravenously. Other medications include phenobarbital, scopolamine, chlorpromazine, metoclopramide, and narcotics. In severe cases, surgery to disrupt the phrenic nerve or to inject the phrenic nerve with a procaine solution may be performed.

Additional Reading: Hiccups. In: Domino F, ed. *The 5-Minute Clinical Consult.* Philadelphia, PA: Lippincott Williams and Wilkins; 2014

Category: Neurologic

76. Which of the following organisms is responsible for the development of pseudomembranous colitis?
A) *Escherichia coli*
B) *Clostridium difficile*
C) *Pseudomonas aeruginosa*
D) Methicillin-resistant *Staphylococcus aureus*
E) *Enterococcus faecalis*

Answer and Discussion

The answer is B. Pseudomembranous colitis is characterized by profuse, watery diarrhea; abdominal cramps; low-grade fevers; and, occasionally, hematochezia. The etiologic agent is *C. difficile,* which produces a toxin that causes the lesions affecting the colon. The condition is thought to be associated with antibiotic use in the preceding 2 to 3 weeks (in some cases up to 6 weeks); however, antibiotic use is not necessary for the condition to occur. The diagnosis may be achieved by a laboratory stool test, which isolates the *C. difficile* toxin. Sigmoidoscopy or colonoscopy usually shows characteristic yellowish-white plaques. Treatment includes the use of metronidazole or vancomycin (which is more expensive). Complications include dehydration, electrolyte imbalances, intestinal perforation, toxic megacolon, and, in severe cases, death. Relapse may occur in up to one-third of patients after treatment.

Additional Reading: Diarrhea, Acute. In: Domino F, ed. *The 5-Minute Clinical Consult.* Philadelphia, PA: Lippincott Williams and Wilkins; 2014

Category: Gastroenterology system

77. Dermatomyositis is associated with which of the following?
A) Generalized morbilliform rash
B) Underlying malignancy
C) Elevated lipids
D) Distal muscle weakness
E) Inflammatory bowel disease

Answer and Discussion

The answer is B. Dermatomyositis is a systemic connective tissue disease that involves inflammation and degeneration of the muscles. Women are affected more than men at a 2:1 ratio. Although the disease may occur at any age, it occurs most commonly in adults 40 to 60 years of age and in children 5 to 15 years of age. The cause is unknown. In adult cases (15% of men older than 50 and a smaller proportion affecting women), there is an underlying malignant tumor, which may give rise to an autoimmune reaction and lead to an attack of tumor antigens with similar muscle antigens. Symptoms include symmetric proximal muscle weakness, muscular pain, violaceous, flat-topped papules over the dorsal interphalangeal joints (Gottron's papules), purple-red discoloration of the upper eyelids (heliotropic rash), polyarthralgia, dysphagia, Raynaud's phenomenon, fever, and weight loss. Interstitial pneumonitis with dyspnea and cough may occur and precedes the development of myositis. Cardiac involvement may be detected when ECG tracings show arrhythmias or conduction disturbances. Laboratory findings include increased erythrocyte sedimentation rate (ESR), positive antinuclear antibodies and/or lupus erythematosus (LE) preparation test, and elevated creatinine kinase (most sensitive and useful marker) and aldolase. Diagnosis is confirmed by electromyography and muscle biopsy. Initial treatment consists of steroids. Patients who fail to respond can be given immunosuppressive agents such as methotrexate, cyclophosphamide, and chlorambucil. After the diagnosis of dermatomyositis is made, an effort should be made to uncover an occult malignancy. Dermatomyositis associated with malignancy often remits once the tumor is removed.

> **Additional Reading:** Polymyositis/Dermatomyositis. In: Domino F, ed. *The 5-Minute Clinical Consult.* Philadelphia, PA: Lippincott Williams and Wilkins; 2014.

Category: Musculoskeletal system

After the diagnosis of dermatomyositis is made, an effort should be made to uncover an occult malignancy.

78. Of the following medications, which is the most effective in relieving premenstrual dysphoric disorder?
A) Spironolactone
B) Bromocriptine
C) Amitryptyline
D) Fluoxetine
E) Oral contraceptives

Answer and Discussion

The answer is D. Premenstrual syndrome is defined as recurrent moderate psychological and physical symptoms that occur during the luteal phase of menses and resolve with menstruation. It affects up to a third of premenopausal women. Women with premenstrual dysphoric disorder experience affective or somatic symptoms that cause severe dysfunction in social or occupational realms. The disorder affects less than 10 percent of premenopausal women. Symptom relief is the goal for treatment of premenstrual syndrome and premenstrual dysphoric disorder. There is limited evidence to support the use of calcium, vitamin D, and vitamin B$_6$ supplementation, and insufficient evidence to support cognitive behavior therapy. Serotonergic antidepressants (citalopram, escitalopram, fluoxetine, sertraline, venlafaxine) are first-line pharmacologic therapy. Fluid retention may be treated by reducing sodium intake and using a thiazide diuretic starting just before symptoms are expected. Benzodiazepines may be used for anxiety, irritability, nervousness, and lack of control, especially if patients cannot alter their stressful environments, but such use should be limited to carefully selected patients because of its dependence, tolerance, and abuse potential. Spironolactone, bromocriptine, and monoamine oxidase inhibitors are not beneficial.

> **Additional Reading:** Premenstrual syndrome and premenstrual dysphoric disorder. *Am Fam Physician.* 2011;84(8):918–924.

Category: Reproductive system

79. A 65-year-old woman presents with glossitis, weight loss, paresthesias, and diarrhea. Laboratory tests show a macrocytic anemia. The most likely cause is
A) Iron-deficiency anemia
B) Thalassemia
C) Pernicious anemia
D) Multiple myeloma
E) Colon cancer

Answer and Discussion

The answer is C. Vitamin B$_{12}$ (cobalamin) deficiency is associated with several different conditions, including pernicious anemia (lack of intrinsic factor required for vitamin B$_{12}$ absorption), celiac sprue, Crohn's disease, and previous gastrectomy. Causes for vitamin B$_{12}$ deficiency include inadequate diet, inadequate absorption, inadequate use, increased requirement, and increased excretion. Symptoms include glossitis, anorexia, weight loss, paresthesias, ataxia, dementia, neuropsychiatric changes, and diarrhea. Signs include a macrocytic anemia, tachycardia, abnormal reflexes, positive Romberg's sign, and abnormal positional and vibratory sensation. Laboratory findings show low vitamin B$_{12}$ levels and reticulocyte counts. Mild thrombocytopenia, leukopenia, elevated lactate dehydrogenase, and indirect bilirubin levels due to ineffective erythropoiesis are seen. The Shilling test is used for additional information in the diagnosis. Treatment consists of removing the underlying cause of vitamin B$_{12}$ deficiency. Vitamin replacement therapy can be used. Iron deficiency, which coexists in up to one-third of patients, should be ruled out. The recommended daily allowance is 2 µg. Vitamin B$_{12}$ is usually used slowly and, unless there is absence of the vitamin for months, there are sufficient stores to prevent deficiency. A strict vegetarian diet avoids the consumption of meat, dairy products, seafood, and poultry (including eggs). Unfortunately, vegetarians often lack adequate vitamin B$_{12}$; physicians should look for deficiencies in this population. Meat substitutes, enriched yeast, and soybean milk are alternative sources for vitamin B$_{12}$.

> **Additional Reading:** Update on vitamin B12 deficiency. *Am Fam Physician.* 2011;83(12):1425–1430.

Category: Hematologic system

80. Which of the following is NOT considered a risk factor for MI?
A) Alcoholism
B) Homocystinemia
C) Type A personality
D) Male sex
E) Obesity

Answer and Discussion

The answer is A. Risk factors for MI include:

- Hypertension
- Hyperlipidemia—particularly high total cholesterol, high LDL cholesterol, and low high-density lipoprotein (HDL) cholesterol
- Cigarette smoking
- Diabetes mellitus
- Obesity (increased weight for height)
- Male gender
- Family history of CAD
- Sedentary lifestyle
- Type A personality
- Increased age
- Postmenopausal
- Homocystinemia

Additional Reading: Myocardial infarction. In: Domino F, ed. *The 5-Minute Clinical Consult*. Philadelphia, PA: Lippincott Williams and Wilkins; 2014.

Category: Cardiovascular system

81. A 55-year-old business executive presents to your office complaining of a 4-week history of daily headaches. He describes the headache as being pronounced in the morning on awakening, associated with nausea and vomiting. The most likely diagnosis is
A) Classic migraine headache
B) Cluster headache
C) Brain tumor
D) Sinus headache
E) Muscle-tension headache

Answer and Discussion

The answer is C. There are several types of headache associated with specific clinical histories. The following are some common types and their distinguishing features:

- *Migraine headaches.* These usually affect young women (but can affect men) and are pulsating and unilateral in location. They occur infrequently, are throbbing, and are associated with photophobia (in some cases an aura preceding the headache), nausea, and vomiting; sleep usually provides relief. They typically last 4 to 72 hours.
- *Headaches associated with tumors.* Pain occurs daily, becomes more frequent and severe as time passes, and may be associated with focal neurologic deficits or visual disturbances.
- Patients may report pain more in the morning on awakening, nausea, vomiting, or the pain may be worse with bending over.
- *Headaches associated with sinus headaches.* These are usually associated with facial pain or pressure in the sinus area, fever, and purulent sinus drainage.
- *Muscle-tension headaches.* These are associated with a bandlike tightness that encircles the scalp area, usually occurring on a daily basis and usually worse at the end of a workday.
- *Cluster headaches.* More common in middle-age men, these headaches are usually described as a unilateral, sharp (i.e., "feels like an ice pick"), agonizing pain located in the orbital area, in many cases occurring 2 to 3 hours after the patient falls asleep; they are associated with tearing, nasal congestion, rhinorrhea, and autonomic symptoms on the same side as the headaches. Frequency of attacks ranges from one to eight daily.

Additional Reading: Approach to acute headache in adults. *Am Fam Physician*. 2013;87(10):682–687.

Category: Neurologic

82. Which of the following statements about sickle cell anemia is true?
A) The disease is a sex-linked, recessive, inherited disorder.
B) The condition is related to a defective β chain with sickling under conditions of low CO_2.
C) Hydroxyurea is contraindicated for patients with sickle cell anemia.
D) Patients with sickle cell should receive pneumococcal vaccination.
E) Individuals with sickle cell should avoid influenza vaccination.

Answer and Discussion

The answer is D. Sickle cell anemia is an autosomal-dominant inherited hemolytic anemia that predominantly affects African Americans (approximately 8% of the African American population). Because of a defective β chain (valine is substituted for a glutamic acid in the sixth position of the β chain), blood cells tend to sickle under conditions of low pO_2. The condition is manifested in a milder heterozygote form (referred to as sickle cell trait) and in the more severe homozygote form. Signs and symptoms include anemia, jaundice, arthralgias, fever, painful aplastic crises that are characterized by severe abdominal and joint pain, poor-healing ulcers associated with the pretibial area, nausea, vomiting, hemiplegia, and cranial-nerve palsies. Other manifestations include pulmonary and renal dysfunction, cardiomegaly, hepatosplenomegaly, cholelithiasis, and aseptic necrosis of the femoral heads. Heterozygous individuals are usually unaffected by these complications. Laboratory findings include normocytic, normochromic anemia with a peripheral smear showing sickled red cells with Howell–Jolly bodies and target cells; leukocytosis with a left shift; thrombocytosis; elevated bilirubin levels; and elevated urinary and fecal urobilinogen. ESRs are usually normal. Diagnosis is usually made by Hb electrophoresis demonstrating HbS chains. Heterozygous individuals usually show HbA and HbS chains. Treatment is symptomatic and may include transfusions in severe cases, hydration, pain control, and possible corticosteroids. More recently, hydroxyurea has been used in the treatment of sickle cell anemia. Most crises are precipitated by infections, and treatment should provide coverage for these infections. Because of splenic dysfunction, those affected are at an increased risk for bacterial infections, particularly pneumococcal and Salmonella infections; therefore, they should receive the pneumococcal (Pneumovax) vaccine. Genetic counseling should also be instituted for those affected. Life spans may be shortened for those affected but have been increasing.

Additional Reading: Anemia, Sickle Cell. In: Domino F, ed. *The 5-Minute Clinical Consult*. Philadelphia, PA: Lippincott Williams and Wilkins; 2014.

Category: Hematologic system

83. Which of the following statements about hereditary angioedema is true?
A) It is related to excessive amyloid deposition.
B) It is caused by a deficiency of the C1 esterase inhibitor.
C) Attacks are triggered by antihistamines.
D) Treatment involves dehydroepiandrosterone (DHEA) administration.

Answer and Discussion

The answer is B. Hereditary angioedema is an autosomal-dominant transmitted genetic disorder that is related to a deficiency of C1 esterase inhibitor or, less commonly, to inactive C1 esterase inhibitor that is involved in the first step of complement activation. Symptoms include pruritus; urticarial rashes; abdominal pain; and, in severe cases, bronchoconstriction, which can be life threatening. Attacks are usually triggered by stress, trauma, or illnesses. Diagnosis is made by detection of low C4 levels or deficiency of the C1 esterase inhibitor by immunoassay. Treatment involves the use of antihistamines, glucocorticoids, and epinephrine (in severe cases). Fresh-frozen plasma given before procedures can be used for short-term prophylaxis. Other medications used to prevent attacks include the androgens: methyltestosterone, danazol, and stanozolol. In addition, the C1 esterase inhibitor concentrate may be given directly in life-threatening cases.

Additional Reading: Angioedema. In: Domino F, ed. *The 5-Minute Clinical Consult*. Philadelphia, PA: Lippincott Williams and Wilkins; 2014.

Category: Nonspecific system

84. Which of the following statements best describes astereognosis?
A) Loss of the ability to carry out movements in the absence of paralysis or sensory deficits
B) Inability to recognize smells
C) Loss of the ability to express oneself by speech
D) Loss of the ability to recognize objects by touch
E) Loss of ocular coordination

Answer and Discussion

The answer is D. *Astereognosis* is the loss of the ability to recognize objects by the sense of touch. The loss of the ability to carry out movements in the absence of paralysis or sensory deficits is called *apraxia*. Inability to recognize sensory stimuli is called *agnosia*; subgroups include auditory, visual, olfactory, gustatory, and tactile agnosias. The loss of the ability to express oneself by speech or written language is called *aphasia*.

Additional Reading: Aphasia, agnosia, apraxia, and amnesia. *Massachusetts General Hospital Handbook of Neurology*. Philadelphia, PA: Lippincott Williams and Wilkins; 2007.

Category: Special sensory

85. Which of the following lung cancers is most commonly associated with the syndrome of inappropriate secretion of antidiuretic hormone (SIADH)?
A) Squamous cell carcinoma
B) Small cell (oat cell) carcinoma
C) Large cell carcinoma
D) Adenocarcinoma
E) Mesothelioma

Answer and Discussion

The answer is B. Lung cancer is often associated with a paraneoplastic syndrome, which occurs as a result of cancer and is extrapulmonary. The following are some common neoplastic syndromes:

- *Squamous cell:* hypercalcemia
- *Small cell:* Cushing's syndrome, SIADH with hyponatremia, myasthenic syndrome, Eaton–Lambert syndrome, peripheral neuropathy, subacute cerebellar degeneration
- *Large cell:* gynecomastia
- *Adenocarcinoma:* clubbing, thrombophlebitis, marantic endocarditis, periostitis, or hypertrophic osteoarthropathy

In addition, all of the previously mentioned lung cancers may be associated with dermatomyositis, disseminated intravascular coagulation, eosinophilia, thrombocytosis, and acanthosis nigricans.

Additional Reading: Overview of the risk factors, pathology, and clinical manifestations of lung cancer. In: Basow DS, ed. *UpToDate*. Waltham, MA: UpToDate; 2013.

Category: Respiratory system

86. The best medication to use in the emergent treatment of supraventricular tachycardia is
A) Digoxin
B) Verapamil
C) Adenosine
D) Diltiazem
E) Isoproterenol

Answer and Discussion

The answer is C. Treatments for stable patients with supraventricular tachycardia (also referred to as regular *narrow QRS tachycardias*) include vagal maneuvers such as Valsalva's maneuver; coughing; activation of gag reflex; carotid sinus massage; and placing an ice bag on the face or swallowing ice-cold water, which can be extremely effective. Unilateral carotid sinus massage, one of the more common methods used, should be given at the angle of the jaw on one side for 3 to 5 seconds. Patients with a history of carotid artery disease are at increased risk for the dislodgment of plaque, which may lead to stroke. Adenosine (Adenocard) and verapamil (Isoptin) administered intravenously are also effective if the previously mentioned measures fail to succeed. Adenosine is preferred because of its rapid onset of action and short half-life. For unstable patients, low-energy electrical cardioversion is the treatment of choice. Most patients troubled by this arrhythmia are candidates for radiofrequency ablation.

Additional Reading: Evaluation and initial treatment of supraventricular tachycardia. *N Engl J Med*. 2012;367:1438–1448.

Category: Cardiovascular system

Adenosine is the preferred treatment of supraventricular tachycardia (SVT) because of its rapid onset of action and short half-life.

87. Which of the following effects distinguishes aspirin from acetaminophen?
A) Analgesic properties
B) Antipyretic properties
C) Anti-inflammatory properties
D) Amnestic properties
E) Antipruritic properties

Answer and Discussion

The answer is C. Aspirin (acetylsalicylic acid) is the drug of choice for mild-to-moderate pain. It has antipyretic and anti-inflammatory properties (unlike acetaminophen, which has no anti-inflammatory properties). The major side effect is gastric irritation, which can be reduced by using an enteric-coated aspirin and taking the medication with meals. Tinnitus has also been associated with chronic aspirin use. Aspirin's mode of action is accomplished by the inhibition of prostaglandin synthesis by permanently acetylating cyclooxygenase. Because platelet function is irreversibly inhibited, bleeding times are prolonged as much as 1 to 2 weeks. Aspirin can evoke an anaphylactic response in some individuals, especially in those with a history of asthma and nasal polyps, and, thus, should be avoided. Aspirin use should also be avoided in children and teenagers with viral febrile illnesses (e.g., chickenpox, IM, viral influenza) because of the risk of Reye's syndrome.

Additional Reading: Drugs for pain. *Treat Guidel Med Lett*. 2013;11(128):31–42.

Category: Nonspecific system

88. A 56-year-old man presents to your office with complaints of "chronic" diarrhea. He states that he has had loose stools for the past 2 days. He denies blood in the stool, fever, and has no weight loss and no recent travel. Appropriate management at this time includes
A) Observation
B) Check stool cultures
C) Colonoscopy
D) Stool fat studies

Answer and Discussion

The answer is A. Chronic diarrhea is a common and sometimes difficult problem encountered by physicians and patients. The condition is defined as diarrhea that continues for >4 weeks. The problem occurs in 1% to 5% of the population. Patients often present late in their course, after other symptoms such as weight loss, rectal bleeding, and abdominal pain have developed. Diarrhea results from incomplete absorption of water from the bowel lumen because of a reduced rate of water absorption or osmotically induced luminal retention of water. Even mild changes in absorption can cause loose stools. It is usually impractical to test for the many causes of chronic diarrhea. Instead a useful approach is to first categorize by type of diarrhea before testing and treating to limit the diagnostic possibilities. Chronic diarrhea can be categorized as watery (secretory vs. osmotic vs. functional), fatty, or inflammatory. Watery diarrhea may be subdivided into osmotic (water retention due to poorly absorbed substances), secretory (reduced water absorption), and functional (hypermotility) types. Osmotic laxatives, such as sorbitol, induce osmotic diarrhea. Secretory diarrhea can be distinguished from osmotic and functional diarrhea by virtue of higher stool volumes (greater than 1 L per day) that continue despite fasting and occur at night. Stimulant laxatives fall into this secretory category because they increase motility. Persons with functional disorders have smaller stool volumes (less than 350 mL per day) and no diarrhea at night. Once the diarrhea is categorized, further testing becomes more specific. The fecal osmotic gap can help distinguish secretory from osmotic diarrhea.

> **Additional Reading:** Evaluation of chronic diarrhea. *Am Fam Physician.* 2011;84(10):1119–1126.

> **Category:** Gastroenterology system

89. A 20-year-old otherwise healthy woman presents with cloudy urine, burning on urination, and urinary frequency. The patient has no allergies. Physical examination shows the patient is afebrile. She has mild suprapubic pain with palpation but no costovertebral angle tenderness. Urinalysis is positive for nitrites and leukocyte esterase. Which of the following is the most appropriate treatment?
A) Hospitalize the patient and administer intravenous antibiotics.
B) Administer macrolide-containing antibiotics on an outpatient basis.
C) Administer sulfa-containing antibiotics plus phenazopyridine (Pyridium) on an outpatient basis.
D) Advise the patient to increase fluid intake, especially with cranberry juice.
E) Arrange for an intravenous pyelogram.

Answer and Discussion

The answer is C. UTIs are more common in sexually active women. Symptoms include dysuria, urinary frequency, enuresis, incontinence, suprapubic tenderness, flank pain, or costovertebral angle tenderness (which usually indicates pyelonephritis). Gram-negative bacteria that originate from the intestinal tract (i.e., *Escherichia coli, Staphylococcus saprophyticus, Klebsiella, Enterobacter, Proteus, Pseudomonas*) are usually the causative organisms. Diagnosis is accomplished by microscopic or dipstick evaluation of a clean-catch midstream urine sample. Urine culture confirms the diagnosis. Treatment is oral (and in most cases sulfa-containing) antibiotics. With no complicating clinical factors, reasonable empiric treatment for presumed cystitis before organism identification is a 3-day regimen of any of the following: oral TMP-SMX, TMP, norfloxacin, ciprofloxacin, ofloxacin, lomefloxacin, or enoxacin. With complicating factors of diabetes, symptoms for more than 7 days, recent UTI, use of diaphragm, and postmenopausal women, a 7-day regimen can be considered using the same antibiotics. Phenazopyridine hydrochloride may be necessary for 1 to 3 days if significant dysuria is present. Affected patients should also be encouraged to increase their fluid intake.

> **Additional Reading:** Diagnosis and management of uncomplicated urinary tract infections. *Am Fam Physician.* 2005;72: 451–456, 458.

> **Category:** Nephrologic system

90. Treatment of severely infected diabetic foot ulcers should involve
A) Topical antibiotics
B) Debridement only
C) Debridement with systemic antibiotics
D) Debridement with topical antibiotics
E) None of the above

Answer and Discussion

The answer is C. Diabetic foot ulcers usually result from large vessel disease, microvascular disease, neuropathies, or a combination of all three. Ulcers associated with large vessel disease tend to affect the distal tips of the toes, whereas those secondary to neuropathy typically occur on the weight-bearing surfaces. Smoking and heavy alcohol abuse can increase the risk of diabetic ulcers. Prevention is the key to treatment. All diabetic patients should be instructed about foot care, and their feet should be examined regularly. Organisms that typically infect diabetic ulcers include *Staphylococcus, Streptococcus*, anaerobes, and gram-negative organisms. Severe infections may involve methicillin-resistant *Staphylococcus aureus* and *Pseudomonas* infections. Cultures should be taken from the debrided ulcer base or from purulent drainage. Oral antibiotics may be adequate for mild infections. However, if the infection is severe, debridement and systemic antibiotics are usually necessary. Topical antibiotics provide little help in the treatment of such infections.

> **Additional Reading:** Diabetes: foot ulcers and amputations. *Am Fam Physician.* 2009;80(8):789–790.

> **Category:** Musculoskeletal system

91. A 19-year-old man with asthma complains of shortness of breath and wheezing when playing sports. Otherwise he has no symptoms. The best preventive treatment is
A) Antileukotrienes before exercise
B) Regular inhaled steroids
C) Inhaled β agonist before exercise
D) Long-acting β agonist
E) Anxiolytic medication

Answer and Discussion

The answer is C. Exercise-induced asthma occurs mainly in patients already diagnosed with asthma. Wheezing usually begins shortly after the initiation of exercise and can be debilitating and limit participation. Short-acting β2 agonists (15 to 30 minutes before exercise) are recommended first-line agents for pharmacologic treatment, although leukotriene-receptor antagonists or inhaled corticosteroids with or without long-acting β2 agonists may be needed in refractory cases. If symptoms persist despite treatment, alternative diagnoses such as cardiac or other pulmonary etiologies, vocal cord dysfunction, or anxiety should be considered. The regular use of inhaled corticosteroids is best in the setting of asthmatic symptoms occurring in addition to exercise. Other preventive measures include a slow warm-up and the avoidance of very warm and very cold conditions.

Additional Reading: Exercise-induced bronchoconstriction: diagnosis and management. *Am Fam Physician.* 2011;84(4): 427–434.

Category: Respiratory system

92. A 30-year-old man with HIV infection and a CD4+ cell count of 150 cells per mm^3 should
A) Start antiviral medication
B) Have additional follow-up tests in 1 month
C) Have additional follow-up tests in 3 months
D) Have additional follow-up tests in 6 months
E) Have tests repeated in 1 year

Answer and Discussion

The answer is A. The CD4+ cell count is a marker for T-helper cells and is used in the treatment of HIV. Once the patient has been diagnosed with HIV, the CD4 cell count should be measured and followed. Typically, there is a diurnal variation in the CD4 cell count; therefore, it should be measured at the same time with each determination. Plasma HIV viral load is used to determine response to treatment in HIV and is no longer used when considering initiation of antiretroviral drug therapy (ART). ART is recommended for all HIV-infected individuals to reduce the risk of disease progression and for the prevention of transmission of HIV. Patients starting ART should be willing and able to commit to treatment and understand the benefits and risks of therapy and the importance of adherence. Patients may choose to postpone therapy, and providers, on a case-by-case basis, may elect to defer therapy on the basis of clinical and/or psychosocial factors.

Without treatment, the vast majority of HIV-infected individuals will eventually develop progressive immunosuppression (as evident by CD4 count depletion), leading to AIDS-defining illnesses and premature death. The primary goal of ART is to prevent HIV-associated morbidity and mortality. This goal is best accomplished by using effective ART to maximally inhibit HIV replication so that plasma HIV RNA levels (viral load) remain below that detectable by commercially available assays. Durable viral suppression improves immune function and quality of life, lowers the risk of both AIDS-defining and non-AIDS-defining complications, and prolongs life. Furthermore, high-plasma HIV RNA is a major risk factor for HIV transmission and use of effective ART can reduce viremia and transmission of HIV to sexual partners.

Historically, HIV-infected individuals have presented for care with low CD4 counts, but increasingly there have been concerted efforts to both increase testing of at-risk patients and to link HIV-infected patients to medical care soon after HIV diagnosis (and before they have advanced HIV diseases). For those with high CD4 cell counts, whose short-term risk for death may be low, the recommendation to initiate ART is based on growing evidence that untreated HIV infection or uncontrolled viremia is associated with development of non-AIDS-defining diseases, including cardiovascular disease (CVD), kidney disease, liver disease, neurologic complications, and malignancies. Furthermore, newer ART regimens are more effective, more convenient, and better tolerated than regimens used in the past. Regardless of CD4 count, the decision to initiate ART should always include consideration of any comorbid conditions, the willingness and readiness of the patient to initiate therapy, and the availability of resources. In settings where resources are not available to initiate ART in all patients, treatment should be prioritized for patients with the lowest CD4 counts and those with the following clinical conditions: pregnancy, CD4 count <200 cells per mm^3, or history of an AIDS-defining illness, including HIV-associated dementia, HIV-associated nephropathy (HIVAN), hepatitis B virus (HBV), and acute HIV infection.

Additional Reading: US Department of Health and Human Services (DHHS). Guidelines for the use of antiretroviral agents in HIV-1-infected adults and adolescents. From: http://aidsinfo.nih.gov/guidelines

Category: Nonspecific system

93. Which of the following factors is associated with dysplastic nevi syndrome?
A) No genetically related transmission
B) Scattered moles with benign appearance
C) Increased risk for malignant transformation
D) The number of lesions noted at birth remaining the same over time
E) Excessive vitamin A ingestion

Answer and Discussion

The answer is C. Dysplastic nevi syndrome is a condition that is inherited as an autosomal-dominant disease. Usually more than two family members are affected; however, sporadic cases do occur. Patients are affected with numerous (in some cases >100) irregular, large moles. These moles are abnormal in appearance and show variegation of color. The moles more commonly occur on covered areas such as the breast, buttocks, and scalp. Unlike common moles, dysplastic nevi continue to appear as the patient ages. These patients are at increased risk for the development of melanoma. Patients should be counseled to avoid sun exposure, and any suspicious lesion or change in nevi should warrant a biopsy. Photographs of the patients can help determine if there are any changes in nevi.

Additional Reading: Atypical moles. *Am Fam Physician.* 2008; 78(6):735–740.

Category: Integumentary

94. The proportion of patients with a disease in whom a test result is positive is referred to as
A) The *p* value
B) Sensitivity
C) Specificity
D) Reliability
E) Variability

Answer and Discussion

The answer is B. *Sensitivity* is defined as the proportion of people who are affected by a given disease and who also test positive for that disease. For example, the proportion of patients who actually have CAD and also test positive with a treadmill exercise test would be defined as the sensitivity. Typically, the sensitivity for treadmill exercise testing is 72% to 96%.

Additional Reading: Terms used in evidence-based medicine. *Am Fam Physician.* From: http://www.aafp.org/journals/afp/authors/ebm-toolkit/glossary.html.

Category: Patient/population-based care

⟲ Sensitivity is defined as the proportion of people who are affected by a given disease and who also test positive for that disease.

95. An intensely pruritic, vesicular rash that is localized to the upper extremity is most likely
A) Herpes zoster
B) Poison ivy
C) *Staphylococcus* infection
D) Atopic dermatitis
E) Varicella

Answer and Discussion

The answer is B. Exposure to poison ivy, poison oak, or poison sumac can cause an intensely pruritic vesicular rash. The patient often recalls an exposure to the plants within 24 to 48 hours, and the extremities are often affected. The condition is a result of a delayed hypersensitivity reaction that may take several days to appear. Management should include thorough washing with soap and water, preferably within 10 minutes of exposure, as this may prevent dermatitis. All contaminated clothes should be removed as soon as possible and cleaned. Frequent baths using colloidal oatmeal also relieve symptoms. Treatment of mild-to-moderate rash includes application of cool compresses or diluted aluminum acetate solution such as Burow's solution or calamine lotion. Use of topical antihistamines and anesthetics should be avoided because of the possibility of increased sensitization. Early application of topical steroids is useful to limit erythema and pruritus. However, occlusive dressings should be avoided on moist lesions. Refractory dermatitis can be treated with oral corticosteroids such as prednisone, with an initial dosage of 1 mg per kg per day, slowly tapering the dosage over 2 to 3 weeks. Shorter courses of steroids may be followed by severe rebound exacerbations shortly after drug therapy is discontinued. Oral antihistamines may help reduce pruritus and provide sedation, when needed.

Herpes zoster may have a similar appearance, but is in a dermatomal distribution and tends to be painful, not pruritic. *Staphylococcus* infection (impetigo) will have crusting and weeping and maybe itchy, but is usually painful as well. Atopic dermatitis can be pruritic, but the skin is usually normal initially and patients presents with scaly excoriations from scratching. Varicella would not be localized to one location.

Additional Reading: Diagnosis and management of contact dermatitis. *Am Fam Physician.* 2010;82(3):249–255.

Category: Integumentary

96. The presence of polymorphonuclear fecal leukocytes in stool samples most likely supports the diagnosis of a
A) Bacterial infection
B) Viral infection
C) Parasitic infection
D) Fungal infection

Answer and Discussion

The answer is A. Acute diarrhea is defined as stools occurring with increased frequency or decreased consistency. There are many different organisms. Bacterial agents include *E. coli*, *Salmonella*, *Shigella*, *Campylobacter*, *Clostridium*, *Yersinia*, and *Vibrio cholerae*. Viral agents include rotavirus, enterovirus, and Norwalk agent. Parasitic infections include *Giardia lamblia*, *Entamoeba histolytica*, *Cryptosporidium*, and *Strongyloides*. Fungal agents include *Candida*, *Histoplasma*, and

Actinomyces. Diagnosis is accomplished with stool culture and sensitivity studies; however, the presence of polymorphonuclear cells supports a bacterial cause. In most cases of acute diarrhea, the use of antibiotics is unnecessary; however, the empiric use of antibiotics, including TMP-SMX, ciprofloxacin, or erythromycin, may be appropriate (although controversial) in severe cases in which stool cultures are pending, especially for those at risk for transmitting the offending organism to others.

Additional Reading: Diarrhea in adults (acute). *Am Fam Physician.* 2008;78(4):503–504.

Category: Gastroenterology system

97. Cafe-au-lait spots are associated with which of the following disorders?
A) Peutz–Jeghers syndrome
B) Neurofibromatosis
C) Dysplastic nevus syndrome
D) Addison's disease

Answer and Discussion

The answer is B. The following are skin abnormalities noted in patients affected with the following disease processes:

Neurofibromatosis (von Recklinghausen's disease)	Cafe-au-lait spots
Peutz–Jeghers syndrome	Hyperpigmentation around the oral cavity, hamartomas of the intestine
Dysplastic nevus syndrome	Multiple pigmented nevi
Hypoadrenocorticism (Addison's disease)	Hyperpigmentation of the gingiva, areola of the nipples, labia, and linea alba of the abdomen

Additional Reading: Neurofibromatosis Type 1. In: Domino F, ed. *The 5-Minute Clinical Consult.* Philadelphia, PA: Lippincott Williams and Wilkins; 2014.

Category: Integumentary

98. Which of the following tests is most helpful in distinguishing fever of unknown origin (FUO) from factitious fever?
A) Urinalysis
B) Chest x-ray
C) Rheumatoid factor
D) Blood cultures
E) Sedimentation rate

Answer and Discussion

The answer is E. FUO is defined as a fever higher than 101°F (38.3°C) on at least three occasions, accompanied by an illness that lasts longer than 3 weeks, and the diagnosis is uncertain after 3 days of hospitalization, although most workups are now done in the outpatient setting. Causes include infection, neoplasm, drugs, collagen vascular disease, vasculitis, and factitious fever. Laboratory tests include complete blood cell count (CBC), urinalysis with culture, blood cultures, chest radiography, HIV testing, serum protein electrophoresis, sedimentation rate, serology tests, antinuclear antibody (ANA), rheumatoid factor, and thyroid tests. The ESR may be helpful in distinguishing real disease from a factitious fever. A good history and physical examination are imperative in the evaluation of a patient with FUO and helps direct further testing. Observing the temperature pattern can be helpful. Disease states such as malaria, babesiosis, Hodgkin's disease, and cyclic neutropenia have patterns, whereas factitious fever often has no pattern.

> **Additional Reading:** Approach to the adult with fever of unknown origin. In: Basow DS, ed. *UpToDate*. Waltham, MA: UpToDate; 2013.

Category: Nonspecific system

99. Which of the following test results supports the diagnosis of Graves' disease?
A) Decreased TSH
B) Increased TSH
C) Decreased thyroxine (T_4) levels
D) Decreased triiodothyronine (T_3) levels
E) None of the above

Answer and Discussion

The answer is A. Graves' disease is the most common form of hyperthyroidism seen predominantly in women between 20 and 40 years of age. The condition, also known as *toxic diffuse goiter*, is characterized by a triad of symptoms, including goiter, exophthalmos, and pretibial edema. Patients affected may report palpitations, tachycardia, heat intolerance with excessive sweating, weight loss, emotional lability, weakness and fatigue, diarrhea, or menstrual irregularities. Laboratory findings include a decreased sensitive TSH (sTSH) and positive thyroid-stimulating antibodies (which are thought to bind to the TSH receptors and stimulate the gland to hyperfunction). T_4 levels are usually elevated, but in rare cases may be normal with increased T_3 levels. Treatment involves the use of propylthiouracil or methimazole, inorganic iodine, propranolol (especially in thyroid storm), radioactive iodine (but not in pregnant patients), and surgery.

> **Additional Reading:** Grave's disease. In: Domino F, ed. *The 5-Minute Clinical Consult*. Philadelphia, PA: Lippincott Williams and Wilkins; 2014.

Category: Endocrine system

100. A 45-year-old man comes to your clinic. The patient has known cirrhosis, diabetes, and complains of multiple joint pain. Examination shows a bronze discoloration of the skin and testicular atrophy. Laboratory values show a serum iron of 500 μg per dL, serum ferritin of 2,000 ng per mL, and a transferrin saturation of 80%. The most likely diagnosis is
A) Alcoholism
B) Hemochromatosis
C) Wilson's disease
D) Gilbert's disease
E) Hepatitis C

Answer and Discussion

The answer is B. Hemochromatosis is a result of excessive iron deposition in the body (hemosiderosis) that leads to damage of bodily tissues. Primary hereditary hemochromatosis is an autosomal-recessive trait. Persons who are homozygous for the HFE gene mutation C282Y comprise 90% of phenotypically affected persons. It is the most common form of hemochromatosis, affecting approximately 5 in 1,000 persons. End-organ damage or clinical manifestations of hereditary hemochromatosis occur in approximately 10% of persons homozygous for C282Y. Complications include

- Cirrhosis
- Diabetes mellitus
- Multiple joint pain

- Abdominal pain
- Chondrocalcinosis
- Bronze discoloration of the skin
- Cardiomyopathy that may result in cardiac enlargement, CHF, and cardiac arrhythmias
- Hepatomas
- Pituitary dysfunction leading to testicular atrophy and decreased sexual drive

The onset is usually in the fourth and fifth decades of life. The condition is rare before middle age. Diagnosis in women usually occurs after menopause because menstrual blood loss helps provide protection from iron overload. Laboratory findings show serum iron >300 mg per dL, serum ferritin >1,000 ng per mL, and transferrin saturation >50%. Liver biopsy confirms the diagnosis when hepatic siderosis and cirrhosis is suspected. Treatment involves phlebotomy (500 mL per week = 200 to 250 mg iron) to remove excess iron from the body and the chelating agent deferoxamine in severe cases, which promotes urinary excretion of iron. Family members of those affected should be screened for hemochromatosis with HLA typing and iron studies.

> **Additional Reading:** Hereditary hemochromatosis. *Am Fam Physician*. 2013;87(3):183–190.

Category: Hematologic system

101. Acromegaly is associated with which of the following factors?
A) Excessive cortisol secretion
B) Lack of adequate parathyroid hormone
C) Excessive growth hormone
D) Thyroid dysfunction
E) Excessive gastrin secretion

Answer and Discussion

The answer is C. The condition of acromegaly is associated with an excessive amount of growth hormone, which in most cases is caused by a pituitary tumor. If there is excessive growth hormone secretion before closure of the epiphyses during childhood, then the condition of excessive skeletal growth is referred to as gigantism. When excessive growth hormone occurs in adulthood, it is usually between the third and fifth decades and is referred to as *acromegaly*. Associated conditions include coarsening of facial features with increased hand, foot, jaw, and cranial size; macroglossia; wide spacing of the teeth; deep voice; excessive coarse hair growth; thickening of the skin; excessive sweating as a result of increased number of sweat glands; and neurologic symptoms, including headaches, peripheral neuropathies, muscle weakness, and arthralgias. Insulin resistance is common; diabetes occurs in 25% of patients. CAD, cardiomyopathy with arrhythmias, left ventricular dysfunction, and hypertension occur in 30% of patients. Sleep apnea occurs in 60%. Acromegaly is also associated with an increased risk of colon polyps and colonic malignancy. The diagnosis is made by detecting elevated levels of growth hormone after the administration of a 100-g glucose load. Because of the pulsatility of growth hormone secretion, a single random growth hormone level is not useful. Further diagnostic tests include MRI and CT scanning. Treatment is usually surgery; however, radiation is considered in some patients to treat pituitary tumors. Bromocriptine and a long-acting somatostatin analog (e.g., octreotide acetate) may also be used as adjuncts to surgery to help shrink the tumor.

> **Additional Reading:** Acromegaly. In: Domino F, ed. *The 5-Minute Clinical Consult*. Philadelphia, PA: Lippincott Williams and Wilkins; 2014.

Category: Endocrine system

102. Which of the following signs is associated with Achilles tendonitis?
A) Hyperpronation
B) Gynecoid pelvis
C) Increased Q angle
D) Lateral collateral ligament instability

Answer and Discussion

The answer is A. Achilles tendonitis occurs with repeated stress to the Achilles tendon. Precipitating factors include brisk walking, running, jumping, or hiking. Although known as *Achilles tendonitis*, it is generally a *tendinosis* involving fibrosis of the tendon. Persons who exercise or compete in low-heel shoes and those who hyperpronate their feet are at increased risk for Achilles tendonitis. Patients report pain in the heel and leg discomfort when the Achilles tendon is used. Physical findings include pain with palpation over the Achilles tendon approximately 3 cm above the insertion site on the calcaneus. Treatment goals are to decrease the inflammation associated with the inflamed structures and to reduce the stress on the Achilles tendon. Treatment includes NSAIDs, 1/2-in. heel lifts, and strengthening and stretching exercises of the gastrocnemius and soleus muscles. For patients with hyperpronation, a soft navicular pad and 1/8-in. medial wedge may help prevent excessive pronation. Eccentric Achilles strengthening exercises have been found to be helpful when there is a thickened nodule present consistent with Achilles tendinosis.

> **Additional Reading:** Busconi BD, Stevenson JH. Approach to the athlete with Achilles tendon injury. *Sports Medicine Consult: A Problem-Based Approach to Sports Medicine for the Primary Care Physician*. Philadelphia, PA: Lippincott, Williams & Wilkins; 2009.

> Category: Musculoskeletal system

103. Which of the following statements about systolic hypertension is true?
A) It represents relatively little risk to the patient.
B) It is defined as a systolic pressure >140 mm Hg with a diastolic pressure >100 mm Hg.
C) It does not increase the risk of stroke.
D) It is often caused by mitral regurgitation.
E) It is more dangerous to elderly patients than an elevated diastolic pressure.

Answer and Discussion

The answer is E. Systolic hypertension is a condition that usually affects the elderly. The condition is defined as a systolic blood pressure >140 mm Hg and diastolic pressure <90 mm Hg. The cause is the loss of elasticity of the arteries that occurs with aging. Other causes include thyrotoxicosis, arteriovenous fistulas, or aortic regurgitation. Untreated systolic hypertension can lead to an increased risk for stroke and CVD. Data from the Framingham study and the Multiple Risk Factor Intervention Trial indicated the importance of isolated systolic hypertension in the development of coronary heart disease (CHD). These trials concluded that elevated systolic blood pressure in the elderly was probably of more significance than elevated diastolic blood pressure. In other words, a systolic blood pressure of 160 mm Hg with a diastolic blood pressure of 85 mm Hg posed a greater risk for CVD than a systolic blood pressure of 135 to 140 mm Hg and a diastolic blood pressure of 95 mm Hg. Isolated systolic hypertension, defined as a blood pressure of >140 mm Hg systolic and <90 mm Hg diastolic, occurs in more than 30% of women older than 65 years and in more than 20% of men of the same age. Treatment involves lifestyle changes (e.g., exercise, sodium restriction, weight loss) and the use of hypertensive medications. In most instances, low-dose diuretic therapy should be used as initial antihypertensive therapy in the elderly. A long-acting dihydropyridine CCB may be used as an alternative therapy in elderly patients with isolated systolic hypertension. Diabetics benefit from ACE inhibitors. In some cases, systolic hypertension may be more difficult to control than essential hypertension.

> **Additional Reading:** Hypertension cardiovascular medicine. *ACP Medicine*. October 2010.

> Category: Cardiovascular system

104. Which of the following statements is true regarding pneumococcal vaccination?
A) Healthy individuals older than 50 years should receive the vaccine.
B) Medicare does not cover the cost of pneumococcal vaccination.
C) Adults with previous splenectomy should not receive pneumococcal vaccination.
D) Children younger than 2 years with sickle cell anemia should receive pneumococcal vaccination.
E) Boosters are recommended for individuals older than 65 years if they received their first dose more than 5 years before their last injection.

Answer and Discussion

The answer is E. The pneumococcal vaccine is made from the polysaccharides of 23 different strains of bacterial pneumonia. The vaccine is recommended for patients older than 65 years, individuals with underlying pulmonary disease or chronic debilitating diseases (e.g., diabetes, liver and renal disease, cardiac disease, lymphoma, transplant patients, HIV patients), and those without a spleen. The vaccine is given intramuscularly or subcutaneously and is not recommended during an acute illness. Antigenic response occurs 2 to 3 weeks after vaccination. Adverse reactions include local irritation or soreness, erythema, induration, low-grade fever, rash, myalgia, and arthralgia; in severe reactions (less than 1%), anaphylaxis or nerve disorders may occur. Children younger than 2 years should not receive the vaccine. Since 1981, Medicare has covered the cost of pneumococcal vaccine. One-time boosters are recommended for individuals older than 65 years if they received their first dose more than 5 years prior. Other individuals at high risk who received pneumococcal vaccination more than 5 to 10 years prior may require boosters. The vaccine has been determined to be cost-effective for all ages.

> **Additional Reading:** Pneumococcal advisory committee on immunization practices (ACIP): vaccine recommendations. *MMWR*. 2012; 61(21).

> Category: Respiratory system

105. The most effective therapy for tobacco cessation is which of the following?
A) Bupropion
B) Nicotine transdermal patch
C) Nicotine polacrilex gum
D) Varenicline
E) Clonidine

Answer and Discussion

The answer is D. Tobacco dependence is a chronic disease that often requires pharmacological therapy, but counseling improves the effectiveness of any treatment for this indication. The greater the number of office visits and the longer the counseling time, the higher the smoking cessation rates have been. The most effective drugs available for treatment of tobacco dependence are bupropion (Zyban and others) and varenicline (Chantix). Varenicline appears to be the most effective single drug for treatment of tobacco dependence, but bupropion has been available much longer and is also well tolerated. Bupropion is a dopamine-norepinephrine reuptake inhibitor used mainly for treatment of depression, but it also has some nicotine-receptor-blocking activity. A partial agonist that binds selectively to $\alpha4/\beta2$ nicotinic acetylcholine receptors, it stimulates receptor-mediated activity, relieving cravings and withdrawal symptoms during abstinence. Since varenicline binds to the $\alpha4/\beta2$ receptor with greater affinity than does nicotine, it also acts as an antagonist to nicotine delivery from active cigarette use, thus reducing the reward of smoking. Both varenicline (Chantix) and bupropion (Zyban and others) are effective in treating tobacco dependence. Varenicline is more effective, but bupropion offers the benefit of mitigating the weight gain that often accompanies smoking cessation. All nicotine-replacement therapies (NRTs) deliver nicotine, which acts as an agonist at the nicotinic acetylcholine receptor, to the CNS in a lower dose and at a substantially slower rate than tobacco cigarettes. All of these products roughly double smoking cessation rates. Nicotine is subject to first-pass metabolism, limiting the effectiveness of oral pill formulations. Nicotine gum, lozenges, and patches are available in the United States without a prescription; these products appear to be as effective as those that require a prescription (the oral inhaler and nasal spray). All of the NRTs appear to be about equally effective, but results may be better with the combination of a patch and a rapid-onset nicotine medication. NRTs should be started 1-4 weeks before the target quit date. The optimum duration of treatment is not clear; 3-6 months is probably the minimum, and some patients may need even longer treatment in order to remain abstinent.

All patients who smoke should be encouraged to stop. The physician should always ask about smoking; if the patient does smoke, there should be an attempt by the physician to motivate the patient to stop. Setting a stop date may be helpful, and follow-up is necessary to provide support and reinforce the patient's commitment to stop.

Although not approved for this indication by the FDA, the antihypertensive drug clonidine, an $\alpha2$-adrenergic agonist available both as tablets (Catapres, and others) and in a patch formulation (Catapres TTS), can be used as a second-line treatment for patients who cannot tolerate or do not wish to use NRTs, bupropion, or varenicline. Clinical trial results have been mixed, but one meta-analysis concluded that clonidine was effective.

Additional Reading: Drugs for tobacco dependence. *Med Lett Drugs Ther.* 2008;6(73):61–66.

Category: Respiratory system

106. A 45-year-old woman presents with persistent nasal symptoms for the last 6 weeks. She has been treated with an extended course of antibiotics but despite therapy her symptoms remain. She is afebrile and otherwise looks well. Appropriate management at this time includes
A) Additional 2-week course of antibiotic therapy
B) Plain films of the sinuses
C) CT scan of the sinuses
D) MRI of the sinuses
E) Laboratory evaluation including a complete blood cell count and blood cultures

Answer and Discussion

The answer is C. Rhinosinusitis is typically divided into four subtypes, namely, acute, recurrent acute, subacute, and chronic, on the basis of patient history and a limited physical examination. In most cases,

therapy is administered on the basis of this classification. Mild rhinosinusitis symptoms of less than 7 days' duration can be managed with supportive care, including analgesics, short-term decongestants, saline nasal irrigation, and intranasal corticosteroids. Antibiotic therapy is recommended for patients with rhinosinusitis symptoms that do not improve within 7 days or that worsen at any time; those with moderate illness (moderate to severe pain or temperature $\geq 101°F$ [38.3°C]); or those who are immunocompromised. Amoxicillin is considered the first-line antibiotic for most patients with acute bacterial rhinosinusitis. Trimethoprim/sulfamethoxazole (Bactrim, Septra) and macrolide antibiotics are reasonable alternatives to amoxicillin for treating acute bacterial rhinosinusitis in patients who are allergic to penicillin. Radiographic imaging in patients with acute rhinosinusitis is not recommended unless a complication or an alternative diagnosis is suspected.

For patients with chronic disease, the same treatment regimen is indicated for an additional 4 weeks or more, and a nasal steroid may also be prescribed if inhalant allergies are suspected as an etiologic agent. Nasal endoscopy and CT of the sinuses are reserved for circumstances that include a failure to respond to therapy as expected, spread of infection outside the sinuses, a question of diagnosis, and when surgery is being considered. Laboratory tests are rarely needed and are reserved for patients with suspected allergies, cystic fibrosis, immune deficiencies, mucociliary disorders, and similar disease states. Findings on endoscopically guided culture obtained from the middle meatus correlate 80% to 85% of the time with results from the more painful antral puncture technique and is performed in patients who fail to respond to the initial antibiotic selection. Surgery is indicated for extranasal spread of infection, evidence of mucocele or pyocele, fungal sinusitis, or obstructive nasal polyposis and is often performed in patients with recurrent or persistent infection not resolved by drug therapy.

Additional Reading: Acute rhinosinusitis in adults. *Am Fam Physician.* 2011;83(9):1057–1063.

Category: Special sensory

107. A 56-year-old smoker with recently diagnosed small cell carcinoma of the lung presents with increasing muscle contraction with repeated nerve stimulation. The most likely diagnosis is
A) Lambert-Eaton myasthenic syndrome (LEMS)
B) Myasthenia gravis
C) Tetanus
D) Polymyalgia rheumatica
E) Parkinson's disease

Answer and Discussion

The answer is A. LEMS is an uncommon neurologic disorder that results from inadequate release of acetylcholine from the presynaptic nerve endings. Often associated with a paraneoplastic syndrome (e.g., small cell or oat cell carcinoma of the lung), the condition causes weakness and sometimes pain associated with the proximal muscles, paresthesia, impotence, and ptosis. Reflexes are usually reduced or absent. Diagnosis is made by showing increasing muscle contraction with repeated nerve stimulation, unlike myasthenia gravis, in which decreased muscle contraction with repeated nerve stimulation is seen. Special care must be taken to rule out underlying malignancy. The treatment is to identify and treat any underlying malignancy. Guanidine has also been shown to help acetylcholine release from the presynaptic membrane; however, side effects (bone marrow suppression) may limit its use. Other treatment includes the use of immunosuppressant medication (e.g., steroids, azathioprine) and plasmapheresis. Anticholinesterase medications (e.g., pyridostigmine, neostigmine) are variably effective.

Additional Reading: Clinical features and diagnosis of Lambert-Eaton myasthenic syndrome. In: Basow DS, ed. *UpToDate*. Waltham, MA: UpToDate; 2013.

Category: Respiratory system

108. Which is *not* generally a characteristic of a suspicious skin lesion?
A) Asymmetric border
B) Bleeding
C) Color change
D) Variegation of color
E) Diameter less than 5 mm

Answer and Discussion
The answer is E. Skin lesions that represent concern usually possess certain characteristics, including

A = Asymmetric and irregular borders
B = Bleeding or ulceration; persistent itching or tenderness
C = Color change or variegation of color
D = Diameter >6 mm

If any of these criteria are met, the lesion should be biopsied and sent for pathologic examination. Large, raised, and pigmented congenital lesions should also be biopsied. Patients who have a history of dysplastic nevi syndrome are at increased risk for the development of melanoma, particularly if a family member has been affected.

Additional Reading: Screening for skin cancer. *Am Fam Physician*. 2010;81(12):1435–1436.

Category: Integumentary

109. Which of the following conditions is a contraindication to influenza vaccination?
A) Allergy to eggs
B) Allergy to red dye
C) Allergy to penicillin
D) Allergy to milk
E) Allergy to dust mites

Answer and Discussion
The answer is A. Influenza immunizations are administered yearly to help prevent outbreaks of different strains of viral influenza. The inactivated vaccine is derived from purified egg protein, which harbors the viral protein. The vaccine is developed on the basis of the preceding year's outbreak of virus, those viruses seen in other parts of the world, and the antibody response of persons previously vaccinated. Persons who are allergic to eggs or neomycin (a component of the vaccine) should not receive the vaccine. In those individuals, amantadine may be considered. Protective vaccine should be administered to immunocompromised individuals; individuals with underlying medical conditions such as asthma, COPD, and diabetes; and individuals older than 50 years. (Other recommendations follow.) Otherwise healthy patients may also elect to receive vaccination. Side effects, including fever, fatigue, cough, and headache, are no more common in those who received a placebo in double-blinded studies; however, arm soreness was reported more frequently in vaccine recipients.

Recommendations for the administration of influenza vaccine include the following categories and specific indications:

Age
- Persons 6 months or older with an underlying medical condition (e.g., cardiac, pulmonary) who are at increased risk for

complications of influenza or who required regular medical follow-up or hospitalization during the preceding year (see Medical conditions as follows)
- Healthy children ages 6 to 23 months and close contacts of healthy children ages 6 to 23 months
- Persons 50 years or older
- Any person 6 months or older to reduce the chance of influenza infection

Occupations
- Physicians, nurses, and other personnel in hospital and outpatient care settings, including emergency response workers
- Employees of health care facilities (e.g., nursing homes, chronic care facilities) who have contact with residents
- Persons who provide home care to people in high-risk groups

Medical conditions
- Alcoholism and alcoholic cirrhosis
- Long-term aspirin therapy in children and teenagers (6 months to 18 years of age) who may be at risk for Reye's syndrome after influenza virus infection
- Chronic cardiovascular disorders in adults and children
- Hemoglobinopathies
- Immunocompromised conditions (e.g., congenital immunodeficiency, malignancy, HIV infection, organ transplantation, immunosuppressive therapy)
- Chronic metabolic diseases (e.g., diabetes)
- Chronic pulmonary diseases, including asthma and COPD
- Chronic renal dysfunction
- Pregnancy beyond 14 weeks of gestation during the influenza season
- Pregnancy in women with medical conditions that increase their risk for complications from influenza, regardless of trimester
- Persons who can transmit influenza to high-risk individuals
- Household members (including children) in close contact with persons who are at high risk for influenza
- Residents of nursing homes and other chronic care facilities, regardless of age, who have chronic medical conditions

Vaccination ideally should occur approximately 2 weeks before chemotherapy or immunosuppressive therapy is started. If a patient is vaccinated during or within 2 weeks before the initiation of immunosuppressive therapy, influenza vaccine should be given again approximately 3 months after treatment ends.

Additional Reading: Prevention and control of influenza: Recommendations of the advisory committee on immunization practices (ACIP) 2013. Centers for disease control and prevention. From: www.cdc.gov/vaccines/.

Category: Respiratory system

110. A 41-year-old business executive presents to your office and complains of palpitations and shortness of breath. After further questioning, he admits to heavy alcohol consumption the previous evening. On examination, he is found to have an irregular heartbeat of 130 bpm. The most likely diagnosis is
A) Ventricular tachycardia
B) Ventricular fibrillation
C) Premature ventricular contractions (PVCs)
D) Atrial fibrillation
E) Wolff–Parkinson–White syndrome

Answer and Discussion

The answer is D. Atrial fibrillation is the most common cardiac arrhythmia. It is characterized on ECG by the absence of P waves and an irregular ventricular rhythm. The atrial rate can range from 400 to 600 bpm, whereas the ventricular rate usually ranges from 80 to 180 bpm in the untreated state. Causes include thyrotoxicosis, rheumatic or ischemic heart disease, hypertension, pericarditis, chest trauma, or excessive alcohol intake. The major risk associated with atrial fibrillation is stroke secondary to embolic complications. Rapid ventricular response of atrial fibrillation requires treatment with rate-controlling CCBs, β-blockers, or digoxin to achieve rate control. Elective medical cardioversion may be considered for stable patients. Patients in whom medical conversion fails or whose conditions are unstable may need electrical cardioversion. Patients with long-standing atrial fibrillation (longer than 6 months) have less chance for success than those who have new or relatively new onset. Anticoagulation therapy with warfarin can decrease the risk of stroke and is recommended before any attempt at cardioversion if there is risk for thrombus formation. Patients with chronic atrial fibrillation who are at low risk for bleeding may be treated with warfarin; others may be treated with aspirin therapy. Antiarrhythmics may be needed to treat resistant cases. The risk of embolism during cardioversion in unanticoagulated patients is 1% to 7%; however, this risk can be minimized with anticoagulation for 4 weeks before and after cardioversion. Recent studies demonstrate no reductions in either mortality or stroke rates between those patients managed with simple rate control and anticoagulation compared with those receiving cardioversion with rhythm maintenance using antiarrhythmic medication.

Additional Reading: Atrial fibrillation: diagnosis and treatment. *Am Fam Physician.* 2011;83(1):61–68.

Category: Cardiovascular system

111. The most common cause of superior vena cava syndrome is
A) Carcinoma of the lung
B) Aortic aneurysm
C) Tuberculosis
D) Metastatic carcinoma from a distant site
E) Constrictive pericarditis

Answer and Discussion

The answer is A. Superior vena cava syndrome results from compression of the superior vena cava by a neoplastic process (90% of cases) and less commonly by inflammatory states. Other causes include benign tumors, aortic aneurysm, thyroid enlargement, thrombosis of a central venous line, and fibrosing mediastinitis. Lung cancer, particularly small cell and squamous cell type, is the most common associated malignancy. The condition causes the obstruction of venous drainage to the heart and leads to dilation of collateral veins of the upper chest and neck. Signs include plethora and swelling of the face, neck, and upper torso. Edema of the conjunctiva, shortness of breath in a supine position, and CNS disturbances, including headache, dizziness, stupor, and syncope, may be seen. Acute development of symptoms indicates a poor prognosis. The diagnosis of superior vena cava syndrome is essentially a clinical one. Chest x-rays may show widening of the mediastinum, particularly on the right, but the best confirmatory test is CT. The MRI has no advantages over CT. The one potentially life-threatening complication of a superior mediastinal mass is tracheal obstruction. Treatment includes steroids, chemotherapy, and radiation to the tumor. Although the most common cause of this syndrome is metastasized carcinoma of the lung, other less common infectious causes include tuberculosis, histoplasmosis, and constrictive pericarditis.

Additional Reading: Superior vena cava syndrome. In: Domino F, ed. *The 5-Minute Clinical Consult.* Philadelphia, PA: Lippincott Williams and Wilkins; 2014.

Category: Respiratory system

112. A construction worker presents with pain over the lateral elbow. He reports that he has been using a hammer more often, and this seems to aggravate his discomfort. The most likely diagnosis is
A) Carpal tunnel syndrome
B) Rotator cuff dysfunction
C) Lateral epicondylitis
D) Ulnar nerve entrapment
E) Biceps tendonitis

Answer and Discussion

The answer is C. Lateral epicondylitis, commonly referred to as "tennis elbow," is usually caused by overuse, repeated trauma, strain, or exercise that involves the upper extremity and a gripping motion. Although associated with playing tennis, it may affect baseball players, golfers, and racquetball enthusiasts, as well as carpenters, assembly-line workers, and electricians, all of whom repeatedly extend the wrist and rotate the forearm. The cause of pain originates at the extensor origin of the extensor carpi radialis brevis in the area of the lateral epicondyle. Symptoms include pain in the area of the lateral epicondyle but may also include the extensor surface of the forearm. In more severe cases, swelling and erythema may be noted. Pain is exacerbated by passively flexing the fingers and wrist with the elbow fully extended. Radiographs are usually negative; however, calcification may be noted in chronic cases. The condition should be distinguished from radial nerve entrapment syndrome (pain with middle finger extension and forearm supination with the elbow fully extended) and posterior interosseous nerve syndrome (pain located more distally over the forearm supinator muscle). Treatment includes use of NSAIDs, rest of the affected arm, ice therapy, and a volar wrist splint that immobilizes the wrist and prevents flexion and extension. If this treatment does not provide relief, a steroid injection of 1 mL of 1% lidocaine and 0.5 mL of corticosteroid should be attempted. Once the inflammation has been controlled, a constricting band can be used over the proximal forearm to help prevent recurrence. In addition, rehabilitation exercises should be instituted. In severe cases, orthopaedic referral may be necessary for possible surgical treatment.

Additional Reading: Busconi BD, Stevenson JH. Approach to the athlete with lateral epicondylitis (tennis elbow). *Sports Medicine Consult: A Problem-Based Approach to Sports Medicine for the Primary Care Physician.* Philadelphia, PA: Lippincott, Williams & Wilkins; 2009.

Category: Musculoskeletal system

113. Which of the following is a characteristic of Marfan's syndrome?
A) Autosomal-recessive transmission
B) Decreased mobility of joints
C) Arm span less than height
D) Aortic dilatation with possible rupture
E) Cafe-au-lait spots

Answer and Discussion

The answer is D. Marfan's syndrome is an autosomal-dominant transmitted disorder that affects the connective tissue and results in abnormalities associated with the eyes, bones, and cardiovascular system. Up to 25% of all cases may develop from spontaneous mutations. Symptoms include tall stature with arm span exceeding height, arachnodactyly, dislocation of the ocular lens, high-arched palate, pectus excavatum, and hyperextensibility of joints. Complications of the condition include myopia; spontaneous detachment of the lens; and cardiac defects, including aortic regurgitation, mitral valve prolapse (MVP), mitral regurgitation, and aortic dilatation with aortic dissection and rupture (the most common cause of cardiovascular death). Patients affected are at increased risk of endocarditis. Treatment is directed toward the cardiovascular findings. An echocardiogram can help determine cardiac involvement. In some cases, β-blockers may help protect the aorta. Surgery is reserved for those with aortic dilatation or aortic valve dysfunction. New DNA diagnostic tests for mutations in fibrillin-1 and fibrillin-2 can help determine which patients affected with Marfan's are at increased risk for aortic aneurysm. Scoliosis may require bracing or surgery for severe cases.

Additional Reading: Dominio F. Marfan syndrome. *The 5-Minute Clinical Consult*. Philadelphia, PA: Lippincott Williams and Wilkins; 2014.

Category: Cardiovascular system

114. Third-generation cephalosporins differ from first-generation cephalosporins in their increased effectiveness against
A) Gram-positive organisms
B) Gram-negative organisms
C) Anaerobic organisms
D) Parasites
E) Fungi

Answer and Discussion

The answer is B. Cephalosporins are antibiotics that have a similar chemical structure as penicillins. They are bacteriocidal and cover gram-positive organisms; second-generation and third-generation cephalosporins also cover gram-negative organisms. As a group, the cephalosporins' mechanism of action is the inhibition of cell wall synthesis. Inflammation increases their absorption, and they are active against a wide spectrum of organisms with relatively few side effects. Some of the cephalosporins, especially third-generation ones, are concentrated enough in the cerebrospinal fluid (CSF) to treat meningitis. Because of their similarity to penicillin, there is a 2% to 3% cross-reactivity in those allergic to penicillin. Unfortunately, there are no predictable skin tests that can test for allergic reactions. Therefore, use of cephalosporins in patients with penicillin allergies should be monitored closely. If the patient has had a severe, immediate reaction to any of the cillintype medications, it is necessary to use extreme caution prescribing cephalosporins; alternative antibiotics should be strongly considered.

Additional Reading: Drugs for bacterial infections. *Treat Guidel Med Lett*. 2013;11(131):65–74.

Category: Nonspecific system

> Because of their similarity to penicillin, there is a 2% to 3% cross-reactivity in those patients taking cephalosporins who are allergic to penicillin.

115. During which of the following stages of sleep does most dreaming occur?
A) Stage 1 non–rapid eye movement (REM) sleep
B) Stage 2 non-REM sleep
C) Stage 3 non-REM sleep
D) Stage 4 non-REM sleep
E) REM sleep

Answer and Discussion

The answer is E. There are two distinct states of sleep: REM sleep and non-REM sleep, which make up 75% to 80% of sleep. Based on electroencephalographic (EEG) patterns, non-REM sleep can be classified into stages 1, 2, 3, and 4. Necessary for survival, sleep is a cyclical phenomenon. There are four to five REM periods nightly that always follow non-REM sleep and end each cycle. REM sleep, which accounts for 25% (or 1.5 to 2 hours) of the night's sleep, is the period of sleep in which most dreaming occurs. The first period of REM sleep occurs approximately 1.5 to 2 hours after sleep has occurred and lasts approximately 10 minutes. A night's sleep cycles through the different stages and reenters REM stage three or four times for longer periods (15 to 45 minutes), usually in the last several hours of sleep. Non-REM sleep is characterized by slow waves on EEG, with stage 4 being the deepest stage of sleep. REM sleep is characterized by low-voltage, fast activity on EEG. Most night terrors, sleep walking, and sleep talking occur during stage 4 sleep. In REM sleep, muscle tone is decreased, but depth of respiration is increased. As patients become older, the length of REM sleep remains the same; however, there are significant decreases in stages 3 and 4 sleep and an increase in wakeful periods during the night. In addition, it takes elderly patients a longer period to fall asleep. Wakefulness is characterized by alpha wave activity on EEG.

Additional Reading: Management of common sleep disorders. *Am Fam Physician*. 2013;88(4):231–238.

Category: Neurologic

116. Treatment for uncomplicated Infectious Mononucleosis (IM) should be
A) Intravenous antiviral medication
B) Oral antiviral therapy (acyclovir or ganciclovir)
C) Oral steroids
D) Empiric antibiotic treatment
E) Symptomatic treatment only

Answer and Discussion

The answer is E. The mainstay of treatment for individuals with IM is supportive care. Acetaminophen or NSAIDs are recommended for the treatment of fever, throat discomfort, and malaise. Provision of adequate fluids and nutrition is also important. It is prudent to get adequate rest, although complete bed rest is unnecessary.

The use of corticosteroids in the treatment of EBV-induced IM has been controversial. In a multicenter, placebo-controlled study of 94 patients with acute IM, the combination of acyclovir and prednisolone reduced oropharyngeal shedding of the virus but did not affect the duration of symptoms or lead to an earlier return to school or work. A subsequent meta-analysis of seven studies found insufficient evidence to recommend steroid treatment for symptom relief; furthermore, two studies reported severe complications in patients assigned to the corticosteroid arm compared with placebo. Corticosteroid therapy is not recommended for routine cases of IM as it is generally a self-limited illness and there are theoretical concerns about immunosuppression during clinical illness with a virus that has been causally linked to a variety of malignancies. However, corticosteroids may be considered in the management of patients with some EBV-associated complications.

The incidence of IM is highest in young adults 15 to 35 years of age. Asymptomatic infections are common, and most adults are seropositive to the EBV. Symptoms include fever, headache, generalized fatigue, and malaise. Signs include lymphadenopathy (especially the posterior cervical chain), splenomegaly, hepatomegaly, jaundice, periorbital edema, exudative pharyngitis, palatine petechiae, and rash. Laboratory findings show a lymphocytosis with 20% or more atypical lymphocytes (Downey lymphocytes), a positive heterophile agglutination (Monospot) test after the second week of illness, and a heterophile titer greater than 1:56. Liver function tests are usually elevated. Other laboratory findings may include granulocytopenia, thrombocytopenia, and hemolytic anemia in complicated cases. No specific treatment is recommended for mild cases, and symptoms usually improve in 2 to 4 weeks. In severe cases in which the pharyngitis threatens to obstruct the patient's airway, a 5-day course of steroids may be beneficial. Specific antiviral therapies (acyclovir or ganciclovir) do not appear to be clinically beneficial. Treatment with amoxicillin or ampicillin may lead to a severe maculopapular rash and should be avoided. If the patient has evidence of spleno- megaly, contact sports should be avoided until the splenomegaly has resolved. Mononucleosis-type infections may occur more than once but are generally caused by sequential infections with differ- ent pathogens rather than by reactivated EBV infections. EBV infec- tions can become reactivated when patients are immunosuppressed (during corticosteroid or cyclosporine therapy) or develop immune deficiencies (e.g., HIV).

> **Additional Reading:** Infectious mononucleosis in adults and adolescents. In: Basow DS, ed. *UpToDate.* Waltham, MA: UpTo- Date; 2013.

> Category: Nonspecific system

117. A 65-year-old man presents with increasing shortness of breath over the previous 5 years. Further history reveals that the patient worked for many years in a factory that produced fluorescent lights. On examination, the patient has granulomas affecting the skin and conjunctivae. A chest radiograph shows evidence of parenchymal in- filtrates and intra-alveolar edema with mediastinal lymphadenopathy. The most likely diagnosis is
A) Coccidioidomycosis
B) Berylliosis
C) Tuberculosis
D) Sarcoidosis
E) Asbestosis

Answer and Discussion

The answer is B. Chronic inhalation of beryllium compounds and their products can result in a disease characterized by granulomas that affect primarily the lungs but also the skin and conjunctivae. Beryllium is found in electronics and chemical plants, aerospace fac- tories, beryllium-mining sites, and industries in which fluorescent lights are manufactured. Changes that occur in the lungs include dif- fuse parenchymal inflammatory infiltrates with the development of intra-alveolar edema. The hallmark finding is a granulomatous reac- tion involving the hilar lymph nodes and pulmonary parenchyma, which is indistinguishable from sarcoidosis. Symptoms of the dis- ease include dyspnea with shortness of breath, cough, and weight loss. Chest radiographs usually show diffuse alveolar consolidation with hilar lymphadenopathy. The prognosis of the disease is variable and ranges from mild pulmonary symptoms to extreme respiratory compromise and even death. Chronic exposure tends to cause a pro- gressive decrease in pulmonary function with the development of right heart failure and cor pulmonale. Treatment is usually support- ive. Steroids have been used with little benefit in chronic cases but may be used for acute berylliosis. Those exposed to beryllium dust should be counseled to protect themselves with masks and should

take measures to avoid exposure. A pulmonary function test may be helpful in determining the extent of damage and the progression of disease.

> **Additional Reading:** Fibrosis, Pulmonary. In: Domino F, ed. *The 5-Minute Clinical Consult.* Philadelphia, PA: Lippincott Williams and Wilkins; 2014.

> Category: Respiratory system

118. Which of the following drugs is associated with drug- induced LE?
A) Hydralazine
B) Azithromycin
C) Metoprolol
D) Digoxin
E) Penicillin

Answer and Discussion

The answer is A. Drug-induced LE is associated with the use of procainamide (most common), hydralazine, INH, penicillamine, sulfonamides, quinidine, thiouracil, methyldopa, and cephalosporins. All patients with drug-induced LE have positive reactions to ANA testing; however, they usually do not have positive reactions to antibodies to double-stranded DNA. Other laboratory findings sup- porting drug-induced lupus include anemia, leukopenia, throm- bocytopenia, positive rheumatoid factor, positive cryoglobulins, positive lupus anticoagulants, false-positive Venereal Disease Research Laboratory (VDRL) test results, and positive results on a direct Coombs' test. Signs and symptoms include polyarthralgias, fever, butterfly rash affecting the facial area, alopecia, photosensitiv- ity, pleurisy, proteinuria, and glomerulonephritis. In most cases, the symptoms disappear when the medication is discontinued. Steroids may be necessary for severe cases.

> **Additional Reading:** Lupus erythematosus. In: Domino F, ed. *The 5-Minute Clinical Consult.* Philadelphia, PA: Lippincott Williams and Wilkins; 2014.

> Category: Nonspecific system

119. Which of the following medications is used for the treatment of pseudomembranous colitis?
A) Metronidazole
B) Amphotericin B
C) Ketoconazole
D) Acyclovir
E) Intravenous vancomycin

Answer and Discussion

The answer is A. Overgrowth of *Clostridium difficile* in the intestine gives rise to a condition known as *pseudomembranous colitis.* The condition results from the use of antibiotics (especially clindamy- cin, ampicillin, and cephalosporins) usually 2 days to 6 weeks after administration. In some cases, it may occur without recent antibiotic use. Symptoms include watery diarrhea, abdominal cramps, tenes- mus, low-grade fever, and, in some cases, hematochezia. Physical findings may include a tender, distended abdomen with hyperactive bowel sounds. *C. difficile* may be present in as much as 3% to 8% of healthy asymptomatic carriers. Diagnosis is made by the detection of *C. difficile* toxin in the stool and sigmoidoscopy or colonoscopy find- ings consisting of yellowish-white plaques of exudate with alternating areas of normal bowel mucosa. If the exudate is removed, bleeding often occurs from the affected mucosa. Not all affected patients have the identifiable lesions. Treatment involves the use of metronidazole.

For infections unresponsive to metronidazole, oral vancomycin can be used. Mild cases can be treated with cholestyramine resin. *Saccharomyces boullardii* yeast may also be helpful in treatment. Complications include dehydration with electrolyte imbalances, intestinal perforation, toxic megacolon, and, in severe cases, death. Relapses may occur in up to 20% of cases.

> **Additional Reading:** Diarrhea, Acute. In: Domino F, ed. *The 5-Minute Clinical Consult*. Philadelphia, PA: Lippincott Williams and Wilkins; 2014.

Category: Gastroenterology system

120. Which of the following is a distinguishing feature between drug-induced and idiopathic SLE?
A) In drug-induced lupus, there is an absence of antibodies to double-stranded DNA.
B) In drug-induced lupus, there are increased levels of complement.
C) In idiopathic SLE, a butterfly facial rash is seen.
D) Renal and CNS involvement are common with drug-induced SLE.
E) There are no differences seen between the two conditions.

Answer and Discussion

The answer is A. Several drugs are known to cause a lupus-like syndrome; two of the most common are procainamide and hydralazine. Most patients with drug-induced SLE do not have antibodies to double-stranded DNA, and they rarely have depressed levels of complement, which can distinguish drug-induced SLE from idiopathic SLE. Other laboratory abnormalities seen with drug-induced SLE include anemia, thrombocytopenia, and leukopenia. Additional findings include a positive rheumatoid factor, false-positive VDRL result, and positive direct Coombs' test. In most cases, the symptoms resolve once the medication is discontinued; however, steroid administration may be needed in severe cases. Most symptoms are completely resolved in 6 months, but ANA test results may remain positive for years. Most affected patients complain of arthralgias, myalgias, fever, and pleuritic chest pain. Renal and CNS involvement are rare with drug-induced SLE. Other medications associated with drug-induced lupus include chlorpromazine, methyldopa, and INH.

> **Additional Reading:** A systematic review of drug-induced subcutaneous lupus erythematosus. *Br J Dermatol*. 2011;164(3): 465–472.

Category: Integumentary

121. The drug of choice to treat a serious methicillin-resistant *S. aureus* (MRSA) skin infection is
A) Penicillin
B) Dicloxacillin
C) Cefuroxime
D) Vancomycin
E) Metronidazole

Answer and Discussion

The answer is D. MRSA has become the predominant cause of suppurative skin infection in many parts of the United States. Community-associated MRSA (CA-MRSA) usually causes furunculosis, cellulitis, and abscesses, but necrotizing fasciitis and sepsis can occur. CA-MRSA strains are usually susceptible to trimethoprim/sulfamethoxazole, clindamycin, and tetracyclines. Patients with serious skin and soft tissue infections suspected to be caused by MRSA

should be treated empirically with vancomycin, linezolid, or daptomycin. The most common reservoir is the nasal mucosa and oropharynx. Isolates are usually resistant to all the cillin-type antibiotics and the cephalosporins. Duration of therapy is based on the patient's response but is usually 2 to 4 weeks. Colonization occurs in approximately 50% of treated patients. Asymptomatic colonization with MRSA does not require systemic treatment.

> **Additional Reading:** Drugs for bacterial infections. *Treat Guidel Med Lett*. 2013;11(131):65–74.

Category: Nonspecific system

122. Ramsay Hunt syndrome is associated with
A) Herpes zoster infection affecting the geniculate ganglion of the facial nerve
B) Spinothalamic disruption leading to loss of motor function in the lower extremities
C) Spontaneous progressive demyelination of motor neurons
D) Autoimmune destruction of norepinephrine receptors in the thalamus

Answer and Discussion

The answer is A. Ramsay Hunt syndrome is a disorder caused by the herpes zoster virus that affects the geniculate ganglion of the facial nerve. The syndrome can give rise to ipsilateral facial nerve palsy and can be distinguished from Bell's palsy by the development of vesicular herpetic lesions that affect the pharynx, external auditory canal, and, occasionally, the eighth cranial nerve. Patients report painful lesions and lose their sense of taste associated with the anterior two-thirds of the tongue.

> **Additional Reading:** Diagnosis of ear pain. *Am Fam Physician*. 2008;77(5):621–628.

Category: Integumentary

> Ramsay Hunt syndrome is a disorder caused by the herpes zoster virus that affects the geniculate ganglion of the facial nerve.

123. A 19-year-old jumped off the high dive at a local swimming pool and presents to your office complaining of severe right-sided ear pain after landing on that side when he hit the water. You have seen him for this problem for the last 12 weeks, but a small perforation remains in the tympanic membrane. There is no sign of infection. Appropriate treatment at this point consists of
A) Continued observation
B) An audiogram to document hearing
C) Steroid otic drops
D) Antibiotic eardrops and no water exposure
E) Referral to an ear–nose–throat specialist

Answer and Discussion

The answer is E. Rupture of the tympanic membrane can be caused by placing objects (e.g., cotton swabs, twigs, pencils) in the ear canal, excessive positive pressure applied to the ear (e.g., explosions, loud noises), swimming, diving, or excessive negative pressure (e.g., kiss over the ear); it can be iatrogenically produced by a ventilating tube. Symptoms of traumatic rupture include a sudden severe pain followed by, in some cases, bleeding from the ear. Hearing loss and tinnitus are also usually present. Vertigo suggests damage to the inner ear. Treatment involves gentle removal of debris and blood from the otic canal and use of earplugs to provide protection when bathing or shampooing. Antibiotic eardrops are indicated only if there has been contamination by water or debris. Oral antibiotics can be used prophylactically to prevent infection but are generally unnecessary. Pain medication may be necessary for the first few days. Persistent perforation for more than 10 to 12 weeks is an indication for otolaryngology referral. An audiogram should be performed after treatment to document the return of hearing.

Additional Reading: Barotrauma of the middle ear, sinuses, and lung. In: Domino F, ed. *The 5-Minute Clinical Consult*. Philadelphia, PA: Lippincott Williams and Wilkins; 2014.

Category: Special sensory

124. A 36-year-old day care worker presents with generalized malaise and "a cold that won't go away." It started a couple of weeks ago with a runny nose and a low-grade fever. She reports that she has now having "coughing fits," which are sometimes so severe that she vomits. She does not smoke and cannot remember when she last had any immunizations. On examination, you note excessive lacrimation and conjunctival injection. Her lungs are clear. Which one of the following is the most likely diagnosis?
A) Pertussis
B) Rhinovirus infection
C) Nonasthmatic eosinophilic bronchitis
D) Cough-variant asthma
E) Gastroesophageal reflux

Answer and Discussion

The answer is A. Pertussis, once a common disease in infants, declined to around 1,000 cases in 1976 as a result of widespread vaccination. The incidence began to rise again in the 1980s, possibly because the immunity from vaccination rarely lasts more than 12 years. The disease is characterized by a prodromal phase that lasts 1 to 2 weeks and is indistinguishable from a viral upper respiratory infection. It progresses to a more severe cough after the second week. The cough is paroxysmal and may be severe enough to cause vomiting or fracture ribs. Patients are rarely febrile, but may have increased lacrimation and conjunctival injection. The incubation period is long compared with a viral infection, usually 7 to 10 days.

Nonasthmatic eosinophilic bronchitis, cough-variant asthma, and gastroesophageal reflux disease cause a severe cough not associated with a catarrhal phase. A rhinovirus infection would probably be resolving within 2 to 3 weeks.

Additional Reading: Prevention and treatment of pertussis. *Med Lett Drugs Ther*. 2012;54(1399):73–74.

Category: Respiratory system

125. A 62-year-old woman presents to your office complaining of unilateral headache, temporal area tenderness, and visual disturbances. Laboratory tests show mild anemia and a sedimentation rate of 110 mm per hour. The most appropriate management includes
A) CT scan of the head
B) Initiation of high-dose steroids
C) Referral to an ophthalmologist
D) MRI of the head
E) Initiation of NSAIDs

Answer and Discussion

The answer is B. Polymyalgia rheumatica is a generalized inflammatory disorder that tends to affect middle-age and elderly patients (usually older than 50 years). Onset of symptoms is usually rapid and includes fever, generalized fatigue, weight loss, and pain and stiffness associated with the shoulder girdle that may extend to involve other areas, including the pelvis. Laboratory tests invariably show signs of anemia and an elevated sedimentation rate usually exceeding 100 mm per hour (especially with temporal arteritis). Creatine phosphokinase levels are normal, ruling out muscle destruction. One-fourth to one-half of patients with polymyalgia rheumatica have temporal arteritis.

In many cases, temporal arteritis coexists with but usually develops after the onset of polymyalgia rheumatica. Symptoms of temporal arteritis (giant cell arteritis) include unilateral headache, temporal area tenderness, visual disturbances, and jaw claudication. Women are more commonly affected than men. Whenever temporal arteritis is suspected, corticosteroids (60 mg per day of prednisone) should immediately be prescribed to prevent blindness, which is secondary to inflammation and occlusion of the ophthalmic arteries. Corticosteroids are also used to treat polymyalgia rheumatica, but in smaller doses (10 to 20 mg per day of prednisone) than that required for temporal arteritis. The diagnosis of polymyalgia rheumatica is usually based on clinical findings supported by the laboratory test; however, temporal arteritis is usually confirmed with a temporal artery biopsy. Treatment usually requires months of a slow, gradual taper of steroids while following the sedimentation rate. In some cases, medication may be needed for extended periods (up to 1 year); relapses requiring extended courses are not unusual.

Additional Reading: Arteritis, Temporal. In: Domino F, ed. *The 5-Minute Clinical Consult*. Philadelphia, PA: Lippincott Williams and Wilkins; 2014.

Category: Nonspecific system

126. Which of the following has been shown in multiple cohort studies to reduce the risk of colon cancer?
A) Folic acid
B) B-complex vitamin
C) Aspirin
D) Vitamin C
E) Vitamin E

Answer and Discussion

The answer is C. Daily intake of aspirin has been demonstrated to decrease the risk of colorectal cancer in multiple cohort and case-control studies, although the benefit varies slightly among the studies. However, the USPSTF recommends against the routine use of aspirin and NSAIDs to prevent colorectal cancer in individuals at average risk for colorectal cancer. This recommendation applies to asymptomatic adults at average risk for colorectal cancer, including those with a family history of colorectal cancer, and not to individuals with familial adenomatous polyposis, hereditary nonpolyposis colon cancer syndromes (Lynch I or II), or a history of colorectal cancer or adenomas.

There is fair to good evidence that aspirin and NSAIDs, taken in higher doses for longer periods, reduces the incidence of adenomatous polyps. There is good evidence that low-dose aspirin does not lead to a reduction in the incidence of colorectal cancer.

There is fair evidence that aspirin used in doses higher than those recommended for prevention of CVD and NSAIDs may be associated with a reduction in the incidence of colorectal cancer and fair evidence that aspirin used over longer periods may be associated with a reduction in the incidence of colorectal cancer.

However, there is poor-quality evidence that aspirin and NSAID use leads to a reduction in colorectal cancer-associated mortality.

The USPSTF also assesses harms when making its recommendation and has found that there is good evidence that aspirin increases the incidence of gastrointestinal bleeding in a dose-related manner and fair evidence that aspirin increases the incidence of hemorrhagic stroke. Likewise there is good evidence that NSAIDs increase the incidence of gastrointestinal bleeding and renal impairment, especially in the elderly. Overall, there is good evidence of at least moderate harms associated with aspirin and NSAIDs.

More than 80% of colorectal cancers arise from adenomatous polyps. However, most adenomatous polyps will not progress to cancer. Age represents a major risk factor for colorectal cancer, with approximately 90% of cases occurring after age 50 years. Thirty to fifty percent of Americans older than age 50 will develop adenomatous polyps. Between 1% and 10% of these polyps will progress to cancer in 5 to 10 years. The risk for a polyp developing into cancer depends on the villous architecture, degree of cytologic dysplasia, size, and total number of polyps.

> **Additional Reading:** Routine aspirin or nonsteroidal anti-inflammatory drugs for the primary prevention of colorectal cancer: 2007 update. US Preventive Service Task Force. From: http://www.uspreventiveservicestaskforce.org/uspstf/uspsasco.htm.

> **Category:** Gastroenterology system

127. Your 52-year-old woman patient who has passed several calcium oxalate kidney stones over the past few years returns for recommendations on her diet. The most appropriate advice would be to
A) Restrict her calcium intake
B) Restrict her intake of yellow vegetables
C) Increase her sodium intake
D) Increase her dietary protein intake
E) Take potassium citrate with meals

Answer and Discussion

The answer is E. Calcium oxalate stones are the most common of all renal calculi. A low-sodium, restricted-protein diet with increased fluid intake reduces stone formation. A low-calcium diet has been shown to be ineffective. Oxalate restriction also reduces stone formation. Oxalate-containing foods include spinach, chocolate, tea, and nuts, but not yellow vegetables. Potassium citrate should be taken at mealtime to increase urinary pH and urinary citrate.

> **Additional Reading:** Medical management of common urinary calculi. *Am Fam Physician.* 2006;74(1):86–94.

> **Category:** Nephrologic system

128. Which of the following statements about Charcot–Marie–Tooth syndrome is true?
A) Decreased pain, temperature, and vibratory sense are usually seen.
B) Symptoms include the development of a foot drop.
C) Symptoms are commonly noted at birth.
D) Hypertrophy of the distal leg muscles is common.
E) Hyperactive reflexes are noted.

Answer and Discussion

The answer is B. Charcot–Marie–Tooth syndrome (or peroneal muscular atrophy) is an inherited disorder, usually autosomal dominant, affecting the peripheral nervous system. Manifestations include weakness and atrophy of the peroneal and distal leg muscles. The condition affects motor and sensory nerves. Other features include impaired sensation and absent or hypoactive deep tendon reflexes. There are two types:

- *Type 1:* Usually occurs in middle childhood. Features include the development of a foot drop; decrease in pain, temperature, and vibratory sense; slow nerve conduction velocities; and loss of reflexes.
- *Type 2:* Usually occurs later in life and is slower in its clinical course than type 1. Nerve conduction velocities are usually normal. Patients with Charcot–Marie–Tooth syndrome typically present with abnormal high-stepped gait with frequent tripping or falling. Despite involvement with sensory nerves, complaints of limb pain and sensory disturbance are unusual. Treatment consists of braces to help prevent the associated foot drop. Surgery is reserved for those with severe foot deformities. Chemotherapeutic agents known to affect peripheral nerves should be used with great caution. Vincristine use should be avoided.

> **Additional Reading:** Charcot-Marie-Tooth Disease Fact Sheet. National Institute of Neurological Disorders and Stroke; 2013. From: http://www.ninds.nih.gov/disorders/charcot_marie_tooth/detail_charcot_marie_tooth.htm

> **Category:** Neurologic

129. Indications for pacemaker placement include which of the following?
A) Asymptomatic bradyarrhythmias
B) Mobitz II AV block
C) Atrial fibrillation
D) Atrial flutter
E) Mobitz I AV block

Answer and Discussion

The answer is B. The use of a permanent pacemaker is indicated if the patient suffers from symptomatic bradyarrhythmias, asymptomatic Mobitz II AV block, and complete heart block. First-degree AV block, thought to be a relatively benign arrhythmia, can be associated with severe symptoms that may benefit from permanent pacing. Specifically, some uncontrolled trials have shown a benefit from pacing in patients with a PR interval longer than 0.3 seconds. Type I second-degree AV block does not usually require permanent pacing because progression to a higher degree AV block is not common. Permanent pacing is known to improve survival in patients with complete heart block, especially if they have had syncope. Single and dual chamber pacemakers are available and can be used depending on the patient's diagnosis. Typically, pacemakers are monitored on a regular basis by the patient's cardiologist with telephonic monitoring.

> **Additional Reading:** Indications for permanent cardiac pacing. In: Basow DS, ed. *UpToDate.* Waltham, MA: UpToDate; 2013.

> **Category:** Cardiovascular system

130. Which of the following statements about AZT (Zidovudine) is true?
A) AZT is a macrolide antibiotic.
B) AZT inhibits cell wall synthesis.
C) AZT administration requires monitoring of complete blood cell counts.
D) AZT is classified as an antifungal medication.
E) AZT does not prevent opportunistic infections in AIDS patients.

Answer and Discussion

The answer is C. AZT was the first drug approved for the treatment of HIV and AIDS. Also known as Retrovir, AZT is a thymidine analog that inhibits reverse transcriptase, an enzyme necessary for retroviral DNA synthesis, as well as viral replication. Side effects of the medication include suppression of blood elements, including erythrocytes, leukocytes (particularly granulocytes), and platelets. Because of this, frequent CBCs are necessary for monitoring; alterations in the dosage of the drug or its discontinuation may be necessary. The drug dramatically reduces perinatal transmission from HIV-infected mothers to their newborn. Combination therapy with other antiviral medications is superior to treatment with AZT alone for HIV individuals. Other side effects of the medication include headache, restlessness, malaise, dizziness, paresthesias, nausea, vomiting, and anorexia. Other drugs metabolized by the liver, including acetaminophen and TMP-SMX, may increase the risk of AZT toxicity.

Additional Reading: Drugs for HIV infection. *Treat Guidel Med Lett.* 2011;9(106):29–40.

Category: Nonspecific system

131. A 54-year-old previously healthy accountant sees you because of a tremor which is most noticeable in his hands when he is holding something or writing. He has noticed that it seems better after having a beer or two at. On examination, you note a very definite tremor when he unbuttons his shirt. His gait is normal and there is no resting tremor. He has a previous history of intolerance to β-blockers. Of the following, which medication would be the best choice for this patient?
A) Levodopa/carbidopa (Sinemet)
B) Amantadine (Symmetrel)
C) Primidone (Mysoline)
D) Lithium carbonate

Answer and Discussion
The answer is C. Parkinson's disease and essential tremors are the primary concerns in a person of this age who presents with a new tremor. A coarse, resting, pill-rolling tremor is characteristic of Parkinson's disease. Essential tremor is primarily an action tremor and is a common movement disorder, occurring in members of the same family with a high degree of frequency. Alcohol intake will temporarily cause marked reduction in the tremor. β-Adrenergic blockers have been the mainstay of treatment for these tremors, but this patient is intolerant to these drugs. Primidone has been effective in the treatment of essential tremor, and in head-to-head studies with propranolol has been shown to be superior after 1 year. Levodopa in combination with carbidopa is useful in the treatment of parkinsonian tremor but not essential tremor.

Additional Reading: Differentiation and diagnosis of tremor. *Am Fam Physician.* 2011;83(6):697–702.

Category: Neurologic

132. A 36-year-old construction worker is brought to the emergency room. He has been working in the sun all day and, on arrival, he exhibits hyperventilation, profuse sweating, normal body temperature, and hypotension. The most likely diagnosis is
A) Heat stroke
B) Hypothermia
C) Heat exhaustion
D) Thyroid storm
E) Organophosphate poisoning

Answer and Discussion
The answer is C. Heat stroke is a medical emergency. Symptoms include headache, vertigo, fatigue, and increased body temperature (>40°C). Sweating is usually absent. The skin is hot and dry. Patients may exhibit bizarre and confused behavior, hallucinations, loss of

consciousness, and seizures. Other manifestations include tachycardia and tachypnea; blood pressure is usually preserved. If circulatory collapse occurs, patients may suffer brain damage and even death. Patients should immediately be treated with cool water or wet dressings. Careful monitoring of body core temperature should be instituted to avoid conversion of hyperpyrexia to hypothermia. Once hospitalized, fluid replacement and further temperature management can be instituted. Complications include renal failure, cardiac failure, and the development of disseminated intravascular coagulopathy.

Heat exhaustion is different in that individuals affected usually exhibit hyperventilation, profuse sweating with substantial bodily fluid loss, and low blood pressure. Body temperature is usually normal and when elevated does not exceed 40°C. Mental status is usually normal, unlike in heat stroke. Treatment for heat exhaustion is similar to heat stroke and consists mainly of fluid resuscitation.

Additional Reading: Heat-related illness. *Am Fam Physician.* 2011;83(11):1325–1330.

Category: Nonspecific system

> Heat exhaustion is different from heat stroke in that individuals affected usually exhibit hyperventilation, profuse sweating with substantial bodily fluid loss, and low blood pressure. Body temperature is usually normal and when elevated does not exceed 40°C. Mental status is usually normal, unlike in heat stroke.

133. Which of the following statements about diabetic retinopathy is true?
A) Proliferative retinopathy is associated with a poorer prognosis than nonproliferative retinopathy.
B) Nonproliferative retinopathy is associated with neovascularization.
C) Symptoms of retinopathy usually begin with eye pain.
D) Diabetics should have eye examinations every 3 years.
E) Unfortunately, there is no treatment for diabetic retinopathy.

Answer and Discussion
The answer is A. Diabetic retinopathy is the leading cause of blindness in middle-age Americans. The degree of retinopathy is highly correlated with the duration of the diabetes. The disease process is divided into the following:

- *Nonproliferative retinopathy:* Characterized by dilated retinal veins, retinal hemorrhages, microaneurysms, retinal edema, and soft exudates (cotton-wool spots). Hard exudates are usually yellow in appearance and caused by chronic edema. Visual symptoms generally do not occur in the early stages of nonproliferative retinopathy.
- *Proliferative retinopathy:* Associated with neovascularization and proliferation of blood vessels into the vitreous with resulting fibrosis and retinal detachment and hemorrhage.

Symptoms of diabetic retinopathy usually begin with a decrease in visual acuity. Diagnosis can be made with ophthalmologic examination and fluorescein angiography. Treatment involves panretinal laser coagulation and vitrectomy, as well as active management to control the diabetes and, if present, hypertension. The prognosis of proliferative retinopathy is worse than that of nonproliferative retinopathy. Diabetics should be encouraged to have yearly eye examinations.

Additional Reading: The visually impaired patient. *Am Fam Physician.* 2008;77(10):1431–1436.

Category: Special sensory

134. Which of the following findings characterize(s) aortic stenosis?
A) Lack of pressure gradient across the aortic valve
B) Angina, dyspnea, and syncope
C) Diastolic murmur that radiates to the axilla
D) Palpitations
E) Crescendo murmur with midsystolic click

Answer and Discussion

The answer is B. Aortic stenosis occurs when there is obstruction in the blood flow through the aortic valve. Typically, there is a pressure gradient >10 mm Hg across the obstruction. The causes for aortic stenosis include previous rheumatic fever with associated damage to the valves, excessive calcification of the valves leading to narrowing, or congenital causes (e.g., bifid aortic valve). Men are more commonly affected than women. Cardiac output is usually maintained until the stenosis is severe. Once the condition becomes severe, symptoms may include the classic triad (i.e., angina, dyspnea, and syncope), especially with physical exertion. The classic symptoms of angina, exertional syncope, and dyspnea generally follow an extended latent period during which the patient is asymptomatic. The survival of patients with aortic stenosis is nearly normal until the onset of symptoms when survival rates decrease sharply. After the onset of symptoms, average survival is typically 5 years or less. Although the rate of progression of aortic stenosis is variable and difficult to predict, approximately 75% of patients with aortic stenosis die within 3 years after the onset of symptoms if the aortic valve is not replaced. Some patients with severe aortic stenosis remain asymptomatic, whereas others with moderate stenosis have symptoms attributable to the condition. The normal aortic valve area averages 2.5 cm², and there should normally be no gradient. A valve area of <0.8 cm² or a gradient of >50 mm Hg represents critical stenosis capable of causing symptoms or death. Severe cases can result in sudden death. Physical findings include a harsh systolic-ejection murmur found at the left sternal border that radiates to the carotids, a palpable left ventricular heave, and delayed carotid pulse upstroke. Some patients may present with findings of CHF. Echocardiography is recommended in patients with classic symptoms of aortic stenosis accompanied by a systolic murmur and in asymptomatic patients with a grade 3/6 or louder systolic murmur. Severe cases should be referred for possible valve replacement. Those patients with severe aortic stenosis should avoid strenuous activity.

Additional Reading: Aortic stenosis: diagnosis and treatment. *Am Fam Physician.* 2008;78(6):717–724.

Category: Cardiovascular system

135. Which of the following signs and symptoms are associated with Sjögren's syndrome?
A) Hepatomegaly, chronic rhinitis, and palmar erythema
B) Keratoconjunctivitis, parotid gland enlargement, and xerostomia
C) Confusion, tremors, and peripheral neuropathies
D) Polycythemia, leukocytosis, and negative rheumatoid factor
E) Hyperextensibility of joints, iriditis, and glossitis

Answer and Discussion

The answer is B. Sjögren's syndrome is a rare chronic inflammatory disorder that leads to dry mouth, dry eyes (keratoconjunctivitis sicca), dryness of other mucous membranes, and joint pain. Women are more commonly affected. The disease is often found in conjunction with autoimmune disorders such as scleroderma, rheumatoid arthritis, and lupus. The cause is unknown, but there has been a genetic link with the HLA-DR3 focus. Signs include keratoconjunctivitis, parotid gland enlargement, xerostomia, and loss of taste and smell. Other complications include alopecia, increased risk of pulmonary infections, pancreatitis, pericarditis, sensory neuropathies, interstitial nephritis, and RTA. Laboratory findings include positive rheumatoid factor (seen in 70% of affected patients), elevated ESR (70% of affected patients), anemia (33% of affected patients), and leukopenia and eosinophilia (25% of affected patients). Diagnosis is accomplished with the Schirmer's test, which measures the quantity of tears secreted in 5 minutes in response to irritation from a filter paper strip placed under each lower eyelid. Many patients affected with Sjögren's are at increased risk for lymphoma and Waldenstrom's macroglobulinemia. Treatment is aimed at control of symptoms. In some cases, steroids and immunosuppressants may be used.

Additional Reading: Diagnosis and management of Sjögren syndrome. *Am Fam Physician.* 2009;79(6):465–470.

Category: Gastroenterology system

136. Which of the following is the most appropriate medication for the treatment of hypertension in a diabetic patient?
A) β-Blocker
B) ACE inhibitor
C) Diuretic
D) CCB
E) α-Blocker

Answer and Discussion

The answer is B. ACE inhibitors (e.g., captopril, enalapril, lisinopril, ramipril) function as afterload reducers by inhibiting the renin–angiotensin–aldosterone system. An ACE inhibitor or ARB is clearly preferred as initial therapy in any hypertensive diabetic patient who has moderately increased albuminuria (formerly called microalbuminuria) or severely increased albuminuria (formerly called macroalbuminuria) to slow renal disease progression. However, most experts begin treating hypertension with an ACE inhibitor or ARB in diabetics even in the absence of proteinuria.

The mechanism of action of ACE inhibitors involves the blockage of angiotensin I to angiotensin II, resulting in a decrease in aldosterone production, which leads to increased sodium and water excretion. Hemodynamic effects include decreased peripheral resistance, increased renal blood flow, and minimal effects on cardiac output and glomerular filtration rate. Adverse effects include headaches, nausea, dizziness, skin rashes, nonproductive irritative cough (10% to 20% of patients), acute renal failure in patients with renal artery stenosis, and angioneurotic edema. ACE inhibitors are generally not associated with depression, sedation, fatigue, or impotence. They can be useful in preserving renal function in patients with diabetes. Those patients with preexisting renal insufficiency or renal artery stenosis require close monitoring of renal function when ACE inhibitors are administered. Patients with CHF, diabetes, peripheral vascular disease, history of recent MI, hyperlipidemia, and renal insufficiency are good candidates for ACE inhibitors.

Additional Reading: Treatment of hypertension in patients with diabetes mellitus. In: Basow DS, ed. *UpToDate.* Waltham, MA: UpToDate; 2013.

Category: Cardiovascular system

137. Which of the following factors is an absolute contraindication for the use of thrombolytics in the treatment of MI?
A) Altered mental status
B) More than 4 hours having elapsed since the onset of the chest pain
C) Current menstruation
D) Patient having renal insufficiency
E) Patient having a history of diabetic retinopathy

Answer and Discussion

The answer is A. Every patient with an evolving MI should be evaluated for thrombolytic therapy. Thrombolytic therapy reduces in-hospital and 1-year mortality by 25%. The criteria for an evolving MI include the following:

- Thirty minutes of cardiogenic chest pain.
- At least 1 mm of ST elevation in at least two adjacent limbs or at least 2 mm elevation of precordial chest leads noted on ECG tracings.
- New left bundle branch block.
- Patients with complete bundle branch block and cardiogenic chest pain may also benefit from thrombolytics.
- Patients with only ST-segment depression do not benefit from thrombolytics, nor do patients with normal ECGs.

Medications such as tissue-type plasminogen activator (tPA), also known as alteplase, tenecteplase (TNK) and reteplase (rPA), and streptokinase, which are fibrin-specific agents, should be administered as soon as possible up to 12 hours after the onset of chest pain. Those who receive medication within the first 6 hours have the best outcome. Absolute contraindications to thrombolytics include recent surgery (within 4 weeks) or biopsy of a noncompressible site within 2 weeks, any history of hemorrhagic stroke, unclear mental status, the possibility of aortic dissection, active bleeding, pericarditis, prolonged (more than 10 minutes) cardiopulmonary resuscitation, and antibodies to streptokinase or its use within the previous 12 months (in which case tissue-type plasminogen activator should be given). Relative contraindications include history of GI or GU hemorrhage within the past 6 months, trauma, history of cardiopulmonary resuscitation within the previous month, uncontrolled hypertension (systolic BP > 180 mm Hg and diastolic BP > 110 mm Hg), intracranial or systemic neoplasm, prior (nonhemorrhagic) stroke, pregnancy, or liver dysfunction. Minor hemorrhage, menstruation, and diabetic retinopathy are not contraindications to fibrinolytic therapy.

> **Additional Reading:** Myocardial infarction. In: Domino F, ed. *The 5-Minute Clinical Consult.* Philadelphia, PA: Lippincott Williams and Wilkins; 2014.

> **Category:** Cardiovascular system

138. Which of the following tests is considered routine (recommended) in the initial evaluation of a patient with hypertension?
A) Chest x-ray
B) TSH
C) Uric acid level
D) 24-hour urine protein
E) ECG

Answer and Discussion

The answer is E. The initial evaluation of a patient with hypertension should include a thorough history and a number of tests, including the following:

Routine tests

- CBC
- Chemistry panel, including fasting, glucose, potassium, creatinine, and BUN
- Cholesterol panel (total cholesterol and HDL/LDL cholesterol)
- 12-lead ECG
- Urinalysis

Optional tests

- Creatinine clearance
- 24-hour urinary protein
- Uric acid
- Glycosylated Hb
- TSH
- Limited echocardiography
- Chest x-ray

Hypertension exists when the diastolic blood pressure is consistently measured >90 mm Hg and a systolic blood pressure remains >140 mm Hg. Initial management should consist of sodium restriction, limitation of alcohol consumption, and a regular exercise program. Overweight patients should be counseled to lose weight. Other tests to assess kidney function, cardiac performance, or endocrine abnormalities (e.g., pheochromocytoma) are usually unnecessary. It is strongly recommended that physicians intervene with lifestyle modifications that can prevent or delay the onset of hypertension in patients.

> **Additional Reading:** Initial evaluation of the hypertensive adult. In: Basow DS, ed. *UpToDate.* Waltham, MA: UpToDate; 2013.

> **Category:** Cardiovascular system

139. A 62-year-old business executive with a history of migraines is noted to have hypertension; otherwise, he is healthy. Which of the following is the best medication for the treatment of his hypertension?
A) β-Blocker
B) ARB
C) α-Blocker
D) ACE inhibitor
E) Thiazide diuretic

Answer and Discussion

The answer is A. β-Blockers are used as first-line therapy for the treatment of uncomplicated hypertension. These agents decrease the heart rate and cardiac output. β1-Adrenergic receptors are located in the cardiac muscle, whereas β2-adrenergic receptors are located in the bronchial musculature. Adverse effects include exacerbation of bronchoconstriction in asthmatics because of β2-receptor blockade, bradycardia, left ventricular failure, nasal congestion, nightmares, Raynaud's phenomenon, fatigue, depression, cold extremities, and impotence. β-Blockers are also associated with elevated triglycerides and decreased HDL cholesterol; however, there is not enough effect on lipids to discourage their use in select cases. These agents are contraindicated in patients with poorly controlled diabetes, second- or third-degree heart block, or moderate-to-severe asthma; however, these agents have been shown to improve survival after MI and in select patients with CHF. These agents have also been used for the treatment of "stage fright" and as migraine prophylaxis. β-Blockers should not be discontinued abruptly because of the risk of rebound hypertension.

Additional Reading: Drugs for migraine. *Treat Guidel Med Lett.* 2011;9(102):7–12.

Category: Cardiovascular system

140. Which of the following combinations would be best utilized in the treatment of diastolic heart failure?
A) CCB + α-blocker
B) β-Blocker + diuretic
C) ACE inhibitor + α-blocker
D) CCB + ARB
E) ARB + CCB

Answer and Discussion
The answer is B. Diastolic heart failure is a major contributor of morbidity and mortality. The condition is defined as symptoms of heart failure in a patient with a normal left ventricular function. It is characterized by a stiff left ventricle with decreased compliance and impaired relaxation, which leads to increased end-diastolic pressure. Signs and symptoms are similar to those of heart failure with systolic dysfunction. The diagnosis of diastolic heart failure is made with transthoracic echocardiography. Treatment of diastolic heart failure should include normalizing blood pressure, promoting regression of left ventricular hypertrophy (LVH), avoiding tachycardia, treating symptoms of congestion, and maintaining normal atrial contraction when possible. Diuretic therapy is the mainstay of treatment for preventing pulmonary congestion, while β-blockers appear to be useful in preventing tachycardia and thereby prolonging left ventricular diastolic filling time. ACE inhibitors and ARBs may be beneficial in patients with diastolic dysfunction, especially those with hypertension.

The European Society of Cardiology recommendations specify the type of therapy for heart failure. In order to reduce heart rate, β-blockers or nondihydropyridine CCB are recommended. In order to eliminate fluid retention, diuretics are used with caution. ACE inhibitors are used to control blood pressure, suppress LVH, and improve relaxation. High doses of ARB are recommended to reduce the risk of hospitalization.

Additional Reading: Management of diastolic heart failure. *Cardiol J.* 2010;17(6):558–565.

Category: Cardiovascular system

141. A 58-year-old man presents to your office 4 weeks after being hospitalized for MI. He is complaining of chest pain, fever, and multiple joint pain. Laboratory tests do not show an increase in cardiac enzymes. The most likely diagnosis is
A) Dressler's syndrome
B) Costochondritis
C) Meigs' syndrome
D) Recurrent MI
E) Pneumonia

Answer and Discussion
The answer is A. Dressler's syndrome, or postmyocardial infarction syndrome, occurs several days to several weeks after MI. The condition is characterized by chest pain, fever, pericarditis with a pericardial friction rub, pericardial effusion, pleurisy, pleural effusions, and multiple joint pain. The cause is thought to be an autoimmune response to the damaged myocardial tissue and pericardium. The difference between Dressler's syndrome and recurrent MI is difficult to determine; however, in Dressler's syndrome, there is minimal or no increase in cardiac enzymes. Treatment includes the use of aspirin, NSAIDs, and, in some cases, corticosteroids.

Additional Reading: Acute pericarditis. *Am Fam Physician.* 2007; 76(10):1509–1514.

Category: Cardiovascular system

142. A patient transferred from an outlying hospital after being involved in a serious motor vehicle accident has a positive dipstick for hemoglobinuria, but erythrocytes are not noted on microscopic examination. The most likely diagnosis is
A) Myocardial contusion
B) Rhabdomyolysis
C) Intravascular hemolysis
D) Renal contusion
E) Laceration of the spleen

Answer and Discussion
The answer is B. A positive urine dipstick for hemoglobin results from free hemoglobin or myoglobin in the urine. Free hemoglobin appears in the urine when there is intravascular hemolysis. Once haptoglobin becomes saturated, free hemoglobin spills into the urine. A common cause is a transfusion reaction. Myoglobinuria is associated with rhabdomyolysis and occurs when there is significant muscle injury with the release of myoglobin into the bloodstream. Causes include electrical shock or massive muscle trauma. Other causes may include toxin exposures, metabolic disorders, inflammatory conditions, and infection. Myoglobinuria causes a positive urine test for blood in the absence of urinary erythrocytes.

Additional Reading: Clinical manifestations and diagnosis of rhabdomyolysis. In: Basow DS, ed. *UpToDate.* Waltham, MA: UpToDate; 2013.

Category: Nephrologic system

> Myoglobinuria causes a positive urine test for blood in the absence of urinary erythrocytes.

143. Positive results for which of the following tests support the diagnosis of de Quervain's tenosynovitis?
A) Allen's test
B) Finkelstein's test
C) Lachman's test
D) Anterior–posterior drawer test
E) Phalen's test

Answer and Discussion
The answer is B. The abductor pollicis longus and the extensor pollicis brevis share a common protective sheath that can become inflamed, giving rise to de Quervain's tenosynovitis. Patients usually report pain with movement of the fibrous bands that make up the first dorsal compartment over the radial styloid. Paresthesia and pain that radiates distally into the thumb and dorsal part of the hand and index finger may occur. In most cases, the patient has a history of repetitive motions of the hand or thumb. A positive Finkelstein's test is the hallmark test finding: Pain occurs when a fist is made over the thumb and the wrist is placed in ulnar deviation. Long-standing inflammation may lead to calcification of the tendon and its sheath and is visible on a radiograph. Treatment options involve rest, anti-inflammatory agents, immobilization of the affected area with a thumb spica splint, and injection of the compartment with 0.5 mL of steroid and 1 mL of 1% lidocaine. The splint is to be worn

for 3 weeks; surgery is rarely necessary but can be considered in refractive cases.

Allen's test is used in the diagnosis of Raynaud's phenomenon. The radial and ulnar arteries are occluded by the examiner while the patient makes a fist. The hand is then opened, and one side of the wrist is released. Blood flow to the hand should be detected by color, which is restored to the hand. If the hand remains pale and cyanotic on either of the two sides, Raynaud's phenomenon should be suspected. During asymptomatic periods, the examination is entirely normal.

Phalen's test is used to diagnose carpal tunnel syndrome. The patient holds his or her wrists in complete and forced flexion (pushing the dorsal surfaces of both hands together) for 30 to 60 seconds. A positive test is when symptoms (e.g., parathsias in the thumb and index finger are reproduced).

The Lachman and anterior–posterior drawer tests are used to assess the integrity of the knee ligaments.

> **Additional Reading:** De Quervain tenosynovitis. In: Domino F, ed. *The 5-Minute Clinical Consult.* Philadelphia, PA: Lippincott Williams and Wilkins; 2014.

> Category: Musculoskeletal system

144. Which of the following statements about testicular tumors is true?
A) Boys ages 10 to 15 years are most commonly affected.
B) African American men are more commonly affected.
C) Seminomas are the most common type.
D) The prognosis is extremely poor.
E) Carcinoembryonic antigen levels are elevated.

Answer and Discussion

The answer is C. Testicular tumors are usually found in men between 20 and 35 years of age. They are relatively uncommon and tend to affect white men more than African American men. Cryptorchidism is associated with a higher incidence of tumor formation. The tumors are categorized as seminomas (most common) or nonseminomatous germ cell tumors. Symptoms include painless swelling or enlargement of the testicle and testicular heaviness. Diagnosis is confirmed with testicular ultrasound examination. Tumor markers, including human chorionic gonadotropin and α-fetoprotein, may be elevated in affected patients. In most cases, treatment involves surgical removal of the testicle or radiation therapy. If diagnosed in the early stages, the prognosis is usually excellent; therefore, young men should perform monthly testicular self-examinations.

> **Additional Reading:** Dominio F. Testicular malignancies. *The 5-Minute Clinical Consult.* Philadelphia, PA: Lippincott Williams and Wilkins; 2014.

> Category: Reproductive system

145. Olecranon bursitis is usually the result of
A) Deposition of negative birefringent crystals in the bursa
B) Repeated trauma to the elbow
C) Autoimmune destruction of the joint leading to a reactive bursitis
D) Referred pain from the wrist
E) Staphylococcal infection

Answer and Discussion

The answer is B. Olecranon bursitis (also known as *miner's elbow*) is an inflammation that affects the olecranon bursa. The inflammation is usually caused by repeated trauma to the affected area, such as repeated weight-bearing on the elbow. Patients usually report pain, discomfort, and swelling of the elbow area. In some cases, the bursa may harbor an infection, which may require antibiotic treatment; in most cases, there is no associated infection. Treatment involves anti-inflammatories, aspiration of the fluid, and, in some cases, steroid injection followed by the use of a pressure dressing to help prevent reaccumulation of fluid. Infection should be excluded before administering steroid medication. The avoidance of trauma to the elbow should also be emphasized for treatment. Surgery may be necessary for resistant and debilitating cases.

> **Additional Reading:** Evaluation of elbow pain in adults. In: Basow DS, ed. *UpToDate*. Waltham, MA: UpToDate; 2013.

> Category: Musculoskeletal system

146. The most effective drug for the treatment of traveler's diarrhea is
A) Metronidazole
B) Tetracycline
C) Ciprofloxacin
D) Trimethoprim-sulfamethoxazole (TMP-SMX)
E) Doxycycline

Answer and Discussion

The answer is C. Travel to the third world countries can be complicated by traveler's diarrhea. The incidence ranges from 4% to >50%. The most common pathogens are enteropathogens (e.g., *E. coli*) in approximately 80% of cases; occasionally, viruses such as the Norwalk agent or rotavirus are causative. Traveler's diarrhea usually is a self-limited disorder and often resolves without specific treatment; however, oral rehydration is often beneficial to replace lost fluids and electrolytes. Clear liquids are routinely recommended for adults. Travelers who develop three or more loose stools in an 8-hour period—especially if associated with nausea, vomiting, abdominal cramps, fever, or blood in stools—may benefit from antimicrobial therapy. Antibiotics are usually given for 3 to 5 days. Currently, fluoroquinolones are the drugs of choice. Commonly prescribed regimens are 500 mg of ciprofloxacin twice a day or 400 mg of norfloxacin twice a day for 3 to 5 days. Trimethoprim-sulfamethoxazole and doxycycline are no longer recommended because of the high level of resistance to these agents. Bismuth subsalicylate also may be used as treatment: 1 fluid ounce or two 262-mg tablets every 30 minutes for up to eight doses in a 24-hour period, which can be repeated on a second day. If diarrhea persists despite therapy, travelers should be evaluated and treated for possible parasitic infection.

The traveler should also take precautions by eating only freshly prepared foods that are adequately cooked, eating freshly peeled fruits, drinking only boiled or bottled water, and avoiding tap water and ice made from tap water (even in alcoholic drinks).

> **Additional Reading:** Travelers' diarrhea. Center for Disease Control and Prevention. From: http://www.cdc.gov/ncidod/dbmd/diseaseinfo/travelersdiarrhea_g.htm#treatment.

> Category: Gastroenterology system

147. Which of the following statements about orthostatic hypotension is true?
A) It is a decrease in systolic blood pressure that occurs when moving from a standing to a sitting position.
B) It is commonly associated with a decrease in pulse rate.
C) In some cases, it is associated with antidepressant medications.
D) It is rarely associated with symptoms.
E) The condition results from volume overload.

Answer and Discussion

The answer is C. *Orthostatic hypotension* is defined as a decrease in blood pressure of at least 20 mm Hg (systolic) and at least 10 mm Hg (diastolic) that occurs when moving from a supine to an upright position. Also, orthostatic tachycardia is defined as an increase in heart rate >27 bpm or to a level >108 bpm. Measurements of blood pressure and pulse rate should be taken after the individual has been in an upright position for 3 minutes. Causes of orthostatic hypotension include volume depletion, medications (e.g., tricyclic antidepressants, antihypertensive agents), and autonomic dysfunction (as seen in diabetic patients). Elderly patients are at increased risk, and syncope may result. Treatment involves volume replacement, discontinuation of offending pharmacologic medications, and slow positional changes.

> **Additional Reading:** Evaluation and management of orthostatic hypotension. *Am Fam Physician*. 2011;84(5):527–536.

> **Category:** Cardiovascular system

148. A 18-year-old woman arrives in the emergency room with carpal-pedal spasms and circumoral paresthesias. She was brought in by paramedics after she fainted at a rock concert. The most likely diagnosis is
A) Cardiac arrhythmia
B) Seizure disorder
C) Hyperventilation
D) Heat exhaustion
E) Cocaine overdose

Answer and Discussion

The answer is C. Hyperventilation can lead to a significant respiratory alkalosis and is frequently the result of anxiety or extreme excitement. Other less common causes include drug effects, CNS dysfunction, alcohol withdrawal, asthma, heart failure, pulmonary embolus, exposure to high altitudes, intense exercise, and chronic pain. Symptoms include carpal-pedal spasms, circumoral and extremity paresthesias, light-headedness, giddiness, and sometimes syncope. Blood gases usually show low CO_2 (20 to 25 mm Hg) and elevated pH. Treatment can be accomplished by breathing into a paper bag. Other efforts should be directed at the treatment of anxiety or underlying contributing factors; relaxation training may be beneficial.

> **Additional Reading:** Dizziness: a diagnostic approach. *Am Fam Physician*. 2010;82(4):361–368.

> **Category:** Nonspecific system

149. Which of the following statements about type 1 herpes infections is true?
A) Type I is most commonly associated with genital infections.
B) Topical acyclovir is used for prophylaxis.
C) Recurrent outbreaks are usually more severe than an initial outbreak.
D) The rash usually consists of pustules, papules, and macules.
E) Multinucleated giant cells are seen with Tzanck smears.

Answer and Discussion

The answer is E. Herpes simplex infections are divided into type 1, which usually affects the oral mucosa, and type 2, which usually affects the genitals. The virus invades the nervous tissue and remains dormant in the skin or nerve ganglia. Symptoms include recurrent, clear vesicles that usually occur in clusters and are extremely painful; fever; arthralgias; and adenopathy. Initial attacks are usually more severe and longer in duration than repeated attacks. Before the appearance of the vesicles, the patient may report paresthesias or tingling at the site of the outbreak. Transmission occurs by direct contact and is usually sexually transmitted, particularly for type 2. Repeated attacks are usually precipitated by excessive sunlight exposure, menstruation, stress, and febrile illnesses. Laboratory tests include positive Tzanck smears (with the presence of multinucleated giant cells), cultures (gold standard for diagnosis), and rapid immunofluorescent antibody tests. The treatment of choice involves the use of topical and oral antiviral medication (acyclovir, valacyclovir, and famciclovir). Oral administration is more effective and should be begun at the initial onset of clinical symptoms. For severe cases, intravenous acyclovir may be used. In some cases, daily prophylactic oral therapy may be necessary.

> **Additional Reading:** Nongenital herpes simplex virus. *Am Fam Physician*. 2010;82(9):1075–1082.

> **Category:** Integumentary

150. A 42-year-old man presents with multiple pigmented skin lesions, ataxia, and decreased hearing. Other family members are similarly affected. The most likely diagnosis is
A) Hemochromatosis
B) Malignant melanoma
C) Neurofibromatosis
D) Sturge–Weber syndrome
E) Measles

Answer and Discussion

The answer is C. Neurofibromatosis type 1 (NF1) and 2 (NF2) are neurocutaneous syndromes (phakomatoses). Although they share a name, they are distinct and unrelated conditions with genes on different chromosomes. NF2 is a rare condition that causes bilateral vestibular schwannomas. As many as 33% of patients are asymptomatic. Symptomatic patients may have blindness, dizziness, ataxia, deafness secondary to acoustic neuromas, or other symptoms related to nerve compression from neuromas. The diagnosis of neurofibromatosis is supported by the detection of more than six pigmented lesions or one lesion larger than 1.5 cm. Asymptomatic patients do not require further therapy; however, those who exhibit symptoms may require surgery or radiation to remove offending neuromas. Genetic counseling is recommended.

> **Additional Reading:** Neurofibromatosis Type 2. In: Domino F, ed. *The 5-Minute Clinical Consult*. Philadelphia, PA: Lippincott Williams and Wilkins; 2014.

> **Category:** Neurologic

151. Guillain–Barre syndrome is most closely associated with
A) Normal electromyogram (EMG) findings found late in the course
B) Descending asymmetric paralysis
C) Previous trauma
D) Symptoms that usually begin in the lower extremities
E) Low levels of protein in the CSF

Answer and Discussion

The answer is D. Guillain–Barre syndrome is an acute or subacute demyelinating polyradiculopathy that often follows an infection (two-thirds of patients recall a recent viral infection), vaccinations (rabies, influenza), malignancy (lymphomas), medications (streptokinase, captopril, danazol), or surgical procedure. Although it is believed to be associated with an immunologic response, the exact mechanism is unknown. The presenting complaint is usually weakness associated with the proximal muscles in a symmetric distribution that varies in severity. Paresthesias of the toes and fingers may also occur. The symptoms usually begin in the lower extremity and may progress to involve the arms and face (ascending symmetric paralysis). In severe cases, the respiratory muscles may be affected, and the patient may require mechanical ventilation. Sensory-related paresthesias are common. Other symptoms include tachycardia, hypotension, hypertension, diaphoresis, hyporeflexia, and loss of sphincter control. Laboratory findings include elevated protein levels and minimal lymphocytic pleocytosis in CSF samples, altered EMG findings, and evidence of demyelination on nerve biopsies. Treatment involving the use of plasmapheresis and intravenous Ig has been shown to be beneficial, particularly early in the course of the disease (i.e., within the first few days). Steroids have not been shown to be beneficial and may actually worsen the outcome. Most cases resolve spontaneously, but recovery may take months. Mortality is approximately 10%. Up to 20% of patients may be left with persisting deficits. Approximately 3% may develop relapses, sometimes years later.

Additional Reading: Guillain–Barré syndrome. *Am Fam Physician.* 2013;87(3):191–197.

Category: Neurologic

> The symptoms of Guillain–Barre syndrome usually begin in the lower extremities and may progress to involve the arms and face (ascending symmetric paralysis).

152. An obese, hypertensive woman is involved in a motor vehicle accident. Skull films show an enlarged sella turcica. Further questioning reveals that the patient has also complained of galactorrhea, and results of a recent prolactin test were abnormal. The most likely diagnosis is
A) Sheehan's syndrome
B) Empty sella syndrome
C) Subdural hematoma
D) Subarachnoid hemorrhage
E) Undetected pregnancy at 12 to 16 weeks' gestation

Answer and Discussion
The answer is B. Empty sella syndrome is a congenital abnormality that results in abnormal formation of the sella turcica, in which the hypothalamus and pituitary gland are found. In many cases, an enlarged sella turcica is seen by chance on a skull radiograph. Diagnosis is confirmed by a CT scan or MRI. Those affected are usually obese women who have hypertension and benign intracranial hypertension. In most cases, the individual is asymptomatic. However, patients may have persistent rhinorrhea or pituitary disorders, including tumors releasing growth hormone, adrenocorticotropic hormone (ACTH), or prolactin. No treatment is required if empty sella syndrome is present without other abnormalities.

Additional Reading: Empty sella syndrome. In: Domino F, ed. *The 5-Minute Clinical Consult.* Philadelphia, PA: Lippincott Williams and Wilkinson; 2014.

Category: Endocrine system

153. Which of the following medications would improve survival following an MI?
A) Metoprolol
B) Hydrochlorothiazide
C) Warfarin
D) Nitroglycerin
E) Morphine

Answer and Discussion
The answer is A. β-Blockers reduce mortality during both acute and long-term management of MI. Administration of intravenous β-blockers within 12 to 24 hours of infarction, followed by oral therapy, has been found to significantly reduce the mortality rate within the first week of infarction. The most marked reduction occurs in the first 2 days after infarction. Initiation of β-blocker therapy within days to weeks after infarction and continuation of therapy has been shown to reduce total mortality, nonfatal MI, and sudden death. This has been shown regardless of the patient's age or sex, infarct location, and initial heart rate, or the presence or absence of ventricular arrhythmias. The greatest benefit occurs in high-risk patients, including the elderly and those with large anterior infarctions, arrhythmias, or left ventricular dysfunction.

Additional Reading: Myocardial infarction. In: Domino F, ed. *The 5-Minute Clinical Consult.* Philadelphia, PA: Lippincott Williams and Wilkinson; 2014.

Category: Cardiovascular system

154. A 72-year-old woman presents to the emergency room with the acute onset of right-sided hemiplegia. She is conscious but confused and agitated. Blood pressure is measured at 210/110. She has no cardiac findings. Appropriate management at this time should be
A) The administration of IV labetolol
B) Oral administration of clonidine
C) Additional dose of her CCB
D) Sublingual nifedipine
E) Observation

Answer and Discussion
The answer is E. Unless systolic blood pressure is >220 mm Hg or diastolic pressure is >120 mm Hg (sustained on repeated measurement), elevated blood pressure should not be treated within the first days after ischemic stroke. The reason is that perfusion is directly linked to mean arterial pressure. Acute elevations in blood pressure are often transient, and spontaneous declines are common. Aggressive treatment of hypertension following acute ischemic stroke can convert vulnerable areas of the brain into an infarct. The two exceptions to this general recommendation are (1) after use of tissue plasminogen activator (tPA), blood pressure should be maintained below 185/110 mm Hg; and (2) in the presence of MI, heart failure, or aortic dissection, elevated blood pressure should be treated aggressively. If antihypertensive therapy is necessary, agents that have a rapid onset and predictable response should be used.

Additional Reading: Stroke. In: Domino F, ed. *The 5-Minute Clinical Consult.* Philadelphia, PA: Lippincott Williams and Wilkinson; 2014.

Category: Neurologic

155. Which of the following medications should be avoided in patients with hypertrophic obstructive cardiomyopathy?
A) Aspirin
B) Digoxin
C) Disopyramide
D) Acetaminophen
E) Atenolol

Answer and Discussion

The answer is B. Hypertrophic obstructive cardiomyopathy is an autosomal-dominant transmitted disorder that is characterized by an enlarged cardiac septum, which obstructs blood flow from the left ventricle. Symptoms include dizziness, light-headedness, palpitations, chest pain, dyspnea, or syncope with physical exertion. The most important complication of the disease is sudden death. The condition has an annual incidence of 4% to 6% in children, and 2% of adults are affected. Signs include pulses that are bifid and brisk in upstroke and a systolic-ejection-type murmur positioned along the left sternal border, which becomes louder with movements that decrease venous return (afterload), such as standing or Valsalva's maneuver. Movements that increase venous return (afterload), such as squatting, reduce the murmur. ECG usually shows evidence of LVH and septal Q waves in the lateral leads. Diagnosis is accomplished by echocardiogram. First-line treatment is accomplished with the use of β-blockers. Disopyramide (Norpace) may be used as an alternative. Verapamil has also been used frequently on an empiric basis especially in atrial fibrillation but its effect is unpredictable, and acute hemodynamic collapse is described in patients with substantial gradients or severe diastolic dysfunction. Digoxin should be avoided. Because of the risk for sudden death, extreme physical exertion should be avoided.

> **Additional Reading:** Cardiomyopathy. In: Domino F, ed. *The 5-Minute Clinical Consult*. Philadelphia, PA: Lippincott Williams and Wilkins; 2014.

> Category: Cardiovascular system

156. Which of the following statements regarding aminoglycosides is true?
A) Liver function should be followed closely during administration.
B) Volume of distribution is increased in obese patients.
C) Nephrotoxic effects can occur with administration.
D) Lupus-like syndrome can occur with prolonged use.
E) Respiratory depression is not associated with aminoglycosides.

Answer and Discussion

The answer is C. Toxicity associated with the use of aminoglycosides (e.g., gentamicin) includes ototoxicity with clinically apparent hearing loss (<1% of cases), tinnitus, and vertigo, as well as nephrotoxic effects (5% to 10% of adults who receive therapy for 10 to 14 days), including renal failure. Rarely, respiratory depression can occur. Drug levels should be followed after a steady state is achieved—every 3 to 5 days or more often if increases in serum creatinine are noted. Patients with decreased renal function may need an adjustment of medication on the basis of their creatinine clearance. Some data suggest that once-daily administration may cause less nephrotoxicity. Aminoglycosides have low solubility in lipids; therefore, the volume of distribution is decreased in obese patients. Patients with trauma, burns, cancer, and postoperative septic shock have increased volumes of distribution. Neuromuscular depression from aminoglycosides is caused by reduced acetylcholine activity at postsynaptic membranes and can result in rare but severe respiratory depression. This can be largely avoided if the aminoglycoside is given intravenously over 30 minutes or by intramuscular injection. If respiratory depression does occur, it can be reversed by the administration of calcium.

> **Additional Reading:** Drugs for bacterial infections. *Treat Guidel Med Lett.* 2013;11(131):65–74.

> Category: Nonspecific system

157. Which of the following best describes migraine headaches?
A) Aura following the resolution of the headache
B) Recurrent headaches lasting less than 4 hours
C) Unilateral, throbbing headache
D) Bilateral, bandlike headache
E) Rhinitis with facial pain

Answer and Discussion

The answer is C. There are basically two types of migraine headaches: those with an aura (classic migraine) and those without an aura (common migraine). A classic migraine is characterized by recurrent attacks of a moderate-to-severe unilateral, throbbing headache that is usually preceded by visual prodrome, which may include scotomata, zigzag lines, photopsia, or visual distortions. Patients also report nausea, vomiting, photophobia, mood swings, food cravings, and heightened perception of smell. The unilateral "throbbing" headache may become generalized and usually lasts 4 to 72 hours. Patients usually report a positive family history. Migraines usually begin at 10 to 40 years of age and are more common in women. The pathophysiology is not fully understood. Whether vasodilation or vasoconstriction is a cause or an effect of the migraine is unclear.

Tryptans such as sumatriptan (Imitrex) that activate serotonin receptors (5-hydroxytryptamine) block neurogenic inflammation and can abort migraine pain in approximately 70% of patients. Additionally, vasoconstrictors, such as ergotamines, have also been used to treat migraines. Other medications used include NSAIDs and narcotic analgesics. Migraine attacks may be triggered by emotional or physical stress, lack of sleep, specific foods (e.g., chocolate, cheese), alcohol, oral contraceptives, or menstruation. Migraines usually disappear during pregnancy. Antiemetics and intravenous hydration may be needed if associated vomiting is severe. β-Blockers, low-dose amitriptyline, topiramate (Topamax) and other antiseizure medications, and CCBs may be used for prophylaxis, particularly if patients have more than one migraine per week. Most patients experience a decrease in the number and intensity of headaches as they age. Common migraines are identical to classic migraines except that the patient does not have an aura, and the headache may last longer.

> **Additional Reading:** Treatment of acute migraine headache. *Am Fam Physician.* 2011;83(3):271–280.

> Category: Neurologic

158. Which of the following can improve survival in patients with severe COPD?
A) Supplemental oxygen
B) β Agonist
C) Inhaled corticosteroids
D) Smoking cessation
E) Pulse antibiotic therapy

Answer and Discussion

The answer is A. For patients with the diagnosis of severe COPD, only the administration of supplemental oxygen has been shown to positively affect survival, reduce dyspnea, and reduce pulmonary artery pressure. β Agonist and inhaled corticosteroids can lower the rate of exacerbations but have no direct effect on survival. Discontinuation of smoking can slow the decline in lung function but has no effect on survival. Pulse antibiotic therapy does not directly affect mortality.

> **Additional Reading:** Chronic obstructive pulmonary disease and emphysema. In: Domino F, ed. *The 5-Minute Clinical Consult.* Philadelphia, PA: Lippincott Williams and Wilkins; 2014.

> Category: Respiratory system

159. Which of the following sequences represents how a typical anteroseptal MI progresses on ECG?
A) Q-wave development, peaked T-waves, ST-segment elevation, T-wave inversion
B) T-wave inversion, Q-wave development, ST-segment elevation, peaked T-waves
C) Peaked T-waves, ST-segment elevation, Q-wave development, T-wave inversion
D) Peaked T-waves, Q-wave development, ST-segment elevation, T-wave inversion
E) ST-segment elevation, T-wave inversion, Q-wave development, peaked T-waves

Answer and Discussion

The answer is C. The natural progression of ECG changes seen with MI include peaked hyperacute T-waves to ST-segment elevation, to Q-wave development, and to T-wave inversion. In anteroseptal infarction, ECG changes are usually noted in leads V1 through V3. Q waves indicate a transmural infarct.

> **Additional Reading:** ECG tutorial: myocardial infarction. In: Basow DS, ed. *UpToDate.* Waltham, MA: UpToDate; 2013.

> Category: Cardiovascular system

160. The presence of a "bamboo spine" on spine radiographs, elevated ESR, and a positive test for HLA-B27 support the diagnosis of
A) Multiple myeloma
B) Reiter's syndrome
C) Ankylosing spondylitis
D) Rheumatoid arthritis
E) Pott's disease

Answer and Discussion

The answer is C. Ankylosing spondylitis is an inflammatory condition that usually affects the axial skeleton of young men. The exact cause is not known. Symptoms include low back pain or stiffness that radiates to the posterior thighs, decreased range of motion in the back or hips, and decreased range of motion of the chest wall. Sacroiliitis is usually one of the earliest manifestations. Other joints may be painful or swollen. Patients often report that the symptoms worsen with rest and improve with activity. Radiographs show periarticular destructive changes, destruction of the sacroiliac joint, development of syndesmophytes on the margins of the vertebral bodies, and bridging of osteophytes between the vertebral bodies, giving rise to the appearance of a "bamboo spine." Acute anterior uveitis (iritis) occurs in approximately 20% of these patients. Laboratory tests show an elevated ESR and a positive test for HLA-B27 antigen in approximately 90% of those affected. The course of the disease is variable. Some patients may have no symptoms or only mild stiffness, whereas others may experience chronic pain and significant disabilities. Most patients with ankylosing spondylitis can remain gainfully employed. Treatment includes the use of NSAIDs and physical therapy. Attacks of iritis are effectively managed with local glucocorticoids in conjunction with mydriatic agents. In severe cases, systemic steroids or immunosuppressive drugs may be used.

> **Additional Reading:** Ankylosing spondylitis. In: Domino F, ed. *The 5-Minute Clinical Consult.* Philadelphia, PA: Lippincott Williams and Wilkins; 2014.

> Category: Musculoskeletal system

161. Which of the following statements is a common feature of fibromyalgia?
A) Men are more commonly affected than women.
B) Alcohol abuse is commonly associated.
C) Joint inflammation and erythema
D) Aggravation of the condition due to lack of sleep, trauma, or cold exposure
E) Normal autonomic and neuroendocrine regulation

Answer and Discussion

The answer is D. Fibromyalgia is an idiopathic, chronic, nonarticular pain syndrome with generalized tender points. It is a multisystem disease characterized by sleep disturbance, fatigue, headache, morning stiffness, paresthesias, and anxiety. Nearly 2 percent of the general population in the United States suffers from fibromyalgia, with women of middle age being at increased risk. The diagnosis is primarily based on the presence of widespread pain for a period of at least 3 months and the presence of 11 tender points among 18 specific anatomic sites. There are certain comorbid conditions that overlap with, and also may be confused with, fibromyalgia. Recently, there has been improved recognition and understanding of fibromyalgia. Although there are no guidelines for treatment, there is evidence that a multidimensional approach with patient education, cognitive behavior therapy, exercise, physical therapy, and pharmacologic therapy can be effective.

Fibromyalgia/fibromyositis is characterized by generalized pain, tenderness, and muscle stiffness. Pain at the point of tendon insertion ("trigger points") and surrounding soft tissue may also be present. Inflammation of joints is not characteristic. Although the etiology remains unclear, characteristic alterations in the pattern of sleep and changes in neuroendocrine transmitters such as serotonin, substance P, growth hormone, and cortisol suggest that dysregulation of the autonomic and neuroendocrine system appears to be the basis of the syndrome.

The condition may be aggravated by stress (both physical and mental), lack of sleep, trauma, exposure to cold, and sometimes infection. Primary fibromyalgia syndrome is more likely to affect young women who are tense, depressed, or anxious. Symptoms of stiffness and pain are usually diffuse and have an "achy" quality that comes on gradually. Localized symptoms tend to occur more abruptly. Other diseases (e.g., rheumatoid arthritis, hypothyroidism, polymyositis, polymyalgia rheumatica) must be excluded before the diagnosis is made. Myofascial pain syndrome is very similar to fibromyalgia/fibromyositis; however, the painful areas are usually regional, and men are as equally affected as women. In addition, fatigue is not a major finding. Treatment for fibromyalgia/fibromyositis includes low-dose tricyclic antidepressants (e.g., amitriptyline), acupuncture, and muscle relaxants (e.g., cyclobenzaprine). NSAIDS, although commonly used, have not been shown to be effective. Stress-reduction counseling, exercise programs, and improved sleep habits can also be beneficial. American College of Rheumatology criteria for classification of fibromyalgia are as follows:

- Widespread pain for at least 3 months, defined as the presence of all of the following:
  - Pain on the right and left sides of the body
  - Pain above and below the waist (including shoulder and buttock pain)
  - Pain in the axial skeleton (cervical, thoracic, or lumbar spine; anterior chest)
  - Pain on palpation with a 4-kg force in 11 of the following 18 sites (9 bilateral sites, for a total of 18 sites):
    - Occiput: at the insertions of one or more of the following muscles: trapezius, sternocleidomastoid, splenius capitis, semispinalis capitis
    - Low cervical: at the anterior aspect of the interspaces between the transverse processes of C5 to C7
    - Trapezius: at the midpoint of the upper border
    - Supraspinatus: above the scapular spine near the medial border
    - Second rib: just lateral to the second costochondral junctions
    - Lateral epicondyle: 2 cm distal to the lateral epicondyle
    - Gluteal: at the upper outer quadrant of the buttocks at the anterior edge of the gluteus maximus muscle
    - Greater trochanter: posterior to the greater trochanteric prominence
    - Knee: at the medial fat pad proximal to the joint line

Additional Reading: Fibromyalgia. *Am Fam Physician.* 2007; 76(2):247–254.

Category: Musculoskeletal system

> Myofascial pain syndrome is similar to fibromyalgia/fibromyositis; however, the painful areas are usually regional, and men are as equally affected as women.

162. A known HIV-positive patient presents to your office with a violaceous skin lesion. Further examination shows generalized lymphadenopathy. Microscopic examination of a skin punch biopsy shows spindle cells mixed with vascular tissue. The most likely diagnosis is
A) Malignant melanoma
B) Kaposi's sarcoma
C) Tina corpora
D) Cherry hemagioma
E) Cryptococcal granuloma

Answer and Discussion
The answer is B. Kaposi's sarcoma is a malignant skin lesion that was once rare but is now seen more commonly in AIDS patients, primarily among men who have sex with men, and remains the most frequent tumor associated with HIV infection. The lesion is characterized histologically by spindle cells mixed with vascular tissue. Before the detection of AIDS, the disease was predominantly found in Eastern Europe, Italy, and equatorial Africa and affected mostly Italian or Jewish men. Symptoms include pink, violaceous, or red papules or plaques that affect any body surface and become widely disseminated with time and give rise to generalized lymphadenopathy. Serious cases can progress to visceral involvement. Treatment is individualized on the basis of the extent and location of lesions, symptoms, comorbid factors, and patient preference. Up to 60% of cases will resolve within up to 1 to 2 years of effective antiretroviral therapy. Direct treatments include excision, cryotherapy, laser ablation, intralesional chemotherapy, external beam radiation, α-interferon, liposomal doxorubicin, or paclitaxel.

Additional Reading: Kaposi's sarcoma. *AAHIVM Fundamentals of HIV Medicine.* Washington, DC: American Academy of HIV Medicine; 2007:405–411.

Category: Integumentary

163. A 31-year-old woman presents with high fever, dysuria, flank pain, nausea, and vomiting. The most appropriate treatment is
A) Hospitalization with administration of intravenous fluids and antibiotics
B) Oral rehydration and oral antibiotics for 10 days
C) Surgical consultation for exploratory laparotomy
D) Extracorporeal shock wave lithotripsy
E) Nothing given orally and nasogastric suction

Answer and Discussion
The answer is A. Acute pyelonephritis is an infection of the upper urinary tract. It affects the kidneys' collecting system and renal parenchyma. The most common causative agent is *E. coli*. Other causative agents include *Proteus*, *Pseudomonas*, *Enterobacter*, *Klebsiella*, *Staphylococcus*, and *Enterococcus*. Symptoms include lower abdominal pain, flank tenderness, fevers, chills, nausea, and vomiting. Physical findings include tenderness of the costovertebral angle and the abdomen. Laboratory findings include elevated white blood cell (WBC) count, elevated ESR, pyuria, bacteriuria, hematuria, proteinuria, and possible WBC cast. Severe cases may cause bacteremia (20% of patients).

Treatment is accomplished with antibiotics directed at gram-negative organisms. For empirical oral therapy, a fluoroquinolone is recommended. Should fluoroquinolone resistance exceed 10%, a single initial IV dose of a long-acting antibiotic such as ceftriaxone 1 g is recommended. Patients with mild-to-moderate symptoms can be managed as outpatients. Hospitalization is required if the patient has a high fever, dehydration, or other complicating medical conditions (e.g., pregnancy, diabetes). For parenteral therapy, a fluoroquinolone, aminoglycoside ± ampicillin, or an extended-spectrum cephalosporin ± an aminoglycoside can be used. Duration of antibiotic therapy depends on clinical response but should be at least 10 to 14 days. Intravenous antibiotics should be continued until the patient is afebrile. Repeat cultures after treatment should be performed; if the patient has had repeated infections, further workup, including an intravenous pyelogram or voiding cystourethrogram, may be necessary.

Additional Reading: Pyelonephritis. In: Domino F, ed. *The 5-Minute Clinical Consult.* Philadelphia, PA: Lippincott Williams and Wilkins; 2014.

Category: Nephrologic system

164. Which of the following is the medication of choice for the treatment of Legionnaire's disease?
A) Penicillin
B) Cefuroxime
C) Azithromycin
D) Gentamicin
E) Amphotericin

Answer and Discussion

The answer is C. Legionnaire's disease is caused by *Legionella pneumophila*. It was discovered after an outbreak in Philadelphia in 1976 that affected many American Legion members. The condition represents one of the atypical pneumonias that usually affects immunocompromised patients, diabetic patients, patients with renal disease, smokers, and patients with chronic lung disease. It is also a relatively common nosocomial infection. Most affected individuals are middle-aged or elderly men. Although the disease can strike healthy individuals, risk factors include immunosuppression, cigarette smoking, COPD, cardiac or renal disease, or diabetes. The *Legionella* bacteria are found in water supplies, air conditioners, showers, condensers, and aerosol nebulizers. Transmission occurs by inhalation of aerosolized bacteria. Symptoms include a nonproductive cough that becomes productive, high fevers with relative bradycardia, pleuritic chest pain, diarrhea, and a toxic appearance. Laboratory tests usually show a moderate leukocytosis (10,000 to 15,000 per mm^3), hyponatremia (50% of patients), hypophosphatemia, and elevated liver function tests. Sputum smears often show many polymorphonuclear neutrophils but do not show organisms. Chest radiographs show patchy infiltrates, which may progress to consolidations in the lobes. Pleural effusions are common. Diagnosis is achieved by culture, serologies, and direct and indirect antibody assays. The treatment of choice is typically oral erythromycin or similar macrolide antibiotic. More severe cases may require intravenous antibiotics and the addition of rifampin. Alternative medication includes clarithromycin, azithromycin, doxycycline, TMP-SMX, tetracycline, and ciprofloxacin.

Additional Reading: Legionnaires' disease and pontiac fever; 2013. From: http://www.cdc.gov/legionella/clinicians.html

Category: Respiratory system

165. Which of the following statements about babesiosis is true?
A) The disease is transmitted by fecal–oral contamination.
B) The disease is caused by a rickettsial organism.
C) Affected patients without spleens usually have a better prognosis.
D) Diagnosis is made with a peripheral blood smear.
E) Generalized paralysis occurs in those affected.

Answer and Discussion

The answer is D. *Babesia* infection can range from subclinical to severe. Symptoms, if any, usually develop within a few weeks or months after exposure but may first appear or recur many months later, particularly in persons who are or become immunosuppressed.

Clinically manifest *Babesia* infection is characterized by the presence of hemolytic anemia and nonspecific flulike symptoms (e.g., fever, chills, body aches, weakness, fatigue). Some patients have splenomegaly, hepatomegaly, or jaundice.

Risk factors for severe babesiosis include asplenia, advanced age, and other causes of impaired immune function (e.g., HIV, malignancy, corticosteroid therapy). Some immunosuppressive therapies or conditions may affect the clinical manifestations (e.g., the patient

might be afebrile). Severe cases can be associated with marked thrombocytopenia, disseminated intravascular coagulation, hemodynamic instability, acute respiratory distress, MI, renal failure, hepatic compromise, altered mental status, and death.

If the diagnosis of babesiosis is being considered, manual (nonautomated) review of blood smears should be requested explicitly. In symptomatic patients with acute infection, *Babesia* parasites typically can be detected by light-microscopic examination of blood smears, although multiple smears may need to be examined. Sometimes it can be difficult to distinguish between *Babesia* and *Plasmodium* (especially *P. falciparum*) parasites and even between parasites and artifacts (such as stain or platelet debris). Consider having a reference laboratory confirm the diagnosis—by blood-smear examination and, if indicated, by other means, such as molecular and/or serologic methods tailored to the setting/species.

For ill patients, babesiosis is usually treated for at least 7 to 10 days with a combination of two prescription medications, typically either

- atovaquone **PLUS** azithromycin; OR
- clindamycin **PLUS** quinine (this combination is the standard of care for severely ill patients).

Babesiosis is a tick-borne disease caused by *Babesia microti* and rarely affects humans. Most reported cases in the United States have been mild and were found on islands off the New York and Massachusetts coasts. Isolated cases have also been reported in Wisconsin, Georgia, and California. The disease is caused by a parasite that attacks the RBCs. The symptoms of the disease resemble *Falciparum malaria* and include high fevers, hemolytic anemia, hemoglobinuria, jaundice, and renal failure. Those patients without spleens have a more severe course of symptoms. The diagnosis is obtained by observing the parasites (tetrad forms) in peripheral blood smears. Serologies can also be used for diagnosis. Treatment is usually unnecessary for those with intact spleens; however, for severe cases or cases that affect splenectomized patients, intravenous clindamycin and oral quinine are used for treatment.

Additional Reading: Parasites—babesiosis. Center for Disease Control and Prevention. From: http://www.cdc.gov/parasites/babesiosis/health_professionals/index.html.

Category: Nonspecific system

166. The drug of choice for cold-induced urticaria is
A) Verapamil
B) Cimetidine
C) Diphenhydramine
D) Cyproheptadine
E) Hydroxyzine

Answer and Discussion

The answer is D. *Urticaria* is defined as an erythematous, pruritic rash that is often raised and occurs as discrete wheals and hives. The condition affects approximately 20% of the population. The rash involves the superficial layers of the skin. The center of the wheal is usually pale, and the rash blanches with pressure. Involvement of the deeper layers is referred to as *angioedema*. The causes include allergen exposure; heat, cold, or sunlight exposure; and trauma. In many cases, a cause is never detected. The response is thought to be mediated by an IgE antibody. Those affected by cold may have cryoglobulins or cryofibrinogen, which become activated. In extreme cases, bronchoconstriction and anaphylaxis can occur. Unfortunately, an underlying cause is identified in only approximately 20% of cases.

Treatment involves avoiding factors that trigger the response. Other treatment involves the use of antihistamine (H1) medications and histamine blockers (H2) such as cimetidine. Doxepin may also be beneficial. The drug of choice for cold-induced urticaria is cyproheptadine. Other causes of urticaria include medication use, malignancy, endocrinopathies, autoimmune diseases, insect bites, and infestations; psychogenic causes should also be investigated in complicated or persistent cases. Severe cases may require systemic steroids or the use of danazol.

Additional Reading: Urticaria. In: Domino F, ed. *The 5-Minute Clinical Consult.* Philadelphia, PA: Lippincott Williams and Wilkins; 2014.

Category: Integumentary

167. In most situations, which of the following screening tests would be recommended by the USPSTF for an otherwise healthy, nonsmoking, sexually active 50-year-old woman?
A) Bone density scan
B) Mammogram
C) Treadmill exercise test
D) Urinalysis
E) CA 125 level

Answer and Discussion

The answer is B. Routine screening tests during general examinations should be focused. The USPSTF has several tools to help determine which screenings to offer according to the patient's age and gender such as the Electronic Preventive Services Selector (ePSS). While controversy exists over younger women, mammograms should be performed for all women starting at age 50. And bone density scanning is recommended to start at age 65 for those at normal risk for developing osteoporosis. Treadmill exercise tests and urinalysis are not cost-effective for screening purposes. CA-125 testing is used in the workup and treatment of ovarian cancer, but is not recommended for routine screening and has a "D" recommendation from the USPSTF. Colorectal cancer screening should be undertaken with either annual FOBT, flexible sigmoidoscopy at 5 intervals or colonoscopy every 10 years in all patients older than 50 years. Cervical cancer screening is recommended every 3 years, or in combination with HPV testing every 5 years for woman between 21 and 65 years of age.

Additional "A" level testing recommendations by the USPSTF to offer for this patient include screening for hypertension and HIV.

Additional Reading: The U.S. Preventive Services Task Force (USPSTF) screening recommendations. From: http://www.uspreventiveservicestaskforce.org/

Category: Patient/population-based care

168. A 28-year-old man with no history of allergy to *Hymenoptera* stings presents to the emergency room after being stung by a yellow jacket. Other than local swelling at the site, he has no other symptoms. The most appropriate treatment involves
A) Administration of epinephrine and antihistamine as well as hospitalization
B) Ice therapy, administration of antihistamine, and observation at home
C) Meat tenderizer sprinkled over the sting site, warm-water soaks, and aspirin
D) Administration of steroids, epinephrine, intravenous hydration, and β2 agonist
E) Immediate removal of the stinger using tweezers

Answer and Discussion

The answer is B. Stings by a *Hymenoptera* (e.g., bees, wasps, yellow jackets, hornets, and ants) may be fatal in a hypersensitive patient. Each year in the United States, more patients die of beestings than of snakebites. Patients with a history of hypersensitivity may experience severe swelling at the site of the sting with the development of shock, often within minutes. Treatment should be immediate and includes application of ice to the sting site, administration of intramuscular epinephrine and oral antihistamine, and prompt transfer to the hospital. Removal of the stinger by tweezers is usually avoided because of the possibility of injecting further venom at the site. All patients with *Hymenoptera*-sting hypersensitivity should receive a prescription for an epinephrine kit and carry this with them whenever they are outdoors. Patients should also be counseled to receive hymenoptera desensitization immunotherapy. Individuals with no history of anaphylaxis may be treated by application of ice to the sting, administration of oral antihistamine, and observation at home. Large local reactions may be treated with glucocorticoids. Application of meat tenderizer containing papain is of no proven value.

Additional Reading: Drugs for allergic disorders. *Treat Guidel Med Lett.* 2013;11(129):43–52.

Category: Nonspecific system

169. A very active and independent 75-year-old man with a history of type II diabetes and hypertension presents to the ED with complaints of palaptions and chest discomfort. His EKG showed atrial fibrillation with rapid ventricular response. The rate is brought under control with metoprolol and you counsel him about anticoagulation. What is the best recommendation for this patient?
A) He should be on aspirin to prevent strokes
B) Warfarin is much better option considering his CHADS score
C) Neither aspirin nor warfarin is recommended since he is well rate controlled on metoprolol
D) Dabigatran (Pradaxa) is safer anticoagulant compared with warfarin and aspirin combined.

Answer and Discussion

The answer is B. Numerous guidelines including those from the American College of Cardiology and American Heart Association recommend that patients with nonvalvular atrial fibrillation who are at low risk of stroke be treated with 81 to 325 mg of aspirin per day, whereas patients at higher risk should be treated with warfarin (at a dosage necessary to achieve a target INR of 2 to 3). To calculate risk, there is general agreement that warfarin should be recommended in patients with atrial fibrillation and a CHADS score of 2 or greater: **C**ongestive heart failure; **H**ypertension; **A**ge 75 years or older; **D**iabetes mellitus; **S**troke or TIA. To assess risk, add one point for each of the first 4 risk factors, and two points for stroke or TIA. This patient's score is 3, so warfarin would be recommended.

Nevertheless, decisions about using warfarin can be challenging in older patients and in those at risk of bleeding. The Outpatient Bleeding Risk Index (OBRI) is a validated tool used to predict the risk of bleeding in patients taking warfarin. The OBRI includes four risk factors, each counting as one point: (1) age older than 65 years; (2) history of stroke; (3) history of gastrointestinal bleeding; and (4) one or more of the following: recent MI, severe anemia (hematocrit < 30%), diabetes, or renal impairment. A score of 0 is considered low risk, a score of 1 or 2 is intermediate risk, and a score of 3 or 4 is high risk. A study evaluating the OBRI found that the risk of major bleeding in low-, intermediate-, and high-risk patients was 3, 12, and 48 percent, respectively. This patients ORBI is 1 (age > 65), placing him at intermediate risk.

The anticoagulation agent dabigatran (Pradaxa), a direct thrombin inhibitor, was recently approved by the FDA for the prevention of stroke and systemic embolism with atrial fibrillation. In a randomized trial, 150 mg of dabigatran twice per day was shown to be superior to warfarin in decreasing the incidence of ischemic and hemorrhagic strokes. Patients assigned to dabigatran had a higher incidence of MI than those assigned to warfarin, but the difference was not statistically significant.

Additional Reading: Atrial fibrillation: diagnosis and treatment. *Am Fam Physician.* 2011;83(1):61–68.

Category: Cardiovascular system

170. A 58-year-old secretary presents with asthenia and hyperpigmented changes on her elbows and inner cheek. She also has noted her blood pressure is low and she is dizzy when she stands. She has lost 10 pounds and has some nausea but no vomiting. A recent test for coccidioidomycosis was positive. Appropriate testing at this time includes
A) CT of the abdomen
B) Esophagoduodenoscopy
C) Glucose tolerance test
D) ACTH stimulation test
E) Colonoscopy

Answer and Discussion

The answer is D. Addison's disease results from a progressive destruction of the adrenal glands, which must involve the majority of the glands before adrenal insufficiency appears. The adrenal is a frequent site for chronic granulomatous diseases, predominantly tuberculosis but also histoplasmosis, coccidioidomycosis, and cryptococcosis. Although infection with tuberculosis at one time was the most common cause of Addison's disease, now the most frequent cause is ideopathic atrophy, related to an autoimmune mechanism. Adrenocortical insufficiency caused by gradual adrenal destruction is characterized by a gradual onset of fatigability, weakness, anorexia, nausea and vomiting, weight loss, skin and mucous membrane pigmentation, hypotension, and in some cases hypoglycemia depending on the duration and degree of adrenal insufficiency. The manifestations vary from mild chronic fatigue to life-threatening shock associated with acute destruction of the glands. Asthenia is the major presenting symptom. Early in the course, it may be sporadic, occurring at times of stress. Late in the course, the patient is continuously fatigued. Hyperpigmentation can occur. It commonly appears as a diffuse brown, tan, or bronze darkening of parts such as the elbows or creases of the hand and pigmented areas such as the areolae around the nipples. Bluish-black patches may appear on the mucous membranes. Some patients develop dark freckles, and a persistent tan following sun exposure can occur. Hypotension with orthostasis is frequent, and blood pressure may be in the range of 80/50 mm Hg or less. Abnormalities of the gastrointestinal tract are often the presenting complaint. Symptoms include anorexia with weight loss to severe nausea, vomiting, diarrhea, and vague and sometimes severe abdominal pain. Patients may also exhibit personality changes, usually consisting of excessive irritability and restlessness. Axillary and pubic hair may be decreased in women due to loss of adrenal androgens. The diagnosis of adrenal insufficiency is made with the ACTH stimulation testing to assess adrenal reserve capacity for steroid production. The best screening test is the cortisol response 60 minutes after cosyntropin is given intramuscularly or intravenously. Cortisol levels should increase appropriately. If the response is abnormal, then primary and secondary adrenal insufficiency can be distinguished by measuring aldosterone levels from the same blood samples. In secondary, but not primary, adrenal insufficiency, the aldosterone level is normal. In primary adrenal insufficiency, plasma ACTH and associated peptides are elevated because of loss of the usual cortisol–hypothalamic–pituitary feedback loop, whereas in secondary adrenal insufficiency, plasma ACTH values are low or "inappropriately" normal.

Additional Reading: Addison disease. In: Domino F, ed. *The 5-Minute Clinical Consult.* Philadelphia, PA: Lippincott Williams and Wilkins; 2014.

Category: Endocrine system

171. A 18-year-old surfer presents to your office complaining of an intensely pruritic, serpinginous-type rash that has formed on the sole of his foot. The rash appears to be spreading and is forming bullae at the affected site. The most likely diagnosis is
A) Tinea pedis
B) Bathing suit dermatitis
C) Leishmaniasis
D) Ascariasis
E) Cutaneous larva migrans

Answer and Discussion

The answer is E. Cutaneous larva migrans, also known as the *creeping eruption,* is a common, self-limited, parasitic infection seen in patients who live in warm climates or have recently traveled to tropical regions, particularly if they have been to beaches and shady areas. The most common infective agent is a dog and cat hookworm, *Ancylostoma caninum* and *Ancylostoma braziliense,* respectively. Familial outbreaks of cutaneous larva migrans have been noted where the infection began with the household pet. When the animal defecates, the hookworms are shed and the larvae are picked up by humans through breaks in the skin, hair follicles, and even through intact skin. The areas most often affected include the feet, hands, buttocks, thighs, and chest. The eruption begins as a pruritic lesion at the site of entry and progresses within a few hours into an inflamed papular or papulovesicular eruption. Serpinginous tracks left by the larvae's migration may also be seen. The eruption may spread up to 1 to 2 cm per day. Severe pruritus, vesicular and bullous lesions, local swelling, erosions, and folliculitis may be seen. Biopsy is generally not useful, and blood tests rarely show eosinophilia or elevated immunoglobulin E levels. Destructive therapies, such as cryotherapy, are often ineffective. Isolated cutaneous cases are treated with topical thiabendazole, especially when applied ahead of the advancing lesions. Because of the risk of systemic infection and the ease of oral treatment, some recommend routine systemic treatment with oral thiabendazole, albendazole, or ivermectin. Although thiabendazole has significant side effects that include nausea, vomiting, diarrhea, and dizziness, albendazole and ivermectin are reliable and have fewer adverse effects. Ivermectin may be given as a single dose with no known toxic side effects.

Additional Reading: Acute pruritic rash on the foot. *Am Fam Physician.* 2010;81(2):203–204.

Category: Integumentary

172. The most common cause of a community-acquired pneumonia in a 45-year-old otherwise healthy man is
A) *Streptococcus pneumoniae*
B) *Haemophilus influenzae*
C) *Mycoplasma pneumoniae*
D) *Legionella pneumoniae*
E) *Klebsiella pneumoniae*

Answer and Discussion

The answer is A. In young adults, causes for pneumonia include *Mycoplasma, Chlamydia pneumoniae,* influenza, adenovirus, *Pneumocystis carinii* (in immunocompromised patients), and other community-acquired organisms including *Streptococcus, Haemophilus,* and, occasionally, *Legionella.* Pneumonia in adults with no underlying disease is usually caused by *S. pneumoniae,* representing more than 50% of community-acquired pneumonias that require hospitalization. Other causes in this patient group include *H. influenzae, Legionella, Mycoplasma* (more commonly seen in young adults), and influenza viruses. If the patient is older than 60 years and has other significant medical problems (e.g., diabetes, COPD, heart disease, alcoholism), the most common pathogens include the previously mentioned organisms as well as *Klebsiella, Enterobacteriaceae, Chlamydia,* and *S. aureus.* For patients with aspiration or nosocomial infections, the causative organisms include the previously mentioned organisms and the gram-negative organisms (including *Pseudomonas*) and anaerobes.

Additional Reading: Drugs for bacterial infections. *Treat Guidel Med Lett.* 2013;11(131):65–74.

Category: Respiratory system

> Pneumonia in adults with no underlying disease is usually caused by *Streptococcus pneumoniae,* representing more than 50% of community-acquired pneumonias that require hospitalization.

173. Which of the following factors is NOT associated with diabetic ketoacidosis?
A) Hyperglycemia
B) Acidosis
C) Dehydration
D) Hyperkalemia
E) Hyperosmolarity

Answer and Discussion

The answer is D. Diabetic ketoacidosis occurs in diabetics when a severe lack of insulin leads to (1) a breakdown of free fatty acids and (2) the production of acetoacetic acid, β-hydroxybutyric acid, and acetone, resulting in severe and life-threatening acidosis. The condition usually occurs in patients with type I diabetes mellitus and is often seen as the initial presentation. Triggering factors include infection, trauma, poor compliance with insulin administration, MI, cerebrovascular accident, alcohol intoxication, or dehydration. Diabetic ketoacidosis is characterized by the following conditions:

- Hyperglycemia
- Acidosis
- Dehydration (secondary to osmotic diuresis)
- Hyperosmolarity
- Potassium loss

Symptoms include mental status changes, tachypnea, fruity breath (secondary to acetones), and nausea and vomiting with abdominal pain. In severe cases, coma may occur. Treatment involves the administration of insulin to lower glucose levels, fluid rehydration (usually >5 L), and replacement of potassium and other electrolyte losses. If the condition is severe, cardiovascular collapse may occur. Close follow-up with frequent monitoring of serum pH, electrolytes, and urine output is necessary during treatment. Further tests should be conducted to rule out infection as a precipitating cause. Unfortunately, the WBC count is not a reliable indicator for the presence of infection in those with diabetic ketoacidosis because the stress of the illness often causes the WBC count to increase to 15,000 to 30,000 cells per μL.

Additional Reading: Clinical features and diagnosis of diabetic ketoacidosis and hyperosmolar hyperglycemic state in adults. In: Basow DS, ed. *UpToDate.* Waltham, MA: UpToDate; 2013.

Category: Endocrine system

174. Which of the following findings is consistent with the SIADH?
A) Hypernatremia
B) Hypertonic urine
C) Hypovolemia
D) Increased glomerular filtration rate
E) Hyperosmolality

Answer and Discussion

The answer is B. SIADH is defined as less than maximally dilute urine in the presence of plasma hypoosmolality and hyponatremia. The condition is associated with a number of disorders, including small cell carcinoma of the lung, Guillain–Barre syndrome, acute intermittent porphyria, other pulmonary disorders (e.g., pneumonia, tuberculosis), and neurologic disorders (e.g., meningitis, tumors, trauma, stroke). In many cases, the condition may be idiopathic. The cause is the inappropriate release of antidiuretic hormone (ADH) with respect to the body's fluid osmolality. Findings include

- Hyponatremia and hypoosmolality of body fluids
- Normal glomerular filtration rate
- Urine hypertonicity (usually >300 mOsmol per kg) despite a subnormal plasma osmolality and serum sodium concentration
- Isovolemia or hypervolemia without the presence of edema
- Urinary sodium wasting that increases with salt loading

Symptoms include confusion, anorexia, lethargy, and muscle cramps. Treatment involves fluid restriction—often <1 L daily. More severe cases may require replacement of sodium and potassium deficits. Care should be taken not to replace deficits too quickly because of the risk of central pontine myelinolysis. Other treatments involve the long-term use of demeclocycline, which antagonizes the effect of antidiuretic hormone on the kidney and produces a nephrogenic diabetes insipidus and helps to correct hyponatremia.

Additional Reading: Management of hyponatremia. *Am Fam Physician.* 2004;69:2387–2394.

Category: Nephrologic system

175. A 40-year-old woman complains of diffuse symmetric joint pain that is worse in the morning but improves as the day progresses. Examination shows inflammation of the proximal interphalangeal and metacarpophalangeal (MCP) joints. The most likely diagnosis is
A) Reiter's syndrome
B) Rheumatoid arthritis
C) Polymyalgia rheumatica
D) LE
E) Osteoarthritis

Answer and Discussion

The answer is B. Rheumatoid arthritis is a chronic, symmetric, and inflammatory condition that may involve multiple joints. Women are affected two to three times more often than are men, and family members of affected individuals are at increased risk. Onset is usually between the fourth and sixth decade, but may occur at any age. Synovial inflammation leads to the destruction of articular and periarticular structures and proliferation of the synovial tissue (termed *pannus*), all of which causes chronic joint pain. In 30% to 40% of patients, subcutaneous rheumatoid nodules may form at sites subject to trauma and are usually associated with more severe conditions. Patients often complain of multiple joint pain, low-grade fever, fatigue, weight loss, and depression. Symmetric swelling of the hands (especially the proximal interphalangeal and MCP joints), wrists, elbows, shoulder, neck, and ankles is typical; however, any joint may be affected. Patients usually report morning stiffness that involves the small joints of the hands. This stiffness improves as the day progresses. Carpal tunnel syndrome may also occur. Other manifestations, including vasculitis, pericarditis, and interstitial fibrosis, may be found in more severe cases. Laboratory findings include elevated ESR (90% of cases), mild anemia, and a positive rheumatoid factor (85% of cases). Radiographs show periarticular osteoporosis, joint-space narrowing, and joint erosion in more severe cases. However, no laboratory test, histologic finding, or radiographic feature confirms the diagnosis. Treatment consists of NSAIDs (first-line therapy), interarticular and systemic steroids, etanercept (Enbrel) (a tumor necrosis factor α-blocker), infliximab (Remicade) and adalimumab (Humira), disease-modifying antirheumatic drugs, and antimalarials (primarily hydroxychloroquine, which requires eye examinations every 6 months because of the risk of vision loss), sulfasalazine, azathioprine, cyclosporine, and methotrexate with folate supplementation (which requires close monitoring of liver and renal function). Other agents (e.g., penicillamine, cyclophosphamide, gold compounds) are less widely used because of side effects. Traditional drug combinations for rheumatoid arthritis commonly include an NSAID, a disease-modifying antirheumatic drug, and short intermittent courses of oral corticosteroids. The use of etanercept and methotrexate has been effective and promising in the treatment of rheumatoid arthritis. Other associated conditions include Eelty's syndrome (arthritis, splenomegaly, lymphadenopathy, anemia, neutropenia, and thrombocytopenia) and Sjögren's syndrome (arthritis; dry eyes and mucous membranes).

Additional Reading: Arthritis, Rheumatoid (RA). In: Domino F, ed. *The 5-Minute Clinical Consult*. Philadelphia, PA: Lippincott Williams and Wilkins; 2014.

Category: Musculoskeletal system

176. β-Type natriuretic peptide (BNP) is used in the diagnosis of
A) PE
B) CHF
C) Chronic renal failure
D) Asthma
E) Acute coronary syndrome

Answer and Discussion

The answer is B. There is no agreed-upon first-line test for the diagnosis of heart failure and no simple method of measuring the adequacy of cardiac output in relation to normal levels of activity. Heart failure usually is diagnosed in persons with known heart disease who present with nonspecific symptoms (e.g., breathlessness, ankle swelling) and signs (e.g., basal lung crackles). To confirm clinically suspected heart failure, physicians rely on surrogate measures of cardiac function such as left ventricular ejection fraction. However, it is clear that a large proportion of patients with heart failure, particularly older patients and women, have preserved systolic function (i.e., diastolic heart failure). The best way to diagnose and treat

these patients is unclear. BNP increases when cardiac myocytes are strained; therefore, BNP is an effective method for detecting heart failure with or without systolic dysfunction.

Additional Reading: ACC and AHA update on chronic heart failure guidelines. *Am Fam Physician*. 2010;81(5):654–665.

Category: Cardiovascular system

177. When comparing Bell's palsy with a CNS lesion (e.g., stroke, tumor), the distinguishing feature of Bell's palsy is
A) Involvement of the forehead muscles
B) Involvement of the extremities
C) Lack of involvement below the eyes
D) Slurred speech

Answer and Discussion

The answer is A. Bell's palsy is characterized by a sudden onset of unilateral facial paralysis. It is thought to be the result of an infection (usually viral) affecting the facial nerve, which involves compression of the nerve within the temporal bone. Symptoms usually develop as pain behind the ear preceding the facial paralysis. In some cases, the patient cannot close the affected eye because of widening of the palpebral fissures. In 80% to 90% of cases, the physical findings resolve completely within weeks to months after onset; however, in some isolated cases, permanent deficits may occur. The distinguishing feature between Bell's palsy and CNS lesions (e.g., strokes, tumors) is that Bell's palsy involves the entire face (including muscles of the forehead), whereas CNS lesions tend to affect the face below the eyes, and other areas including the arms and legs. Treatment involves the use of steroids, but they are somewhat controversial and are of questionable proven benefit. If the patient has difficulty closing the affected eye, it should be patched for protection against excessive drying.

Additional Reading: Bell palsy. In: Domino F, ed. *The 5-Minute Clinical Consult*. Philadelphia, PA: Lippincott Williams and Wilkins; 2014.

Category: Neurologic

178. A 30-year-old woman from Minneapolis presents to your office complaining of paresthesias, weakness, lack of coordination, and difficulty with gait. Her symptoms are worse after a hot shower. Examination of the cerebral spinal fluid shows oligoclonal bands of immunoglobulin G (IgG). The most likely diagnosis is
A) Multiple sclerosis
B) Huntington's disease
C) Parkinson's disease
D) Neurofibromatosis
E) Amyotrophic lateral sclerosis (ALS)

Answer and Discussion

The answer is A. Multiple sclerosis is a slowly demyelinating disease that affects the CNS. It is characterized by remissions and exacerbations that are separated in time and involve different areas of the CNS. A second form identified is progressive. The cause is unknown but may be related to a combination of genetic factors and perhaps infection with a slow or latent virus. Women are affected more than men (2:1), and there appears to be a geographic predominance, with those in the northern United States affected more than those in the southern United States. The onset is usually between 20 and 40 years of age, and the geographic factor is present even if the individual relocates to a tropical climate (as long as they spent their first 15 years in the north). The pathology involves multiple plaques of demyelination that are found throughout the CNS. Symptoms include paresthesias, including Lhermitte's symptom (sensation of a momentary electrical current or shock when the neck is flexed), weakness, loss of coordination, or visual disturbances (monocular visual loss), initially followed by emotional lability, gait disturbances, and spasticity in more severe cases. Signs include optic neuritis, speech difficulties, cranial-nerve palsies, increased deep tendon reflexes, nystagmus, tremor, urinary incontinence, and impotence. Symptoms increase with exposure to heat. Diagnosis is usually made by the history, appearance of oligoclonal bands of IgG in the CSF, and MRI scans showing plaques of demyelination in the paraventricular white matter. Evoked potential nerve tests may also be abnormal. Treatment is usually supportive; however, steroids and immunosuppressive drugs have been used. Newer medications include interferon β-1b (Betaseron), interferon β-1a (Avonex), and glatiramer acetate (Copaxone), which are interferon-type medications used in the relapsing-remitting forms. In addition, antispasmodic drugs such as baclofen have been used to treat the spasticity.

> **Additional Reading:** Multiple sclerosis. In: Domino F, ed. *The 5-Minute Clinical Consult.* Philadelphia, PA: Lippincott Williams and Wilkins; 2014.

Category: Neurologic

179. A 19-year-old man is seen in the emergency room. He has miosis, bronchoconstriction, and diarrhea. He is also sweating, excessively salivating, and vomiting. His breath has a garlic odor. The most likely diagnosis is
A) Alcohol overdose
B) Organophosphate poisoning
C) Cyanide ingestion
D) Diabetic ketoacidosis
E) Cocaine overdose

Answer and Discussion

The answer is B. Organophosphate insecticides are inhibitors of acetylcholinesterase and result in an accumulation of acetylcholine at the synaptic junction. Organophosphate poisoning is characterized by miosis, bronchoconstriction, sweating, salivation, headache, vomiting, diarrhea, muscle weakness, and convulsions. The patient's breath typically has a garlic odor. Treatment involves gastric lavage followed by activated charcoal or adequate cleansing if skin exposure occurs. Parasympathetic stimulation can be counteracted by the administration of atropine sulfate until symptoms disappear or until signs of atropine use occur (e.g., dilated pupils, dry mouth). Also, pralidoxime helps remove the organophosphate from the cholinesterase.

> **Additional Reading:** Organophosphate and carbamate poisoning. In: Basow DS, ed. *UpToDate.* Waltham, MA: UpToDate; 2013.

Category: Nonspecific system

180. Which of the following statements about polycythemia vera is true?
A) It is a chronic myeloproliferative disorder that is associated with increased levels of hemoglobin (Hb) concentration and RBC mass (erythrocytosis).
B) It is associated with a neurodegenerative condition of the thalamus.
C) Physical examination usually shows decreased peripheral reflexes.
D) Leukopenia and thrombocytopenia are common.
E) The disease is associated with an increased life span of the RBC.

Answer and Discussion

The answer is A. Polycythemia vera is a rare, chronic myeloproliferative disorder that is associated with increased levels of hemoglobin concentration and increased RBC mass (erythrocytosis). The cause is unknown, and the condition is seen more commonly in men older than 60 years and in the Jewish population. The condition is associated with an increased production and turnover of RBCs. As many as one-fourth of those affected develop a reduction in the RBC life span, an associated anemia, and sometimes myelofibrosis. Symptoms are associated with an increased viscosity and volume of blood and include headaches, visual disturbances, shortness of breath, weakness, and fatigue. Patients may also report generalized pruritus, particularly after bathing in warm water. Hepatosplenomegaly is common. Associated conditions include peptic ulcer disease, thrombosis, bone pain, renal lithiasis, and gout. The diagnosis should be considered when the hematocrit is >54% for men and >49% for women. Elevations in all three blood components (i.e., RBCs, WBCs, and platelets) are common. If the condition goes untreated, as many as 50% of those affected die within 1.5 years. Thrombosis is the most common cause of death, followed by complications of myeloid dysplasia, hemorrhage, and leukemia. With therapy, survival time is between 7 and 15 years. Treatment involves phlebotomy (especially for pregnant women and individuals younger than the age of 40 years) and, in some cases, myelosuppressive agents, including hydroxyurea. Hyperuricemia may also be treated with allopurinol.

> **Additional Reading:** Polycythemia vera. In: Domino F, ed. *The 5-Minute Clinical Consult.* Philadelphia, PA: Lippincott Williams and Wilkins; 2014.

Category: Hematologic system

181. Which of the following drugs is commonly used in the treatment of CHF related to systolic dysfunction?
A) Verapamil
B) Diltiazem
C) Ramipril
D) Nifedipine
E) Isoproterenol

Answer and Discussion

The answer is C. The causes of CHF are numerous and include CAD (most common), dilated cardiomyopathy arising from toxins such as alcohol and doxorubicin, idiopathic causes, infection, and collagen vascular disorders. Other causes include hypertension, cardiac arrhythmias, cardiac valvular disorders, hypertrophic cardiomyopathy, and restrictive cardiomyopathies (caused by disorders such as amyloidosis, hemochromatosis, and sarcoidosis). CHF occurs when there is a decrease in cardiac contractility, which leads to decreased cardiac output that does not keep up with the body's physiologic demands. Initially, this inability to keep up with physiologic demands may only be seen with exercise. However, as the disease progresses, signs may also occur at a resting state. Symptoms include shortness of breath; paroxysmal nocturnal dyspnea, which awakens the patient and causes severe shortness of breath and diaphoresis, causing the patient to sit up for prolonged periods; orthopnea (dyspnea in the recumbent position); and peripheral swelling. Signs include jugular venous distention more than 4 cm elevated from the sternal angle with the patient's head elevated at a 45-degree angle, hepatomegaly, hepatojugular reflux, S_3 heart sound, peripheral edema, and pulmonary rales (the most common finding).

Treatment consists of a low-sodium diet, diuretics, ACE inhibitors (ramipril, enalapril, lisinopril) or angiotensin II-receptor blockers (losartan, candesartan) if unable to tolerate ACE inhibitors, β-blockers (carvedilol, long-acting metoprolol succinate), digoxin (particularly in CHF complicated with atrial fibrillation), and other afterload-reducing medications (e.g., hydralazine, isosorbide dinitrate). CCBs, especially verapamil, should be avoided because of their negative inotropic effect on the heart; however, they are useful in cases of CHF caused by diastolic dysfunction and hypertrophic cardiomyopathy.

Additional Reading: Drugs for chronic heart failure. *Treat Guidel Med Lett*. 2012;10(121):69–72.

Category: Cardiovascular system

182. Which of the following statements about influenza is true?
A) Symptoms usually include cough and coryza.
B) Influenza C is the most common cause of the epidemic flu.
C) Diagnosis requires acute and convalescent titers.
D) Immunization for healthy adults should begin at 65 years of age.
E) A lacy rash is usually seen on the trunk and back.

Answer and Discussion

The answer is A. Influenza is an acute viral illness characterized by fever, cough, coryza, headache, myalgias, and fatigue. The usual symptoms last 3 to 7 days. On average, illnesses tend to cause 5 to 6 days of restricted activity, 3 to 4 days in bed, and 3 days lost from work or school. Residual symptoms (nonproductive cough, weakness) may last for several weeks. Epidemics usually occur in the winter months. The disease usually spreads through school-age children first. Those with underlying medical problems (e.g., diabetes, COPD, CHF, chronic renal disease, immunodeficiencies) are at higher risk. The causative agent is an RNA orthomyxovirus. There are three different types of influenza:

1. Influenza A is the most common cause of the flu.
2. Influenza B is usually caused by Paramyxovirus, Rhinovirus, or Echovirus.
3. Influenza C is an endemic virus that occasionally causes mild respiratory disease.

Only types A and B cause epidemics.

Diagnosis is usually made clinically; however, rapid tests are available. Treatment is usually symptomatic. In severe cases, Amantadine (Symmetrel) and rimantadine (Flumadine) are older antiviral agents (M2 inhibitors). Oseltamivir (Tamiflu) and zanamivir (Relenza) are chemically related antiviral medications known as neuraminidase inhibitors that have activity against both influenza A and B viruses. Both are also approved for prophylaxis. For antiviral agents to be effective, they must be initiated within 48 hours of the onset of influenza symptoms. Antiviral agents reduce the duration of fever and illness by 1 day and also reduce the severity of some symptoms.

Additional Reading: Influenza antiviral medications. Centers for disease control and prevention. From: http://www.cdc.gov/flu/professionals/antivirals/summary-clinicians.htm. Accessed: 8/22/2013

Category: Respiratory system

183. Which of the following medications is the most appropriate to use in the emergent treatment of anaphylaxis?
A) Diphenhydramine
B) Isoproterenol
C) Epinephrine
D) Prednisone
E) Atropine

Answer and Discussion

The answer is C. Anaphylaxis may be caused by a variety of factors, including ingestion of certain foods, insect bites or stings, drugs, and contrast dyes. Symptoms include urticaria, angioedema, dyspnea, cough, hoarseness, wheezing, a sense of impending doom, abdominal pain, hypotension, and syncope. Death occurs in 3% of patients. The cause is a massive IgE-mediated response, which results in the release of large amounts of histamine from mast cells. Treatment must be prompt and includes

1. Securing the patient's airway
2. Administering intravenous fluids
3. Administering epinephrine, 0.2 to 0.5 mL of 1:1,000 subcutaneously, every 15 to 20 minutes, repeated three times if the patient is stable; if the patient is unstable, epinephrine should be administered intravenously.

After the administration of epinephrine, diphenhydramine (H1-receptor blocker) should also be initiated; in severe reactions, cimetidine or ranitidine (H2-receptor blockers) should be initiated. All patients with anaphylaxis should be hospitalized and monitored for 24 hours. Corticosteroids have no role in the acute treatment of anaphylaxis but should be initiated to prevent a late-phase reaction. Bronchodilators such as albuterol and theophylline (if necessary) should also be used. Studies show that atopic individuals are not at increased risk for the development of IgE-mediated anaphylaxis as a result of drug reactions or insect stings.

Additional Reading: Anaphylaxis. In: Basow DS, ed. *The 5-Minute Clinical Consult*. Philadelphia, PA: Lippincott Williams and Wilkins; 2014.

Category: Nonspecific system

184. A 37-year-old man requests testing for infertility as his wife has undergone testing, and told that her results were normal. He has recently undergone a semen analysis, which revealed azoospermia. Suspecting hypogonadism, you order morning follicle-stimulating hormone (FSH) and total testosterone levels to help distinguish between primary and secondary causes. Which one of the following would you expect with primary hypogonadism?
A) Normal levels of both FSH and testosterone
B) Low levels of both FSH and testosterone
C) Low FSH and increased testosterone
D) High FSH and low testosterone
E) High levels of both FSH and testosterone

Answer and Discussion

The answer is D. When semen analysis shows severe oligospermia or azoospermia, it is important to distinguish between primary and secondary causes of hypogonadism. Low total serum testosterone levels correlate with hypogonadism. High levels of morning FSH in the presence of low testosterone levels correlate with primary hypogonadism, while low levels of both hormones suggest secondary hypogonadism. High testosterone levels are unlikely to be associated with hypogonadism.

Additional Reading: Infertility. *Am Fam Physician*. 2007;75(6):849–856.

Category: Reproductive system

185. A 63-year-old woman presents with a 2-day history of a sensation of pressure and hearing loss in her left ear. She has been in good health and the physical examination, including your neurologic examination, is normal. While both tympanic membranes are normal, a vibrating tuning fork in the midline of the forehead reveals sound lateralizing to the right ear. Her audiogram shows a 30-decibel hearing loss at three consecutive frequencies in the left ear, with normal hearing on the right. Which one of the following would be most appropriate at this point?

A) CT
B) A CBC, metabolic profile, and thyroid studies
C) Nifedipine (Procardia)
D) Acyclovir (Zovirax)
E) Oral corticosteroids

Answer and Discussion

The answer is E. It is important to distinguish between a sensorineural or a conductive hearing loss when a patient presents with sudden hearing loss. Patients should be asked about previous episodes, and the workup should include an assessment for bilateral hearing loss and a neurologic examination. Sudden sensorineural hearing loss is diagnosed by audiometry demonstrating a 30-decibel hearing loss at three consecutive frequencies, with no other cause indicated from the exam. Evaluation for retrocochlear pathology may include auditory brainstem response, MRI, or follow-up audiometry. Routinely prescribing antiviral agents, thrombolytics, vasodilators, vasoactive substances, or antioxidants is not recommended. Oral corticosteroids may be offered as initial therapy, and hyperbaric oxygen therapy may be helpful within 3 months of diagnosis. Guidelines strongly recommend against routine laboratory tests or CT of the head as part of the initial evaluation.

> **Additional Reading:** Clinical practice guideline: sudden hearing loss. *Otolaryngol Head Neck Surg.* 2012;146(3 suppl):S1–S35.

> **Category:** Special sensory

186. Which of the following relationships between toxin exposure and symptoms is correct?
A) Vinyl chloride—behavioral changes
B) Mercury, lead, and pesticides—acroosteolysis
C) Iron, lithium, and lead—pulmonary fibrosis
D) Chromate and cocaine—nasal septal perforations

Answer and Discussion

The answer is D. Ingestion of toxins can cause a multitude of symptoms. However, there are specific symptoms particularly associated with specific toxins. The following are some toxins and their common identifiable symptoms:

- Mercury, lead, and pesticides—change of behavior
- Asbestos exposure—pulmonary fibrosis
- Vinyl chloride—acroosteolysis
- Chromate and cocaine—nasal septal perforations

> **Additional Reading:** Pulmonary complications of cocaine abuse. In: Basow DS, ed. *UpToDate.* Waltham, MA: UpToDate; 2013.

> **Category:** Nonspecific system

187. Side effects of 3-hydroxy-3-methylglutaryl coenzyme A (HMG CoA) reductase inhibitors include
A) Chronic rhinitis
B) Infertility
C) Rhabdomyolysis
D) Orthostatic hypotension
E) Cataracts

Answer and Discussion

The answer is C. HMG CoA reductase inhibitors (also referred to as *statins*) are used for the treatment of moderate-to-severe

hypercholesterolemia. The drugs (atorvastatin, pravastatin, cerivastatin, fluvastatin, lovastatin, simvastatin) inhibit HMG CoA reductase, the rate-limiting step in cholesterol production. Statin drugs decrease the patient's total and LDL cholesterol and increase the patient's HDL cholesterol. The drugs can cause elevation of liver function tests; therefore, serum transaminases should be performed before the initiation of treatment, and 12 weeks after initiation of therapy, or at increase of dose and periodically thereafter. Elevations more than three times the normal levels are an indication to discontinue the drug. Statin drugs should be used with caution in patients with underlying liver dysfunction and heavy alcohol use. Rhabdomyolysis with renal failure is also a potential side effect. Routine eye examinations for the detection of lens opacities are no longer recommended.

> **Additional Reading:** Which statin? *Med Lett Drugs Ther.* 2008;50(1284):29–31.

> **Category:** Nephrologic system

188. A 29-year-old female college soccer coach presents with anxiety, fatigue, and insomnia. The symptoms began after a heart murmur was discovered on her preemployment physical. An echocardiogram revealed mild MVP. A male athlete at her school recently died suddenly on the playing field because of undiagnosed idiopathic hypertrophic cardiomyopathy, and she is afraid she will die in a similar manner. She is anxious, sleepless, and fearful of physical activity. Your physical exam is normal and her EKG shows no abnormalities. Which one of the following would be most appropriate at this point?
A) Reassurance regarding the benign course of her condition
B) A stress test
C) Clonazepam (Klonopin)
D) Referral to a cardiologist
E) Referral for group psychotherapy

Answer and Discussion

The answer is A. Much of the psychological distress caused by the diagnosis of MVP is related to a lack of information and a fear of heart disease, which may be reinforced by the death of a friend or relative. A clear explanation of MVP, along with printed material, is a powerful aid in relieving the patient's emotional distress. The American Heart Association publishes a helpful booklet about this condition, which can be given to these patients. It is important to avoid reinforcing illness behavior with unnecessary testing, medications, or referrals to specialists.

> **Additional Reading:** Mitral valve prolapse. In: Domino F, ed. *The 5-Minute Clinical Consult.* Philadelphia, PA: Lippincott Williams and Wilkins; 2014.

> **Category:** Cardiovascular system

189. Gilbert's disease is associated with
A) Overproduction of glucuronyl transferase
B) Mild (benign) elevations of indirect (unconjugated) bilirubin
C) Intravascular hemolysis
D) Increased risk for liver disease

Answer and Discussion

The answer is B. Gilbert's disease is a persistent, lifelong condition that involves the deficiency of glucuronyl transferase. It affects as much as 5% of the population. There may be a familial component. Patients exhibit a persistent elevation in indirect (unconjugated) bilirubin. Stressful states and fasting may increase bilirubin levels. Patients do not exhibit symptoms, and there is no evidence of hemolysis. Gilbert's syndrome can be distinguished from hepatitis by normal liver function tests, absence of urinary bile, and predominantly unconjugated bilirubin fractionation. Hemolysis is differentiated by the absence of anemia or reticulocytosis. Liver histology is normal but biopsy is not needed for the diagnosis. No treatment is required, and no untoward effects are noted. Patients should be reassured that they do not have liver disease.

Additional Reading: Gilbert disease. In: Domino F, ed. *The 5-Minute Clinical Consult*. Philadelphia, PA: Lippincott Williams and Wilkins; 2014.

Category: Gastroenterology system

190. Which of the following drugs used in the treatment of CHF has been shown to increase survival?

A) Digoxin
B) Furosemide
C) Hydralazine
D) Enalapril
E) Isosorbide dinitrate

Answer and Discussion

The answer is D. Medications for the treatment of CHF (related to systolic failure) include the following:

- *Diuretics.* Thiazide diuretics have been shown to be useful in decreasing fluid overload in patients with mild CHF by inhibiting sodium chloride reabsorption at the distal tubule; however, they are not usually effective in patients with advanced symptomatology. In moderate and severe cases, the loop diuretics (e.g., furosemide, bumetanide) are indicated; these agents inhibit solute resorption in the loop of Henle. Spironolactone (a potassium-sparing diuretic) can also be used in the treatment of CHF. Electrolytes should be monitored because of changes in serum potassium, as well as in sodium, magnesium, and calcium.
- *ACE inhibitors* (captopril, enalapril, lisinopril, ramipril). These medications serve as preload and afterload reducers by blocking (1) the production of angiotensin II, a potent vasoconstrictor, and (2) the release of aldosterone. ACE inhibitors are effective in the treatment of CHF and have been shown to increase survival in affected patients. Electrolytes should be monitored because of the possibility of hyperkalemia and renal insufficiency (especially in patients with renal artery stenosis). ACE inhibitors have also been shown to be beneficial in promoting renal blood flow in diabetes.
- *Angiotensin II-receptor blockers* (losartan, valsartan, candesartan) have similar effects to those of ACE inhibitors, although conclusive trials have not been reported regarding equal effectiveness.
- *Digoxin.* This medication has been shown to be effective in severe CHF and in CHF complicated by atrial fibrillation. Its mechanism of action involves the energy-dependent sodium-potassium pump, leading to increased intracellular calcium and a positive inotropic effect. Elderly patients and those taking other medication (e.g., quinidine, amiodarone) are at increased risk for toxicity and need close follow-up with monitoring of digoxin levels. Potassium levels should also be monitored closely; hypokalemia can precipitate arrhythmias in patients taking digoxin.
- β-*Blockers* (carvedilol, metoprololol) can reduce mortality in select patients—especially in patients with idiopathic dilated cardiomyopathy. With slower heart rates, diastolic function improves. Ventricular filling improves and the ejection fraction may improve over 6 to 12 months, giving rise to improved exercise capacity. Randomized control trials have shown significant reduction in all-cause mortality and cardiac events in patients taking carvedilol with mildly symptomatic CHF and an ejection fraction less than or equal to 35%.
- *Vasodilators* (e.g., hydralazine, isosorbide dinitrate) can be used if patients are unable to tolerate ACE inhibitors. They work by decreasing preload as a result of vasodilation.

Additional Reading: Drugs for chronic heart failure. *Treat Guidel Med Lett.* 2012;10 (121):69–72.

Category: Cardiovascular system

191. Which of the following statements regarding pneumococcal vaccination is true?

A) Immunosuppressed patients should not be immunized.
B) Indian populations are at high risk for complications and should be avoided.
C) Revaccination should occur every 10 years.
D) A one-time booster is given to patients above age 65 if they were vaccinated more than 5 years previously and they were above 65 at the time of their primary vaccination.
E) Sickle cell patients should be revaccinated every 5 years.

Answer and Discussion

The answer is D. Medical indications for pneumococcal vaccination include chronic disorders of the pulmonary system; CVDs; diabetes mellitus; chronic liver diseases, including liver disease as a result of alcohol abuse (e.g., cirrhosis); chronic renal failure or nephrotic syndrome; functional or anatomic asplenia (e.g., sickle cell disease, splenectomy); immunosuppressive conditions (e.g., congenital immunodeficiency, HIV infection, leukemia, lymphoma, multiple myeloma, Hodgkin's disease, generalized malignancy, organ or bone marrow transplantation); chemotherapy with alkylating agents, antimetabolites, or long-term systemic corticosteroids; or cochlear implants. Geographic and other indications include Alaska Natives and certain American Indian populations. Other indications include residents of nursing homes and other long-term-care facilities. A one-time revaccination after 5 years is recommended for persons with chronic renal failure or nephrotic syndrome; functional or anatomic asplenia (e.g., sickle cell disease or splenectomy); immunosuppressive conditions (e.g., congenital immunodeficiency, HIV infection, leukemia, lymphoma, multiple myeloma, Hodgkin's disease, generalized malignancy, or organ or bone marrow transplantation); or chemotherapy with alkylating agents, antimetabolites, or long-term systemic corticosteroids. For persons older than 65 years, a one-time revaccination is recommended if they were vaccinated <5 years previously and were younger than 65 years at the time of primary vaccination.

Additional Reading: Updated recommendations for prevention of invasive pneumococcal disease among adults using the 23-valent pneumococcal polysaccharide vaccine (PPSV23). *MMWR.* 2010;59(34):1093–1096.

Category: Respiratory system

192. A 24-year-old poorly controlled diabetic patient presents to your emergency room with ketoacidosis, fever, pain, and purulent drainage of the sinuses with black eschar formation affecting the nasal septum. The most likely diagnosis is

A) Mucormycosis
B) Cocaine use
C) Chronic sinusitis
D) *Pseudomonas* infection
E) *Staphylococcus* infection

Answer and Discussion

The answer is A. Mucormycosis (phycomycosis) is a fungal infection that can be fulminant and lethal. It affects the nose, sinus, and orbit and is seen in patients with poorly controlled diabetes, diabetic ketoacidosis, or immunodeficiency. Symptoms include dull sinus pain, fever, orbital cellulitis, proptosis, nasal congestion and purulent or bloody nasal discharge, and gangrenous destruction of the nasal septum, orbits, or palate. In many cases, a black eschar is formed in the nasal area. If the fungus invades the cerebral vessels, then convulsions, blindness, and death can result. Diagnosis almost always involves biopsy. CT or MRI can help evaluate the extent of the disease. Treatment is accomplished with diabetic control, amphotericin B, and surgical debridement. The prognosis is poor, with up to a 50% mortality rate in disseminated cases.

> **Additional Reading:** Mucormycosis (Zygomycosis). From: http://www.cdc.gov/fungal/mucormycosis/

Category: Special sensory

> Mucormycosis affects the nose, sinus, and orbit and is seen in patients with poorly controlled diabetes, diabetic ketoacidosis, or immunodeficiency.

193. Pterygium is associated with
A) An increased risk of glaucoma
B) Involvement of the pupillary area, which may require surgical excision if affected
C) Improvement with the use of topical anesthetics
D) Trauma to the retina
E) Macular degeneration

Answer and Discussion

The answer is B. Pinguecula are hyaline, elastic nodules that appear yellow and affect both sides of the cornea but usually more on the nasal side. Occasionally, they become inflamed and require treatment with topical steroids. However, in most cases no treatment is required. Pterygium is a fleshy, triangular growth of a pinguecula that involves the cornea. In some cases, it may involve the pupillary area and requires surgical removal. The causes include irritation from UV sunlight, allergens, and excessive drying, sandy, or windy conditions that cause chronic irritation. In most cases, treatment is supportive with topical vasoconstrictors, saline drops, and protection from sunlight. Surgery is reserved for more severe cases in which vision is compromised.

> **Additional Reading:** Acute red eye. *Am Fam Physician*. 2007; 76(6):857–858.

Category: Special sensory

194. Which of the following statements about Hodgkin's disease is true?
A) Lymphocyte-predominant disease has a better prognosis than mixed-cellularity type.
B) Lymphocyte-depleted Hodgkin's disease is the most common type.
C) Stages A and B are distinguished by the presence of metastatic disease to regional lymph nodes.
D) The disease most commonly affects patients between 40 and 50 years of age.
E) Treatment for stages 1A and 2A involves chemotherapy.

Answer and Discussion

The answer is A. Hodgkin's disease is a type of lymphoma that involves the presence of Reed–Sternberg cells. This type of cell is a large, abnormal macrophage-like one with two prominent nuclei and surrounding halos that look like owl eyes. The disease has a bimodal distribution with a peak in individuals in their mid-20s and another peak in individuals older than 50 years. Symptoms include fever, weight loss, night sweats, and occasionally pain associated with involved lymph nodes with the ingestion of alcohol. Most patients affected present with painless lymphadenopathy in the neck. Metastasis is usually to local lymph nodes, with hematogenous spread late in the course of the disease. Chest radiographs may show asymmetric mediastinal lymphadenopathy (compared with sarcoidosis, which usually involves symmetric lymphadenopathy). The disease is classified into four different types:

1. Lymphocyte predominant
2. Nodular sclerosis (most common type)
3. Mixed cellularity
4. Lymphocyte depleted

Once the diagnosis is made, the disease is staged based on extent. Staging determines the modality of treatment:

Stage 1: one lymph node region involved
Stage 2: two areas of lymph nodes involved on the same side of the diaphragm
Stage 3: lymph node involvement on both sides of the diaphragm
Stage 4: disseminated disease with bone marrow or liver involvement

Further criteria involves stages of symptoms:

Stage A: lack of constitutional symptoms
Stage B: weight loss, fever, and night sweats are present

Treatment of stages 1A and 2A involves radiation. Stages 3B and 4 are treated with combination chemotherapy (i.e., the use of mechlorethamine vincristine [Oncovin], procarbazine, and prednisone). Treatment of stages 2B and 3A is controversial, but usually involves combined chemotherapy and radiotherapy. The prognosis is variable. Those with localized disease have excellent prognoses, whereas those with disseminated disease have poorer prognoses. In addition, those who have lymphocyte-predominant and nodular-sclerosing type fare better than those with mixed-cellularity and lymphocyte-depleted forms.

> **Additional Reading:** Hodgkin disease. In: Domino F, ed. *The 5-Minute Clinical Consult*. Philadelphia, PA: Lippincott Williams and Wilkins; 2014.

Category: Hematologic system

195. Gamekeeper's thumb is associated with a sprain of the
A) Extensor pollicis brevis tendon
B) Extensor pollicis longus tendon
C) Ulnar collateral ligament
D) Flexor carpi ulnaris tendon
E) Flexor retinaculum

Answer and Discussion

The answer is C. Gamekeeper's thumb (also known as *skier's thumb*) occurs when there is a sprain or traumatic rupture of the ulnar collateral ligament in the area of the thumb MCP joint. The injury occurs when there is hyperextension and hyperabduction of the thumb, usually as the result of a fall. The injury results in ulnar laxity of the MCP joint and often dorsal subluxation of the proximal thumb at the MCP joint. Patients often complain of weakness and pain when using the thumb to pinch and to perform activities such as opening car doors or jars or turning the key in a door lock. Other physical findings include swelling, erythema, ecchymosis, and tenderness over the MCP joint of the thumb on the ulnar side. As much as 95% of the injuries to the MCP joint occur on the ulnar side. Radiographs may show ulnar deviation of the proximal thumb and avulsion fracture of the ulnar collateral ligament at the base of the proximal phalanx. If the avulsed fragment is displaced more than 1 mm or involves more than 10% of the articular surface, surgery is indicated for repair. Also, if stress radiographs show laxity of the ulnar collateral ligament greater than 35 degrees on an anteroposterior radiograph, patients should be referred to an orthopaedist. However, in less severe cases, immobilization in a thumb spica cast for 4 to 6 weeks is indicated.

> **Additional Reading:** Ulnar collateral ligament injury (gamekeeper's or skier's thumb). In: Basow DS, ed. *UpToDate*. Waltham, MA: UpToDate; 2013.

> **Category:** Musculoskeletal system

196. Chronic alcohol consumption is associated with which of the following laboratory findings?
A) Increased HDL cholesterol
B) Decreased aspartate transaminase
C) Decreased γ-glutamyl transferase
D) Increased testosterone
E) Microcytic anemia

Answer and Discussion

The answer is A. Fifteen percent of patients seen in family practice and 10% to 20% of patients in the hospital have an alcohol problem requiring at least minimal intervention. Chronic alcohol consumption can lead to a number of laboratory findings, including increased levels of HDL cholesterol; mild elevations of aspartate transaminase and, more specifically, γ-glutamyl transferase; megaloblastic anemia as a result of folate deficiency; thiamine deficiency; decreased serum calcium; and decreased testosterone levels. In most cases, cessation of alcohol consumption corrects the abnormal laboratory results, except in cases in which permanent damage has occurred. Screening for alcohol abuse may be accomplished quickly in the office setting with the CAGE questions. This acronym is used to remind the examiner of the following questions:

- Have you ever felt the need to **C**ut down on your drinking?
- Have you ever been **A**nnoyed by others' criticism of your drinking?
- Have you ever felt **G**uilty about your drinking?
- Have you ever had an "**E**ye opener" in the early morning?

A positive response to any of these questions should alert the examiner to ask more questions about the patient's alcohol consumption.

> **Additional Reading:** Alcohol abuse and dependence: epidemiology, clinical manifestations, and diagnosis. In: Basow DS, ed. *UpToDate*. Waltham, MA: UpToDate; 2013.

> **Category:** Patient/population-based care

197. A 55-year-old patient with a history of hypertriglyceridemia and severe abdominal pain with vomiting over the previous 6 hours is transferred from the emergency room to the hospital ward with the following laboratory findings:

- WBC count: 20,000
- Glucose: 295 mg per dL
- Aspartate aminotransferase: 333 IU per L
- Lactate dehydrogenase: 375 IU per L

The most likely diagnosis is
A) Acute cholecystitis
B) Acute pancreatitis
C) Hepatitis
D) IM
E) Diabetic ketoacidosis

Answer and Discussion

The answer is B. Acute pancreatitis is caused by biliary tract disease, alcoholism, hyperlipidemia, hypercalcemia, hyperparathyroidism, trauma, medications (e.g., furosemide, valproic acid, sulfasalazine), infections, and structural abnormalities of the biliary tract. Symptoms include constant, boring, abdominal pain that radiates to the back; nausea; and repeated vomiting with a low-grade fever. Physical examination shows a distended rigid abdomen with positive peritoneal signs, tachycardia, tachypnea, and signs of dehydration and shock. Laboratory tests show an elevation in serum lipase (more sensitive) and amylase, elevated WBC count (12,000 to 20,000 per mm^3), elevated liver function tests, increased bilirubin, hyperglycemia, and hypocalcemia. Chest radiographs may show pleural effusions. Abdominal films may show the presence of a sentinel loop (ileus of the transverse colon). Ultrasound or CT examination may show evidence of gallstones, dilation of the common bile duct, or edema of the pancreas. Pancreatitis associated with hemorrhage or necrosis of the pancreas has a mortality rate that approaches 50%. Hemorrhage is suspected if there is a grayish-blue discoloration of the back or flanks of the patient's body (Grey Turner's sign) or affecting the periumbilical area (Cullen's sign). Treatment involves bowel rest with nasogastric suction and fluid resuscitation with correction of electrolyte disturbances. Ranson's criteria are used to predict outcome at the time of admission:

- Older than 55 years
- WBC count >16,000 per mm^3
- Serum glucose >200 mg per dL
- Lactate dehydrogenase >350 IU per L
- Aspartate aminotransferase level >250 IU per L 48 hours after admission
- Greater than 10% decrease in hematocrit
- Elevation in BUN >5 mg per dL
- Serum calcium levels <8 mg per dL
- Base deficit >4 mEq per L
- Arterial PO_2 <60 mm Hg
- Greater than an estimated 6 L of fluid deposition in the body's interstitial spaces

If less than three signs are present at the time of admission, the mortality rate is <5%. The presence of three or more signs on admission has an associated mortality rate of 15% to 20%. If seven or more signs total are present, the mortality rate approaches 100%.

> **Additional Reading:** Pancreatitis, Acute. In: Domino F, ed. *The 5-Minute Clinical Consult*. Philadelphia, PA: Lippincott Williams and Wilkins; 2014.

> **Category:** Gastroenterology system

198. A 40-year-old florist presents to your office complaining of a nontender nodule that formed on his hand, then enlarged, and finally ulcerated. In the days that followed, the patient developed similar nodules in the area of the axillary lymphatics. Otherwise he has had no other symptoms. The most likely diagnosis is
A) Cat-scratch fever
B) Sporotrichosis
C) Tuberculosis
D) Blastomycosis
E) Histoplasmosis

Answer and Discussion

The answer is B. Sporotrichosis is a disease caused by inoculation of the plant *Sporothrix schenckii* when patients prick themselves with a thorn. The condition is associated with the formation of nodules, ulcers, and abscesses affecting the skin and lymphatic system. Farm workers and those who work around plants (i.e., florists, gardeners, nursery workers, and horticulturists) such as sphagnum moss, rosebushes, and barberry bushes are the most likely to be affected. Most patients present with a nontender nodule that forms on an arm or hand. The nodule enlarges, becomes erythematous (blush red), and finally ulcerates. In the following days, other nodules may form in the area of the draining lymphatics. Local pain and constitutional symptoms are usually absent. Other areas such as lungs, spleen, liver, kidney, genitalia, muscle, joints, and eyes may become involved. Diagnosis is usually achieved by culturing the organism from the nodules. Treatment is accomplished with itraconazole and extended courses of saturated solution of potassium iodide; in severe disseminated cases, intravenous amphotericin B or ketoconazole (less effective) is used.

> **Additional Reading:** Sporotrichosis. In: Domino F, ed. *The 5-Minute Clinical Consult*. Philadelphia, PA: Lippincott Williams and Wilkins; 2014.

> **Category:** Nonspecific system

199. A hemodynamically unstable patient is noted to have supraventricular tachycardia. The most appropriate treatment is
A) Electrical synchronized cardioversion
B) Carotid massage
C) Adenosine
D) Verapamil
E) Digoxin

Answer and Discussion

The answer is A. Supraventricular tachycardia is characterized by a rapid regular rhythm with a narrow QRS complex and abnormal P waves. The heart rate is usually 100 to 200 bpm. Some patients may be asymptomatic; others may experience chest pain, palpitations, and shortness of breath. Hemodynamically unstable patients with supraventricular tachycardia require immediate treatment with electrical synchronized cardioversion. For those patients who are stable, vagal stimulation can be attempted with carotid massage (but not in patients with previous cerebrovascular accidents or carotid bruits), Valsalva's maneuver, activation of the gag reflex, or placing a cold ice bag on the face. If these measures are unsuccessful, medication including adenosine, verapamil, diltiazem, or a β-blocker, can be used. Untreated supraventricular tachycardia may lead to heart failure.

> **Additional Reading:** Clinical manifestations, diagnosis, and evaluation of narrow QRS complex tachycardias. In: Basow DS, ed. *UpToDate*. Waltham, MA: UpToDate; 2013.

> **Category:** Cardiovascular system

200. The most common cause of tinnitus is
A) Infection (otitis media)
B) Chronic use of salicylates
C) Sensorineural hearing loss
D) Hypertension
E) Acoustic neuroma

Answer and Discussion

The answer is C. Tinnitus is a common condition that is characterized by a ringing, roaring, rushing, buzzing, or whistling sound in the ears. The condition may be continuous or pulsatile with each heartbeat. In most cases, there is an associated hearing loss. In fact, the major cause of tinnitus is a sensorineural hearing loss. The list of associated conditions is extensive and includes obstruction of the canals, eustachian tube dysfunction, otosclerosis, Meniere's disease, aminoglycoside toxicity, chronic use of salicylates, anemia, hypertension, hypothyroidism, hyperlipidemia, noise-induced hearing loss, and tumors associated with the inner ear (e.g., acoustic neuroma). The evaluation of a patient with tinnitus includes an audiogram and CT scan or MRI of the head, with special emphasis given to the temporal area. Pulsatile tinnitus may require vascular studies to rule out aneurysm formation. Treatment depends on the diagnosis, but in most cases if the underlying disease is controlled, the tinnitus disappears. If no underlying disease process is present, background music or amplification may help to relieve symptoms.

> **Additional Reading:** Tinnitus. In: Domino F, ed. *The 5-Minute Clinical Consult*. Philadelphia, PA: Lippincott Williams and Wilkins; 2014.

> **Category:** Special sensory

201. All the following medication can reduce the β-type natriuretic peptide (BNP) level except
A) Spironolactone
B) Lisinopril
C) Valsartin
D) Digoxin

Answer and Discussion

The answer is D. Many medications used to treat heart failure (e.g., diuretics such as spironolactone [Aldactone], ACE inhibitors, angiotensin II-receptor blockers) reduce BNP concentrations. Therefore, many patients with chronic stable heart failure will have BNP levels in the normal diagnostic range (i.e., BNP level less than 100 pg per mL [100 ng per L]). However, digoxin and some β-blockers appear to increase natriuretic peptide concentrations. Exercise causes a short-term increase in BNP levels, although only small changes are detectable one hour after exercise. No circadian variation has been reported when BNP is measured every three hours for 24 hours, and there is less hourly variation with BNP than with ANP.

> **Additional Reading:** The role of BNP testing in heart failure. *Am Fam Physician*. 2006;74(11):1893–1900.

> **Category:** Cardiovascular system

202. Which of the following toxin exposure–antidote associations is correct?
A) Cyanide–calcium carbonate
B) Ethylene glycol–ethanol and pyridoxine
C) Magnesium–amyl nitrite
D) Organic phosphates–epinephrine

Answer and Discussion

The answer is B. Toxin exposure is often treated by family physicians. The following are the drugs of choice for treating the associated toxin exposures:

Toxin	Treatment
Atropine	Physostigmine
Cyanide	Amyl nitrite
Magnesium	Calcium carbonate
Ethylene glycol	Ethanol and pyridoxine
Organic phosphates	Atropine

> **Additional Reading:** General approach to drug poisoning in adults. In: Basow DS, ed. *UpToDate.* Waltham, MA: UpToDate; 2013.

Category: Nonspecific system

203. Guttate psoriasis are
A) Thick, scaly plaque-like lesions that are commonly identified as psoriasis
B) Not associated with respiratory illnesses
C) Not usually associated with skin creases
D) Insidious in their outbreak with large "bull's-eye" type lesions

Answer and Discussion

The answer is C. The condition of guttate psoriasis is characterized by numerous small, oval (teardrop-shaped) lesions that develop after an acute upper respiratory tract infection. These lesions are often not as scaly or as erythematous as the classic lesions of plaque-type psoriasis. Usually, guttate psoriasis must be differentiated from pityriasis rosea, another condition characterized by the sudden outbreak of red scaly lesions. Compared with pityriasis rosea, psoriatic lesions are thicker and scalier, and the lesions are not usually distributed along skin creases.

> **Additional Reading:** Psoriasis. *Am Fam Physician.* 2013;87(9): 626–633.

> The condition of guttate psoriasis is characterized by numerous small, oval (teardrop-shaped) lesions that develop after an acute upper respiratory tract infection.

Category: Integumentary

204. In the treatment of external genital warts, it is important to
A) Biopsy the visible lesions
B) Aceto-white stain the areas to identify the affected lesions
C) Obtain viral-typing of the lesions
D) Remove visible warts

Answer and Discussion

The answer is D. Genital warts caused by human papillomavirus infection are frequently seen in primary care. Evidence-based treatment recommendations are limited. Biopsy, viral-typing, aceto-white staining, and other diagnostic measures are not routinely required. The goal of treatment is removal of visible warts; some evidence exists that treatment reduces infectivity, but there is no evidence that treatment reduces the incidence of cervical and genital cancer. The choice of therapy is based on the number, size, site, and appearance of lesions, as well as patient preferences, cost, convenience, adverse effects, and clinician preference. Patient-applied therapies include imiquimod cream (Zyclara, Aldara), podofilox (Condylox), and sinecatechins ointment (Veregen). Trichloroacetic acid, cryotherapy, and surgical excision are used in the office.

> **Additional Reading:** Drugs for sexually transmitted infections. *Treat Guidel Med Lett.* 2013;11(133):75.

Category: Integumentary

205. Silo filler's disease is caused by chronic inhalation of
A) Carbon monoxide
B) Nitrogen dioxide
C) Nitrogen mustard
D) Nitrous oxide
E) Carbon dioxide

Answer and Discussion

The answer is B. Silo filler's disease is a pulmonary disease that is caused by the inhalation of nitrogen dioxide. Those affected are usually farmers who are exposed to the toxic gas, which is produced from moldy hay found in silos and grain bins. Because of the irritant effects, the gas can lead to the development of pulmonary edema, usually 10 to 12 hours after exposure to the gas. In severe cases, exposure can lead to bronchiolitis obliterans with associated respiratory failure and death. Symptoms include irritation to the mucous membranes and eyes, cough, hemoptysis, wheezing, nausea, vomiting, and dyspnea. Chest radiographs usually show alveolar infiltrates and pulmonary edema. Bacterial superinfections can occur and can lead to serious complications. Treatment usually involves bronchodilators, intravenous fluids, mechanical ventilation, and steroids. Chronic exposure may lead to chronic bronchitis.

> **Additional Reading:** Nitrous dioxide toxicity; 2013. From: http://emedicine.medscape.com/article/302133-overview

Category: Respiratory system

206. Which of the following is an effect of niacin use?
A) Increased LDL cholesterol
B) Increased triglyceride levels
C) Increased HDL cholesterol
D) Hypoglycemia
E) Decreased uric acid levels

Answer and Discussion

The answer is C. Niacin (nicotinic acid) is used to treat hyperlipidemia. It lowers LDL cholesterol and triglyceride levels and increases HDL cholesterol levels. The medication is available without a prescription. Side effects include flushing, pruritus, hepatotoxicity, elevated glucose and uric acid levels, and GI irritation. Doses range from 500 mg per day to a maximum of 3 g per day. Aspirin taken approximately 45 minutes before the administration of niacin may help to decrease flushing episodes. Liver function tests should be periodically monitored when patients are taking the medication.

> **Additional Reading:** What about niacin? *Med Lett Drugs Ther.* 2011;53(1378):94.

Category: Cardiovacular system

207. Tourette's syndrome is associated with which one of the following comorbidities?
A) Cardiac arrhythmias
B) Partial or complex seizures
C) Hypertension
D) Attention-deficit disorder
E) Hypothyroidism

Answer and Discussion

The answer is D. Tourette's syndrome is often associated with psychiatric comorbidities, mainly attention-deficit/hyperactivity disorder and obsessive-compulsive disorder. The other conditions listed are not associated with Tourette's syndrome.

Additional Reading: Tourette's syndrome. *Am Fam Physician.* 2008;77(5):651–658; 782–783.

Category: Neurologic

208. Which of the following statements best describes a case-control study?
A) It is an observational design-type study that begins with an outcome and then looks for common aspects among those who are affected.
B) It is a study that categorizes subjects into groups and observes outcomes.
C) It is a study that identifies outcomes and predictors of outcomes simultaneously.
D) It is a study that records information, activities, and observations but does not provide explanations.

Answer and Discussion

The answer is A. The following are types of studies encountered in the medical literature:

- *Case-control study:* This is an observational design-type study that begins with an outcome and then looks for common aspects among those who are affected.
- *Cohort study:* This is a prospective design study. Subjects with similar characteristics are categorized into groups and then researchers observe the outcome.
- *Cross-sectional study:* This is an observational design-type study that takes a subject group and identifies outcomes and their predictors simultaneously.
- *Clinical series study:* This is a descriptive-type study that records information, activities, and observations but provides no explanations. These studies usually lead to further explanatory-type studies.

Additional Reading: Terms used in evidence-based medicine. *Am Fam Physician.* From: http://www.aafp.org/journals/afp/authors/ebm-toolkit/glossary.html.

Category: Patient/population-based care

209. A 50-year-old man complains of gradual increasing shortness of breath, and evidence of honeycombing of pulmonary architecture is seen on a chest radiograph. Pulmonary function tests show both decreased vital and diffusing capacities as well as reduced total lung volumes with a normal forced expiratory volume in 1 second to forced vital capacity ratio. The most likely diagnosis is
A) COPD
B) Tuberculosis
C) Asthma
D) Idiopathic pulmonary fibrosis
E) Chronic PE

Answer and Discussion

The answer is D. Idiopathic pulmonary fibrosis, a form of interstitial lung disease, results when there is inflammation of the lung tissue with resulting fibrosis. A toxic exposure or antigenic response is thought to precipitate the inflammatory process. Affected patients may report a gradual, increasing shortness of breath; a dry cough; and generalized fatigue with lack of endurance with physical exercise.

Physical examination shows bibasilar dry rales, clubbing, and, occasionally, cyanosis. In advanced disease, chest radiographs show honeycombing, and pulmonary function tests show a restrictive pattern with reduced vital capacity, diffusing capacity for carbon monoxide, and total lung volume. In addition, there is a normal or increased forced expiratory volume in 1 second to forced vital capacity ratio. Arterial blood gases may show mild hypoxemia, but hypercarbia is rare. The patient's ESR may be increased. Transthoracic or transbronchial biopsy is usually needed for a definitive diagnosis. The treatment of idiopathic pulmonary fibrosis is controversial because of a lack of understanding of the natural history of the disease. Only 10% to 15% of patients improve with corticosteroid therapy, and 26% of patients develop serious complications from the steroid therapy. Indicators of good response to steroid therapy include young age, female gender, ground-glass lesions on CT scan, and active inflammation on lung biopsy samples. Azathioprine, cyclophosphamide, and other cytotoxic drugs have been used as second-line agents or in combination with steroids as first-line therapy. Although the general prognosis was poor, combined treatment improved 3-year survival rates. Selected patients with idiopathic pulmonary fibrosis have been treated with lung transplantation.

Additional Reading: Causes and evaluation of chronic dyspnea. *Am Fam Physician.* 2012;86(2):173–180.

Category: Respiratory system

210. A 52-year-old man who is otherwise healthy is found to have a DVT affecting his left lower extremity below the knee. Appropriate management includes
A) Administration of clopidogrel
B) Initiation of aspirin as an outpatient
C) Observation
D) Intravascular thrombolysis
E) Administration of LMW heparin as an outpatient

Answer and Discussion

The answer is C. DVT is a condition that involves thrombus formation, usually in the lower-extremity veins. Predisposing conditions include lack of activity; previous DVT; recent surgery; smoking; and hypercoagulable states, including antithrombin III deficiency, protein C or S deficiency, lupus, cancer, and estrogen use. Symptoms include pain and swelling, as well as erythema and warmth of the lower extremity. Physical examination may be normal, and a positive Homans' sign is not a reliable predictor for DVT. Diagnosis is usually made with Doppler ultrasound (duplex) studies, which is operator-dependent and does not detect thrombi below the knee very well. The gold standard test is contrast venography. A d-dimer is often elevated in patients with venous thrombosis. It is sensitive but not specific. Impedance plethysmography is highly sensitive for thrombi above the knee, but less sensitive if the thrombosis is below the knee. Treatment for DVT above the knee involves intravenous heparin or LMW heparin and oral warfarin. It is important to overlap heparin treatment with oral warfarin for at least 4 to 5 days because the full anticoagulant effect of warfarin is delayed. Warfarin should be continued for at least 3 to 6 months, although the optimal treatment time is controversial. Age and a history of thromboembolic events are strong risk factors for recurrence.

Treatment of DVT below the knee is controversial. Calf vein thrombosis should be either treated with anticoagulants or followed with serial Doppler studies to rule out propagation. DVT prophylaxis regimens depend on the level of risk:

- *Low risk.* Individuals who are at low risk include those who have major surgery requiring anesthesia for at least 30 minutes, immobilized patients, patients with MI or CHF, and women after cesarean section. The prophylaxis is heparin at 5,000 U (given subcutaneously every 12 hours) and intermittent compressive devices (at least once per minute).

- *High risk.* Individuals who are at high risk include those who have pelvic or lower-extremity surgery, including hip or knee replacement, or a previous DVT or PE. The prophylaxis is a combination of compression devices plus LMW heparin or warfarin.

The use of LMW heparin is becoming more common in the treatment of DVT because it offers the advantages of having a more predictable anticoagulant effect, avoids the need for anticoagulation testing, and allows the patient to be treated at home. It is also associated with less antibody formation, a lower risk of heparin-induced thrombocytopenia, and a decreased overall mortality. Patients being treated at home must learn to give themselves subcutaneous injections and should have close follow-up. Warfarin therapy should be initiated on day 1 when using unfractionated or LMW heparin. After 4 to 5 days and when the INR is greater than 2 for 2 consecutive days, the heparin therapy can be discontinued.

Patients who are at risk for bleeding may be candidates for inferior vena caval filter placement. There is little use in aggressive cancer workup in patients after an initial episode of DVT. A thorough history, physical examination, and age-appropriate cancer screening are adequate.

Additional Reading: Deep vein thrombophlebitis (DVT). In: Basow DS, ed. *The 5-Minute Clinical Consult.* Philadelphia, PA: Lippincott Williams and Wilkins; 2014.

Category: Cardiovascular system

211. Which of the following statements is true regarding ulcerative colitis?
A) There is transmural involvement of the bowel wall.
B) There are skipped areas of inflammation that may have a cobblestone appearance on colonoscopy.
C) There is a smaller risk of developing intestinal cancer in comparison with Crohn's disease.
D) The area of involvement is localized to the colon and rectosigmoid area.
E) Aminosalicylic acid compounds are not effective in the treatment of ulcerative colitis.

Answer and Discussion

The answer is D. Ulcerative colitis is characterized by inflammation of the bowel that is limited to the mucosal surface and submucosa of the bowel wall (i.e., it is not transmural like Crohn's disease). The area of involvement is localized to the colon and rectosigmoid area in a continuous fashion; this is unlike Crohn's disease, which shows skipped areas of involvement. Symptoms include bloody diarrhea, abdominal pain, fever, and tenesmus. Complications include intestinal perforation, development of toxic megacolon, and development of cancer (which is more commonly seen in patients with ulcerative colitis than in those with Crohn's disease). Extracolonic involvement affects the skin, eyes, joints, and liver; however, the kidneys are not involved (as they are in Crohn's disease). Diagnosis is accomplished in the same manner as in Crohn's disease (i.e., colonoscopy or flexible sigmoidoscopy with biopsy or with x-ray contrast studies). Treatment of ulcerative colitis is similar to that for Crohn's disease; however, the oral forms of 5-aminosalicylic acid (e.g., sulfasalazine, olsalazine, mesalamine) are more effective in controlling recurrences and the severity of outbreaks in ulcerative colitis. Close follow-up is necessary for ulcerative colitis and Crohn's disease because of the increased risk of developing bowel cancer.

Additional Reading: Ulcerative Colitis. In: Basow DS, ed. *The 5-Minute Clinical Consult.* Philadelphia, PA: Lippincott Williams and Wilkins; 2014.

Category: Gastroenterology system

212. A 60-year-old man presents with pain, swelling, and redness of the first metatarsal phalangeal joint. His cardiologist recently prescribed hydrochlorothiazide for his hypertension. The most likely diagnosis is
A) Podagra
B) Degenerative joint disease
C) Rheumatoid arthritis
D) Osteomyelitis
E) Morton's neuroma

Answer and Discussion

The answer is A. Gout (also known as podagra when it involves the big toe) is a condition characterized by recurrent pain associated with peripheral joints. The cause is attributed to the development of monosodium urate crystals, which cause acute arthritis. Longstanding gout can lead to chronic, deforming arthritis. The greater the degree of hyperuricemia, the more likely is the development of gouty attacks. Most hyperuricemia is asymptomatic. Hyperuricemia may result from disorders of purine metabolism, which may be genetic or acquired. Disorders causing hyperuricemia include proliferative hematologic disorders, psoriasis, myxedema, parathyroid disorders, enzyme deficiencies, and renal disease; obesity and medications such as thiazide diuretics are also causative. Middle-age and elderly men are usually affected more frequently than women; however, menopause is associated with a sharp increase in incidence in women (especially in those using thiazides and those with renal impairment). Symptoms include severe, throbbing pain with redness and swelling that is usually monoarticular and affects the metatarsophalangeal joint of the great toe (podagra). However, other joints, including the ankle, knee, wrist, and elbow, may also be affected. Other symptoms include fever and malaise. Later attacks may become more frequent and affect multiple joints with resolution between attacks less complete. Precipitating factors include trauma, overindulgence of foods (processed meats), alcohol, surgery, fatigue, stress, infection, or the administration of medications (e.g., penicillin, insulin, thiazide diuretics). Diagnosis is usually made on the basis of history and physical exam. Absolute confirmation involves joint aspiration with the detection of needle-shaped urate crystals that are negatively birefringent under a polarizing microscope. Asymptomatic treatment of hyperuricemia is generally not treated with medication. Treatment of gout involves the use of ice, rest, NSAIDs (e.g., indomethacin, naproxen, ibuprofen), colchicine (which may provide dramatic relief in the acute phase), and allopurinol (xanthine oxidase inhibitor) for patients who have chronically elevated uric acid levels after the acute attack has resolved (low-dose colchicine can also be used). In addition, uricosuric agents, including probenecid and sulfinpyrazone, may be helpful but should be used with caution in patients with renal problems. Prednisone may also be helpful in patients who cannot tolerate other medications. Transplantation recipients and those undergoing chemotherapy are usually protected with the use of allopurinol.

Additional Reading: Gout. In: Domino F, ed. *The 5-Minute Clinical Consult.* Philadelphia, PA: Lippincott Williams and Wilkins; 2014.

Category: Musculoskeletal system

213. The use of proton pump inhibitors (PPIs) can result in
A) Vitamin C deficiency
B) Vitamin D deficiency
C) Vitamin B_{12} deficiency
D) Folate deficiency

Answer and Discussion

The answer is C. Vitamin B_{12} (cobalamin) deficiency is a common cause of macrocytic anemia and has been implicated in a host of neuropsychiatric conditions. The widespread use of gastric acid-blocking agents, which can lead to decreased vitamin B_{12} levels, may contribute to the development of vitamin B_{12} deficiency. Given the widespread use of these agents and the aging of the U.S. population, the actual prevalence of vitamin B_{12} deficiency may be even higher than statistics indicate. Vitamin B_{12} deficiency is associated with hematologic, neurologic, and psychiatric symptoms. Neurologic manifestations from vitamin B_{12} deficiency include paresthesias, peripheral neuropathy, and demyelination of the corticospinal tract and dorsal columns (subacute combined systems disease). Vitamin B_{12} deficiency also has been linked to psychiatric disorders, including impaired memory, irritability, depression, dementia, and, rarely, psychosis. Dietary sources of vitamin B_{12} are primarily meats and dairy products. In a typical Western diet, a person obtains approximately 5 to 15 µg of vitamin B_{12} daily, which is far greater than the recommended daily allowance of 2 µg. Normally, individuals maintain a large vitamin B_{12} reserve, which can last 2 to 5 years even in the presence of severe malabsorption. However, nutritional deficiency can occur in specific populations. Elderly patients and chronic alcoholics are at especially high risk. The dietary restrictions of strict vegans make them another, less common at-risk population. The role of B_{12} deficiency in hyperhomocysteinemia and the promotion of atherosclerosis are under investigation. Diagnosis of vitamin B_{12} deficiency is based on measurement of serum vitamin B_{12} levels; however, about half of patients with subclinical disease have normal B_{12} levels. A more sensitive method of screening for vitamin B_{12} deficiency is measurement of serum methylmalonic acid and homocysteine levels, which are increased early in vitamin B_{12} deficiency. Use of the Schilling test for detection of pernicious anemia has been replaced for the most part by serologic testing for parietal cell and intrinsic factor antibodies. Contrary to prevailing medical practice, supplementation with oral vitamin B_{12} is a safe and effective treatment for the B_{12} deficiency state. Even when intrinsic factor is not present to aid in the absorption of vitamin B_{12} (pernicious anemia) or in other diseases that affect the usual absorption sites in the terminal ileum, oral therapy remains effective.

Additional Reading: Update on vitamin B_{12} deficiency. *Am Fam Physician.* 2011;83(12):1425–1430.

Category: Gastroenterology system

214. A 32-year-old man presents to your office. Approximately 5 days ago, he was cleaning out his dark, undisturbed attic. That day he noticed an erythematous lesion with a clear center on his arm. Since then the lesion has necrosed in the center, giving rise to a crater-like eschar lesion. The most likely diagnosis is
A) Lyme disease
B) Brown recluse spider bite
C) Psittacosis
D) Black widow spider bite
E) Scorpion sting

Answer and Discussion

The answer is B. The brown recluse spider (violin spider) may be identified by a dark, violin-shaped design on its back. These

spiders are usually found in dark areas, woodpiles, attics, and other undisturbed locations. The bite is initially mild (burning at site) and goes unnoticed, although some localized pain develops within 30 to 60 minutes. Within 1 to 4 hours, an erythematous, pruritic area with an ischemic pale center develops, giving the appearance of a bull's-eye target lesion. The central zone may progress to form a pustule that eventually fills with blood and ruptures; within 3 to 4 days, a crater-like lesion with necrosis develops. Large tissue defects may occur and include muscle. Healing usually requires extended periods; if large areas are involved, skin grafting may be necessary in some cases. Symptoms include headache, nausea and vomiting, low-grade fever, chills and sweats, generalized pruritus, malaise, arthralgias, severe pain (late in the course), and rash. Rare fatalities (none in the United States) have been reported with complications such as massive intravascular hemolysis with hemoglobinuria, renal failure, and disseminated intravascular coagulopathy. Treatment with dapsone has been recommended. Because dapsone can cause agranulocytosis and hemolytic anemia, which may be exaggerated in patients with G6PD deficiency, a G6PD test and CBC should be done before starting therapy. Systemic corticosteroids have shown no consistent or reliable benefit. Surgical debridement should be delayed until the area of necrosis is fully demarcated. Incision and suction is not recommended. Most bites require only local treatment. Ice therapy to the site may help reduce pain.

Additional Reading: Common spider bites. *Am Fam Physician.* 2007;75(6):869–873.

Category: Integumentary

215. A 60-year-old alcoholic man, currently being treated for gastritis, presents to the office with painful breasts that appear enlarged. The most likely cause is
A) Breast cancer
B) Excessive calcium carbonate ingestion
C) Omeprazole use
D) Trauma
E) Prolactinoma

Answer and Discussion

The answer is C. Gynecomastia is a condition characterized by enlargement of the breasts in men. It occurs when there is hypertrophy of breast tissue beneath the areola. In young adolescents, it is a natural response to the body's hormones. During this time, the breast may be tender. Patients and their parents should be reassured this is a natural response and will eventually resolve (usually within 3 years). Gynecomastia in older men can result from medication use (e.g., omeprazole and cimetidine, INH, digitalis, phenothiazine, testosterone), substance abuse (e.g., alcohol; illegal drugs, including marijuana and heroin), endocrine disorders (e.g., hypogonadism, hyperthyroidism), Klinefelter's syndrome, liver disease, and neoplasm. The workup of gynecomastia should include a chest radiograph, β-human chorionic gonadotropin determination, luteinizing hormone, β-FSH, estrogen and testosterone levels, liver function tests, and thyroid function tests. Typically, the estrogen:testosterone ratio is high. If the human chorionic gonadotropin is elevated, then a testicular ultrasound should be performed to look for testicular tumor. Additionally, if the testes are small, a karyotype should be obtained to look for Klinefelter's syndrome. Other testing may be necessary, if indicated. Treatment involves stopping any offending medications and correcting the underlying abnormality. If the condition does not resolve, suppressive medication or surgery may be indicated.

Additional Reading: Gynecomastia. *Am Fam Physician.* 2012;85(7):716–722.

Category: Integumentary

> Gynecomastia in older men can result from medication use (e.g., spironolactone, common contributors include antipsychotics, antiretrovirals, prostate cancer therapies), substance abuse (e.g., alcohol; illegal drugs, including marijuana and heroin), endocrine disorders (e.g., hypogonadism, hyperthyroidism), Klinefelter's syndrome, liver disease, and neoplasm.

216. Which of the following can distinguish atrial flutter from sinus tachycardia?
A) Carotid sinus massage
B) Administration of diltiazem
C) Administration of isoproterenol
D) Temporal artery massage
E) Administration of adenosine

Answer and Discussion

The answer is A. Atrial flutter is a regular, rapid cardiac rhythm characterized by an ectopic focus that gives rise to atrial rates from 280 to 350 impulses per minute. Usually, impulses are only transmitted to the ventricles every second, third, or fourth impulse. The heart rate is usually approximately 150 bpm. In many cases, atrial flutter is difficult to distinguish from sinus tachycardia; however, carotid sinus massage or Valsalva's maneuver may help distinguish the characteristic (sawtooth) flutter waves seen with atrial flutter. ECG shows flutter waves best in the inferior leads II, III, aVF, and in V1. RR interval may be regular, reflecting a fixed-ratio AV block (2:1, 3:1), or may be variable, reflecting a Wenckebach periodicity. Limited data suggest that the risk of thromboembolism, although smaller than with atrial fibrillation, is increased, suggesting anticoagulation should be considered. Treatment consists of verapamil, diltiazem, β-blockers, or digoxin, which slows conduction through the AV node. Electric cardioversion (low energy) is indicated for patients who are unstable and show signs of CHF (e.g., pulmonary rales, hepatojugular reflux, distended neck veins).

Additional Reading: Common types of supraventricular tachycardia: diagnosis and management. *Am Fam Physician.* 2010;82(8):942–952.

Category: Cardiovascular system

217. The drug of choice for the treatment of trigeminal neuralgia is
A) Naproxen
B) Prednisone
C) Carbamazepine
D) Valproic acid
E) Phenobarbital

Answer and Discussion

The answer is C. Trigeminal neuralgia is a disorder that involves the trigeminal nucleus of the trigeminal nerve. This disorder is characterized by severe, unilateral, sharp, lancinating-type pain that occurs in the distribution of the trigeminal nerve. Most patients are of middle age or elderly. The symptoms usually occur in recurrent bouts and can be incapacitating. Women tend to be more frequently affected than men. Precipitating factors include touching the affected area and movement of the face (as with eating, talking, and brushing one's teeth), shaving, or feeling a cool breeze on the face. Patients afflicted with trigeminal neuralgia show no physical signs. If deficits are noted during neurologic examination, then alternative diagnosis, including masses impinging on the trigeminal nerve, demyelinating processes, or vascular malformation, should be considered. In most cases, the momentary bouts of pain become more and more frequent and remissions become shorter and shorter. A dull ache that is persistent between the episodes of severe stabbing pain may develop. Remissions may occur and last weeks or even months. The treatment of choice is carbamazepine, which requires monitoring of serial blood counts and liver function tests. Alternative medications include phenytoin and baclofen. Other treatments include injecting glycerol into the offending nerve, surgery to decompress nerve fibers from blood vessels and bony structures, and radiofrequency rhizotomy if medical therapy fails.

Additional Reading: Drugs for pain. *Treat Guidel Med Lett.* 2013;11(128):31–42.

Category: Neurologic

> The treatment of choice for trigeminal neuralgia is carbamazepine, which requires monitoring of serial blood counts and liver function tests.

218. A 27-year-old woman reports a previous reaction to penicillin. She has had recurrent sinus and respiratory infections that frequently require antibiotic treatment. Appropriate management would consist of
A) Having the patient tested for penicillin allergies
B) Using a cephalosporin if patient has had previous anaphylactoid response
C) Administering amoxicillin instead of penicillin
D) Administering diphenhydramine with penicillin
E) Substituting imipenem for penicillin

Answer and Discussion

The answer is A. An allergy to penicillin is related to penicilloic acid—a breakdown product—and other degradation products that are involved in the metabolism of penicillin. All penicillins are cross-reactive and cross-sensitizing. Results of studies have shown that 80 to 90 percent of patients who report a penicillin allergy are not actually allergic to the drug. Therefore, it is obvious that many patients are labeled with a penicillin allergy when, in fact, they can take penicillin safely. The incidence of penicillin allergy is approximately 1% to 10% of adults. Symptoms include characteristic anaphylactoid symptoms with shock and bronchoconstriction in type 1 hypersensitivity reactions. Other symptoms include rashes, oral lesions, fever, joint swelling, pruritus, and respiratory distress. Methicillin and nafcillin have caused interstitial nephritis with RTA. The decision to use penicillin in patients with previous reactions should be based on the severity of previous reactions. If the patient has had a severe anaphylactic reaction in the past, penicillins should be avoided. In addition, there is a 2% cross-reactivity between cephalosporins in patients with penicillin allergies; thus, cephalosporins should be avoided in patients who have had an immediate reaction to penicillin. The same is true for imipenem. Skin tests that use penicilloyl-polylysine and undegraded penicillin may be used to detect patients who have true penicillin allergies.

Additional Reading: The clinical evaluation of penicillin allergy: what is necessary, sufficient and safe given the materials currently available? *Clin Exp Allergy.* 2011;41:1498–1501.

Category: Nonspecific system

219. Which of the following would best help to stop bleeding in a patient with von Willebrand's disease?
A) Fresh-frozen plasma
B) Cryoprecipitate
C) Vitamin K
D) Platelets
E) Protamine sulfate

Answer and Discussion

The answer is B. von Willebrand's disease is an autosomal-dominant transmitted disorder that can lead to abnormal bleeding tendencies. Men and women are equally affected. It is the most common congenital bleeding disorder. The disease is due to a lack of production of von Willebrand factor (type 1) or when the von Willebrand factor is not synthesized properly and is nonfunctional (type 2). The result is a decreased ability of platelets to adhere to collagen. Symptoms include mild-to-moderate bleeding from small cuts, bruising, epistaxis, excessive menstrual blood loss, GI blood loss, and excessive bleeding during surgery. Laboratory results show an increased bleeding time with a slightly prolonged partial thromboplastin time (PTT) if factor VIII is below 25% to 30%. In most cases, the PT, PTT, and platelet count are normal. Definitive diagnosis for von Willebrand's disease type 1 is made by measuring the levels of (1) von Willebrand factor, (2) antibody response to von Willebrand's antigen, (3) factor VIII, and (4) ristocetin cofactor activity. In patients with type 1 disease, all four measurements are decreased; in patients with type 2 disease, electrophoresis studies may be needed for the diagnosis. Treatment involves the administration of cryoprecipitate, which replaces the von Willebrand factor and stops bleeding. A pasteurized intermediate-purity factor VIII concentrate contains large multimers of von Willebrand factor and is a safe (no HIV or hepatitis) alternative cryoprecipitate. Desmopressin acetate, a synthetic analog of vasopressin, stimulates the release of von Willebrand factor from endothelial cells and can be used in the treatment of mild type 1 disease (but not of type 2). Oral contraceptives can also increase the levels of factor VIII and may be beneficial for women with menorrhagia.

> **Additional Reading:** Diagnosis and management of Von Willebrand disease: guidelines for primary care. *Am Fam Physician.* 2009;80(11):1261–1268.

> **Category:** Hematologic system

220. Which of the following values is acceptable for a 65-year-old man who had a previous coronary artery bypass graft?
A) Total cholesterol of 215 mg per dL
B) HDL cholesterol of 32 mg per dL
C) LDL cholesterol of 68 mg per dL
D) Triglycerides of 228 mg per dL
E) Blood glucose of 130 mg per dL

Answer and Discussion

The answer is C. Guidelines have been published to help treat patients with hyperlipidemia. Total cholesterol levels should be kept <200 mg per dL, with HDL cholesterol (good cholesterol) >40 mg per dL. Further recommendations are divided into those patients with CHD and those without CHD. CHD equivalents include peripheral arterial disease, AAA, symptomatic carotid arterial disease, and diabetes mellitus. For patients without CHD and fewer than two risk factors, LDL cholesterol should be kept <160 mg per dL. For those with two or more risk factors and no CAD, the goal is an LDL level <130 mg per dL. For patients who have CAD, the new recommendations give a goal for LDL cholesterol <100 mg per dL with <70 mg per dL as being optimal. Triglyceride levels are not as strongly associated with CAD but should be kept <150 mg per dL. Risk factors for CHD include the following:

- Age: men older than 45 years; women older than 55 years or with premature menopause without estrogen replacement
- Family history of premature CHD in first-degree relative
- Smoking
- Hypertension
- HDL cholesterol <35 mg per dL
- Diabetes
- Obesity
- History of cerebral or peripheral vascular disease

A negative risk factor includes an HDL cholesterol level higher than 60 mg per dL.

> **Additional Reading:** National Cholesterol Education Program: Third report of the expert panel on detection, evaluation, and treatment of high blood cholesterol in adults (Adult Treatment Panel III). From: http://www.nhlbi.nih.gov/guidelines/cholesterol/index.htm.

> **Category:** Cardiovascular system

221. Which of the following statements about Still's murmur is true?
A) It is benign and resolves over time.
B) It is common in the elderly and results from decreased ventricular compliance.
C) It is associated with severe chronic aortic regurgitation.
D) It should always be assessed with an echocardiogram.
E) CHF is usually coexistent.

Answer and Discussion

The answer is A. Some murmurs are specific to certain cardiac conditions:

- *Austin Flint murmur* is associated with severe chronic aortic regurgitation and may be middiastolic or presystolic. The murmur occurs when there is backflow of blood from the aorta into the left ventricle and flow into the left ventricle from the left atrium. The regurgitant stream often prevents the full opening of the mitral valve, thus obstructing flow into the ventricle.
- *Still's murmur* affects children and is described as a humming or musical-sounding systolic murmur that is loudest at the left sternal border. It is a benign murmur. The murmur is usually heard in children 3 to 7 years of age and disappears before the onset of puberty.
- *Physiologic S_3 murmur* affects approximately 33% of children younger than 16 years who have a physiologic S_3 heart sound that disappears before 30 years of age. The sound is best heard with the patient in the left lateral decubitus position, with the bell of the stethoscope over the point of maximal impulse. The sound is usually a low-frequency thud that occurs in early diastole.

> **Additional Reading:** Evaluation and management of heart murmurs in children. *Am Fam Physician.* 2011;84(7):793–800.

> **Category:** Cardiovascular system

> *Still's murmur* affects children and is described as a humming or musical-sounding systolic murmur that is loudest at the left sternal border. It is a benign murmur. The murmur is usually heard in children 3 to 7 years of age and disappears before the onset of puberty.

222. A hospitalized patient is receiving a blood transfusion. The floor nurse reports that the patient is flushed, is complaining of abdominal discomfort, and has a temperature of 101°F. The most appropriate management is to
A) Give the patient acetaminophen and continue the transfusion at a slower rate
B) Administer diphenhydramine and continue the transfusion
C) Administer 100 mg of hydrocortisone intravenously and reduce the rate of the transfusion
D) Stop the transfusion and increase intravenous fluids
E) Administer intravenous ranitidine and order an abdominal series x-ray

Answer and Discussion

The answer is D. Many hemolytic transfusion reactions are caused by human error in the laboratory during the matching process or during the administration of blood. Symptoms may include anxiety, dyspnea, tachycardia, flushing, headache, chest or abdominal pain, nausea, vomiting, and shock with an acute decrease in blood pressure. In most cases, the severity of symptoms and the prognosis depend on the amount of transfusion, rate of delivery, degree of incompatibility, and overall health of the patient. The laboratory evaluation for hemolysis consists of measurements of serum haptoglobin, lactate dehydrogenase, and indirect bilirubin levels. The immune complexes that result in RBC lysis can cause renal dysfunction and failure. Treatment consists of stopping the transfusion as soon as possible, vigorous diuresis with furosemide or mannitol, and possible dialysis if renal failure occurs. With multiple transfusions, the patient may develop antibodies to WBC antigens, which cause febrile reactions that are manifested by chills and temperatures higher than 100.4°F. Using washed RBCs helps prevent these reactions.

> **Additional Reading:** Transfusion of blood and blood products: indications and complications. *Am Fam Physician.* 2011;83(6):719–724.

> Category: Hematologic system

223. A 52-year-old patient who is hypertensive presents to your office after an episode of transient weakness in his right arm that occurred several days ago. The episode lasted about five minutes and was not accompanied by speech difficulty. His blood pressure has been well controlled and measures 130/78 mm Hg during the office visit. You diagnose him with possible TIA. Which of the following is correct about recurrent stroke?
A) Five to 10 percent of patients presenting with TIA will have a stroke within the following week.
B) The ABCD (Age, Blood pressure, Clinical features, Duration of symptoms) rule for predicting stroke risk after TIA is not helpful in predicting recurrent stroke.
C) The risk of stroke within 90 days after a TIA has been reported at 50%.
D) Approximately one-half of strokes occurring within 90 days after the initial presentation will need surgical intervention.

Answer and Discussion

The answer is D. The risk of stroke within 90 days after a TIA has been reported at 10% to 20%, with approximately one-half of these strokes occurring within the first 48 hours after initial presentation. Early initiation of treatment after a TIA, including medication and surgical intervention, can significantly reduce the risk of early stroke. Advantages of admission include the opportunity for complete diagnostic evaluation, confirmation of the diagnosis, and early treatment to reduce the risk of stroke. The potential administration of tissue plasminogen activator may be optimized if an early stroke occurs while the patient is hospitalized and should be considered in any patients with lesions on MRI. Urgent access to tissue plasminogen activator and management of TIA can reduce subsequent stroke risk. Of those presenting with TIA or minor stroke, 50% to 80% have elevated blood pressure on initial evaluation. Patients with systolic blood pressure greater than 140 mm Hg or diastolic blood pressure greater than 90 mm Hg are at higher risk of stroke after TIA (OR = 2.1, 1.9, and 1.6 at 2, 7, and 90 days, respectively).

> **Additional Reading:** Transient ischemic attack: Part II. Risk factor modification and treatment. *Am Fam Physician.* 2012;86(6):527–532.

> Category: Neurologic

224. A 24-year-old presents to your office with numbness noted in her feet bilaterally. She also complains of severe premenstrual syndrome (PMS) symptoms. The most likely cause for her symptoms related to her feet is
A) Excessive use of ibuprofen
B) Hysterical psychosis
C) Folate deficiency
D) Iron-deficiency anemia
E) Excessive vitamin B_6 intake

Answer and Discussion

The answer is E. Women frequently take large daily doses of vitamin B_6 for PMS, even though nutritional deficiency of this vitamin is rare. However, supplementation with 50 to 100 mg of vitamin B_6 per day may improve PMS symptoms. The recommended dietary allowance is about 2 mg per day; high intake has been associated with severe toxicity, including neuropathy. An intake of 200 mg per day may cause reversible damage, and an intake of 2,000 mg per day or greater is associated with peripheral neuropathy. In some European countries, the quantity of vitamin B_6 that may be purchased or prescribed has been restricted to reduce the risk of toxicity from excessive use.

SSRIs have been shown to be effective in relieving PMS symptoms; however, paroxetine (Paxil) should be avoided because of its increased risk for congenital abnormalities when taken in the first trimester of pregnancy.

> **Additional Reading:** Premenstrual syndrome and premenstrual dysphoric disorder. *Am Fam Physician.* 2011;84(8):918–924.

> Category: Neurologic

225. A 71-year-old presents to the emergency room with shortness of breath, hemoptysis, and chest pain. Further tests include an ECG with findings of right-axis deviation, an S1-Q3-T3 pattern, and a right bundle branch block. The most likely diagnosis is
A) Acute MI
B) Community-acquired pneumonia
C) Bronchogenic carcinoma
D) PE
E) Pericarditis

Answer and Discussion

The answer is D. A PE is a thrombus that lodges in the pulmonary vasculature and may give rise to a pulmonary infarction. In most cases, the thrombus forms in the leg or pelvic veins. The most dangerous thrombi form in the iliofemoral vein. Other causes of emboli include fat emboli after fractures and amniotic fluid emboli, which are rare. Risk factors for PE include malignancy, hereditary impaired coagulation, estrogen therapy, obesity, CHF, orthopaedic or pelvic surgery, and prolonged anesthesia. Signs and symptoms include tachypnea, cough, hemoptysis, chest pain, fever, and cyanosis (in severe cases). Diagnosis is based on the clinical history and supportive tests, including a ventilation-perfusion scan and pulmonary arteriogram. Arterial blood tests show hypoxia (PO_2 <60 mm Hg), and ECG findings are nonspecific (T-wave abnormalities in the precordial leads and sinus tachycardia). In addition, right-axis deviation, an S1-Q3-T3 pattern, and a right bundle branch block may be observed. Further testing may include venous studies of the lower extremities to look for thrombus; however, >20% of patients may have no evidence of venous embolism. Chest radiographs are usually normal; however, a homogenous, wedge-shaped density based in the pleura and pointing to the hilum (Hampton's hump) is highly suggestive of PE. Treatment involves anticoagulation for 3 to 6 months with oral warfarin or thrombolytic therapy and embolectomy if the patient has hypotension and continuing hypoxemia while receiving high fractions of inspired oxygen. Thrombolytic therapy is not indicated for the routine treatment of patients with PE. A stepwise approach to the diagnosis of pulmonary embolus consists of a ventilation-perfusion scan. A high-probability ventilation-perfusion scan provides sufficient evidence for the initiation of treatment for PE. Likewise, a normal scan should be considered sufficient to exclude PE. Unfortunately, 50% to 70% of scans are indeterminate (low or intermediate probability). If the results show a high probability of PE, treatment with anticoagulants is indicated. If the ventilation-perfusion scan is normal, treatment is not indicated. If the lung scan shows intermediate or low probability of pulmonary embolus, a noninvasive leg test (ultrasound) for proximal DVT should be obtained. If the leg test is positive, then treatment is indicated. If the leg test is negative and suspicion is high, then a pulmonary angiogram or another ultrasound and d-dimer test can be repeated in 5 to 7 days. If the test is negative, the risk for pulmonary embolus is low. A spiral CT of the chest can also be used for rapid diagnosis.

Additional Reading: Diagnosis of deep venous thrombosis and pulmonary embolism. *Am Fam Physician.* 2012;86(10):913–919.

Category: Cardiovascular system

226. Which of the following statements about macular degeneration is true?
A) The wet form is usually more severe than the dry form.
B) Neovascularization is typically associated with drusen and the dry form.
C) It typically affects only peripheral vision.
D) The condition is more common in African American individuals.
E) The condition is rarely progressive.

Answer and Discussion

The answer is A. Macular degeneration associated with aging is a leading cause of blindness in the elderly. The condition is more common in whites, appears to be hereditary, and is associated with atrophy or degeneration of the macular disc. There are basically two types: atrophic or dry and exudative or wet. Both types usually occur bilaterally and are progressive. The dry form usually progresses slowly and affects the outer retina, retinal pigment epithelium, choriocapillaries, and Bruch's membrane. The wet form of macular degeneration is more severe and progressive, usually affects the eyes sequentially, and is responsible for approximately 90% of blindness in those affected with macular degeneration. The wet form occurs when there is drusen (i.e., degeneration of the pigment epithelium and Bruch's membrane) and accumulation of serous fluid or blood in the retina that produces elevation of the retinal pigment membrane from Bruch's membrane. Neovascularization may then occur, giving rise to a subretinal neovascular membrane that causes permanent vision loss. There is no specific treatment for macular degeneration; however, laser photocoagulation may help stop neovascularization in select cases, and vision aids may help acuity. Macular degeneration affects central vision and does not affect peripheral vision.

Additional Reading: Vision loss in older persons. *Am Fam Physician.* 2009;79(11):963–970.

Category: Special sensory

227. Hypersplenism is associated with all of the following *except*
A) Lymphoma
B) Polycythemia vera
C) Infectious Mononucleosis (IM)
D) Hereditary spherocytosis
E) CHF

Answer and Discussion

The answer is E. Hypersplenism is associated with a number of disorders that lead to a reduction in one or more blood constituents, leading to leukopenia, thrombocytopenia, or a combination of both. Most cases of chronic hemolytic anemias are associated with splenomegaly. Causes of splenomegaly include lymphoma, leukemia, polycythemia vera, myelofibrosis, IM, psittacosis, subacute bacterial endocarditis, tuberculosis, malaria, syphilis, kala-azar, brucellosis, sarcoidosis, amyloidosis, SLE, Felty's syndrome, hereditary spherocytosis, thalassemias, cirrhosis, Gaucher's disease, Niemann–Pick disease, Schüller–Christian disease, Letterer–Siwe disease, and thrombosis or compression of the portal or splenic veins. Patients may exhibit bleeding disorders, palpable splenomegaly, left-upper abdominal discomfort, or splenic bruits. Management usually involves treatment of the underlying disorder; elective splenectomy is reserved for refractory cases. Asplenic patients are at increased risk for infection secondary to encapsulated bacteria and should receive pneumococcal immunization.

Additional Reading: Epocrates Online: Evaluation of splenomegaly. From: https://online.epocrates.com/u/2932895/Evaluation+of+splenomegaly/References/Credits.

Category: Hematologic system

228. Which of the following laboratory results best support the diagnosis of subclinical hypothyroidism?
A) Normal T_4, low TSH
B) Normal T_4, high TSH
C) Low T_4, high TSH
D) Normal T_4, normal TSH
E) Low T_4, borderline low TSH

Answer and Discussion

The answer is B. The following are laboratory findings associated with thyroid dysfunction:

Diagnosis	Laboratory Findings
Overt hypothyroidism	Low T_4, high TSH
Subclinical hypothyroidism	Normal T_4, high TSH
Hypothyroidism secondary to hypopituitarism	Low T_4, normal or borderline low TSH
Euthyroid	Normal T_4, normal TSH
Subclinical hyperthyroidism	Normal T_4, low TSH

Additional Reading: Hypothyroidism: an update. *Am Fam Physician.* 2012;86(3):244–251.

Category: Endocrine system

229. The proportion of disease-free patients in whom a test result is negative is referred to as
A) The *p* value
B) Sensitivity
C) Specificity
D) Reliability
E) Variability

Answer and Discussion

The answer is C. *Specificity* is defined as the proportion of people who are not affected by a given disease and who also test negative for that disease. For example, the proportion of patients who do not have CAD and also test negative with a treadmill exercise test would be defined as the specificity. This specificity, as mentioned in the answer to question 234, is up to 95%. If this percentage is high, it is a highly specific test.

Additional Reading: Terms used in evidence-based medicine. *Am Fam Physician*. From: http://www.aafp.org/journals/afp/authors/ebm-toolkit/glossary.html.

Category: Patient/population-based care

> Specificity is defined as the proportion of people who are not affected by a given disease and who also test negative for that disease.

230. Inflammation and necrosis of the muscular tissue supplied by small- and medium-size arteries is known as
A) Polyarteritis nodosa
B) Pyoderma gangrenosum
C) Polymyositis
D) Giant cell arteritis
E) Dermatomyositis

Answer and Discussion

The answer is A. Polyarteritis nodosa is a condition characterized by inflammation and necrosis of the muscular tissue supplied by small- and medium-size arteries. The cause is unknown but may be associated with an autoimmune response, medication (e.g., sulfonamides, iodide, thiazides, bismuth, penicillins), and infections. Involvement of the renal and visceral arteries is characteristic, but pulmonary arteries are usually spared. Affected individuals are usually between 40 and 50 years of age; men are more commonly affected. Symptoms include fever, abdominal pain, peripheral neuropathy, headaches, seizures, weakness, and weight loss. Those with renal involvement may show hypertension, edema, azotemia, and oliguria. Other symptoms include angina, nausea, vomiting, diarrhea, myalgias, and arthralgias. Palpable subcutaneous lesions that sometimes necrose may be found in the area of an affected artery. Laboratory studies show leukocytosis, proteinuria, microscopic hematuria, thrombocytosis, and an elevated ESR. Diagnosis is usually made with a biopsy of affected tissue, which shows necrotizing arteritis. Treatment involves avoidance of the offending agent and often long-term, high-dose steroid therapy and cyclophosphamide for severe cases and steroids alone for milder cases. The disease can be fatal if untreated.

Polymyositis is an idiopathic inflammatory myopathy with symmetrical, proximal muscle weakness. Histopathology demonstrates endomysial mononuclear inflammatory infiltrate and muscle fiber necrosis.

Dermatomyositis is clinically similar to polymyositis, an idiopathic, inflammatory myopathy associated with characteristic skin findings that include a violet or dusky red rash seen on the face and eyelids and on skin around the nails, knuckles, elbows, knees, chest, and back. The rash can be patchy with bluish-purple discolorations and is often the first sign of dermatomyositis.

Giant cell arteritis, also known as temporal arteritis, is a vasculitis of the large and medium arteries of the head and neck. Giant cell arteritis typically presents with a headache and nonspecific systemic symptoms. The temporal artery is tender to palpations, and a high ESR is detected. The diagnosis is confirmed by patchy inflammation of arterial walls, characterized by the infiltration of mononuclear cells and the presence of giant cells from a temporal artery biopsy.

Pyoderma gangrenosum causes deep leg ulcers, with necrotic tissue, and they can lead to chronic wounds. Ulcers initially present as small papules and progress to larger ulcers, causing pain and scarring.

Additional Reading: Systemic vasculitis. *Am Fam Physician*. 2011;83(5):556–565.

Category: Integumentary

231. A 55-year-old man with past medical history of diabetes mellitus, HTN and dyslipidemia presented to the ED with a day of left-sided weakness. MRI brain was consistent with acute ischemic stroke in the middle cerebral territory. What is the best medical management for this patient?
A) Clopidogrel
B) Coumadin
C) Heparin
D) Aspirin
E) Ibuprofen

Answer and Discussion

The answer is D. Aspirin in a daily dose of 160 to 300 mg initiated within 48 hours of symptom onset results in a net decrease in morbidity and mortality caused by acute ischemic stroke regardless of the availability of CT. Aspirin is as effective as anticoagulants such as Coumadin and heparin in this regard and causes less harm, but it should not be used in patients receiving thrombolytic therapy.

Ibuprofen (Motrin) may decrease aspirin's effectiveness in acute ischemic stroke. A Cochrane systematic review summarizing 15 trials ($n = 16,558$) comparing anticoagulants (unfractionated heparin or LMW heparin) versus aspirin in acute ischemic stroke. No significant difference was found in rates of death or dependency, recurrent stroke, neurologic deterioration, or DVT/PE. However, anticoagulants were associated with higher rates of symptomatic intracranial hemorrhage (OR = 2.27; 95% CI, 1.49 to 3.46), major extracranial hemorrhage (OR = 1.94; 95% CI, 1.20 to 3.12), and all-cause mortality (OR = 1.10; 95% CI, 1.01 to 1.29).

Two trials have evaluated the use of clopidogrel for secondary stroke prevention. One trial compared clopidogrel with aspirin alone, and the other with combination aspirin/dipyridamole. Results from both trials found that rates of primary outcomes were similar between treatment groups. Adverse effects of clopidogrel include diarrhea and rash, although gastrointestinal symptoms and hemorrhage are less common than in persons taking aspirin. PPIs have been shown to reduce the effectiveness of clopidogrel and may also increase the risk of major cardiovascular events when taken with clopidogrel.

Compared with clopidogrel alone, the combination of clopidogrel and aspirin for prevention of vascular effects in persons with a recent TIA or ischemic stroke was not found to have a significant benefit. There was a significantly increased risk of major hemorrhage in persons taking combination therapy compared with those taking clopidogrel alone. When compared with aspirin alone, combination clopidogrel and aspirin did not have a statistically significant benefit but did increase the risk of bleeding in patients who had previously had a stroke.

Additional Reading: Aspirin in patients with acute ischemic stroke. *Am Fam Physician*. 2009;79(3):226–227.

AHA/ASA guidelines on prevention of recurrent stroke. *Am Fam Physician*. 2011;83(8):993–1001.

Category: Neurologic

232. Which one of the following is not a risk factor for stroke?
A) Hypertension
B) Obesity and physical inactivity
C) DM
D) Dyslipidemia
E) Alcohol consumption

Answer and Discussion

The answer is E. Patients with hypertension have an increased risk of stroke, and blood pressure control reduces this risk. Blood pressure control after TIA is associated with a 30% to 40% Relative Risk Reduction (RRR), with larger blood pressure decreases conferring a greater decrease in stroke risk. Variable blood pressure readings in a patient with hypertension may be an important predictor of cerebral ischemia, as well as the effects of antihypertensive agents. In a cohort of patients with TIA, increased visit-to-visit variability of systolic blood pressure and maximum systolic blood pressure reached were strong predictors of subsequent stroke. CCBs have been shown to reduce this variability, thus lowering the risk of stroke.

Current smoking has been shown to increase blood pressure, augment atherosclerosis, and increase the risk of stroke two- to fourfold compared with not smoking. There is a dose–response relationship between smoking and cerebral ischemia, with the heaviest smokers at the highest risk. Smokers with new medical diagnoses, such as TIA and stroke, are three times more likely to successfully change their lifestyle habits.

More than one in four persons will become clinically obese, and increased waist-to-hip ratio increases the risk of stroke. Regular physical activity has been shown to reduce the risk of TIA and stroke. High-intensity activity leads to an RRR of 64%, compared with inactivity. Diets rich in fruits and vegetables, such as the Mediterranean diet, can help control body weight and have been shown to reduce the risk of stroke and MI by at least 60%. The American Heart Association/American Stroke Association recommends weight reduction, at least 30 minutes of moderate to intensity physical activity daily, and a diet low in sodium and high in fruits, vegetables, and low-fat dairy products, such as the DASH (Dietary Approaches to Stop Hypertension) diet.

Diabetes is a well-established risk factor for CVD and confers a hazard ratio of 2.27 for ischemic stroke. Patients with newly diagnosed diabetes have double the rate of stroke compared with the general population, making early intervention and risk factor modification imperative. In most patients who have had a TIA, the A1C target is less than 7% as A1C reduction to targets of less than 6% has not been shown to decrease cardiovascular deaths or all-cause mortality.

Dyslipidemia has also been shown to be a significant risk factor for ischemic stroke. A large prospective cohort study showed a strong association between serum cholesterol levels and cerebral ischemia, with risk increasing proportionally to serum levels. In addition, a large meta-analysis studying the effect of statins on stroke reduction showed that the larger the reduction in low-density lipoprotein (LDL) cholesterol levels, the greater the reduction in stroke risk.

Some studies have suggested that 1 alcoholic drink a day may lower a person's risk for stroke, and recommendations are for moderate alcohol consumption range from 1 to 2 drinks per day. However, heavier drinking (>3 drinks per day) may increase stroke risk.

> Additional Reading: Transient ischemic attack: Part II. Risk factor modification and treatment. *Am Fam Physician*. 2012;86(6):527–532.

Category: Neurologic

233. The most common location for the development of Morton's neuroma is
A) The trigeminal nerve
B) Interdigital nerves between the fourth and fifth metacarpal heads
C) Interdigital nerves between the third and fourth metatarsal heads
D) The median nerve
E) The sural nerve

Answer and Discussion

The answer is C. Morton's neuroma is a common type of forefoot pain. The condition arises from entrapment of the common interdigital nerves between the metatarsal heads. This nerve entrapment leads to inflammation, edema, pain, and the formation of perineural fibrosis and demyelination, which causes a neuroma. The most common location for the neuroma is between the third and fourth metatarsal heads; they also commonly occur between the second and third metatarsal heads. Women are more commonly affected than men (5:1 ratio). Patients report pain, paresthesias, or occasionally a catching sensation in these locations, which may extend distally to the toes or proximally to the midfoot. Many patients report their symptoms are worse when wearing shoes. The distinguishing feature in the differential between metatarsalgia and Morton's neuroma is pain between the metatarsal heads. Radiographs are normal; however, MRIs may show the offending neuroma but are rarely necessary to make the diagnosis. Treatment involves NSAIDs, metatarsal footpads, wide shoes, and steroid injections (using a dorsal approach between the metatarsals); in severe cases, surgical excision of the neuroma is indicated, although persistent pain remains for approximately 33% of patients after surgery.

> Additional Reading: Busconi BD, Stevenson JH. Approach to the Athlete with Morton's Neuroma. *Sports Medicine Consult: A Problem-Based Approach to Sports Medicine for the Primary Care Physician*. Philadelphia, PA: Lippincott, Williams & Wilkins; 2009.

Category: Musculoskeletal system

234. Which of the following is associated with chronic fatigue syndrome?
A) Temporal artery tenderness
B) Minimal (less than 10%) impairment of normal activity
C) High incidence of associated psychiatric disorders
D) Muscle weakness
E) Recent EBV infection

Answer and Discussion

The answer is C. Fatigue is a common complaint heard in a family physician's office. Broadly defined, the chronic fatigue syndrome is described as long-standing severe fatigue without substantial muscle weakness and without proven psychologic or physical causes. Various criteria have been published. The Centers for Disease Control and Prevention Diagnostic Criteria for Chronic Fatigue Syndrome include the following:

- Severe fatigue for longer than 6 months, and at least four of the following symptoms:
  - Headache of new type, pattern, or severity
  - Multijoint pain without swelling or erythema
  - Muscle pain
  - Postexertional malaise for longer than 24 hours
  - Significant impairment in short-term memory or concentration
  - Sore throat
  - Tender lymph nodes
  - Unrefreshing sleep

Symptoms may develop acutely. Typically, there are no signs of muscle weakness, arthritis, neuropathy, or organomegaly. Women are more often affected than men. The syndrome has not been proven to be associated with EBV; however, some believe it may be linked to a viral infection. Persons with chronic fatigue should be evaluated with a comprhensive history and physical examination. Initial laboratory testing would include urinalysis, complete blood count, comprehensive metabolic panel, TSH, C-reactive protein, and phosphorus levels.

There appears to be a high incidence of associated psychiatric disorders, and patients with chronic fatigue syndrome should be evaluated for concurrent depression, pain, and sleep disturbances. Persons diagnosed with chronic fatigue syndrome should be treated with cognitive behavior therapy, graded exercise therapy, or both. Cognitive behavior therapy and graded exercise therapy have been shown to improve fatigue, work and social adjustment, anxiety, and postexertional malaise. Although no placebo-controlled trials have supported the treatment, antidepressants have shown some anecdotal benefits in those affected. Antiviral medication, immunologic treatments (steroids, immunoglobin, interferon), and vitamin therapy are used, but their effectiveness has not been proved. Psychological therapy may be beneficial. Patients should be encouraged to maintain a gradually increasing program of activity.

Additional Reading: Chronic fatigue syndrome: diagnosis and treatment. *Am Fam Physician.* 2012;86(8):741–746.

Category: Nonspecific system

235. Which of the following statements about premature ventricular complexes (PVCs) is correct?
A) They are narrow electrocardiographic wave (QRS) complexes that are preceded by P waves.
B) In most cases, they disappear with exercise.
C) They are treated with type IC antiarrhythmics.
D) They may represent a risk for sudden death in healthy patients.
E) Caffeine use is not associated with PVCs.

Answer and Discussion

The answer is B. PVCs are abnormal ventricular beats that are characterized by wide QRS complexes, which are usually not preceded by P waves. In patients with normal hearts, PVCs usually disappear with exercise. If the patient remains asymptomatic and there is no organic heart disease, no further treatment is necessary. If PVCs are frequent, electrolyte abnormalities and heart disease should be excluded. Patients with frequent, repetitive, or multiform PVCs and underlying heart disease are at increased risk for sudden death because of cardiac arrhythmia (particularly ventricular fibrillation). Without underlying cardiac disease, bigeminy and trigeminy are considered benign rhythms. Treatment of PVCs is controversial but

should be reserved for symptomatic patients. If MVP, hypertrophic obstructive cardiomyopathy, prolonged QT interval, LVH, or CAD is present, a trial of β blockers can be used. Types IA (quinidine, procainamide) and IB (lidocaine, mexiletine) antiarrhythmic agents may be used; however, they are associated with a high incidence of side effects and can make the arrhythmias worse. Type IC agents (flecainide, propafenone) should not be used because of their potential for increased mortality rates. Elimination of exogenous catecholamines, sympathomimetic amines, alcohol, and caffeine may decrease symptoms. In general, antiarrhythmic drug therapy is rarely necessary.

Additional Reading: Clinical significance and treatment of ventricular premature beats. In: Basow DS, ed. *UpToDate*. Waltham, MA: UpToDate; 2013.

Category: Cardiovascular system

236. Which of the following statements about lung cancer is true?
A) Squamous cell and small cell tumors are rarely associated with smoking.
B) Squamous cell tumors typically arise in central bronchi and may be diagnosed with sputum cytology.
C) Large cell tumors are common, arise centrally, and typically metastasize locally.
D) Small cell carcinoma is usually located peripherally and rarely metastasizes.
E) Yearly chest x-rays are recommended for smokers above age 50.

Answer and Discussion

The answer is B. Lung cancer caused by tobacco abuse is a significant health problem that accounts for approximately 150,000 deaths yearly in the United States. Most cases appear between 50 and 70 years of age. Unfortunately, at the time of diagnosis, only approximately 20% of patients have localized disease. The following are the most common types (typically the cancers are divided into small cell cancers and non–small cell cancers):

- *Squamous cell (epidermoid).* As much as 30% to 35% of lung cancers. One of the most common types seen in men, these tumors tend to arise from the central (larger) bronchi and are the most easily diagnosed with sputum cytology. Most of these tumors metastasize locally to the regional lymph nodes and are more localized at the time of diagnosis.

- *Large cell.* As much as 10% to 15% of lung cancers. Less common in incidence, these tumors usually metastasize through the bloodstream. Approximately 20% of patients may develop cavitary lesions. These tumors are usually located peripherally.

- *Adenocarcinoma.* As much as 25% to 35% of lung cancers. One of the more common types, these tumors are usually located peripherally and are usually advanced at the time of diagnosis. It spreads through the bloodstream and lymphatics. A subset of tumors referred to as *bronchoalveolar* is growing in incidence.

- *Small cell (oat cell).* Approximately 15% of lung cancers. This type also tends to occur centrally and is usually widespread at the time of diagnosis.

Additional Reading: Lung, primary malignancies. In: Domino F, ed. *The 5-Minute Clinical Consult.* Philadelphia, PA: Lippincott Williams and Wilkins; 2014.

Category: Respiratory system

237. Which of the following is a potentially severe complication of using warfarin that is unrelated to excessive bleeding?
A) Pancreatic neoplasm
B) Hepatitis
C) Skin necrosis
D) Peripheral neuropathy
E) Pulmonary fibrosis

Answer and Discussion

The answer is C. Warfarin is classified as an anticoagulant. Its mechanism of action is the inhibition of vitamin K-dependent clotting factors (i.e., factors II, VII, IX, and X). The medication is used in stroke prophylaxis for patients with prior neurologic events, atrial fibrillation, mechanical heart valves, or previous DVT or PE. Warfarin interacts with many medications, so concomitant use with other drugs should be monitored carefully. Most complications are related to bleeding; however, other side effects, including nausea, vomiting, fever, burning of the feet, and rashes, may occur. The most common complication unrelated to excessive bleeding is skin necrosis, which usually occurs within the first week of therapy. Some cases may be severe enough to require surgical debridement or even amputation. Patients treated with warfarin should have their PTs and INRs followed to ensure proper levels of anticoagulation.

Additional Reading: Warfarin-induced skin necrosis. *J Am Acad Dermatol.* 2009;61(2):325–332.

Category: Cardiovascular system

> Warfarin's mechanism of action is the inhibition of vitamin K-dependent clotting factors (i.e., factors II, VII, IX, and X).

238. Which of the following is a diagnostic criterion for the presence of diabetes mellitus?
A) Random plasma glucose >200 mg per dL
B) Fasting plasma glucose of 140 mg per dL
C) Abnormal glucose tolerance test
D) Hemoglobin A1C (HbA$_{1c}$) of 7.5
E) All of the above

Answer and Discussion

The answer is E. American Diabetes Association (ADA) consensus guidelines lowered the blood glucose thresholds for the diagnosis of diabetes. This increased the number of patients diagnosed at an earlier stage, although no studies have demonstrated a reduction in long-term complications. Data suggest that as many as 5.7 million persons in the United States have undiagnosed diabetes.

Blood glucose measurements. The diagnosis of diabetes is based on one of three methods of blood glucose measurement. Diabetes can be diagnosed if the patient has a fasting blood glucose level of 126 mg per dL (7.0 mmol per L) or greater on two separate occasions. Diabetes can also be diagnosed with a random blood glucose level of 200 mg per dL (11.1 mmol per L) or greater if classic symptoms of diabetes (e.g., polyuria, polydipsia, weight loss, blurred vision, fatigue) are present.

Lower random blood glucose values (140 to 180 mg per dL have a fairly high specificity of 92% to 98%; therefore, patients with these values should undergo more definitive testing. A low sensitivity of 39% to 55% limits the use of random blood glucose testing.

The oral glucose tolerance test is considered a first-line diagnostic test. In 2003, the ADA lowered the threshold for diagnosis of

impaired fasting glucose to include a fasting glucose level between 100 and 125 mg per dL (5.6 and 6.9 mmol per L). Impaired glucose tolerance continues to be defined as a blood glucose level between 140 and 199 mg per dL 2 hours after a 75-g load. Patients meeting either of these criteria are at significantly higher risk of progression to diabetes and should be counseled on effective strategies to lower their risk, such as weight loss and exercise.

A1C. A1C measurement has recently been endorsed by the ADA as a diagnostic and screening tool for diabetes. One advantage of using A1C measurement is the ease of testing because it does not require fasting. An A1C level of greater than 6.5% on two separate occasions is considered diagnostic of diabetes. Lack of standardization has historically deterred its use, but this test is now widely standardized in the United States. A1C measurements for diagnosis of diabetes should be performed by a clinical laboratory because of the lack of standardization of point-of-care testing. Limitations of A1C testing include low sensitivity, possible racial disparities, and interference by anemia and some medications.

Additional Reading: Diabetes mellitus: diagnosis and screening. *Am Fam Physician.* 2010;81(7):863–870.

Category: Endocrine system

239. Which of the following is indicated in the treatment of chronic CHF?
A) Atenolol
B) Metoprolol
C) Propanolol
D) Acebutolol
E) Timolol

Answer and Discussion

The answer is B. Unless there is a specific contraindication, all patients with heart failure and systolic dysfunction (Left Ventricular Ejection Fraction (EF) ≤40%) should take both an ACE inhibitor and a β-blocker, and if volume overloaded, a diuretic as well. An ARB is recommended for patients who cannot tolerate an ACE inhibitor. Addition of an aldosterone antagonist can be beneficial for patients with symptomatic heart failure or for patients with left ventricular dysfunction after an MI. A combination of hydralazine and isosorbide dinitrate added to standard therapy has been effective in African American patients with class III to IV heart failure. Digoxin can decrease symptoms and lower the rate of hospitalization for heart failure, but does not decrease mortality. There is no evidence that any drug improves clinical outcomes in patients with heart failure with preserved systolic function.

Most guidelines recommend use of a β-blocker in addition to an ACE inhibitor for patients with symptomatic systolic heart failure and for asymptomatic patients with a decreased LVEF. Use of bisoprolol, carvedilol, or sustained-release metoprolol succinate consistently leads to a 30% to 40% reduction in mortality and hospitalization in adults with New York Heart Association (NYHA) class II to IV heart failure. β-Blockers should be started at a low dose and increased gradually to the highest tolerated dose. Full clinical benefits may not occur for 3 to 6 months or more. β-Blockers should be used cautiously, if at all, in patients with asthma or severe bradycardia.

There is no published evidence supporting the effectiveness of β-blockers other than bisoprolol, carvedilol, sustained-release metoprolol succinate, or nebivolol for treatment of heart failure. Bisoprolol and nebivolol are not approved for treatment of heart failure by the FDA, and nebivolol appears to be the least effective of the four.

Additional Reading: Drugs for chronic heart failure. *Treat Guidel Med Lett.* 2012;10(121):69–72.

Category: Cardiovascular system

240. Which of the following would best help to prevent shin splints?

A) Change in running surfaces
B) Ice therapy
C) Running on inclined surfaces
D) More intensive training schedule
E) Stretching before exercise

Answer and Discussion

The answer is E. Shin splints (medial tibial stress syndrome) are a common condition caused by overuse of the lower-extremity muscles. The condition is caused by a periosteitis of the tibia. They typically occur when an athlete's running surface (e.g., hills, inclines, stairs) is changed, when a different type of shoe is used, when an athlete's running style is altered, or when excessive training that does not allow adequate time for the muscles to recover is undertaken. Most affected athletes report pain over the lower tibial area that may be referred to the foot or knee. Any type of movement or exercise that works these muscle groups tends to make the pain worse. In addition to pain, mild diffuse swelling or redness may be noted over the tibia. The differential diagnosis includes stress fractures, exertional compartment syndrome, and tenosynovitis. Diagnosis is usually based on history and physical examination. In severe cases that are refractive to ice, rest, and NSAIDs, plain radiographs and perhaps a bone scan should be performed to rule out a stress fracture. If fractures are not noted, there may be diffuse increased uptake of technetium along the tibia in the area of the periosteum. If the patient is only mildly affected, exercise can be continued; however, more severe cases may require restriction of activity. When the pain and inflammation subsides, the athlete should be instructed in stretching exercises for the muscles of the lower extremity. If shin splints are recurrent, examination to rule out excessive pronation should be performed; if present, orthotics should be used to correct hyperpronation. It is now thought that medial tibial stress syndrome represents one end of a continuum of bony stress injury, with a focal stress fracture representing the other.

> **Additional Reading:** Busconi BD, Stevenson JH. Approach to the athlete with a tibial stress fracture. *Sports Medicine Consult: A Problem-Based Approach to Sports Medicine for the Primary Care Physician.* Philadelphia, PA: Lippincott, Williams & Wilkins; 2009.

Category: Muscoloskeletal system

241. Which of the following is the treatment of choice for pyoderma gangrenosum?

A) Steroid therapy
B) Topical antibiotics
C) Oral antibiotics that treat methicillin-resistant *S. aureus*
D) Methotrexate
E) Plasmapheresis

Answer and Discussion

The answer is A. Pyoderma gangrenosum is a rapidly evolving and severely debilitating skin disease that is characterized by a painful hemorrhagic pustule that breaks down to form a chronic ulcer. The ulcer is associated with pus production, and there is usually a dusky red or purple halo around the ulcer. The cause of the lesions is unknown, but they tend to form at the sites of trauma (most commonly the legs). The borders of the lesions are usually irregular, and the lesions are boggy and usually quite painful. Although as many as 50% of cases have no associated underlying abnormality, other diseases associated with pyoderma gangrenosum include Crohn's disease, ulcerative colitis, leukemia, paraproteinemia, multiple myeloma, rheumatoid arthritis, hepatitis, and Behcet's disease. The diagnosis of pyoderma gangrenosum is usually made by the history and clinical findings. Laboratory tests show elevated ESR and leukocytosis. Treatment involves correction of underlying disease and the use of high-dose oral steroids or intravenous pulse steroid therapy. Additional findings in these patients include cutaneous anergy and benign monoclonal gammopathy.

> **Additional Reading:** Pyoderma gangrenosum: treatment and prognosis. In: Domino F, ed. *UpToDate.* Waltham, MA: UpToDate; 2013.

Category: Integumentary

242. Which of the following is an acceptable treatment for *Helicobacter pylori* infection?

A) Bismuth, amoxicillin, metronidazole, and omeprazole
B) TMP-sulfamethoxazole, sucralfate, and metronidazole
C) Omeprazole, clindamycin, and sucralfate
D) Docusate, tetracycline, and metronidazole
E) Ranitidine, metronidazole, and ampicillin

Answer and Discussion

The answer is A. *Helicobacter pylori* is a bacteria found in the stomach that is present in >80% of patients with duodenal ulcers and up to 60% of those with gastric ulcers. The incidence appears to increase with increasing age. Most *H. pylori* colonization is asymptomatic. Test sensitivity is reduced if the patient is taking Proton Pump Inhibitors (PPIs), bismuth or antibiotics. Tests include urea breath testing. The patient ingests a urea solution with a carbon isotope and then breathes into a container; in the presence of *H. pylori*, urease hydrolyzes the urea to release labeled CO_2, which can be detected by a mass spectrometer. A stool antigen enzyme immunoassay is reliable in confirming successful treatment, but should not be used to test for eradication of *H. pylori* until at least 4 weeks after completion of therapy. Serology antibody tests for *H. pylori* are useful in ruling out the diagnosis, but they lack specificity and are not reliable (because of persisting antibodies) for documenting eradication. The gold standard for diagnosis is biopsy and histologic examination.

In large clinical trials, combinations of antimicrobial drugs have been successful in eradicating the organism in up to 90%, but in practice, eradication rates are lower due to increasing resistance to clarithromycin and metronidazole and poor patient adherence to the multidrug regimens. Eradication rates with commonly prescribed triple therapy regimens have fallen below 80%. Quadruple therapy and sequential therapy have higher rates of eradication. A recent study found no difference between sequential therapy and quadruple therapy, with both achieving eradication rates of 92% to 93%. Quadruple therapy should be considered for initial treatment in areas with a high rate (>20%) of clarithromycin-resistant *H. pylori*. Triple therapy includes clarithromycin, plus amoxicillin or metronidazole, plus a PPI. Quadruple treatment includes bismuth subsalicylate (PeptoBismol), plus metronidiazole, plus tetracycline plus a PPI.

Patients should be tested for successful eradication of *H. pylori* and those still infected after treatment with two different regimens should receive salvage therapy with a different regimen, such as a PPI, amoxicillin, and levofloxacin (Levaquin and others), if needed.

> **Additional Reading:** Drugs for peptic ulcer disease and GERD. *Treat Guidel Med Lett.* 2011;9(109):55–60.

Category: Gastroenterology system

243. Which of the following treatments is the treatment of choice for chronic allergic rhinitis?
A) Systemic antihistamines
B) Intranasal steroids
C) Topical decongestants
D) Cromolyn sodium
E) Bee pollen extract

Answer and Discussion

The answer is B. Allergic rhinitis is characterized by nasal congestion, clear rhinorrhea, mucosal thickening, and conjunctivitis with the absence of fever or sinus tenderness. Patients may exhibit a bluish discoloration below the eyelids ("allergic shiners") as a result of venous congestion. Constant nose rubbing is known as the "allergic salute" and can result in a crease across the bridge of the nose. Treatment involves avoiding the triggering factors such as pollens, molds, cigarette smoke, animal dander, and dust mites. Many patients report symptoms related to seasons (spring, summer, or fall). The best treatment is the administration of intranasal steroids, which have few associated side effects. Other treatment options include montelukast (Singulair), azelastine (Astelin nasal spray), cromolyn sodium, ipratropium bromide, and second-generation (nonsedating) systemic antihistamines such as loratadine (Claritin), fexofenadine (Allegra), and cetirizine (Zyrtec). The chronic use of topical decongestants can lead to rebound congestion known as rhinitis medicamentosa and should be used only on a temporary basis (i.e., no more than 3 days). Immunotherapy may also be an alternative treatment for debilitating symptoms.

Additional Reading: Drugs for allergic disorders. *Treat Guidel Med Lett.* 2013;11(129):43–52.

Category: Respiratory system

244. A 24-year-old intravenous drug abuser presents with fever, night sweats, chest pain, and arthralgias. On examination, painless erythematous lesions are noted on the palms of the hands; round, erythematous lesions with central clearing are noted in the retina; and splinter hemorrhages are noted on the fingernails. The most likely diagnosis is
A) HIV infection
B) Bacterial endocarditis
C) Syphilis
D) Infectious hepatitis
E) Lyme disease

Answer and Discussion

The answer is B. Bacterial endocarditis is an infection of the endocardium and heart valves. It is characterized by fever, anemia, valvular dysfunction, cardiac murmurs, petechiae, emboli, and cardiac vegetations that may result in valve incompetence, abscesses, or aneurysms. The most serious complication is CHF. The aortic and mitral valves are the most commonly affected. Infections are usually caused by *S. aureus* or *Streptococcus* species (e.g., *Streptococcus viridans, S. pneumoniae*). Infections of prosthetic valves are of particular concern and usually require removal of the artificial valve. Splenomegaly is often seen in conjunction with endocarditis. Other symptoms include night sweats, malaise, weight loss, arthralgias, and chest pain. Painful erythematous nodules at the distal tips of the fingers are called *Osler's nodes*. Round, erythematous lesions with central clearing (Roth spots) can affect the retina. Painless erythematous lesions (Janeway lesions) can affect the palms or soles. Subungual "splinter hemorrhages" can affect the fingernails. Laboratory findings are usually nonspecific and may show anemia, reticulocytopenia, hypergammaglobulinemia, circulating immune complexes,

and positive rheumatoid factor. The patient's ESR may be elevated. Urinalysis frequently shows proteinuria and microscopic hematuria.

Intravenous drug abuse is a major cause of endocarditis, which usually affects the right side (tricuspid valve) of the heart. If treated early, the prognosis is usually good. Echocardiography is the best diagnostic test for bacterial endocarditis. Transthoracic echocardiography detects vegetations in 50% of patients with endocarditis, whereas transesophageal echocardiography detects vegetations in >90% of cases. Blood cultures can determine the causative organism; however, 15% to 20% of patients with clinical endocarditis may test negative, usually as a result of recent antibiotic therapy.

Additional Reading: Infectious endocarditis: diagnosis and treatment. *Am Fam Physician.* 2012;85(10):981–986.

Category: Cardiovascular system

245. In diagnosing a PE, which of the following tests is considered the diagnostic test of choice?
A) Ventilation-perfusion (V/Q) lung scan
B) Venous compression ultrasonography of the legs
C) Pulmonary angiography
D) Spiral CT of the chest
E) Multidetector computed tomography (MDCT) angiography

Answer and Discussion

The answer is E. PE is usually a consequence of DVT and is associated with greater mortality. MDCT angiography is the diagnostic test of choice when the technology is available and appropriate for the patient. MDCT is a form of CT scan, where the two-dimensional array of detector elements replaces the linear array of detector elements used in typical conventional and helical CT scanners. The development of MDCT has resulted in the development of high-resolution CT applications such as CT angiography and CT colonoscopy. It is warranted in patients who may have a PE and a positive d-dimer assay result, or in patients who have a high pretest probability of PE, regardless of d-dimer assay result.

For patients with contraindications to CT, including contrast allergy, renal disease, and pregnancy, ventilation-perfusion scanning is the preferred imaging modality for evaluation of possible PE.

Pulmonary angiography is needed only when the clinical suspicion for PE remains high, even when less invasive study results are negative. In unstable emergent cases highly suspicious for PE, echocardiography may be used to evaluate for right ventricular dysfunction, which is indicative of but not diagnostic for PE.

In patients with a low pretest probability of DVT or PE, a negative result from a high-sensitivity d-dimer assay is sufficient to exclude venous thromboembolism.

Additional Reading: Diagnosis of deep venous thrombosis and pulmonary embolism. *Am Fam Physician.* 2012;86(10): 913–919.

Category: Cardiovascular system

246. Which of the following findings is associated with chronic myelocytic leukemia (CML)?
A) Leukopenia
B) Philadelphia chromosome
C) Elevated leukocyte alkaline phosphatase level
D) Thrombocytopenia
E) Decreased vitamin B_{12} levels

Answer and Discussion

The answer is B. CML is a clonal myeloproliferative disorder that results in the overproduction of granulocytes from the bone marrow, liver, and spleen. The average age of onset is approximately 45 years. In most cases, the CML clone has the potential to progress into an accelerated phase and final blast crisis but usually remains stable for years before transformation. Symptoms are usually nonspecific and include low-grade fever, weight loss, night sweats, fatigue, anorexia, and, in some cases, abdominal fullness secondary to splenomegaly. Physical examination may show significant splenomegaly and generalized lymphadenopathy (ominous signs). Laboratory findings include significant elevation in the WBC count (200,000 at the time of diagnosis) and thrombocytosis. Bone marrow studies show hypercellularity with a significant left shift and low leukocyte alkaline phosphatase value. Vitamin B_{12} levels and serum vitamin B_{12}–binding capacity are usually elevated as a result of increased granulocyte production of transcobalamin I, and there is almost always a Philadelphia chromosome (translocation of a part of chromosome 9 to chromosome 22) present.

Treatment involves the use of chemotherapy medications such as hydroxyurea. In most cases, the patient may be kept asymptomatic for long periods while maintaining the WBC count at <50,000. True remission does not occur because of the persistence of the Philadelphia chromosome in the bone marrow. Median survival after the clinical onset is approximately 3 to 4 years. If a blast crisis occurs, the average survival is approximately 2 months but can be improved with adequate treatment. α-Interferon produces remission in 20% to 25%. Bone marrow transplantation has been shown to improve survival in select patients.

Additional Reading: Clinical manifestations and diagnosis of chronic myeloid leukemia. In: Basow DS, ed. *UpToDate*. Waltham, MA: UpToDate; 2013.

Category: Hematologic system

247. A 63-year-old smoker (35 pack years) presents for follow-up after a recent bout of acute bronchitis. He reports having a productive cough for several months and states that every time he gets a cold, it settles into his chest and lasts for "ever." He also reports dyspnea on exertion. On lung exam, you hear scattered rhonchi. A chest x-ray done 3 months ago when he went to the ER for the last similar episode was negative except for hyperinflation and flattened diaphragms. Which one of the following would be best for making the diagnosis?
A) A chest radiograph
B) CT of the chest
C) Peak flow measurement
D) Spirometry
E) A BNP level

Answer and Discussion
The answer is D. Distinguishing between COPD and asthma is important because of the differences in treatment. Patients with COPD are usually in their sixties when the diagnosis is made. Symptoms of chronic cough (sometimes for months or years), dyspnea, or sputum production are often not reported because the patient may attribute them to smoking, aging, or poor physical condition. Spirometry is the best test for the diagnosis of COPD. The presence of outflow obstruction that is not fully reversible is demonstrated by postbronchodilator spirometry showing an FEV/FVC ratio of 70% or less.

Additional Reading: Management of COPD exacerbations. *Am Fam Physician.* 2010;81(5):607–613.

Category: Respiratory system

> Emphysema is a condition associated with the destruction of lung tissue and the development of blebs (coalescence of alveoli).

248. A 72-year-old smoker with a positive history of severe degenerative arthritis, diabetes, and CVD presents to your office complaining of bilateral leg pain that occurs after walking 200 yards. He reports that rest improves his symptoms. Which of the following would be appropriate?
A) Ankle/brachial indices
B) MRI of the lumbar spine
C) Ultrasonography of the lower extremities
D) EMG of the lower extremities
E) Arteriogram of the lower extremities

Answer and Discussion
The answer is A. Claudication occurs when there is arterial insufficiency of the lower extremities. It usually occurs in the calf muscles, thighs, and buttocks and is bilateral and progressive. Symptoms include pain, fatigue, or weakness associated with the lower legs that typically occurs after walking predictable distances, and, occasionally, impotence in men. If the pain or discomfort occurs with varying distances, a workup for other causes is necessary. Patients who experience significant restriction in their activities may be considered for surgery; however, their overall health status should be considered first. Many patients have underlying CVD that may put them at surgical risk. Ankle/brachial indices (usually <0.90 with peripheral arterial disease) are the simplest method to estimate blood flow to the lower extremities. The use of arteriogram is not necessary unless the patient is considering surgery.

The Eighth American College of Chest Physicians Conference on Antithrombotic and Thrombolytic Therapy recommends lifelong use of aspirin at a dosage of 75 to 100 mg per day in all patients with intermittent claudication. Clopidogrel (Plavix) is recommended in patients who cannot take aspirin. Cilostazol is recommended only in patients with disabling intermittent claudication who do not respond to risk factor modification and exercise and who are not surgical candidates. The guidelines also recommend against the use of pentoxifylline, prostaglandins, and anticoagulants in patients with intermittent claudication.

The American College of Cardiology/American Heart Association 2005 guidelines for the management of peripheral arterial disease recommend statins, antiplatelet therapy, risk factor modification, and supervised exercise training (30 to 45 minutes at least three times per week) for all patients with peripheral arterial disease. They recommend a trial of cilostazol for patients with lifestyle-limiting claudication. They also recommend surgical interventions in persons with functional disability from claudication symptoms that are unresponsive to exercise or pharmacotherapy but that have a reasonable likelihood of improvement.

Additional Reading: Effective therapies for intermittent claudication. *Am Fam Physician.* 2011;84(6):699–704.

Category: Cardiovascular system

249. A 65-year-old man presents complaining of back pain and generalized fatigue. Laboratory findings include anemia with Rouleau formation, a monoclonal spike seen with serum protein electrophoresis, and hypercalcemia. Radiographs of the lumbar spine show lytic lesions. The most likely diagnosis is
A) Metastatic prostate cancer
B) Paget's disease
C) Osteitis fibrosa cystica
D) Multiple myeloma
E) Colon cancer

Answer and Discussion

The answer is D. Multiple myeloma is a malignancy associated with plasma cells and involves replacement of the bone marrow, bone destruction, and the formation of paraproteins that are found in the blood and urine. It is the most common primary malignancy that affects the spine. Affected patients are usually older than 60 years and present with anemia, bone pain, and an elevated sedimentation rate. Other manifestations include renal failure; spinal cord compression; or symptoms of hyperviscosity, including mucosal bleeding, vertigo, visual abnormalities, and alterations in mental status. Laboratory abnormalities include an anemia with Rouleau formation, abnormal serum and urine protein electrophoresis with a monoclonal spike in the β or γ region, hypercalcemia as a result of bone destruction, and radiographs showing lytic lesions associated with the skeletal bones (bone scans are inferior to conventional radiographs). Diagnosis is made by bone marrow biopsy showing more than 10% of plasma cells in the bone marrow. Treatment is aimed at palliation and involves chemotherapy and correction of hypercalcemia. Patients are at increased risk of infection caused by encapsulated organisms, such as *S. pneumoniae* and *H. influenzae*, because of impaired immune response. The median survival time is 3 to 5 years.

> **Additional Reading:** Multiple Myeloma. In: Domino F, ed. *The 5-Minute Clinical Consult*. Philadelphia, PA: Lippincott Williams and Wilkins; 2014.

> **Category:** Hematologic system

250. Which one of the following patients is eligible for the Medicare hospice benefit?
A) A patient with end-stage COPD with a life expectancy of 6 months
B) A patient with ALS with a life expectancy of 9 months
C) A patient on hemodialysis with a life expectancy of 12 months
D) A patient with stage IV breast cancer with a life expectancy of 18 months

Answer and Discussion

The answer is A. Patients with a life expectancy of 6 months or less are eligible for the Medicare hospice benefit. This benefit allows patients to receive hospice care in either the home or hospital setting. In addition to patients with terminal cancer, patients with end-stage cardiac, pulmonary, and chronic debilitating diseases are eligible. Approximately two-thirds of patients enrolled in hospice die from non–cancer-related diagnoses, and approximately 60% of Medicare patients are not enrolled in hospice at the time of their death.

> **Additional Reading:** The use of hospice care for patients without cancer. *Am Fam Physician.* 2010;82(10):1196.

> **Category:** Patient/population-based care

251. The anticoagulation effects associated with heparin therapy are best reversed with the use of
A) Vitamin K
B) Fresh-frozen plasma
C) Cryoprecipitate
D) Protamine sulfate
E) Platelet administration

Answer and Discussion

The answer is D. Heparin is an anticoagulant used to prevent thrombosis. Heparin works by binding to and activating antithrombin III, an extremely potent anticoagulant that prevents thrombin generation and fibrin formation. The drug is administered intravenously and subcutaneously. The major side effect is bleeding. If needed, protamine sulfate may be administered to rapidly reverse heparin's anticoagulant effect; in most cases, this measure is unnecessary and the discontinuation of heparin is adequate. Other complications include heparin-induced thrombocytopenia, which occurs in 10% of patients taking the medication. The thrombocytopenia can actually lead to a paradoxical arterial thrombosis, which can be life threatening. Discontinuation of the medication usually reverses the thrombocytopenia. When administering intravenous heparin, the PTT should be monitored. Any increase in heparin dose is usually detected 4 hours later (as noted with a prolonged PTT) and vice versa with decreased doses of heparin. The goal for anticoagulation is usually 1.5 to 2.0 times the normal value, but may depend on the individual case. Patients should not take aspirin while taking heparin; intramuscular injections should also be avoided. Chronic use of heparin may increase the risk of osteoporosis. LMW heparin is now available and is used for anticoagulation. PTT and thrombin times are minimally affected by typical therapeutic doses. Therefore, laboratory monitoring is not required.

> **Additional Reading:** Antithrombotic drugs. *Treat Guidel Med Lett.* 2011;9(110):61–66.

> **Category:** Cardiovascular system

252. A 36-year-old runner presents with pain associated with the anterior heel. The patient reports his symptoms are worse on awakening and improve as the day progresses. The most likely diagnosis is
A) Achilles tendonitis
B) Plantar fasciitis
C) Calcaneal fracture
D) Calcaneal bone spur
E) Anterior talotibial impingement syndrome

Answer and Discussion

The answer is B. Plantar fasciitis is caused by inflammation, fibrosis, or tearing (microtears) of the plantar fascia at the attachment site to the os calcis. It is a common complaint in runners. Symptoms include pain at the attachment of the plantar fascia at the calcaneus. The pain is usually worse in the morning on standing or standing after prolonged sitting. The pain may improve early in the day but usually worsens toward the end of the day and is relieved when the patient lies or sits down. Calcaneal spurs, visible on radiographs, may occur in chronic cases but are not responsible for evoking pain and discomfort. Treatment involves NSAIDs, stretching exercises (e.g., rolling a tennis ball under the foot), heel pads (Viscoheel), orthotics, rest, and ice therapy. In more severe cases that are refractory to these measures, night splints or steroid injection (0.5 mL of steroid and 1.0 mL of 1% lidocaine) can be used. In addition, surgery may be indicated for severe cases that are unresponsive to conservative therapy.

> **Additional Reading:** Busconi BD, Stevenson JH. Approach to the athlete with plantar fasciitis. *Sports Medicine Consult: A Problem-Based Approach to Sports Medicine for the Primary Care Physician.* Philadelphia, PA: Lippincott, Williams & Wilkins; 2009.

> **Category:** Musculoskeletal system

253. A 52-year-old man is seen for fevers and weight loss. A chest radiograph shows mediastinal lymphadenopathy. Laboratory findings show hypercalcemia, elevated alkaline phosphatase, and an elevated level of ACE. The most likely diagnosis is

A) Small cell carcinoma of the lung
B) Pulmonary tuberculosis
C) Sarcoidosis
D) Histoplasmosis
E) Asbestosis

Answer and Discussion

The answer is C. Sarcoidosis is a systemic granulomatous disease that is characterized by noncaseating granulomas that may affect multiple organ systems. The condition occurs mainly in persons ages 20 to 40 years and is most common in Northern Europeans and African Americans. Symptoms are variable and the etiology is unknown. Fever, weight loss, arthralgias, and erythema nodosum (more commonly seen in Europeans) are the usual initial presenting symptoms. Cough and dyspnea may be minimal or absent. Other manifestations include mediastinal lymphadenopathy seen on chest radiograph (hallmark finding in 90% of cases), hepatic granulomas, granulomatous uveitis, polyarthritis, cardiac symptoms (including angina, CHF, and conduction abnormalities), cranial-nerve palsies, and diabetes insipidus. Laboratory findings include leukopenia, hypercalcemia, hypercalciuria, and hypergammaglobulinemia (particularly in African American patients). Other abnormalities include elevated uric acid (not usually associated with gout), elevated alkaline phosphatase, elevated gamma glutamyl transpeptidase, elevated levels of ACE, and pulmonary function tests showing restriction and impaired diffusing capacity. Diagnosis can be made with biopsy of peripheral lesions or fiber-optic bronchoscopy for central pulmonary lesions. Whole-body gallium scans can be used to show useful sites for biopsy and, in some cases, to follow disease progression. Serial pulmonary function tests are important for assessing disease progression and guiding treatment. The prognosis depends on the severity of the disease. Spontaneous improvement is common; however, significant disability can occur with multiorgan involvement. Pulmonary fibrosis is the leading cause of death. Treatment for symptomatic patients consists of corticosteroids, methotrexate, and other immunosuppressive medications if steroid therapy is not helpful.

Additional Reading: Sarcoidosis. *The 5-Minute Clinical Consult*, 21st ed. Philadelphia, PA: Lippincott Williams and Wilkins; 2014.

Category: Nonspecific system

254. A cytomegalovirus infection has developed in a patient with AIDS. The most appropriate treatment is

A) Ganciclovir
B) Amphotericin B
C) Amantadine
D) Metronidazole
E) Ciprofloxacin

Answer and Discussion

The answer is A. Cytomegalovirus is a viral infection that may occur congenitally or at any age. The severity of the infection varies. The virus is a variant of the herpes virus and is ubiquitous. Manifestations of the illness include fever, hepatitis, pneumonitis, and neurologic damage to brain tissue in the newborn (hearing losses or perinatal death in severe cases). The infection may be acquired in utero from an infected mother or by contact with infected secretions, including urine, saliva, breast milk, feces, blood, and semen. Patients with AIDS or immunocompromised conditions such as transplant patients and those living in institutions (such as nursing homes) or attending day care centers are at increased risk. The infection is very common (as much as 90% of the population is affected) and in most cases is represented by mild symptoms. More severe cases can produce a mononucleosis-type illness, retinitis, or pneumonitis in adults. Congenital cytomegalovirus may include jaundice, hepatosplenomegaly, petechial rash, microcephaly, and cerebral calcifications. Diagnosis is achieved with the detection of the virus by immunofluorescence with monoclonal antibodies. Treatment is usually supportive; however, ganciclovir can be used in more severe cases and particularly in AIDS patients. Foscarnet sodium (Foscavir) is also effective, especially in ganciclovir-resistant cases.

Additional Reading: Antiviral drugs. *Treat Guidel Med Lett.* 2013;11(127):19–30.

Category: Nonspecific system

255. Which of the following ECG findings is associated with hypothermia?

A) J (Osborne) wave
B) Tachycardia
C) Atrioventricular dissociation
D) Atrial fibrillation
E) First-degree AV block

Answer and Discussion

The answer is A. Hypothermia is caused by prolonged exposure to a cold environment, causing the body's core temperature to fall below 35°C (or 95°F). Infants, the elderly, and those with altered mental status or debilitating illnesses are at increased risk. Others at increased risk include trauma and burn victims and those with malnutrition. Symptoms include shivering, decreased mental status with confusion, impaired coordination, drowsiness, bradycardia, and, in more severe cases, loss of the shivering reflex and coma. ECG tracings may show a characteristic J (Osborne) wave, a positive deflection after the QRS complex in the lateral leads. Death usually results from the progression of severe bradycardia to ventricular fibrillation. Treatment involves slow central body warming (over 2 to 3 hours to prevent shock) with warmed intravenous fluids, warmed oxygen, and warming blankets or warm baths. Life-sustaining measures should always be continued until the normal core body temperature is achieved.

Additional Reading: Hypothermia. In: Domino F, ed. *The 5-Minute Clinical Consult*. Philadelphia, PA: Lippincott Williams and Wilkins; 2014.

Category: Nonspecific system

256. Which of the following toxin–antidote associations is correct?

A) Organophosphates–atropine and pralidoxime
B) Carbon monoxide–nitrous oxide
C) Opioids–benzodiazepines
D) Methanol–isopropyl alcohol
E) Arsenic–flumazenil

Answer and Discussion

The answer is A. Organophosphates are potent cholinesterase inhibitors that result in severe cholinergic toxicity following cutaneous exposure, inhalation, or ingestion. One of the common smells associated with poisonings is a garlic smell that may represent arsenic, dimethyl sulfoxide, organophosphates, and selenium toxicities. There is a cluster of symptoms that is associated with organophosphates represented by the acronym SLUDGE: *S*alivation, *L*acrimation, *U*rinary frequency, *D*efecation, *G*astric hypersecretion, *E*mesis.

The treatment for organophosphate poisoning is the concomitant use of atropine and pralidoxime. The treatment of choice for arsenic poisoning is penicillamine or dimercaprol. Sodium nitrite and sodium thiosulfate are antidotes for poisoning with cyanide amyl nitrate. Oxygen is used for carbon monoxide poisoning. Anticholinergic overdoses with medication such as atropine, scopolamine, and antihistamines are usually associated with symptoms in which the patient is described as "Dry as a bone, red as a beet, and mad as a hatter." Treatment involves the use of physostigmine as an antidote. Methanol overdoses are treated with ethanol, and opioid overdoses are treated with naloxone. Flumazenil (Romazicon) is used to treat benzodiazepine overdoses. Acetylcysteine is the treatment of choice for acetaminophen overdose.

Additional Reading: Organophosphate and carbamate poisoning. In: Basow DS, ed. *UpToDate*. Waltham, MA: UpToDate; 2013.

Category: Nonspecific system

> The treatment for organophosphate poisoning is the concomitant use of atropine and pralidoxime.

257. A BUN:creatinine level greater than 20 is associated with
A) Dehydration
B) Renal stones
C) Bladder outlet obstruction
D) Hypercalcemia
E) Renal artery stenosis

Answer and Discussion

The answer is A. Acute renal failure is divided into the following categories:

- *Prerenal.* This is due to inadequate renal perfusion. It can be caused by volume depletion (dehydration), cardiac or hepatic failure, and sepsis. Laboratory tests reveal a low urinary sodium (<20 mEq per L) and a high urine-to-plasma creatinine ratio (>20:1). The BUN-to-serum creatinine ratio is higher than 20.
- *Intrarenal.* This was previously known as acute tubular necrosis. Causes include ischemia, hypertension, vasculitis, metabolic disorders (e.g., hypercalcemia, hyperuricemia), toxins, x-ray dyes, myoglobinuria, and medications (e.g., aminoglycosides, penicillins, anesthetic agents). Laboratory tests show results similar to postrenal azotemia.
- *Postrenal.* This is usually caused by obstruction by renal calculi or bladder outlet obstruction (prostate enlargement). Laboratory tests show a high urinary sodium (>40 mEq per L) and a low urine-to-plasma creatinine ratio (<20:1). The BUN-to-serum creatinine ratio is lower than 20.
- Prerenal and postrenal causes for acute renal failure are potentially reversible. If caught early, some forms of intrarenal azotemia (e.g., drug effects, infections, hypertension) can be reversed.

Additional Reading: Acute kidney injury: a guide to diagnosis and management. *Am Fam Physician.* 2012;86(7):631–639.

Category: Nephrologic system

258. Which of the following tests is used in the initial evaluation of persistent hemoptysis?
A) Fiber-optic bronchoscopy
B) Chest radiograph
C) Upper gastrointestinal (GI)
D) MRI of chest
E) CT scan of chest

Answer and Discussion

The answer is B. Hemoptysis is the presence of blood in the expectorate. Intrapulmonary causes include infections (e.g., bronchitis, pneumonia, tuberculous, fungal infections), neoplasm, bronchiectasis, pulmonary embolus, AV malformations, Goodpasture's disease, vasculitis, trauma, or the presence of a foreign body. Extrapulmonary causes include GI bleeding, CHF with pulmonary edema, severe mitral stenosis, epistaxis, or other conditions (including disseminated intravascular coagulation). Most cases are self-limited and require no additional workup; however, persistent or severe hemoptysis should be evaluated with sputum collection for Gram's stain and culture, cytology, acid-fast bacillus stains, CBC, PT, PTT, chest radiograph, and flexible bronchoscopy. If a lower respiratory tract source is suspected, the patient should undergo a chest x-ray first, and if a mass is noted, bronchoscopy should be performed. A high-resolution CT may be helpful in the diagnosis. It is important to distinguish between GI blood loss (which has a dark red color and acidic pH) and true hemoptysis (which is typically bright red in color and alkaline).

Additional Reading: Etiology and evaluation of hemoptysis in adults. In: Basow DS, ed. *UpToDate*. Waltham, MA: UpToDate; 2013.

Category: Respiratory system

259. Thyroid replacement therapy can be assessed by measuring the patient's
A) T_3 level
B) T_4 level
C) TSH level
D) Thyroid-releasing hormone level
E) None of the above

Answer and Discussion

The answer is C. Patients diagnosed with hypothyroidism should receive replacement therapy with levothyroxine. These patients can be monitored for effective replacement by evaluating their serum sTSH levels. A low-level TSH usually results from overreplacement, and adjustments should be made in the dose of medication; monitoring is repeated in 6 to 8 weeks. Underreplacement is represented by an increased TSH level and can be corrected by increasing the dose of thyroxine; monitoring is repeated in 6 to 8 weeks. Checking TSH levels earlier usually does not provide enough time for the levels to stabilize.

Additional Reading: Hypothyroidism, Adult. In: Domino F, ed. *The 5-Minute Clinical Consult*. Philadelphia, PA: Lippincott Williams and Wilkins; 2014.

Category: Endocrine system

260. Which of the following is true regarding breast cancer screening?
A) Teaching breast self-examination reduces breast cancer mortality.
B) Teaching breast self-examination should start at as early as 15 years of age.
C) The goal of the breast self-examination is to detect breast cancer.
D) Mammography is the only screening test shown to reduce breast cancer–related mortality.

Answer and Discussion

The answer is D. Teaching self breast examination (SBE) does not reduce breast cancer mortality and may increase false-positive rates. Two large randomized international trials did not demonstrate a mortality benefit from teaching SBE. A review of eight other studies did not show a benefit from SBE in the rate of breast cancer diagnosis, tumor stage, or the rate of breast cancer. However, the number of times that women find lumps that lead to a breast cancer diagnosis warrants educating patients to recognize and report changes in their breasts. Thus, although there are no studies to support breast self-awareness, some organizations recommend encouraging women 20 years and older to recognize the normal feel of their breasts (rather than teaching formal SBE), and to report any changes to their physician.

Screening mammography has been shown to reduce breast cancer mortality. A meta-analysis found a 26% reduction in the relative risk of breast cancer–related mortality when women 50 to 74 years of age received screening mammography. Although there is general agreement that screening mammography should be offered routinely to women 50 to 74 years of age, there are conflicting guidelines for its use in younger women. In 2009, the USPSTF recommended against routine screening mammography in women younger than 50 years on the basis of the analysis of closely balanced benefits and harms. They noted that the rates of false-positive results in young women were nearly double those in women 50 years and older; that the number needed to screen for women 39 to 49 years of age to prevent one breast cancer death was much higher than that for women 50 to 59 and 60 to 69 years of age (1,904, 1,339, and 377, respectively); and that the risks of over diagnosis (e.g., ductal carcinoma in situ that may not grow or become invasive) and overtreatment were additional potential harms.

Additional Reading: Breast cancer screening update. *Am Fam physician*. 2013;87(4):274–278.

Category: Integumentary

261. Which of the following statements about ALS, or Lou Gehrig's disease, is true?
A) It is a progressive motor neuron disease that affects the corticospinal tracts.
B) The onset is usually before 20 years of age.
C) It typically destroys sensory function.
D) It may respond to high-dose steroid administration.
E) Dementia is common.

Answer and Discussion

The answer is A. ALS, or Lou Gehrig's disease, is a progressive motor neuron disease that affects the corticospinal tracts and/or the anterior horn cells and/or bulbar motor nuclei. Onset of the disease is usually after 40 years of age, and the disease is more common in men. Approximately 5% to 10% of cases are familial and are associated with an autosomal-dominant mode of transmission. The hands are usually affected first with cramps, followed by weakness. Other manifestations include atrophy, muscle fasciculations, spasticity, and increased reflex response. There is usually a combination of upper and lower motor neuron signs. Dysarthria and dysphagia may occur; however, extraocular muscles, sensory function, sexual function, and urinary continence are usually not affected. Dementia is usually not present. Late in the illness, inappropriate, involuntary, and uncontrollable laughter or crying may occur. Diagnosis is usually made with EMG findings that correlate with the clinical presentation. Unfortunately, there is no treatment other than supportive care. Baclofen has been used to treat muscular spasticity and cramping. Death as a result of respiratory failure usually occurs within 5 years.

Additional Reading: Amyotrophic lateral sclerosis. In: Domino F, ed. *The 5-Minute Clinical Consult*. Philadelphia, PA: Lippincott Williams and Wilkins; 2014.

Category: Neurologic

262. A 32-year-old man presents with recurrent oral and genital ulcers. He also has had arthralgias. Recently, he was administered a tetanus vaccination and developed a sterile abscess at the site of the injection. The most likely diagnosis is
A) Behçet's disease
B) Systemic herpes
C) Syphilis
D) Gonorrhea
E) Lyme disease

Answer and Discussion

The answer is A. Named after a famous Turkish dermatologist, Behcet's syndrome is an inflammatory disorder that may involve ocular, genital, articular, mucocutaneous, vascular, and CNS structures. Symptoms usually develop when patients are in their 30s. Men are more severely affected than women. Symptoms include episodic and recurrent oral and genital apthous-type ulcers, uveitis, arthritis (usually affecting the knees and ankles), skin lesions, thrombophlebitis, and vasculitis. Signs include cranial-nerve palsies, seizures, mental disturbances, and spinal cord lesions. The disease is usually chronic and is characterized by remissions and exacerbations. The syndrome is usually benign; however, severe ocular involvement can lead to blindness. Steroids and immunosuppressive medication (interferon, azathioprine, cyclosporine) have been used for treatment, especially in cases of severe uveitis and CNS involvement. Other medications used in treatment include thalidomide, chlorambucil, and colchicine. The disease is more commonly seen in Japan and Korea, as well as the eastern Mediterranean countries. Sterile abscesses or pustules at the site of an injection are hallmark findings for the disease.

Additional Reading: Behcet syndrome. In: Domino F, ed. *The 5-Minute Clinical Consult*. Philadelphia, PA: Lippincott Williams and Wilkins; 2014.

Category: Gastroenterology system

263. The pneumococcal vaccine should be administered to healthy individuals beginning at age
A) 50 years
B) 55 years
C) 60 years
D) 65 years
E) 70 years

Answer and Discussion

The answer is D. There are currently 2 types of pneumococcal vaccines: pneumococcal conjugate vaccine (PCV13) and pneumococcal polysaccharide vaccine (PPSV23). PCV13 is recommended for all children younger than 5 years and for adults with certain risk factors, including

- CSF leaks
- Cochlear implant(s)
- Sickle cell disease and other hemaglobinopathies
- Functional or anatomic asplenia
- Congenital or acquired immunodeficiencies
- HIV infection
- Chronic renal failure
- Nephrotic syndrome
- Leukemia
- Hodgkin disease
- Generalized malignancy
- Long-term immunosuppressive therapy
- Solid organ transplant
- Multiple myeloma

PPSV23 is indicated for children 2 years or older who are at high risk of pneumococcal disease; all adults 65 or older; and all residents of nursing homes or long-term care facilities. Any adult 19 through 64 years of age who is a smoker or has asthma should also be vaccinated. Additionally, anyone 2 through 64 years of age who has a long-term health problem (e.g., heart or lung disease, sickle cell disease, diabetes, alcoholism, cirrhosis, leaks of CSF or cochlear implant) or if immunocompromised due to illness (e.g., Hodgkin's disease; lymphoma or leukemia; kidney failure; multiple myeloma; nephrotic syndrome; HIV infection or AIDS; splenectomy; organ transplant) or secondary to medication or treatment (e.g., long-term steroids, chemotherapy or radiation therapy).

The pneumococcal vaccine is typically a single, lifetime immunization; however, if the patient received their first dose before age 65 years and it has been more than 5 years they should receive a one-time booster. In addition, immunocompromised individuals or those with chronic underlying conditions should be considered for booster vaccination after 5 years.

Additional Reading: Pneumococcal vaccination: who needs it? Center for Disease Control and Prevention. From: http://www.cdc.gov/vaccines/vpd-vac/pneumo/vacc-in-short.htm.

Category: Respiratory system

264. MVP is associated with
A) Elderly, obese men
B) Diastolic click that disappears with Valsalva's maneuver
C) Chest pain, dyspnea, and syncope
D) Rheumatic heart disease
E) Myxomatous transformation of the valve leaflet

Answer and Discussion
The answer is E. MVP (systolic-click syndrome, Barlow's syndrome, and floppy valve syndrome) is usually asymptomatic but may cause chest pain, palpitations, anxiety, dyspnea, or fatigue. The condition is common and associated with myxomatous transformation of the valve leaflet. MVP usually affects healthy, young (15 to 30 years of age), thin women. MVP is determined by the detection of a midsystolic click that is followed by a late systolic murmur and becomes louder with Valsalva's maneuver. A high-pitched late systolic crescendo–decrescendo murmur heard best at the apex may also be present. Presence of both murmur and click is not necessary for the diagnosis. In patients with MVP, cardiac arrhythmias, including PVCs, paroxysmal supraventricular tachycardia, and ventricular tachycardia, may cause palpitations and may need treatment (usually with β-blockers).

Rarely, MVP may progress to mitral insufficiency because of rupture of the chordae tendineae and may require valve replacement.

Additional Reading: Mitral valve prolapse. In: Domino F, ed. *The 5-Minute Clinical Consult.* Philadelphia, PA: Lippincott Williams and Wilkins; 2014.

Category: Cardiovascular system

MVP is determined by the detection of a midsystolic click that is followed by a late systolic murmur and becomes louder with Valsalva's maneuver.

265. Which of the following statements about Peutz–Jeghers syndrome is true?
A) The condition is sex linked and usually skips a generation.
B) The condition involves the development of multiple polyps in the stomach and the small and large intestine that commonly show malignant change.
C) There is associated hyperpigmentation around the oral cavity lips, soles of the feet, and dorsum of the hands.
D) The condition is associated with inflammatory bowel disease.
E) The condition is identified by elevation in carcinoembryonic antigen levels.

Answer and Discussion
The answer is C. Peutz–Jeghers syndrome is a familial autosomal-dominant condition that involves the development of multiple, benign, hamartomatous polyps in the stomach and in the small and large intestine. Malignant change has occurred but is rare. Those affected also have melanin-associated brownish-black hyperpigmentation around the oral cavity, lips, soles of the feet, and dorsum of the hands. The condition usually causes no problems except in severe cases in which abdominal pain, intestinal obstruction, or bleeding can occur. In these severe cases, surgery may be considered.

Additional Reading: Peutz–Jeghers syndrome. *GeneReviews.* From: http://www.ncbi.nlm.nih.gov/books/NBK1266/

Category: Gastroenterology system

266. Which of the following statements about angina pectoris is true?
A) It typically lasts 1 to 2 hours.
B) It may be associated with epigastric pain.
C) It causes predictable ECG changes.
D) It is typically associated with chest wall tenderness.
E) It rarely radiates to the neck, jaw, or left arm.

Answer and Discussion
The answer is B. Angina pectoris is typically described as substernal chest pain or pressure that may radiate to the neck, jaw, or left arm. Patients usually also experience shortness of breath, dizziness, nausea, and vomiting with diaphoresis. Symptoms are usually precipitated by physical exertion or stress and are relieved with rest. Episodes usually last 2 to 10 minutes and rarely last longer than 30 minutes. Atypical presentations include epigastric pain, indigestion, right-arm pain, light-headedness, nausea, or shortness of breath. These occurring alone are referred to as anginal equivalents. There are several types of angina:

- *Stable:* Intensity, character, and frequency of episodes are predictable; angina occurs in response to a known amount of exercise or stress.
- *Unstable:* Intensity, frequency, and duration are different and unpredictable; pain is precipitated by a lesser amount of exercise or the angina is longer in duration. Angina at rest or new-onset angina is unstable.
- *Variant:* Pain that may occur at rest and is secondary to spasm of the coronary arteries is variant angina.

Typically, the pain is relieved with the administration of sublingual nitroglycerin. ECG may show T-wave inversion or ST-segment depression, but in many cases is normal and should not be discounted if normal. Exercise stress testing can be used to determine coronary insufficiency. Treatment of angina is accomplished with the use of nitrates, β-blockers, and CCBs.

Additional Reading: Pathophysiology and clinical presentation of ischemic chest pain. In: Basow DS, ed. *UpToDate.* Waltham, MA: UpToDate; 2013.

Category: Cardiovascular system

267. Which of the following best describes Ludwig's angina?
A) Substernal chest pain that radiates to the right arm.
B) An infection involving the sublingual and submaxillary space.
C) Abdominal pain secondary to an enlarging AAA.
D) A tonsillar infection that leads to chronic abscess formation.
E) Ischemic pain related to insufficient blood flow to an extremity.

Answer and Discussion

The answer is B. Ludwig's angina usually develops from a periodontal or dental infection and is one of the most common neck space infections. The condition is usually a rapidly developing, bilateral cellulitis that affects the sublingual and submaxillary space, without involvement of the lymph nodes or formation of abscesses. The infection usually rapidly arises from the second and third mandibular molars as a result of poor dental hygiene, tooth extraction, or trauma. Symptoms include edema and erythema of the upper neck (under the chin) and floor of the mouth, trismus, drooling, dysphonia, dysphagia, and dyspnea. Fever, chills, and tachycardia are usually present. Tongue displacement upward may also occur and threaten the airway. In severe cases, the condition may be fatal. Treatment includes protection of the airway in severe cases and intravenous antibiotics (e.g., penicillin, wide-spectrum cephalosporins) in high doses to cover anaerobic organisms (*Bacteroides*). Incision and drainage may be required.

Additional Reading: Ludwig angina. In: Basow DS, ed. *The 5-Minute Clinical Consult.* Philadelphia, PA: Lippincott Williams and Wilkins; 2014.

Category: Respiratory system

268. Vitamin A toxicity is associated with
A) Peripheral neuropathy
B) Renal stones
C) Increased intracranial pressure and vomiting
D) Night blindness
E) Pulmonary fibrosis

Answer and Discussion

The answer is C. Excessive ingestion of vitamin A may cause acute or chronic toxicity. Acute toxicity especially in children may result from taking large doses (>100,000 µg or 300,000 IU). The condition is associated with increased intracranial pressure and vomiting, which may lead to death. After discontinuation, recovery is usually spontaneous, with no residual damage. Infants who are given 6,000 to 20,000 µg (20,000 to 60,000 IU) per day of water-soluble vitamin A may show evidence of toxicity within a few weeks. Birth defects have been reported in the children of women receiving 13-cis-retinoic acid (isotretinoin) for skin conditions during pregnancy. Megavitamin tablets containing vitamin A have occasionally induced acute toxicity when taken long term. Chronic toxicity usually affects older children and adults after doses of >33,000 µg (100,000 IU) per day have been taken for an extended course (i.e., months).

Additional Reading: Overview of vitamin A. In: Basow DS, ed. *UpToDate.* Waltham, MA: UpToDate; 2013.

Category: Neurologic

269. A 65-year-old woman is undergoing a general examination. On your exam, you note a fullness in the left adnexa. Which of the following conditions would be reassuring that the finding is benign?
A) A multiloculated cyst noted on ultrasound
B) Elevated CA 125 level
C) Simple cyst measured at 2.5 cm as seen on ultrasound
D) Elevated CEA level

Answer and Discussion

The answer is C. Adnexal masses are commonly encountered in women. In premenopausal women, physiologic follicular cysts and corpus luteum cysts are the most common adnexal masses. Ectopic pregnancy can occur and should be considered. Other causes for masses in this age group include endometriomas, polycystic ovaries, tubo-ovarian abscesses, and benign neoplasms. Malignant neoplasms become more frequent with increasing age. In postmenopausal women with adnexal masses, neoplasms must be considered, along with leiomyomas, ovarian fibromas, and other lesions such as diverticular abscesses. Measurement of serum CA 125 is an appropriate test for assessing postmenopausal women with pelvic masses. Asymptomatic premenopausal patients with simple ovarian cysts <10 cm in diameter can be observed or placed on suppressive therapy with oral contraceptives. Postmenopausal women with simple cysts <3 cm in diameter may also be followed, provided the serum CA 125 level is not elevated and the patient has no signs or symptoms suggestive of malignancy. If the cyst is >3 cm or the CA 125 is elevated, further evaluation is necessary.

Additional Reading: Ovarian cancer: an overview. *Am Fam Physician.* 2009;80(6):609–616.

Category: Reproductive system

270. Which of the following factors is associated with a cause of impotence?
A) Masturbation
B) Alcohol dependence
C) Nocturnal tumescence
D) Vacuum erection devices
E) Excessive testosterone levels

Answer and Discussion

The answer is B. Impotence (often referred to as *erectile dysfunction*) was for the most part attributed to psychogenic factors such as life stressors and performance anxiety. However, current studies show that up to 90% of men with erectile dysfunction have underlying organic pathology. Organic causes of impotence include diabetes, drug or alcohol dependency, vascular and neurogenic compromise, and medications (e.g., hypertension medications). Most causes are multifactorial in nature. Nocturnal tumescence studies have been advocated as a method to distinguish psychogenic versus organic impotence; however, there is no consensus on the use and validity of these studies. Most urologists now initiate diagnostic testing by injecting alprostadil (Caverject), with resultant increase in penile flow. The ability to obtain an erection with pharmacologic injection, for the most part, rules out significant vascular causes of impotence. Initial laboratory testing should include only basic tests (however, this is controversial); hormonal testing should be based on clinical suspicion. Many experts feel serum testosterone determination should only be obtained in cases of low sexual desire or abnormal physical findings. Serum prolactin measurements should be obtained only in patients with low sexual desire, gynecomastia, visual symptoms, and/or testosterone levels <4 ng per mL. Others advocate serum testosterone and prolactin levels for all those affected. If pituitary abnormalities are suspected, brain imaging to rule out pituitary tumors should be performed. Treatment may involve the use of phospodiesterase 5 inhibitors (PDE5) including oral sildenafil (Viagra), vardenafil (Levitra), and tadalafil (Cialis), testosterone patches or injections, penile injections (phentolamine, alprostadil), vacuum devices, or penile implants.

> **Additional Reading:** Management of erectile dysfunction. *Am Fam Physician.* 2010;81(3):305–312.

> **Category:** Reproductive system

271. Cephalosporins are contraindicated for which of the following groups?
A) Patients allergic to eggs
B) Patients who have had a mild rash as a result of penicillin administration
C) Patients with G6PD deficiency
D) Patients suspected of bacterial meningitis
E) None of the above

Answer and Discussion

The answer is E. Hypersensitivity reactions to cephalosporins may occur and include rash, urticaria, and, in severe cases, anaphylaxis. Because of the similar chemical structure, there is a small proportion (<2%) of patients with penicillin allergy who cross-react with cephalosporins. Therefore, cephalosporins should be avoided in patients with a history of an immediate reaction to penicillin. Cephalosporins are used in patients with a history of mild reactions to penicillins.

> **Additional Reading:** Cephalosporins for patients with penicillin allergy. *Med Lett Drugs Ther.* 2012;54(1406):101.

> **Category:** Nonspecific system

272. A 21-year-old man presents to your office complaining that his left testicle feels abnormal. On examination, the area adjacent to the left testicle feels like a "bag of worms" that gets larger with a Valsalva's maneuver. The most likely diagnosis is
A) Hydrocele
B) Varicocele
C) Left inguinal hernia
D) Spermatocele
E) Testicular cancer

Answer and Discussion

The answer is B. Varicoceles are a collection of veins (pampiniform plexus) usually associated with the left scrotum, which are separate from the testicle. They are found in up to 15% of adult men. On clinical examination, a varicocele feels like a bag of worms that becomes larger with a Valsalva's maneuver. Some cases may be associated with decreased sperm counts and infertility. In these cases or if the patient has testicular pain or discomfort, surgical correction should be considered; otherwise, no further therapy is needed. Varicoceles are found most commonly on the left side, but up to 20% may be bilateral. Diagnosis should be made in a warm room by palpation of the spermatic cord with the patient in the standing position. Varicoceles are graded 1+ (palpable with Valsalva's maneuver only), 2+ (palpable), and 3+ (visible through the scrotal skin). An isolated right-sided varicocele or a lesion on either side that does not disappear when the patient assumes the supine position should prompt imaging of the retroperitoneum to evaluate for inferior vena caval or renal vein obstruction.

> **Additional Reading:** Evaluation of scrotal masses. *Am Fam Physician.* 2008;78(10):1165–1170.

> **Category:** Reproductive system

> An isolated right-sided varicocele or a lesion on either side that does not disappear when the patient assumes the supine position should prompt imaging of the retroperitoneum to evaluate for inferior vena caval or renal vein obstruction.

273. Exposure to radon gas has been associated with the development of
A) Renal cell carcinoma
B) Pancreatic cancer
C) Lung cancer
D) Bladder cancer
E) Esophageal cancer

[the development ...sure are asso- ...he soil and in ...sk to inhabit- ...ay be present ...oncrete block ...an do cinder ...s also impor- ...nmental Pro- ...s 4 pCi per L. ...en houses are ...re considered ...the problem ...don particles ...inhaled.

In: Domino ...A: Lippincott Williams and Wilkins; 2014.

> **Category:** Respiratory system

274. A 28-year-old man with a history of sex with men presents to your office complaining of a nonproductive cough, shortness of breath, fever, and chills. A chest radiograph shows bilateral interstitial infiltrates. The best treatment is
A) Oral azithromycin
B) Intravenous penicillin
C) Oral TMP-SMX
D) Intravenous amphotericin
E) Observation only

Answer and Discussion

The answer is C. *Pneumocystis jirovecii* (formerly *P. carinii*) is an opportunistic infection that often affects patients with profound immune suppression; the abbreviation of PCP is still used to designate this infection. Prior to the introduction of prophylaxis for PCP and the advent of potent antiretroviral therapy for HIV, 70% to 80% of patients with AIDS presented with PCP. Symptoms include fever, progressive dyspnea, nonproductive cough, and chest discomfort. Most common physical exam findings are tachypnea, tachycardia, and dry rales with exertion; pulmonary exam may be normal at rest. Chest radiograph classically shows diffuse bilateral symmetrical infiltrates in a butterfly pattern, but x-ray may be normal in early disease. Definitive diagnosis involves demonstration of the organism in tissue obtained either through inducted sputum collection or bronchoalveolar lavage. Treatment involves TMP-SMX for 21 days; intravenous therapy is indicated if patient is unable to tolerate oral medication. Oral prednisone or intravenous methylprednisolone may also be added once tuberculosis is ruled out if the PaO_2 is <70 mm Hg. Prophylactic therapy should be initiated for all patients with CD4 counts <200 cells per mm^3 or with a previous infection with PCP or oral thrush. For patients who cannot tolerate TMP-SMX due to allergy or adverse effects, alternatives include dapsone, aerosolized pentamidine, or atovaquone. Prophylaxis against PCP can be discontinued once the CD4 count is > 200 cells per mm^3 for > 3 months.

Additional Reading: Panel on opportunistic infections in HIV-infected adults and adolescents. Guidelines for the prevention and treatment of opportunistic infections in HIV-infected adults and adolescents: recommendations from the Centers for Disease Control and Prevention, the National Institutes of Health, and the HIV Medicine Association of the Infectious Diseases Society of America. May 2013. From: http://aidsinfo.nih.gov/contentfiles/lvguidelines/

Category: Respiratory system

275. A 59-year-old woman who has a 16-year history of diabetes mellitus reports weakness of her lower left leg, giving way of the knee, and discomfort in her anterior thigh for the last week. She has no recent injuries that she can recall. On examination, you find decreased sensation to pinprick and light touch over the left anterior thigh and reduced strength on hip flexion and knee extension. The straight leg raising test is normal. The most likely cause of this condition is
A) Femoral neuropathy
B) Diabetic polyneuropathy
C) Meralgia paresthetica
D) Spinal stenosis
E) Iliofemoral atherosclerosis

Answer and Discussion

The answer is A. Femoral neuropathy is a mononeuropathy commonly seen with diabetes mellitus, although it has been found to be secondary to a number of conditions that are common in diabetics and not specifically to the diabetes. Diabetic polyneuropathy is characterized by symmetric and distal limb sensory and motor deficits. Meralgia paresthetica, or lateral femoral cutaneous neuropathy, may be secondary to diabetes mellitus, but is manifested by numbness and paresthesia over the anterolateral thigh with no motor dysfunction. Spinal stenosis causes pain in the legs, but is not associated with the neurologic signs seen in this patient, nor with knee problems. Iliofemoral atherosclerosis, a relatively common complication of diabetes mellitus, may produce intermittent claudication involving one or both calf muscles but would not produce the motor weakness noted in this patient.

Additional Reading: Evaluation and prevention of diabetic neuropathy. *Am Fam Physician.* 2005;71(11):2123–2128.

Category: Neurologic

276. Which one of the following is associated with testosterone replacement for men with hypogonadism?
A) Osteoporosis
B) Depression
C) Reduced cognitive function
D) Increased fat deposition
E) Infertility

Answer and Discussion

The answer is E. Testosterone-replacement therapy is not appropriate in men who are interested in maintaining fertility, as exogenous testosterone will suppress the hypothalamic-pituitary-thyroid axis and cause infertility. However, replacement therapy can improve many of the effects of hypogonadism, including improvements in mood, energy level, sexual functioning, sense of well-being, lean body mass and muscle strength, erythropoiesis, bone mineral density, and cognition. In addition to infertility, other risks associated with testosterone use include a possible increased risk for prostate cancer, worsening of symptoms of benign prostatic hyperplasia, liver toxicity and tumor, worsening of sleep apnea and heart failure, gynecomastia, and skin diseases.

Additional Reading: Adverse events associated with testosterone administration. *N Engl J Med.* 2010;363:109.

Category: Reproductive system

277. Which of the following treatments should be used for a patient suspected of having Wernicke–Korsakoff syndrome?
A) Intravenous administration of glucose followed by administration of thiamine
B) Administration of folic acid followed by intravenous administration of dextrose
C) Administration of haloperidol with psychotherapy
D) Administration of thiamine followed by intravenous administration of dextrose
E) Lactated Ringer's solution with naloxone

Answer and Discussion

The answer is D. *Wernicke–Korsakoff syndrome* refers to the coexistence of Wernicke's encephalopathy and Korsakoff's psychosis. Wernicke's encephalopathy is characterized by gait ataxia, mental confusion, nystagmus, vomiting, fever, and ophthalmoplegia. The disease is primarily seen in alcoholics but can also occur in hyperemesis gravidarum or the use of vitamin-free nutrition (e.g., fad diets). The cause is thiamine deficiency (also known as *beriberi*). Wernicke's encephalopathy is a medical emergency and deserves prompt attention; otherwise, permanent brain damage or even death may occur. If Wernicke's encephalopathy is suspected, thiamine should always be administered before dextrose. Administration of glucose solution before thiamine administration may exhaust a patient's reserve of B vitamins and worsen his or her condition. Korsakoff's psychosis is also related to thiamine deficiency and may follow Wernicke's disease. Symptoms include retrograde amnesia, impaired learning ability, and confabulation. Treatment also involves the administration of thiamine.

Additional Reading: Evaluation of suspected dementia. *Am Fam Physician.* 2011;84(8):895–902.

Category: Neurologic

278. Which of the following laboratory findings is *not* associated with Graves' disease?
A) Thyroid-stimulating antibodies
B) Increased TSH
C) Increased T_4 level
D) Increased T_3 level

Answer and Discussion

The answer is B. The following are thyroid conditions and their associated laboratory findings:

- Euthyroid sick syndrome: decreased serum T_3, increased reverse T_3, decreased total T_4, and normal serum TSH
- Primary thyroid gland failure (hypothyroidism): marked elevation of serum TSH with decreased serum T_3 and T_4 levels
- Thyrotoxicosis: increased T_4 and T_3
- T_3 toxicosis: increased T_3 and normal T_4
- Graves' disease: increased T_4 and T_3, decreased TSH, and thyroid-stimulating antibodies present
- Plummer's disease (toxic multinodular goiter): increased T_3 and T_4, decreased TSH, thyroid-stimulating antibodies absent, and increased radioimmunoassay uptake in the hyperfunctioning nodule

Additional Reading: Hypothyroidism: an update. *Am Fam Physician.* 2012;86(3):244–251.

Category: Endocrine system

279. Benign positional vertigo is most easily confirmed by
A) Orthostatic blood pressures
B) Dix–Hallpike maneuvers
C) Cover–uncover test
D) MRI
E) Cold–warm water calorics

Answer and Discussion

The answer is B. Benign positional vertigo is a condition characterized by severe episodes of vertigo that usually last less than 1 minute and are precipitated by certain head positions. The vertiginous symptoms are accompanied by nystagmus, and there is no tinnitus or hearing loss (as is seen in Meniere's disease). The diagnosis is usually based on the history and reproduction of symptoms by the Dix–Hallpike maneuver: The patient's head is turned to the side and the patient goes from a sitting to a lying position with the head positioned beneath the level of the bed. A positive response is noted when the patient reports vertigo and there is evidence of nystagmus. Most cases are self-limited, and repeating the position that causes the vertigo usually fatigues the vertiginous response. Vestibular-type exercises performed several times daily may help eliminate the symptoms, especially for younger patients. Labyrinthine sedatives are of little help for this condition. Canalith repositioning can also be attempted and is beneficial for select patients. If fatigability of symptoms does not occur, further workup may be indicated to rule out a central cause for the vertigo.

Additional Reading: Dizziness: a diagnostic approach. *Am Fam Physician.* 2010;82(4):361–368.

Category: Special sensory

> Benign positional vertigo is a condition characterized by severe episodes of vertigo that usually last less than 1 minute and are precipitated by certain head positions. The vertiginous symptoms are accompanied by nystagmus, and there is no tinnitus or hearing loss (as is seen in Meniere's disease). The diagnosis is usually based on the history and reproduction of symptoms by the Dix–Hallpike maneuver.

280. A 72-year-old woman presents to your office with left-sided headaches, visual disturbances, low-grade fevers, generalized malaise, anorexia, and weight loss. Laboratory testing reveals a mild normocytic anemia, ESR of 120 mm per hour, and a mild leukocytosis. Appropriate management at this time consists of
A) MRI of the brain
B) Colonoscopy
C) Neurology referral
D) Visual field testing
E) High-dose steroid therapy

Answer and Discussion

The answer is E. Temporal arteritis is an inflammatory disease that predominantly affects the temporal and occipital arteries, although other arteries of the aortic arch may be involved. Systemic symptoms include low-grade fever, malaise, weakness, anorexia, weight loss, painful joints, headaches in the temporal distribution, and visual disturbances. Most cases occur in patients older than 50 years, and women are more commonly affected than men. Although the cause is unknown, it is believed to be autoimmune in origin. Granulomatous inflammatory lesions involving the arteries are seen. The diagnosis is made by the clinical history and an elevated ESR (usually greater than 100 mm per hour). Leukocytosis and mild normochromic normocytic anemia are also usually seen. A biopsy of the temporal artery showing inflammation provides the definitive diagnosis. If left untreated, the major and most serious complication of temporal arteritis is blindness. If temporal arteritis is suspected, high doses of corticosteroids (at least 40 mg per day) should be initiated immediately to prevent blindness. Monitoring the patient's ESR can determine dose reduction of steroid therapy. Significant improvement is usually seen within 4 weeks of therapy. Extended therapy (up to 2 years) may be necessary to control the disease. Polymyalgia rheumatica occurs in 40% to 60% of patients with temporal arteritis.

Additional Reading: Arteritis, temporal. In: Domino F, ed. *The 5-Minute Clinical Consult.* Philadelphia, PA: Lippincott Williams and Wilkins; 2014.

Category: Neurologic

281. A 55-year-old man with a history of difficult-to-control hypertension treated with chlorthalidone 25 mg, lisinopril (Zestril) 40 mg, amlodipine (Norvasc) 10 mg, and doxazosin (Cardura) 8 mg daily presents for follow-up with a complaint of weakness of several weeks' duration. On examination, his blood pressure is 160/109 mm Hg, with a normal cardiac examination, no abdominal bruits, and normal pulses. A CBC is normal, and a blood chemistry panel is also normal except for a serum potassium level of 3.1 mmol per L (N 3.5 to 5.5). Which one of the following would be best for confirming the most likely diagnosis in this patient?
A) Magnetic resonance angiography of the renal arteries
B) A renal biopsy
C) 24-hour urine for metanephrines
D) Early morning fasting cortisol
E) A plasma aldosterone/renin ratio

Answer and Discussion

The answer is E. Difficult-to-control hypertension has many possible causes, including nonadherence or the use of alcohol, NSAIDs, certain antidepressants, or sympathomimetics. Secondary hypertension can be caused by relatively common problems such as chronic kidney disease, obstructive sleep apnea, or primary hyperaldosteronism, as in the case described here. It is more common in women and often is asymptomatic. A significant number of these individuals will not be hypokalemic. Screening can be done with a morning plasma aldosterone/renin ratio. If the ratio is 20 or more and the aldosterone level is >15 ng per dL, then primary hyperaldosteronism is likely and referral for confirmatory testing should be considered.

Additional Reading: Education and management of the patient with difficult-to-control or resistant hypertension. *Am Fam Physician.* 2009;79(10):863–869.

Category: Cardiovascular system

282. Which of the following statements regarding enoxaparin (Lovenox) is true?
A) Its use has not been shown to be cost-effective in an outpatient setting.
B) The medication does not require laboratory monitoring.
C) The incidence of thrombocytopenia is the same as with heparin.
D) It must be given through an intravenous route.
E) It is safe to use in renal failure patients.

Answer and Discussion

The answer is B. Enoxaparin was the first LMW heparin approved by the U.S. FDA for the treatment of DVT in a dosage of 1 mg per kg twice daily or 1.5 mg once daily. LMW heparin offers distinct advantages over unfractionated heparin: It can be administered subcutaneously once or twice daily, it has a longer biologic half-life, dosing is fixed, and laboratory monitoring is not required. In addition, thrombocytopenia appears to be less likely. In patients with DVT, subcutaneous administration of heparin is as effective as continuous infusion of unfractionated heparin in preventing complications and reducing the risk of recurrence. Outpatient management of DVT using LMW heparin for short-term anticoagulation until warfarin is at a therapeutic level is considered safe and cost-effective. Candidates for outpatient therapy must be hemodynamically stable, without renal failure, and not at high risk for bleeding. Additionally, they must have an appropriate supportive home environment and be capable of daily monitoring until the INR is therapeutic. LMW heparin is typically given in combination with warfarin for 4 to 5 days. Simultaneous initiation of warfarin and unfractionated heparin or LMW heparin has not been associated with adverse outcomes. Dalteparin (Fragmin), another LMW heparin, is approved only for prophylaxis of DVT. The FDA has also approved the use of tinzaparin (Innohep) for the treatment of DVT.

Additional Reading: Updated guidelines on outpatient anticoagulation. *Am Fam Physician.* 2013;87(8):556–566.

Category: Cardiovascular system

283. A 59-year-old man presents to your office with complaints of "allergies" as he is having rhinorrhea. Which of the following would treat this symptom, but is not effective against other symtoms of allergic rhinitis?
A) Topical corticosteroid
B) Topical anticholinergic
C) Topical antihistamine
D) Oral antihistamine
E) Topical decongestant

Answer and Discussion

The answer is B. Allergic rhinitis may be seasonal or perennial. Seasonal allergic rhinitis is caused by seasonal allergens. Perennial allergic rhinitis may be caused by dust mites, molds, animal allergens, occupational allergens, or pollen. Risk factors for allergic rhinitis include a family history of atopy, serum immunoglobulin E (IgE) levels greater than 100 IU per mL before 6 years of age, higher socioeconomic class, and a positive allergy skin prick test. The diagnosis of rhinitis includes a history of symptoms and a physical examination. Skin testing for specific IgE antibody is the preferred diagnostic test to provide evidence of an allergic cause of the patient's symptoms.

There are numerous topical (intranasal) and oral agents available to treat allergic rhinitis such as antihistamines, decongestants, corticosteroids, and anticholinergics. Ipratropium (Atrovent) is a topical anticholinergic that reduces rhinorrhea but not other allergic rhinitis symptoms. It is recommended for episodic rhinitis because of its rapid onset of action and minimal side effects, although dryness of nasal membranes may occur.

Additional Reading: Practice parameters for managing allergic rhinitis. *Am Fam Physician.* 2009;80(1):79–85.

Category: Special sensory

284. Postpolio syndrome typically occurs
A) Immediately after the primary infection
B) 3 to 6 months after the initial infection
C) 2 to 3 years after the initial infection
D) 5 to 10 years after the initial infection
E) 15 to 30 years after the initial infection

Answer and Discussion

The answer is E. Postpolio syndrome is a constellation of symptoms that affects patients previously infected with the poliovirus. Typically, symptoms occur 15 to 30 years after the initial infection and include progressive generalized weakness, muscle pain, cramps, fasciculations, and atrophy. Other findings include cold, cyanotic extremities that have adequate pulses, and diffuse joint pain. Typically, the areas that were affected during the original infection are the same areas affected with the postpolio syndrome. In most, new symptoms are not due to progression of remote polio but due to a superimposed second condition such as diabetes, disk herniation, or degenerative joint disease. Treatment is supportive and involves rest.

Additional Reading: Post-polio syndrome. In: Basow DS, ed. *UpToDate.* Waltham, MA: UpToDate; 2013.

Category: Neurologic

285. Clubbing is thought to be a result of
A) Chronic hypercarbia
B) Chronic hypoxemia
C) Excess nitrogen production
D) Malignancy
E) Protein storage disease

Answer and Discussion

The answer is B. Clubbing has interested physicians for years. The cause is thought to be related to chronic hypoxemia. The condition is evident when the patient has an enlargement and softness of the nail beds and a reduction in the angle between the nail and the distal phalanx. The ratio of the anteroposterior diameter of the finger at the nail bed to that at the distal interphalangeal joint is a simple measurement of finger clubbing. If the ratio is more than 1, clubbing is present. Causes include pulmonary processes such as bronchogenic carcinoma, chronic pulmonary tuberculosis, COPD, and bronchiectasis; cyanotic congenital heart disease; subacute bacterial endocarditis; inflammatory bowel disease; and biliary cirrhosis. Clinical evidence of clubbing should be further evaluated with a chest radiograph because of the possibility of underlying lung disease.

Additional Reading: Evaluation of nail abnormalities. *Am Fam Physician.* 2012;85(8):779–787.

Category: Respiratory system

286. Which of the following statements about myasthenia gravis is true?
A) Symptoms usually improve with administration of norepinephrine-inhibiting medications.
B) Symptoms include ptosis, diplopia, dysarthria, dysphagia, and proximal muscle weakness of the limbs.
C) Symptoms are aggravated by the administration of edrophonium.
D) Symptoms rarely fluctuate and usually spare the facial nerves.

Answer and Discussion

The answer is B. Myasthenia gravis is a neuromuscular transmission disorder. It may occur at any age and may be associated with thymic tumors, thyrotoxicosis, lupus, or rheumatoid arthritis. It is more commonly seen in young women and appears to be linked to the HLA-DR3 genetic focus. If the patient is an elderly man, there is often an associated thymoma. Episodic muscle weakness is a symptom that often fluctuates in intensity, particularly in muscles associated with the cranial nerves; this includes ptosis, diplopia, dysarthria, dysphagia, and proximal muscle weakness in the limbs. These symptoms improve when cholinesterase-inhibiting medication is administered. Sensory function and deep tendon reflexes are unaffected. The disease is thought to be associated with an autoimmune-mediated attack on the postsynaptic acetylcholine-receptor sites, which prevents neurosynaptic transmission.

Diagnosis is usually confirmed by the edrophonium (Tensilon) test, which involves administration of an anticholinesterase medication. This test can help distinguish between a myasthenic and a cholinergic crisis. The patient is given 2 mg of edrophonium intravenously. If the patient's symptoms improve, the diagnosis of myasthenia gravis is confirmed. If symptoms become worse, a cholinergic crisis should be suspected. Because of the potential for respiratory arrest, atropine must be available as an antidote. Other findings that support the diagnosis of myasthenia gravis include the detection of acetylcholine-receptor antibodies in the patient's serum and the detection of thymomas by chest CT scans. Treatment is accomplished with the use of anticholinesterase medications (e.g., pyridostigmine, neostigmine), thymectomy, corticosteroids, immunosuppressive agents, and plasmapheresis.

> **Additional Reading:** Myasthenia graves. In: Domino F, ed. *The 5-Minute Clinical Consult.* Philadelphia, PA: Lippincott Williams and Wilkins; 2014.

> **Category:** Neurologic

287. Coenzyme Q10 appears to be most promising in the treatment of
A) Parkinson's disease
B) Diabetes mellitus
C) CHF
D) Hyperthyroidism

Answer and Discussion

The answer is A. Coenzyme Q10 is a supplement used in the treatment of a variety of medical conditions primarily related to low cellular energy metabolism and oxidative injury. Coenzyme Q10 appears most promising for neurodegenerative disorders such as Parkinson's disease and certain encephalomyopathies for which coenzyme Q10 has been used. Results in other areas of research, including treatment of CHF and diabetes, appear to be contradictory or need further clarification before proceeding with recommendations. Coenzyme Q10 appears to be a safe supplement with minimal side effects (e.g., gastrointestinal) and low drug interaction potential.

> **Additional Reading:** Coenzyme Q10. *Am Fam Physician.* 2005;72(6):1065–1070.

> **Category:** Neurologic

288. A 60-year-old woman presents with complaints of diffuse proximal muscle pain, low-grade fevers, and generalized fatigue. Laboratory findings include an elevated ESR and mild anemia. The most likely diagnosis is
A) Influenza
B) Dermatomyositis
C) Polymyalgia rheumatica
D) SLE
E) Rheumatoid arthritis

Answer and Discussion

The answer is C. Polymyalgia rheumatica is an inflammatory disease characterized by pain and stiffness associated with the proximal muscle groups. The condition is more common in women and usually occurs in patients older than 50 years. As many as 25% of patients may have associated giant cell arteritis, which can lead to blindness if not treated immediately with steroids. Symptoms include symmetric pain and morning stiffness associated with the proximal muscles such as the neck, shoulders, and hips. Patients may also report fever, generalized fatigue, anorexia, and weight loss. Laboratory findings include an elevated ESR (usually >50 mm per hour and often >100 mm per hour) and anemia of chronic disease. The physical examination is unremarkable with no evidence of synovitis or true muscle weakness. Diagnosis is made on the basis of the clinical findings and confirmed with response to therapy. Treatment involves the use of orally administered corticosteroids (prednisone 10 to 20 mg per day); usually the patient responds immediately. Once the ESR returns to normal and the patient's symptoms are improved, the steroids may be slowly tapered. In some cases, it may take months to years to completely taper the medication.

> **Additional Reading:** What is the best treatment for polymyalgia rheumatica? *Am Fam Physician.* 2010;81(6):788.

> **Category:** Musculoskeletal system

289. Which of the following statements best describes the rash associated with Rocky Mountain spotted fever?
A) It usually develops first on the extremities and spreads centrally.
B) It usually develops first on the trunk and spreads to the extremities.
C) It typically affects only the face.
D) It appears as bull's-eye lesions with central clearing.
E) The lesions are erythematous, raised papules that are intensely pruritic.

Answer and Discussion

The answer is A. The causative agent of Rocky Mountain spotted fever is *Rickettsia rickettsii*, which is transmitted by the bite of the wood tick or the dog tick. The disease is usually found in the southern United States and is more commonly seen during the summer months. It is the most common rickettsial disease in the United States. The wood tick (*Dermacentor andersoni*) is the principal vector in the Western United States, whereas the dog tick (*Dermacentor variabilis*) is the most common vector in the eastern and southern United States. Transmission from person to person is not thought to occur. The incidence of Rocky Mountain spotted fever is highest in children 5 to 9 years of age. A tick bite is recalled by only 50% to 70% of patients.

The onset of symptoms of Rocky Mountain spotted fever usually begins 5 to 7 days after inoculation. Common symptoms include generalized malaise, myalgias (especially in the back and leg muscles), fever, frontal headaches, nausea, and vomiting. Other symptoms may include nonproductive cough, sore throat, pleuritic chest pain, and abdominal pain. The classic presenting symptoms include sudden onset of headache, fever, and chills accompanied by an exanthem appearing within the first few days of symptoms. Initially, lesions appear on the palms, soles, wrists, ankles, and forearms. The lesions are pink and macular and fade with applied pressure. The rash then extends to the axilla, buttocks, trunk, neck, and face, becoming maculopapular and then petechial. The lesions may then coalesce to form large areas of ecchymosis and ulceration. Respiratory and circulatory failure, as well as neurologic compromise, may occur. Patients with glucose-6-phosphate dehydrogenase (G6PD) deficiency are at especially high risk for complications and poor outcomes.

Diagnosis is based primarily on clinical signs and symptoms. If a rash is present, the use of skin biopsy and immunofluorescent staining for *Rickettsia* is highly specific, although with only slightly more than 60% sensitivity. Laboratory testing is of limited usefulness but may include thrombocytopenia and hyponatremia. Elevation of specific ELISA and latex agglutination titers is usually delayed until the convalescence period. Fever and headache during peak months of tick exposure in endemic areas should suggest Rocky Mountain spotted fever. Rash, thrombocytopenia, and hyponatremia make immediate treatment imperative. Doxycycline is the recommended treatment for Rocky Mountain spotted fever, given for a minimum of 7 days. For optimal effect, it is critical to treat patients early in the course of their illness. Treatment should not be delayed until laboratory confirmation is obtained. Mortality rates for the elderly can approach 70%, whereas mortality rates for children are less than 20%.

Additional Reading: Rocky mountain spotted fever. In: Domino F, ed. *The 5-Minute Clinical Consult*. Philadelphia, PA: Lippincott Williams and Wilkins; 2014.

Category: Nonspecific system

In most cases of Rocky Mountain Spotted Fever, a rash develops on the wrist and ankles, sparing the face, and spreads centrally after the first few days of the fever. The rash, initially erythematous and macular, often becomes petechial.

290. Which of the following is associated with pseudogout?
A) Calcium pyrophosphate crystal deposition in the large joints
B) Lack of response with the use of colchicine
C) High uric acid levels
D) Lack of response with the use of anti-inflammatory medication
E) Negative birefringence seen with polarized microscopy

Answer and Discussion

The answer is A. Pseudogout is a condition that results from the deposition of calcium pyrophosphate crystals in the large joints (principally the knees) and leads to a reactive synovitis. Affected patients are usually older than 60 years. Men and women are affected equally, except in some studies that show women are more affected than men. Pseudogout is associated with trauma, surgery, amyloidosis, hemochromatosis, and hyperparathyroidism. Diagnosis is made by joint aspiration and examination of the fluid under a polarized microscope. Calcium pyrophosphate exhibits a positive birefringence in contrast to a negative birefringence seen with urate crystals in gout. Laboratory tests do not show elevated uric acid levels. Radiographs of the affected joints usually show degenerative changes and calcification of the surrounding cartilaginous structures. Treatment involves the use of anti-inflammatory agents and colchicine. Intra-articular steroid injection is occasionally helpful in resistant cases.

Additional Reading: Gout: an update. *Am Fam Physician*. 2007;76(6):801–808.

Category: Musculoskeletal system

291. Diabetic foot ulcers
A) Are typically polymicrobial
B) Rarely become infected
C) Require topical antibiotics
D) Should not be debrided because of the risk of bacteremia

Answer and Discussion

The answer is A. Foot ulcers in diabetic patients result from a diminished sensation associated with peripheral neuropathy and peripheral vascular disease (which is also usually present). Persistent pressure from ill-fitting shoes or skin cracking secondary to tinea pedis may predispose the patient's feet to infection. Diabetics who smoke should be encouraged to stop, and alcohol use should be discouraged. Infections associated with the feet are usually caused by *Staphylococcus*, *Streptococcus*, anaerobes, and gram-negative organisms. Aerobic and anaerobic cultures should be taken when signs of infection, such as purulence or inflammation, are present. Cultures are best taken from purulent drainage or curetted material from the ulcer base. Because all ulcers are contaminated, culture of noninfected wounds is generally not recommended. Polymicrobial infections predominate in severe diabetic foot infections and include a variety of aerobic gram-positive cocci, gram-negative rods, and anaerobes. Treatment involves debridement of nonvital and necrotic tissue, as well as oral or intravenous antibiotics. In severe cases, amputation may be necessary. Topical antibiotics are of little help and may delay healing. Osteomyelitis should always be considered in severe and persistent cases. Periodic examinations and treatment by a podiatrist are recommended.

Additional Reading: Diabetic foot infections. *Am Fam Physician*. 2013;88(3):177–184.

Category: Endocrine system

292. What is the threshold BMI for obesity?
A) 25
B) 27
C) 30
D) 35
E) 40

Answer and Discussion

The answer is C. The BMI is an approximate measure of body fat. It is based on height and weight. A BMI between 19 and 25 is considered normal. If a patient's BMI is 25 to 29.9, that individual is considered to be overweight. A person is categorized as obese if his or her BMI is 30 or higher.

Additional Reading: Obesity. In: Domino F, ed. *The 5-Minute Clinical Consult*. Philadelphia, PA: Lippincott Williams and Willkins; 2014.

Category: Endocrine system

293. A 65-year-old man complains of gynecomastia and galactorrhea with erectile dysfunction. The most likely diagnosis is
A) Breast cancer
B) Testicular cancer
C) Prolactinoma
D) Adrenal adenoma
E) Diabetes mellitus

Answer and Discussion

The answer is C. Prolactinomas are the most common functioning, secreting pituitary tumors. Galactorrhea, oligomenorrhea, primary and secondary amenorrhea, and infertility are seen in women with prolactinomas. Men may experience impotence, infertility, and, less commonly, gynecomastia and/or galactorrhea. Prolactin levels >300 μg per L usually indicate a pituitary adenoma. Patients with hypogonadism, impotence, or galactorrhea may have abnormal prolactin levels associated with prolactinomas. Some medications, including oral contraceptives, phenothiazines, tricyclic antidepressants, antihypertensives (e.g., α-methyldopa), and opioid-type medications, may increase prolactin levels. Other causes for hyperprolactinemia include nipple stimulation, pregnancy, stress, sexual intercourse, sleep, hypoglycemia, hypothyroidism, sarcoidosis, paraneoplastic syndromes (bronchogenic carcinoma and hypernephroma), and chronic renal failure. Treatment (controversial) for larger tumors involves the use of bromocriptine (dopamine agonist), which lowers the serum prolactin level. If residual tumor remains, surgery or radiotherapy may be necessary. With small tumors, close observation may be instituted if the patient is asymptomatic.

> **Additional Reading:** Hyperprolactinemia. In: Domino F, ed. *The 5-Minute Clinical Consult*. Philadelphia, PA: Lippincott Williams and Wilkins; 2014.

> Category: Endocrine system

294. Which of the following statements about clonidine is true?
A) Rapid withdrawal may precipitate a hypertensive crisis.
B) It is classified as an ACE inhibitor.
C) Concomitant use with β-blockers decreases the risk of hypertensive crisis when both medications are discontinued.
D) The mechanism of action involves the increased release of renin and α-receptor activation.
E) Use of the drug can exacerbate RLS.

Answer and Discussion

The answer is A. Clonidine is a second-line drug used in the treatment of hypertension, RLS, nicotine withdrawal, prophylaxis for vascular headaches, and opiate withdrawal. Clonidine works by decreasing vascular resistance through α-receptor blockade and inhibiting renin release. Rapid withdrawal of the medication may precipitate a hypertensive crisis, which can be life threatening. Symptoms of hypertensive crisis include tachycardia, diaphoresis, headache, nervousness, and abdominal pain. Concomitant use with β-blockers may also increase the risk of hypertensive crisis when both medications are discontinued.

> **Additional Reading:** Drugs for hypertension. *Treat Guidel Med Lett*. 2012;10(113):1–10.

> Category: Cardiovascular system

295. A 62-year-old woman presents complaining of joint pain, polyuria, polydipsia, and generalized fatigue. The woman reports a history of recurrent kidney stones and depression. Radiographs show osteopenia and subperiosteal resorption on the phalanges. Which of the following blood tests may best help determine the cause of her symptoms?
A) ACE level
B) Parathyroid hormone level
C) ANA test
D) Sedimentation rate (ESR)
E) Bone densitometry

Answer and Discussion

The answer is B. Primary hyperparathyroidism is a disorder caused by excessive secretion of parathyroid hormone. Findings include hypercalcemia (ionized), hypophosphatemia (hyperphosphatemia suggests secondary hyperparathyroidism), an excessive bone loss leading to cystic bone lesions, and osteitis fibrosa cystica. Most patients are asymptomatic; however, some may present with renal lithiasis, joint or back pain, polyuria and polydipsia, constipation, and fatigue. It is the most common cause of hypercalcemia in the general population. Familial cases are often related to endocrine tumors. The condition is more common in women and in patients older than 50 years. It also

occurs in high frequency three or more decades after neck irradiation. It is usually caused by an adenoma of the parathyroid (90% of cases); carcinoma is rare (3% of cases). Radiographs may show subperiosteal resorption of the phalanges and osteopenia. Treatment usually involves surgical exploration and removal of parathyroid adenoma. For patients with mild, asymptomatic primary hyperparathyroidism, the recommendations for surgery are controversial.

> **Additional Reading:** Hyperparathyroidism. In: Domino F, ed. *The 5-Minute Clinical Consult*. Philadelphia, PA: Lippincott Williams and Wilkins; 2014.

> Category: Endocrine system

296. The most common cause of chronic cough is
A) Postnasal drip
B) Bronchiectasis
C) Gastroesophageal reflux
D) Asthma
E) ACE inhibitors

Answer and Discussion

The answer is A. Coughing is part of the body's infection protective system and helps remove particles and material from the airway. In some cases, the patient may experience a chronic cough that can be attributed to a number of different problems, including postnasal drip (most common cause), gastroesophageal reflux, and bronchoconstriction as seen in cough-variant asthma patients. Other common associated conditions include the use of ACE inhibitors, chronic bronchitis seen in smokers, and bronchiectasis. Treatment involves eliminating the underlying cause. Treatment of conditions, such as asthma and COPD, may involve the use of bronchodilators (β agonist or theophylline), cromolyn sodium, and inhaled steroids; the treatment of postnasal drip may involve the use of antihistamines and topical nasal steroids. Patients should be informed that it may take 8 to 12 weeks before their cough improves when using inhaled steroids. Treatment of gastroesophageal reflux involves the use of antacids, H_2-receptor blockers, and PPIs. Eliminating a cough caused by ACE inhibitors usually takes several days before improvement is seen. Unfortunately, it is more difficult to treat patients with chronic bronchitis. The use of antibiotics with the absence of supporting symptoms suggestive of infection is not useful and should be avoided. Mucolytics have not been shown to be beneficial.

> **Additional Reading:** Evaluation of the patient with chronic cough. *Am Fam Physician*. 2004;69:2159–2166, 2169.

> Category: Respiratory system

297. A 26-year-old single man presents to your office complaining of a painless ulcer that formed on his penis approximately 3 months ago. The ulcer healed, but an erythematous rash on the palms and soles of his feet has recently developed. He also reports generalized fatigue, malaise, fever, headache, and arthralgias. The most likely diagnosis is
A) Gonorrhea
B) Chancroid
C) Syphilis
D) Reiter's syndrome
E) Lyme disease

Answer and Discussion

The answer is C. Syphilis, also known as lues, is a disease caused by the spirochete *Treponema pallidum*. The disease is characterized by differing clinical stages that may affect multiple organ systems and is transmitted primarily by sexual contact. The usual incubation period is approximately 4 to 5 weeks. The following are the different stages associated with the disease:

- Primary syphilis is the initial stage of syphilis and is marked by the appearance of a chancre, which is a papule that ruptures and develops into a painless ulcer. In most cases, the ulcer heals in 4 to 6 weeks. Chancres occur on the penis, vulva, cervix, anus, and also the lips, tongue, oral mucosa, fingers, and other body parts. In addition to the ulcer, there may be associated lymphadenopathy but usually no other symptoms.
- Secondary syphilis is the second stage of syphilis and is characterized by cutaneous rashes that usually affect the volar surfaces of extremities, such as the palms of the hands and soles of the feet. They appear 6 to 12 weeks after the initial infection and are usually circular macules, papules, or pustules that are not pruritic. Other areas can be affected, and uveitis, periostitis, hepatitis, meningitis, and glomerulitis can occur. Additional symptoms include flulike symptoms such as generalized fatigue, anorexia, malaise, fever, headache, anemia, lymphadenopathy, and arthralgias. Mucous membranes often become ulcerated and form circular ulcerated lesions. The secondary stage may last up to 1 year.
- Latent syphilis is characterized by the resolution of the rashes seen during the secondary stage and may last for many years after the initial infection. During this period, the patient is usually completely asymptomatic but has a positive treponemal antibody test.
- Late or tertiary syphilis occurs 10 or more years after the initial infection and is characterized by benign tertiary syphilis involving the skin and giving rise to gummas (granulomatous lesions that lead to fibrosis, necrosis, and scarring), cardiovascular syphilis (giving rise to thoracic aortic aneurysms and aortic insufficiency), and neurosyphilis (causing a multitude of neurologic disorders including headaches, insomnia, blurred vision, confusion, seizures, and decreased motor function with paralysis). Tabes dorsalis presents as symptoms and signs of demyelination of the posterior columns, dorsal roots, and dorsal root ganglia. Symptoms include an ataxic wide-based gait, paresthesias, bladder dysfunction, impotence, areflexia, and loss of pain, temperature, and position sensation.

Screening tests for syphilis include a VDRL test and the rapid plasma reagin test. If positive, a confirming fluorescent treponemal antibody–absorption test should be performed. In addition, microscopic examination of fluid taken from lesions can be examined with dark-field microscopy to look for spirochetes. The treatment of choice is penicillin given in the long-acting benzathine form intramuscularly. In many cases, there is a reaction to treatment after 6 to 12 hours called the Jarisch–Herxheimer reaction; symptoms include fatigue, headaches, low-grade fever, sweating, and more severe reactions, including seizures in patients with neurologic involvement. It is important to distinguish these reactions from allergic reactions to penicillin. A repeated VDRL or rapid plasma reagin can be assessed to ensure adequate treatment. In most cases, they become negative 1 year after treatment. Sexual contacts should also be treated appropriately. Any patient suspected of having syphilis more than 1 year should have a CSF examination.

Additional Reading: Syphilis. In: Domino F, ed. *The 5-Minute Clinical Consult.* Philadelphia, PA: Lippincott Williams and Wilkins; 2014.

Category: Neurologic

Screening tests for syphilis include a VDRL test and the rapid plasma reagin test. If positive, a confirming fluorescent treponemal antibody–absorption test should be performed.

298. Which one of the following has been shown to be effective for improving symptoms of varicose veins?
A) Horse chestnut seed extract
B) Vitamin B
C) Ephedra
D) Milk thistle
E) St. John's wort

Answer and Discussion

The answer is A. Horse chestnut seed extract has been shown to be effective when used orally for symptomatic treatment of chronic venous insufficiency, such as varicose veins. It may also be useful for relieving pain, tiredness, tension, and swelling in the legs. It contains a number of anti-inflammatory substances, including escin, which reduces edema and lowers fluid exudation by decreasing vascular permeability. Milk thistle may be effective for hepatic cirrhosis. Ephedra is considered unsafe, as it can cause severe life-threatening or disabling adverse effects in some people. St. John's wort may be effective for treating mild-to-moderate depression. Vitamin B is used to treat pernicious anemia.

Additional Reading: Management of varicose veins. *Am Fam Physician.* 2008;78(11):1289–1294.

Horse chestnut seed extract for chronic venous insufficiency. *Cochrane Database Syst Rev.* 2006;(1):CD003230.

Category: Cardiovascular system

299. A 16-year-old surfer presents with an erythematous, maculopapular rash that was noted in the area of his bathing suit. Initial treatment includes
A) Cryotherapy
B) Clotrimazole cream
C) Ice packs
D) Application of vinegar
E) Zinc oxide

Answer and Discussion

The answer is D. Swimmers or surfers with seabather's eruption present with an urticarial maculopapular rash on areas of the body that were covered by the swimsuit. The rash may appear while the bather is in the water or up to 1.5 days later. The rash may last for 2 to 28 days; most reactions resolve within 1 to 2 weeks. Systemic symptoms include fever, nausea, vomiting, and headache and are more likely to affect children. Initial treatment involves the topical application of heat or vinegar. Further treatment is symptomatic and may include topical corticosteroids, oral antihistamines, and oral steroids. Twice-daily application of thiabendazole (Mintezol) can be beneficial. The swimsuit should be cleaned thoroughly because larvae can persist and reenvenomate.

Additional Reading: Health issues for surfers. *Am Fam Physician.* 2005;71:2313–2317.

Category: Integumentary

300. A 33-year-old woman presents for an office visit after passing a 4-mm calcium oxalate stone. This was his first episode of nephrolithiasis, but he is worried and wants to know how he can prevent developing more kidney stones in the future, as this was a painful experience for him. You would advise which of the following:
A) Drink up to 2 L of water per day.
B) Increase his consumption of meats and grains.
C) Increase the level of fructose in his diet.
D) Restrict foods high in oxalate, such as spinach and rhubarb.

Answer and Discussion

The answer is A. Recommendations to prevention recurrent nephrolithiasis include increasing fluid intake up to 2 L of water daily (larger amounts are not recommended as they may lead to electrolyte disturbances). Dietary changes depend on the composition of the passed stone. If no stone is available for analysis, a 24-hour urine collection is advised for calcium, phosphorus, magnesium, uric acid, and oxalate. Approximately 60% of all stones are calcium oxalate. Uric acid stones account for up to 17% of stones and, like cystine stones, form in acidic urine. Alkalinization of the urine to a pH of 6.5 to 7.0 may reduce stone formation in patients with these types of stones. This includes a diet with plenty of fruits and vegetables, and limiting acid-producing foods such as meat, grains, dairy products, and legumes. Drinking mineral water, which is relatively alkaline with a pH of 7.0 to 7.5, is also recommended. Restriction of dietary oxalates has not been shown to be effective in reducing stone formation in most patients. Acidification of the urine to a pH < 7.0 is recommended for patients with the less common calcium phosphate and struvite stones. This can be accomplished by consumption of at least 16 oz of cranberry juice per day, or by taking betaine, 650 mg three times daily.

Additional Reading: Treatment and prevention of kidney stones: an update. *Am Fam Physician.* 2011;84(11):1234–1242.

Category: Nephrologic system

301. A 66-year-old woman presents for a follow-up visit a month after you had prescribed enalapril (Vasotec) for her heart failure. She is felling okay, but feels that her ankles are swollen. Her serum creatinine level is 2.6 mg per dL (N 0.6 to 1.5) and potassium level is 5.8 mEq per L (N 3.4 to 4.8). Her baseline values were normal 2 months ago. Which one of the following is a side effect of ACE inhibitors that is the most likely cause of these changes in renal function?
A) Toxicity to the proximal renal tubules
B) Impaired autoregulation of glomerular blood flow
C) Microangiopathic arteriolar thrombosis
D) Rhabdomyolysis
E) Interstitial nephritis

Answer and Discussion

The answer is B. Renal blood flow is autoregulated so to sustain pressure within the glomerulus, by angiotensin II–related vasoconstriction. ACE inhibitors impair renal autoregulatory function, resulting in a decreased glomerular filtration rate and can cause acute renal injury. This is usually reversible if recognized and the offending medication stopped. NSAIDs can exert a similar effect, but they can also cause glomerulonephritis and interstitial nephritis. Statins, haloperidol, and drugs of abuse (cocaine, heroin) can cause rhabdomyolysis with the release of myoglobin, which causes acute renal injury. Thrombotic microangiopathy is a rare mechanism of injury to the kidney and may be caused by clopidogrel, quinine, or certain chemotherapeutic agents.

Additional Reading: Drug-induced nephrotoxicity. *Am Fam Physician.* 2008;78(6):743–750.

Category: Nephrologic system

302. Which of the following infections causes tabes dorsalis?
A) Gonorrhea
B) Tuberculosis
C) Syphilis
D) Bacterial meningitis
E) ALS

Answer and Discussion

The answer is C. Tabes dorsalis is the result of syphilitic lesions that affect the posterior columns of the spinal cord. Symptoms include the insidious onset of pain, loss of sensation, proprioception and vibratory sense, loss of reflexes, and ataxia. The main symptom is an insidious, sharp, stabbing pain that is periodic and recurrent and affects the lower extremities. Over time, the patient may experience increasing difficulty with gait, particularly in poorly illuminated areas. Paresthesias and loss of sensation are commonly associated with the soles of the feet. Other findings include a thin appearance with sad- or depressed-appearing facies, Argyll Robertson pupils (react poorly to light but well to accommodation), positive Romberg's sign, loss of reflexes in the lower extremities, bladder disturbances, and visible ataxia. Acute abdominal pain with vomiting (visceral crisis) can occur in 15% to 30%. In tabes dorsalis, the rapid plasma reagin and VDRL tests may not be positive; however, the fluorescent treponemal antibody–absorption test is usually positive. Treatment involves the administration of a prolonged course of high-dose penicillin to treat syphilis. Pain medications along with chlorpromazine and carbamazepine may be helpful for the control of pain. Unfortunately, tabes dorsalis often progresses despite treatment.

Additional Reading: Syphilis treatment and care. From: http://www.cdc.gov/std/syphilis/treatment.htm

Category: Neurologic

303. A 21-year-old otherwise healthy woman is seen in your office with a recent purified protein derivative tuberculin skin test that is positive. The woman has never had a positive test before. A chest radiograph is negative, and there are no signs of disease. The most appropriate treatment is
A) Reassurance
B) INH and rifampin for 6 months
C) INH for 6 months
D) INH, rifampin, and streptomycin (or ethambutol) for 12 months
E) Streptomycin for 6 months

Answer and Discussion

The answer is C. Tuberculosis is caused by *Mycobacterium tuberculosis*, a nonmotile acid-fast rod that is spread primarily by inhalation. The organism can affect many different systems but usually affects the lungs. There has been a recent increase in incidence, particularly in the immunocompromised and elderly populations. Symptoms include fever, fatigue, weight loss, a productive cough, dyspnea, and, occasionally, hemoptysis. Diagnosis is usually accomplished with a chest radiograph, which shows apical infiltrates and mediastinal lymphadenopathy, and microscopic examination of sputum, which shows acid-fast rods. A definitive diagnosis is achieved with a culture of early morning sputum growing *M. tuberculosis*. A Mantoux tuberculin skin test using purified protein derivative injected intradermally is also used to support the diagnosis. In most cases, an area of induration >10 mm (with risk factors), 15 mm (without risk factors), or 5 mm (in HIV patients) 48 hours after administration is a positive response. A negative response does not exclude the diagnosis. A calcified focus of infection seen on chest radiograph is referred to as a *Ghon complex*.

Treatment for active disease is accomplished with INH, rifampin, and pyrazinamide. In some cases, a fourth drug (e.g., streptomycin or ethambutol) is necessary. Most treatment regimens require extended courses lasting at least 6 to 9 months. Patients younger than 35 years who have a positive skin test but no evidence of disease (including a negative chest radiograph) are usually treated with INH for 6 to 9 months. All patients who have a positive skin test, no evidence of active disease, and a negative chest radiograph are diagnosed with latent tuberculosis infection (LTBI), regardless of prior BCG vaccination history, and should be treated with INH 300 mg per day for 9 months, or an alternative regimen if needed. Prior guidance to avoid LTBI treatment in patients older than 35 years due to a higher risk of INH hepatotoxicity have been abandoned in favor of screening targeted to high-risk individuals and treatment of all positives, with careful monitoring for drug toxicity. Compliance is a critical factor in ensuring adequate treatment for both active and latent tuberculosis and is often followed by the local department of public health. Other sites affected by tuberculosis include the kidneys, pericardium, and spine. All patients with a new diagnosis of tuberculosis should be tested for HIV and vice versa.

> **Additional Reading:** Latent tuberculosis infection: a guide for primary health care providers. From: http://www.cdc.gov/tb/publications/LTBI/default.htm.

> **Category:** Respiratory system

304. A 32-year-old woman reports frequent bouts of constipation alternating with diarrhea. She frequently experiences abdominal discomfort, which is relieved with bowel movements. Stress tends to aggravate her symptoms. The most appropriate treatment includes
A) Steroid enemas
B) Mesalamine enemas
C) Peppermint oil
D) Metoclopramide
E) None of the above

Answer and Discussion

The answer is C. Irritable bowel syndrome is defined as abdominal discomfort or pain associated with altered bowel habits for at least 3 days per month in the previous 3 months, with the absence of organic disease. Cramping abdominal pain is the most common symptom along with diarrhea, constipation, or alternating diarrhea and constipation. The goals of treatment are symptom relief and improved quality of life. Exercise, antibiotics, antispasmodics, peppermint oil, and probiotics appear to improve symptoms. Over-the-counter laxatives and antidiarrheals may improve stool frequency but not pain. Treatment with antidepressants and psychological therapies are also effective for improving symptoms compared with usual care. Lubiprostone is effective for the treatment of constipation-predominant irritable bowel syndrome.

> **Additional Reading:** Diagnosis and management of IBS in adults. *Am Fam Physician.* 2012;86(5):419–426.

> **Category:** Gastroenterology system

305. Which of the following statements about treadmill exercise testing is true?
A) Women have a low incidence of false-positive results.
B) It is recommended for patients who experience angina at rest to document ECG changes.
C) It is contraindicated in patients with moderate-to-severe aortic stenosis.
D) The appearance of a bundle branch block on ECG represents no concern.
E) A positive result requires >3 mm of ST-segment depression.

Answer and Discussion

The answer is C. Exercise stress testing is used to evaluate chest pain in patients with suspected CVD. The sensitivity ranges from 56% to 81%, and the specificity ranges from 72% to 96%. With this in mind, the exercise stress test has relatively low sensitivity and specificity. Because of this, a patient with a high pretest likelihood of ischemic heart disease still has a high probability of developing significant disease even in the face of a normal (negative test). Furthermore, a patient with a low probability of ischemic heart disease still has a low chance of significant disease even if the test is positive. The optimal use of diagnostic testing is for those patients with moderate pretest probabilities. Women tend to have a higher incidence of false-positive results. There are two basic protocols: the Bruce protocol and the Ellestad protocol. In the standard exercise stress test (Bruce protocol), the patient is asked to exercise for 3-minute intervals on a motorized treadmill device while being monitored for the following: heart rate and blood pressure response to exercise, symptoms during the test, ECG response (specifically ST-segment displacement), dysrhythmias, and exercise capacity. A positive test is defined as an ST-segment depression of at least 1 mm below baseline. Contraindications to exercise stress testing include the following:

- Recent MI within the preceding 4 to 6 weeks (except for a submaximal exercise stress test [65% of predicted maximum heart rate] that is often performed before hospital discharge for patients with a recent MI)
- Angina at rest
- Rapid ventricular or atrial arrhythmias
- High-grade AV block or bradyarrhythmias
- Uncompensated CHF
- Recent acute illness (noncardiac in origin)
- Moderate-to-severe aortic stenosis
- Uncontrolled blood pressure (systolic >200 or diastolic >110 mm Hg before onset of exercise)
- Active myocarditis/pericarditis
- Acute PE
- Systemic illness
- Noncompliant patient
- Criteria for stopping an exercise stress test include
- Predicted heart rate is achieved
- Patient complains of excessive fatigue, claudication, or dyspnea
- PVCs that increase in frequency or ventricular tachycardia
- High-grade AV block appears on ECG
- Significant ST changes seen on ECG (>3 mm depression)
- Severe angina
- Systolic blood pressure >220 or diastolic blood pressure >120 during exercise or a decrease in systolic blood pressure with exercise
- Appearance of a bundle branch block
- Equipment malfunction or technical failure

The following are considered to be parameters associated with poor prognosis or increased disease severity: failure to complete stage 2 of a Bruce protocol, failure to achieve a heart rate >120 bpm (off β-blockers), onset of ST-segment depression at a heart rate of <120 bpm, ST-segment depression more than 2 mm, ST-segment depression lasting >6 minutes into recovery, ST-segment depression in multiple leads, poor systolic blood pressure response to exercise, ST-segment elevation, angina with exercise, and exercise-induced ventricular tachycardia.

Additional Reading: Noninvasive cardiac imaging. *Am Fam Physician.* 2007;75(8):1219–1228.

Category: Cardiovascular system

306. Anemia of chronic disease is associated with which of the following?
A) Macrocytic, normochromic anemia
B) Increased serum ferritin
C) Increased TIBC
D) High serum iron level
E) Hemoglobin of 5 to 8 mg per dL

Answer and Discussion

The answer is B. Anemia of chronic disease can be caused by

- Chronic infections, such as osteomyelitis and subacute bacterial endocarditis
- Chronic disorders, including rheumatoid arthritis, lupus, renal failure, sarcoidosis, and polymyalgia rheumatica
- Other disorders, including neoplasm, liver disorders, and hypothyroidism

Symptoms include typical complaints associated with anemia such as generalized fatigue, malaise, decreased mentation, and those symptoms associated with the primary disorder. Laboratory tests show a mild, normocytic normochromic anemia with an Hb at approximately 10 mg per dL. Microcytic indices are also possible. Serum ferritin is also usually increased, with a low TIBC and low serum iron level. The only therapy is treatment of the underlying disorder. The administration of iron, folic acid, or vitamin B_{12} is ineffective. Transfusion should only be considered in advanced cases in patients with severe symptoms.

Additional Reading: Anemia, chronic disease. In: Domino F, ed. *The 5-Minute Clinical Consult.* Philadelphia, PA: Lippincott Williams and Wilkins; 2014.

Category: Hematologic system

307. Which of the following would be best in the short- and long-term treatment of back pain?
A) To stay active with regular physical activity
B) Back supports
C) Work site modification
D) Back education school

Answer and Discussion

The answer is A. Patient education to stay active, avoid aggravating movements, and return to normal activity as soon as possible and a discussion of the often benign nature of acute low back pain is effective in patients with nonspecific acute back pain. Bed rest is not helpful for nonspecific acute low back pain and although regular exercises may not be beneficial in the treatment of nonspecific acute low back pain, physical therapy (McKenzie method and spine stabilization) may lessen the risk of recurrence and need for health care services. Neither lumbar supports nor back belts appear to be effective in reducing the incidence of low back pain. Work site modifications, including educational interventions, have some short-term benefit in reducing the incidence of low back pain. However, their applicability to the primary care setting is unknown. Back (educational) schools may prevent further back injury for persons with recurrent or chronic low back pain, but their long-term effectiveness has not been well studied.

Additional Reading: Diagnosis and treatment of acute low back pain. *Am Fam Physician.* 2012;85(4):343–350.

Category: Musculoskeletal system

Neither lumbar supports nor back belts appear to be effective in reducing the incidence of low back pain.

308. A 75-year-old presents with a painful erythematous and vesicular rash that is developing on the forehead in the periorbital area. The rash began yesterday. The patient has had some generalized myalgias and low-grade fevers. Appropriate management at this time includes
A) Antiviral medication and follow-up in 3 to 5 days
B) Antibiotics plus antiviral medications and follow-up in 3 to 5 days
C) Reassurance
D) Hospitalization with IV antibiotics
E) Antiviral medication and ophthalmology referral

Answer and Discussion

The answer is E. The most common complication of herpes zoster is postherpetic neuralgia (i.e., pain along cutaneous, dermatomal nerves persisting >30 days after the lesions have healed). The incidence of postherpetic neuralgia increases with age and is not commonly seen in patients younger than 60 years. Herpes zoster lesions can become secondarily infected with staphylococci or streptococci, and cellulitis may develop. Herpes zoster involving the ophthalmic division of the trigeminal nerve can lead to ocular complications and visual loss. In these cases, immediate referral to an ophthalmologist is recommended. Other less common complications include motor paresis and encephalitis.

Additional Reading: Herpes zoster and postherpetic neuralgia: prevention and management. *Am Fam Physician.* 2005;72:1075–1080.

Category: Integumentary

309. Addison's disease (primary adrenal insufficiency) is associated with
A) Increased ACTH production
B) Decreased ACTH production
C) Increased urine 17-hydroxysteroids and 17-ketosteroids
D) Hypernatremia
E) Hypothalamic dysfunction

Answer and Discussion

The answer is A. Primary adrenal insufficiency (Addison's disease) is a condition resulting from adrenocortical insufficiency. Secondary adrenal insufficiency is secondary to a lack of ACTH production from the pituitary gland. The primary disease results in electrolyte disturbances, such as hyponatremia, hyperkalemia, low bicarbonate, and elevated BUN. The plasma renin and ACTH are increased with primary adrenal insufficiency. Other laboratory findings include moderate neutropenia, lymphocytosis, eosinophilia, low plasma cortisol, decreased urine 17-hydroxysteroids, and decreased 17-ketosteroids. There is also a failure of plasma cortisol to rise after administration of ACTH (corticotropin). Symptoms include weakness, fatigue, anorexia with nausea, vomiting, and diarrhea. Physical findings include hypoglycemia, sparse axillary hair, and increased pigmentation of the gingival mucosa, nipples, labia, and linea alba. Treatment involves the replacement of glucocorticoids and mineralocorticoids. Symptoms of adrenal crisis include severe abdominal pain, generalized muscle weakness, hypotension, and shock. Severe cases may result in death.

Additional Reading: Addison disease. In: Domino F, ed. *The 5-Minute Clinical Consult*. Philadelphia, PA: Lippincott Williams and Wilkins; 2014.

Category: Endocrine system

310. Which of the following tests is the most appropriate to diagnose carbon monoxide (CO) poisoning?
A) Arterial blood gas
B) Chest radiograph
C) Carboxyhemoglobin levels
D) CBC
E) Lactic acid levels

Answer and Discussion

The answer is C. CO poisoning is a dangerous but relatively common occurrence. It usually occurs during the winter months in cold regions of the United States. The affinity of CO for hemoglobin is 240 times greater than that of oxygen; it shifts the oxygen dissociation curve to the left, which impairs hemoglobin release of oxygen to tissues and inhibits the cytochrome oxidase system. Symptoms include headache, confusion, fatigue, and nausea; in more severe cases, seizures, rhabdomyolysis, parkinsonian-type symptoms, coma, and death may occur. In many cases, the initial symptoms are attributed to a flulike illness, and CO poisoning is overlooked. The diagnosis is usually made by obtaining a history of exposure (usually a fuel oil furnace or exhaust fumes in a poorly ventilated enclosure) and laboratory testing, which shows elevated carboxyhemoglobin levels. Treatment involves the use of 100% oxygen and, in severe cases, hyperbaric oxygen. Prolonged exposures usually have a worse prognosis. Patients with CO poisoning necessitating treatment need follow-up neuropsychiatric examinations.

Additional Reading: Carbon monoxide poisoning. In: Domino F, ed. *The 5-Minute Clinical Consult*. Philadelphia, PA: Lippincott Williams and Wilkins; 2014.

Category: Respiratory system

311. Barrett's esophagus is associated with
A) Overuse of PPIs
B) Tracheoesophageal fistula
C) Trauma associated with prior esophagogastroduodenoscopy
D) Transformation of columnar epithelium to squamous epithelium
E) Adenocarcinoma of the esophagus

Answer and Discussion

The answer is E. Barrett's esophagus is the result of chronic gastroesophageal reflux. The condition causes metaplasia and transformation of squamous to columnar epithelium in the areas affected. Patients usually report symptoms of pyrosis and, occasionally, dysphagia if strictures develop. Men are more commonly affected than women. The diagnosis is made with esophagoscopy and biopsy of suspected areas. Treatment is accomplished with H2-blockers and PPIs. PPIs strongly inhibit gastric acid secretion. They act by irreversibly inhibiting the H+–K+ adenosine triphosphatase pump of the parietal cell. By blocking the final common pathway of gastric acid secretion, the PPIs provide a greater degree and duration of gastric acid suppression compared with H2-receptor blockers. Clinical trials have clearly shown that the PPIs provide better symptom control, esophageal healing, and maintenance of remission than H2-receptor blockers or prokinetic agents. Long-term use of PPIs in humans has not been associated with an increased risk of gastric carcinoma, although this was initially a concern. Prolonged use of the drugs has been associated with gastric atrophy; however, atrophy is more likely to be a problem in patients infected with *H. pylori*. The PPIs are fairly well tolerated. The most common side effects are nausea, diarrhea, constipation, headache, and skin rash. PPIs are more expensive than standard-dose H2-receptor blockers or prokinetic agents. However, when prescribed appropriately to patients with severe symptoms or refractory disease, the PPIs are more cost-effective because of their higher healing and remission rates and the consequent prevention of complications. Occasionally, severe cases of Barrett's esophagitis are treated with surgery. Because of a 10% increased risk for the development of adenocarcinoma in the affected areas, follow-up with endoscopy every 3 to 5 years is indicated, although screening endoscopy time frames are controversial. Treatment of gastroesophageal reflux disease associated with Barrett's esophagus has not been shown to eliminate the metaplasia of that condition or the risk of malignancy. Consequently, patients with Barrett's esophagus require periodic endoscopic biopsy to assess esophageal tissue for malignant changes.

Additional Reading: Barrett's esophagus. *Am Fam Physician*. 2004;69:2113–2118, 2120.

Category: Gastroenterology system

312. Type I diabetes mellitus is associated with
A) Hypersensitivity to glucose
B) Overproduction of glucagon
C) Lack of insulin production by the pancreas
D) Tissue resistance to insulin
E) Excessive growth hormone secretion

Answer and Discussion

The answer is C. Diabetes mellitus type I (juvenile diabetes) tends to occur in individuals younger than 30 years. The cause is complete failure of the β islet cells in the pancreas to produce insulin. A genetic predisposition and perhaps a viral or autoimmune reaction that destroys the insulin-producing β cells are believed to be the cause. The incidence among schoolchildren is reported to be 1 in 500. Symptoms include polydipsia, polyphagia, polyuria, dry mouth, nausea, vomiting and abdominal pain, weight loss, and fatigue. In severe cases, the patient may present in diabetic ketoacidosis with stupor, coma, dehydration, labored Kussmaul-type respirations, abdominal distention, and pain. The treatment is aggressive fluid and electrolyte replacement along with exogenous insulin administration. Diabetic complications include retinopathy, nephropathy, macrovascular disease, and diabetic foot ulcers. Judicious control of glucose may help to prevent these complications. Typically, patients require 0.5 to 1.0 U per kg per day of insulin. This daily dose is divided as follows:

- *Morning dose.* Two-thirds of the total daily dose is administered in the morning. The morning dose is composed of two-thirds intermediate-acting insulin and one-third short-acting regular insulin.
- *Evening dose.* One-third of the total daily dose is administered in the evening; 50% is short-acting regular insulin, which the patient takes before the evening meal, and 50% is intermediate-acting insulin, which the patient takes at bedtime.

Additional Reading: Diabetes mellitus, type I. In: Domino F, ed. *The 5-Minute Clinical Consult.* Philadelphia, PA: Lippincott Williams and Wilkins; 2014.

Category: Endocrine system

313. Which of the following is a common ophthalmologic finding in patients with HIV infection?
A) Retinal tears
B) Cataracts
C) Retinitis
D) Glaucoma
E) Conjunctivitis

Answer and Discussion

The answer is C. HIV syndrome can affect many different organ systems. Ophthalmologic findings include toxoplasmic and cytomegalovirus retinitis, herpes infections, syphilis, and pneumocystic infections of the eye. The most common ophthalmologic finding is cotton-wool spots caused by retinal ischemia secondary to microvascular disease. All patients with HIV should undergo complete eye examinations to rule out associated conditions.

> **Additional Reading:** Pathogenesis, clinical manifestations, and diagnosis of AIDS-related cytomegalovirus retinitis. In: Basow DS, ed. *UpToDate.* Waltham, MA: UpToDate; 2013.

Category: Special sensory

314. Which of the following statements is true regarding insulin injections?
A) Absorption from the buttock is rapid and can be used as a site just before eating.
B) Rotation of injections to different zones of the body can cause wide variations in serum glucose levels.
C) Injection in the arm often leads to exercise-induced hypoglycemia.
D) The thigh is the best site for reliable and predictable absorption.

Answer and Discussion

The answer is B. The abdomen is the best site for insulin administration, because the insulin is more reliably and predictably absorbed. Injection in exercised areas (e.g., the thigh) may lead to development of exercise-induced hypoglycemia. However, insulin injection at the arm does not cause as much exercise-induced hypoglycemia and thus can be used as an alternative injection site. Absorption from the buttocks is the slowest and is a good site to use at bedtime to avoid nocturnal hypoglycemia. Rotation of injection sites can lead to erratic absorption of insulin with wide variations in serum glucose levels. Thus, injection sites should remain within the same zone (abdomen, arm, or buttock) but rotated at different sites within the zones to prevent lipohypertrophy.

> **Additional Reading:** Insulin Routines American Diabetes Association. From: http://www.diabetes.org/living-with-diabetes/treatment-and-care/medication/insulin/insulin-routines.html

Category: Endocrine system

315. The treatment of choice for adult respiratory distress syndrome (ARDS) is
A) Loop diuretics
B) Corticosteroids
C) Positive end-expiratory pressure
D) β2 agonist
E) High-dose immunosuppressive drugs

Answer and Discussion

The answer is C. ARDS is characterized by respiratory distress that may be caused by different insults. Most cases of ARDS in adults are associated with pulmonary sepsis (46%) or nonpulmonary sepsis (33%). Risk factors include those causing direct lung injury (e.g., pneumonia, inhalation injury, pulmonary contusion) and those causing indirect lung injury (e.g., nonpulmonary sepsis, burns, transfusion-related acute lung injury). The mechanism of injury involves damage of capillary endothelial cells and alveolar epithelial cells, which leads to pulmonary edema with decreased pulmonary compliance and decreased functional residual capacity. Symptoms include rapid onset of dyspnea usually 12 to 48 hours after the insult, with wheezing and intercostal retractions. Laboratory tests show hypoxemia that responds poorly to oxygen administration, requiring frequent monitoring of arterial blood gases. Radiographs show diffuse or patchy alveolar and interstitial infiltrates without cardiomegaly or pulmonary vascular redistribution.

When treatment with mechanical ventilation is required, the use of low-volume ventilation with higher positive end-expiratory pressure values (12 to 18 or more cm H_2O) for the initial mechanical ventilation is recommended. Fluids should be minimized. Patients are usually paralyzed with pancuronium. Antibiotics are unnecessary, but nosocomial infections may develop. Most patients with the development of ARDS also have multiple organ failure, which is the major cause of death. Mortality rates approach 50%.

> **Additional Reading:** Acute respiratory distress syndrome: diagnosis and management. *Am Fam Physician.* 2012;85(4):352–358.

Category: Respiratory system

> **The predominate medical risk factor for ARDS is sepsis.**

316. Which of the following is associated with rebound hypertension?
A) Oral contraceptives
B) Hyperthyroidism
C) Excessive alcohol consumption
D) Abrupt withdrawal of β-blockers
E) Pheochromocytoma

Answer and Discussion

The answer is D. Causes for secondary hypertension are numerous and include the use of oral contraceptives, excessive alcohol consumption, disorders of the renal parenchyma associated with malfunction of the renin–aldosterone system, Cushing's syndrome, pheochromocytoma, primary aldosteronism, hyperthyroidism, myxedema, renal vascular disease, and coarctation of the aorta. In many cases, blood pressure may be difficult to control. Physical examination may reveal abdominal bruits, suggestive of renovascular hypertension, or other findings suggestive of contributing disease. Adequate treatment is necessary to prevent the long-term detrimental effects of hypertension. Abrupt discontinuation of β-blockers is associated with rebound hypertension.

> **Additional Reading:** Drugs for hypertension. *Treat Guidel Med Lett.* 2012;10(113):1–10.

Category: Casrdiovascular system

317. A 27-year-old patient with asthma presents to your office complaining of shortness of breath with wheezing. Which of the following medications is indicated in the initial treatment of this patient?

A) Salmeterol
B) Albuterol
C) Cromolyn sodium
D) Ipratropium bromide
E) Theophylline

Answer and Discussion

The answer is B. Asthma is a reversible obstructive lung disorder that is characterized by reactive airways. The condition is thought to be inherited; however, some individuals may be affected without a family history. Many factors may precipitate an attack, including infections, smoke, cold weather, exercise, toxic fumes, and stress. Symptoms include wheezing, shortness of breath, tachypnea, cough (particularly in children), and tightness or pressure in the chest. The mainstay of acute treatment (rescue therapy) is an inhalant form of a β2-adrenergic agonist, such as albuterol. Inhaled corticosteroids and salmeterol (a long-acting β2-adrenergic agonist) are used in chronic therapy. For patients who have more severe asthmatic attacks, short courses of oral corticosteroids may be necessary, particularly with upper respiratory infections. Theophylline, once readily prescribed, is used less frequently, and its benefits are controversial. Cromolyn sodium, a mast-cell stabilizer; ipratropium bromide, an anticholinergic medication; and the leukotriene modifiers can be used for chronic asthmatic conditions. Pulmonary function tests in patients affected with asthma usually show a normal or decreased vital capacity, decreased forced expiratory volume in 1 second, increased residual volume, increased total lung capacity, and a positive response to inhaled bronchodilators. In children, rescue β2-adrenergic agonists are the treatment of choice for mild intermittent asthma.

Additional Reading: Management of acute asthma exacerbations. *Am Fam Physician.* 2011;84(1):40–47.

Category: Respiratory system

318. A 22-year-old sexually active woman presents with a 24-hour history of dysuria. She is otherwise healthy and has no other symptoms. Appropriate management includes

A) Urine culture followed by antibiotics until culture result is determined
B) Empiric antibiotic for 3 days
C) Continued observation
D) Midstream urinalysis followed by microscopic evaluation and treatment if positive

Answer and Discussion

The correct answer is B. UTI is typically classified as "complicated" in pregnant women and in those with comorbidities (e.g., diabetes mellitus, recent urinary tract instrumentation, chronic renal disease, urinary tract abnormalities, immunosuppression). For these women, urine culture and empiric therapy are recommended to confirm UTI diagnosis and to determine antibiotic sensitivities. Women with complicated UTIs require longer courses of broader-spectrum antibiotics. Women with uncomplicated UTIs can be treated empirically with a 3-day course of trimethoprim/sulfamethoxazole (Bactrim, Septra), or with a 3-day course of a quinolone antibiotic if resistance to *Escherichia coli* is greater than 10% to 20%.

It is unclear whether age alone increases the risk of a complicated infection, and few studies have evaluated shorter antibiotic courses in older patients. Physicians should use their own judgment to decide if otherwise healthy women older than 65 years with uncomplicated infections can be treated for only 3 days or whether a longer course is indicated. Physicians should follow up with patients after 3 days by telephone or in person to ensure clinical improvement.

Additional Reading: Point-of-care guides: treating adult women with suspected UTI. *Am Fam Physician.* 2006;73(2):293–296.

Category: Nephrologic system

319. Based on the USPSTF recommendation, screening DEXA in all woman without fracture risk factors should start

A) At age 50
B) At age 55
C) At age 60
D) At age 65
E) At age 70

Answer and Discussion

The answer is D. The USPSTF guideline, based on a systematic review of the evidence, recommends screening DEXA in all women 65 years and older, as well as in women 60 to 64 years of age who have increased fracture risk. The USPSTF states that the evidence is insufficient to recommend for or against screening in postmenopausal women younger than 60 years.

Additional Reading: Screening for osteoporosis; 2011. From: http://www.uspreventiveservicestaskforce.org/uspstf/uspsoste.htm

Category: Endocrine system

320. Which of the following statements about use of ticlopidine is true?

A) The drug inhibits von Willebrand factor.
B) Side effects include peripheral neuropathy and tremor.
C) Liver function tests and blood counts should be monitored initially.
D) The drug is associated with gastric ulceration.
E) The drug inhibits vitamin K-dependent clotting factors.

Answer and Discussion

The answer is C. Ticlopidine (Ticlid) and clopidogrel are used as an alternative to aspirin when selecting an anticoagulant for stroke prophylaxis. Ticlopidine works by inhibiting platelet aggregation by blocking adenosine diphosphate–induced aggregation. Major side effects include diarrhea, nausea, dyspepsia, rash, an abnormal liver function test, and severe neutropenia and thrombocytopenia. Most side effects, including blood dyscrasias, occur within the first 3 months. Blood tests, including CBCs and liver function tests, should be monitored every 2 weeks for the first 3 months of drug therapy. Abnormalities may necessitate the discontinuation of the medication. Unlike aspirin, ticlopidine is not associated with gastric ulceration. Because of safety and tolerance issues associated with ticlopidine, clopidogrel is the more widely used second-line antiplatelet agent. Neutropenia, rash, diarrhea, and thrombotic thrombocytopenic purpura (TTP) occur less frequently with clopidogrel than with ticlopidine. The incidence of ticlopidine-related TTP is estimated to be 1 case per 1,600 to 5,000 patients treated. Although clopidogrel and aspirin have similar safety profiles, there have been rare reports of clopidogrel-related TTP, with the majority of cases occurring within 2 weeks of initiation of the drug.

Additional Reading: Antithrombotic drugs. *Treat Guidel Med Lett.* 2011;9(110):61–66.

Category: Neurologic

321. Which of the following positive test results supports the diagnosis of Raynaud's phenomenon?

A) Allen's test
B) Finkelstein's test
C) Phalen's test
D) Reverse Phalen's test

Answer and Discussion

The answer is A. Raynaud's phenomenon is secondary to spasm of the arterioles that usually supply the hands but can also affect the nose and other appendages. It is usually idiopathic (termed *Raynaud's disease*), but has been associated with emotional stress, connective tissue diseases (e.g., lupus, rheumatoid arthritis, scleroderma), arterial obstructive diseases, medications (e.g., ergots, β-blockers, clonidine, methysergide), and endocrine disorders. Idiopathic Raynaud's phenomenon occurs more frequently in women and frequently occurs in patients with migraines or variant angina. Symptoms include blanching, cyanosis, and paresthesias that affect the distal extremities. Diagnosis can be determined by performing Allen's test. The radial and ulnar arteries are occluded by the examiner while the patient makes a fist. The hand is then opened, and one side of the wrist is released. Blood flow to the hand should be detected by color, which is restored to the hand. If the hand remains pale and cyanotic with either of the two sides, Raynaud's phenomenon should be suspected. During asymptomatic periods the examination is entirely normal. Treatment for mild-to-moderate cases should only involve avoiding triggering factors (e.g., cold, stress, nicotine, previously listed medications). The medication of choice for the treatment of severe Raynaud's phenomenon includes the CCBs nifedipine and diltiazem. Other medications include reserpine, phenoxybenzamine, methyldopa, terazosin, doxazosin, and prazosin. Surgical treatment for resistant, severe cases involves sympathectomy. Finkelstein's test is used to diagnose DeQuervain's tenosynovitis by grasping the thumb, while the hand is deviated in the ulnar direction. A positive test is when pain is reproduced along the distal radius.

Phalen's test is used to diagnose carpal tunnel syndrome. The patient holds their wrists in complete and forced flexion (pushing the dorsal surfaces of both hands together) for 30 to 60 seconds. A positive test is when symptoms (e.g., parathsias in the thumb and index finger) are reproduced. The Reverse Phalen's test adds to the sensitivity of the first test and is performed by having the patient in full wrist and finger extension for 2 minutes.

Additional Reading: Raynaud phenomenon. In: Domino F, ed. *The 5-Minute Clinical Consult*. Philadephia, PA. Lippincott Williams and Wilkins; 2014.

Category: Cardiovascular system

322. Which of the following statements about the diagnosis of SLE is true?

A) The ANA test is specific.
B) The LE prep test is a confirmatory test.
C) The LE prep test should be used as a screening test.
D) The anti-double-stranded DNA test is a confirmatory test.

Answer and Discussion

The answer is D. SLE is an autoimmune disorder affecting all major organ systems. Symptoms wax and wane and include diffuse joint pain, facial rashes (butterfly distribution), cardiac involvement (including pericarditis, myocarditis, and endocarditis), renal involvement (proteinuria, hypertension, and uremia), pulmonary involvement (pleuritis, pleural effusions), CNS findings (depression, TIAs, strokes, chorea, and psychosis), and vasculitis. GI involvement is less common. Women are more commonly affected than men.

Antibody testing plays an important role when assessing patients, but should not be used alone to diagnose SLE. The ANA test is the most commonly used screening test for SLE, which is sensitive but not specific and requires confirmatory testing. The presence of anti-DNA, anti-Sm, and antiphospholipid antibodies are more specific for diagnosing SLE.

Because of the high rate of false-positive ANA titers, testing for SLE with an ANA titer or other autoantibody test is not recommended in patients with isolated myalgias or arthralgias in the absence of specific clinical signs. At least 4 of the 11 American College of Rheumatology criteria are present, serially or simultaneously, during any interval of observation for the diagnosis:

1. Malar rash
2. Discoid rash
3. Photosensitivity
4. Oral ulcers
5. Nonerosive arthritis
6. Serositis *or* Pericarditis
7. Renal
8. Neurologic disorder: Seizures *or* Psychosis
9. Hematologic disorder: Hemolytic anemia *or* Leukopenia *or* Thrombocytopenia
10. Immunologic disorder: Anti-DNA *or* Anti-Sm *or* Antiphospholipid antibodies, others.
11. ANA

Additional Reading: Antibody testing for systemic lupus erythematosus. *Am Fam Physician*. 2011;84(12):1407–1409.

Category: Nonspecific system

323. Recurrent vertigo, tinnitus, and hearing loss are hallmark findings of

A) Meniere's disease
B) Cholesteatoma
C) Vestibular neuronitis
D) Benign positional vertigo
E) Acoustic neuroma

Answer and Discussion

The answer is A. Meniere's disease is a peripheral cause of vertigo. Symptoms include the hallmark findings of recurrent vertigo, tinnitus, and hearing loss. The cause is thought to arise from endolymphatic hydrops. In most cases, the vertigo lasts for several hours, up to an entire day. Although at first hearing may be little affected, over time it deteriorates. Tinnitus is usually constant and may become worse during the acute attacks. Vertigo may be severe and accompanied by nausea and vomiting. Treatment consists of salt restriction (i.e., no more than 2 g per day) and the use of hydrochlorothiazide, anticholinergics, antihistamines, and antiemetics. Resistant cases may require referral to an ear–nose–throat specialist.

Additional Reading: Dizziness: a diagnostic approach. *Am Fam Physician*. 2010;82(4):361–368, 369.

Postural orthostatic tachycardia syndrome: a clinical review. *Pediatr Neurol*. 2010;42(2):77–85.

Category: Special sensory

324. Primary hypothyroidism is associated with a deficiency of
A) T_4
B) TSH
C) Thyroid-releasing hormone
D) Thyroid-stimulating antibodies
E) None of the above

Answer and Discussion
The answer is A. There are basically two types of hypothyroidism:

5. Primary hypothyroidism (most common form), which is a deficiency of T_4 that is caused by thyroid gland disease.
6. Secondary hypothyroidism, which is associated with a deficiency in TSH from the pituitary gland or deficient thyroid-releasing hormone by the hypothalamus.

Hypothyroidism is seen more commonly in patients older than 55 years and in women. The most common form occurs as a result of Hashimoto's thyroiditis followed by posttherapeutic hypothyroidism, especially after radioactive iodine therapy or surgery for hyperthyroidism. Symptoms include fatigue, weakness, cold intolerance, constipation, hair loss, menorrhagia, carpal tunnel syndrome, dry skin, nonpitting edema (also referred to as *myxedema*) caused by deposition of mucopolysaccharides, weight gain, memory impairment, depression, hoarseness, delayed relaxation of reflexes, altered mental status, and bradycardia. A low free T_4 with a high TSH is seen in primary hypothyroidism, whereas a low free T_4 with a low TSH is indicative of secondary or tertiary hypothyroidism. In congenital hypothyroidism, the deficiency of thyroid hormone is severe and symptoms usually develop in the early weeks of life. Affected infants may show hypotonia and developmental delay. In the United States, mandatory newborn routine testing includes tests to rule out hypothyroidism, which has made the complications of neonatal hypothyroidism rare. Mental retardation may occur if infants are not identified and treated.

> Additional Reading: Hypothyroidism: an update. *Am Fam Physician*. 2012;86(3):244–251.

> Category: Endocrine system

325. Which of the following statements about Osler–Weber–Rendu disease is true?
A) The condition is not associated with hereditary transmission.
B) It is associated with telangiectasia lesions of the face, lips, nasal and oral mucosa, and GI mucosa.
C) The pulmonary system is unaffected.
D) Treatment involves high-dose prednisone.
E) Laboratory studies show pernicious anemia.

Answer and Discussion
The answer is B. Osler–Weber–Rendu disease (also known as *hereditary hemorrhagic telangiectasia*) is a hereditary disorder that is associated with telangiectasia lesions on the face, lips, nasal and oral mucosa, and GI mucosa. The mode of transmission is autosomal dominant. The condition can lead to significant GI hemorrhage or epistaxis. Some patients may have pulmonary arteriovenous malformations and may experience hemoptysis or dyspnea. Cerebral or spinal arteriovenous malformations may cause subarachnoid hemorrhage, seizures, or paraplegia. Laboratory findings may indicate an iron-deficiency anemia. Treatment is nonspecific and involves topical hemostatics and laser ablation of accessible lesions. In severe cases, blood transfusions may be necessary. Iron supplementation is also recommended.

> Additional Reading: Hereditary hemorrhagic telangiectasia. *GeneReviews 2012*. From: http://www.ncbi.nlm.nih.gov/books/NBK1351/

> Category: Integumentary

Osler–Weber–Rendu (also known as hereditary hemorrhagic telangiectasia) is a hereditary disorder that is associated with telangiectasia lesions on the face, lips, nasal and oral mucosa, and GI mucosa.

326. β-type natriuretic peptide (BNP) is used in the diagnosis of
A) PE
B) CHF
C) Type 1 diabetes mellitus
D) Asthma
E) Amyloidosis

Answer and Discussion
The answer is B. BNP has shown sensitivity and specificity in the diagnosis of heart failure. This peptide is released by ventricular myocytes when heart failure causes increased wall stretch. It is a simple and rapid test that reliably predicts the presence or absence of left ventricular dysfunction on an echocardiogram. A BNP level of 100 pg per mL or below is unlikely to support the diagnosis of CHF, and an elevation >400 to 500 pg per mL is indication that heart failure is likely present. Intermediate values require physicians to rely on other standard evaluation measures to decide whether heart failure was present.

> Additional Reading: ACC and AHA update on chronic heart failure guidelines. *Am Fam Physician*. 2010;81(5):654–665.

> Category: Cardiovascular system

327. A 48-year-old woman with type 1 diabetes mellitus receives a corticosteroid injection for osteoarthritis of her right knee. Which one of the following is true regarding monitoring of his blood glucose levels?
A) Glucose levels should be closely monitored for 48 hours.
B) Glucose levels should be closely monitored for 7 days.
C) Glucose levels should be closely monitored for 14 days.
D) No additional monitoring is necessary.

Answer and Discussion
The answer is D. While a single intra-articular steroid injection has little effect on glycemic control, soft tissue or peritendinous steroid injections can affect blood glucose levels for several days after the injection. Insulin-dependent diabetics should be advised to closely monitor their blood glucose levels for 2 weeks following such injections.

> Additional Reading: Musculoskeletal injections: a review of the evidence. *Am Fam Physician*. 2008;78(8):971–976.

> Category: Cardiovascular system

328. Which of the following conditions is often the first sign of amyloidosis?
A) Proteinuria
B) CHF
C) Cardiac arrhythmias
D) Rheumatoid arthritis
E) Night blindness

Answer and Discussion
The answer is A. Amyloidosis is a condition characterized by excessive protein deposition in tissues, which interferes with normal organ functioning. Common forms include the following:

• Primary idiopathic amyloidosis, or that associated with multiple myeloma. This condition is also referred to with the designation *AL*, which denotes amyloidosis involving Ig light chains. Fewer than 20% of patients with AL have myeloma. Approximately 15% to 20% of patients with myeloma have amyloidosis. AL is a systemic disease that has the capability of affecting multiple organ systems.

- Secondary amyloidosis (designated *AA*, reactive or acquired amyloidosis) is associated with chronic inflammatory diseases such as tuberculosis, osteomyelitis, and leprosy. It more commonly affects the liver, spleen, kidneys, adrenal glands, and lymph nodes. Vascular involvement may be widespread. Effective treatment of the underlying chronic inflammatory disease has reduced the incidence in developed countries.

Diagnosis is usually accomplished after the point of irreversible organ damage and involves biopsy of the abdominal fat or rectal mucosa. Tissue is then examined under a polarizing microscope using Congo red stain to look for a characteristic green birefringence of amyloid. Proteinuria is often the first symptom associated with systemic amyloidosis, particularly the AA and AL types. Nephrotic syndrome may be severe and lead to renal failure. Myocardial amyloidosis–causing arrhythmias and CHF are two common forms of death in those affected with amyloidosis. Generalized amyloidosis is usually a slowly progressive disease that leads to death in several years, but, in some instances, prognosis is improving. The most effective form of treatment (for the AL form) is stem-cell transplantation and immunosuppressive drugs (melphalan). Cardiac transplantation has also been used.

Additional Reading: Amyloidosis. In: Domino F, ed. *The 5-Minute Clinical Consult.* Philadelphia, PA: Lippincott Williams and Wilkins; 2014.

Category: Nonspecific system

329. Which of the following statements is true regarding acyclovir?
A) The medication is not effective for the treatment of herpes zoster.
B) The drug effectively prevents the transmission of herpes from those affected.
C) Topical acyclovir is less effective than oral acyclovir.
D) The medication is most effective after the onset of vesicles.
E) Seizures are not associated with the use of acyclovir.

Answer and Discussion

The answer is C. Acyclovir is a purine compound used as an antiviral agent against the herpes virus. The medication is incorporated into the viral DNA and inhibits DNA polymerase, thus preventing replication of the virus. Available in topical, oral, and intravenous (IV) formulations, acyclovir is used to treat herpes simplex virus (HSV) and varicella zoster virus (VZV) infections. Topical acyclovir cream reduces the duration of orolabial herpes by about 0.5 days. Oral acyclovir can shorten the duration of symptoms in primary orolabial, genital, and anorectal HSV infections, and to a lesser extent in recurrent orolabial and genital HSV infections. Long-term oral suppression with acyclovir decreases the frequency of symptomatic genital HSV recurrences and asymptomatic viral shedding. Oral acyclovir begun within 24 hours after the onset of rash decreases the severity of primary varicella infection and can also be used to treat localized zoster. Suppression with acyclovir for 1 year reduced VZV reactivation in immunocompromised patients. IV acyclovir is the drug of choice for treatment of HSV infections that are visceral, disseminated, or involve the CNS and for serious or disseminated VZV infections.

The medication is generally well tolerated but should be used with caution in patients with underlying renal disease or dehydration. Adverse reactions include headache, encephalopathic signs (e.g., lethargy, obtundation, hallucinations, seizures), hypotension, rash, pruritus, nausea, vomiting, diarrhea, renal dysfunction, and arthralgias. The patient must be informed that the medication helps

decrease the number and severity of occurrences but does not cure the virus. Patients should also be counseled that there is risk of herpes transmission even when there is no visible evidence of the virus.

Additional Reading: Drugs for non-HIV viral infections. *Treat Guidel Med Lett.* 2010;(98):71.

Category: Nonspecific system

330. Which of the following tests is used to detect hepatitis B infection during the "window period"?
A) Hepatitis B surface antigen
B) Hepatitis B surface antibody
C) Hepatitis B core antibody (IgM)
D) Hepatitis B e antigen
E) Hepatitis B antibody to the delta agent

Answer and Discussion

The answer is C. The following are specific tests used when assessing a patient infected with HBV:

- *Hepatitis B surface antigen (Australian antigen).* This test detects the surface antigen of the HBV. It is usually detected 1 to 4 months after exposure to the virus. Its presence represents infection with the virus. In approximately 10% of cases, this test remains positive and no antibodies are formed. This state denotes the chronic carrier state.
- *Hepatitis B antibody.* This test detects the presence of antibodies to the hepatitis B surface antigens. It usually occurs 5 months after exposure to the virus and persists for life. Its presence represents past infection and relative immunity to hepatitis B. It can also be used to check for antibodies after immunization for the HBV.
- *Hepatitis B core antibody IgM and IgG.* Anti-hepatitis B core antibody IgM is useful when trying to determine infection with the virus during the "window period" (i.e., the time between the disappearance of the surface antigen and the development of the antibody). Its presence indicates a current infection with hepatitis B. Anti-hepatitis B core antibody IgG indicates a previous hepatitis B infection, and its presence remains indefinitely.
- *Hepatitis B e antigen.* The presence of the e antigen indicates that the blood is highly infectious. It is associated with more severe cases and the development of the chronic carrier state. Its persistence for longer than 8 weeks indicates that a chronic carrier state has developed. In 90% of cases, hepatitis B e antigen–positive mothers infect their fetuses.
- *Hepatitis B antibody to the delta agent.* Conversion from the hepatitis B e antigen to the anti-hepatitis B e indicates a lower infectivity rate and improvement in the patient's liver function status. It usually reflects a benign outcome.

Additional Reading: Hepatitis B: diagnosis and treatment. *Am Fam Physician.* 2010;81(8):965–972.

Category: Gastroenterology system

331. In which of the following clinical situations is digoxin best used?
A) CHF in the setting of diastolic dysfunction
B) Idiopathic hypertrophic subaortic stenosis
C) Recent MI with CHF
D) Supraventricular arrhythmia with the development of CHF
E) Emergent treatment of ventricular fibrillation

Answer and Discussion

The answer is D. The use of cardiac glycosides, such as digoxin, is not disputed and is generally recommended if there is a supraventricular arrhythmia present, such as atrial fibrillation in the presence of CHF. Digoxin is also used in cases of CHF in which the heart is dilated and the systolic function is significantly impaired. In patients with normal systolic function but with decreased ventricular compliance (diastolic dysfunction) that gives rise to CHF, the use of digoxin is not recommended. Digoxin is recommended for symptomatic patients with stage C or D heart failure. Digoxin should be used only as a second-line therapy for controlling the heart rates of patients with atrial fibrillation associated with heart failure and is not recommended for the treatment of diastolic heart failure.

Digoxin should also not be used in patients with idiopathic, hypertrophic, subaortic stenosis; the medication is also usually withheld in patients with an acute MI and CHF, unless diuretics and vasodilators fail to improve cardiac failure.

Unless there is a specific contraindication, all patients with CHF and systolic dysfunction should take both an ACE inhibitor and a β-blocker, and if volume overloaded, a diuretic as well. An ARB is recommended for patients who cannot tolerate an ACE inhibitor. Addition of an aldosterone antagonist can be beneficial for patients with symptomatic heart failure or for patients with left ventricular dysfunction after an MI. A combination of hydralazine and isosorbide dinitrate added to standard therapy has been effective in African American patients with class III to IV heart failure. Digoxin can decrease symptoms and lower the rate of hospitalization for heart failure, but does not decrease mortality. There is no evidence that any drug improves clinical outcomes in patients with heart failure with preserved systolic function.

Additional Reading: Digoxin therapy for heart failure: an update. *Am Fam Physician.* 2006;74(4):613–618.

Category: Cardiovascular system

332. A 48-year-old man presents with complaints of dyspnea that tends to occur with exercise. He has a 40-pack-year history of smoking and has been diagnosed with exercise-induced asthma in the past, but denies any other medical problems. On spirometry, his expiratory loop is normal, but he has a flattened inspiratory loop. What is the most likely diagnosis?
A) Vocal cord dysfunction
B) COPD
C) Asthma
D) Restrictive lung disease

Answer and Discussion

The answer is A. Vocal cord dysfunction occurs when the vocal cords move toward midline during inspiration or expiration, leading to varying degrees of obstruction. It is often misdiagnosed as exercise-induced asthma. Precipitating factors, including exercise, psychological conditions, irritants, sinusitis, and gastroesophageal reflux disease. Spirometry generally will show a normal expiratory loop with a flattened inspiratory loop. In asthma and COPD, the FEV1/FVC ratio is decreased, resulting in a concave shape in the expiratory portion of the flow-volume curve. The inspiratory loops are generally normal. Patients with restrictive lung disease have a normal FEV1/FVC ratio with a reduced FVC.

Additional Reading: Vocal cord dysfunction. *Am Fam Physician.* 2010;81(2):156–159.

Category: Respiratory system

333. The treatment of choice for cryptococcal meningeal infection is
A) Amphotericin B and flucytosine
B) Metronidazole
C) Acyclovir
D) Amantadine
E) Penicillin G

Answer and Discussion

The answer is A. Cryptococcus is an infection caused by the fungus *Cryptococcus neoformans* that usually involves the lungs with spread to the meninges and occasionally to other sites, including the kidneys, bones, and skin. The disease is found worldwide and tends to affect immunodeficient patients with lymphoma and AIDS or those chronically taking steroids. Symptoms include headaches (usually the first symptom), blurred vision, and mental status changes seen with meningeal involvement. In addition, the patient usually reports a persistent cough, which reflects pulmonary involvement. The disease is acquired by respiratory transmission. Skin lesions and the development of osteomyelitis are infrequent; however, as many as 33% of patients with meningeal involvement also have renal involvement. Laboratory tests show CSF with an increased protein, a white cell count that is mostly lymphocytes, and a decreased glucose level with meningeal involvement. Culture of sputum, blood, urine, or other areas of involvement is diagnostic. The diagnosis is also supported with the evidence of budding yeast seen with India ink preparation. The treatment of choice for cryptococcal meningitis is the administration of intravenous amphotericin B and oral flucytosine until lumbar cultures are clear, followed by lifelong prophylaxis with fluconazole; amphotericin and itraconazole are alternatives. Nonprogressive pulmonary cryptococcus may not require treatment in patients who are not immunocompromised.

Additional Reading: Antifungal drugs. *Treat Guidel Med Lett.* 2012;10(120):61–68.

Category: Neurologic

334. A 28-year-old active runner presents to your office complaining of lateral knee and hip pain. The patient reports she has been training intensely for an upcoming marathon. On physical examination, tenderness of the lateral portion of the thigh at the level of the femoral epicondyle are noted. The most likely diagnosis is
A) Patellofemoral syndrome
B) Iliotibial Band (ITB) friction syndrome
C) Tibial plateau fracture
D) Pes anserine bursitis
E) Stress fracture

Answer and Discussion

The answer is B. ITB friction syndrome is characterized by lateral knee pain and, occasionally, lateral hip pain. The pain is caused by inflammation of the distal portion of the ITB band or at the point in which the ITB crosses the lateral femoral epicondyle. Runners, hammer throwers, and racket sport enthusiasts are those usually affected. The condition usually affects runners when there is an increase in the running distance, increased speed or hill running, change in running surface, or consistent running on a banked surface. These activities lead to increased friction of the ITB and cause inflammation. Associated conditions include genu valgum, prominent lateral epicondyle, trochanteric bursitis, leg-length discrepancy, excessive foot pronation, and quadriceps weakness. Testing may show an excessively tight ITB or gluteus maximus. Treatment involves relative rest, anti-inflammatory medication, ice massage, and electronic galvanic stimulation. Prevention is aimed at proper stretching techniques (e.g., quadriceps strengthening) and measures to correct underlying abnormalities (e.g., excessive pronation).

Additional Reading: Busconi BD, Stevenson JH. Approach to the athlete with iliotibial band friction syndrome. *Sports Medicine Consult: A Problem-Based Approach to Sports Medicine for the Primary Care Physician.* Philadelphia, PA: Lippincott, Williams & Wilkins; 2009.

Category: Musculoskeletal system

335. A 67-year-old obese woman with CAD presents with chest pain worse when taking a deep breath. She does not feel well and reports a low-grade fever. Her medications include simvastatin (Zocor), lisinopril (Zestril), spironolactone (Aldactone), furosemide (Lasix), isosorbide mononitrate (Imdur), hydralazine, carvedilol (Coreg), and nitroglycerin as needed. A chest radiograph is normal. The workup is negative for an MI, pulmonary embolus and there are no signs of pneumonia. You make a diagnosis of pleurisy. Which one of the patient's medications could be related to this condition?

A) Hydralazine
B) Simvastatin
C) Lisinopril
D) Spironolactone
E) Carvedilol

Answer and Discussion

The answer is A. Drug-induced pleuritis is one cause of pleurisy. Several drugs are associated with drug-induced pleural disease or drug-induced lupus pleuritis. Drugs that may cause lupus pleuritis include hydralazine, procainamide, and quinidine. Other drugs known to cause pleural disease include amiodarone, bleomycin, bromocriptine, cyclophosphamide, methotrexate, minoxidil, and mitomycin.

> **Additional Reading:** Pleurisy. *Am Fam Physician.* 2007;75(9): 1357–1364.

> **Category:** Respiratory system

336. Which of the following statements about rapid streptococcal screening tests (enzyme immunoassays) is true?

A) Their accuracy is generally unreliable.
B) They are less accurate than latex agglutination tests.
C) They are expensive and difficult to perform.
D) They are rarely used when compared with cultures.
E) They may be avoided if the criteria for strep pharyngitis is met.

Answer and Discussion

The answer is E. Rapid *Streptococcus* screen tests are quick, easy to perform, and approximately as accurate as the latex agglutination tests. Their sensitivity approaches 80%, whereas their specificity is 85% to 100%; thus, a positive test is fairly predictive of a streptococcal infection and a culture is unnecessary. If negative, cultures can be performed to confirm the results.

In adults, the use of clinical decision rules for diagnosing GABHS (Group A beta-hemolytic strep) pharyngitis improves quality of care while reducing unwarranted treatment and overall cost. Treatment can be started or avoided without a strep test. The criteria include history of fever, tonsillar exudates, absence of cough, and tender anterior cervical lymphadenopathy. Patients who have 0 or only 1 criterion are unlikely to have strep pharyngitis and do not need to be tested. Patients who have 2 to 3 criteria can be tested. Those with 4 criteria can be tested or treated empirically.

> **Additional Reading:** Diagnosis and treatment of streptococcal pharyngitis. *Am Fam Physician.* 2009;79(5):383–390.

> **Category:** Respiratory system

337. The treatment of choice for mucormycosis is

A) Amphotericin
B) Ketoconazole
C) Clotrimazole
D) Miconazole

Answer and Discussion

The answer is A. Mucormycosis infections are usually fulminant and can be fatal. Necrotic lesions usually appear on the nasal mucosa or sometimes the palate. Vascular invasion by hyphae leads to progressive tissue necrosis that may involve the nasal septum, palate, and bones surrounding the orbit or sinuses. Findings include pain, fever, orbital cellulitis, proptosis, purulent nasal discharge, and mucosal necrosis. Extension of the infection to involve the brain can cause cavernous sinus thrombosis, convulsions, aphasia, or hemiplegia. Patients with diabetic ketoacidosis are most commonly affected, but opportunistic infections may also develop in chronic renal disease or with immunosuppression, particularly with neutropenia or high-dose corticosteroid therapy. Pulmonary infections resemble invasive aspergillosis. Diagnosis requires a high index of suspicion and careful examination of tissue samples for large nonseptate hyphae with irregular diameters and branching patterns because much of the necrotic debris contains no organisms. Cultures usually are negative, even when hyphae are clearly visible in tissues. CT scans and x-rays often underestimate or miss significant bone destruction. Effective antifungal therapy requires that diabetes be controlled or, if at all possible, immunosuppression reversed. IV amphotericin B must be used because azoles are ineffective. Posaconazole is an alternative for those who cannot tolerate amphotericin. Surgical debridement of necrotic tissue may be indicated because amphotericin B cannot penetrate into these avascular areas to clear remaining organisms.

> **Additional Reading:** Antifungal drugs. *Treat Guidel Med Lett.* 2012;10(120):61–68.

> **Category:** Nonspecific system

338. Cardiac troponins may remain elevated up to

A) 24 hours
B) 48 hours
C) 72 hours
D) 1 week
E) 2 weeks

Answer and Discussion

The answer is E. The term *acute coronary syndrome* refers to a range of thrombotic CADs, including unstable angina and both ST-segment elevation and non-ST-segment elevation MI. Symptoms of acute coronary syndrome include chest pain, referred pain, nausea, vomiting, dyspnea, diaphoresis, and light-headedness. Pain may be referred to the arms, the jaw, the neck, the back, or even the abdomen. Pain radiating to the shoulder, left arm, or both arms increases the likelihood of acute coronary syndrome. Typical angina is described as pain that is substernal, occurs on exertion, and is relieved with rest. Diagnosis utilizes an ECG and a review for signs and symptoms of cardiac ischemia. In acute coronary syndrome, common electrocardiographic abnormalities include T-wave tenting or inversion, ST-segment elevation or depression (including J-point elevation in multiple leads), and pathologic Q waves. Most high-risk patients should be hospitalized. Intermediate-risk patients should undergo further evaluation, often in a chest pain unit. Many low-risk patients can be discharged with appropriate follow-up.

Troponins are regulatory proteins found in skeletal and cardiac muscle. Three subunits have been identified: troponin I (TnI), troponin T (TnT), and troponin C (TnC). The skeletal and cardiac subforms for TnC are similar but TnI and TnT are distinct. According to the American College of Cardiology guidelines, any elevated measure of troponin above the 99th percentile upper reference limit in the appropriate clinical setting is defined as an MI.

Troponin T and I have similar sensitivity and specificity for the detection of myocardial injury. Unlike troponin I levels, troponin T levels may be elevated in patients with renal disease, polymyositis, or dermatomyositis. The cardiac troponins may remain elevated up to 2 weeks after symptom onset, which makes them useful as late markers of recent acute MI. An elevated troponin T or I level is helpful in identifying patients at increased risk for death or the development of acute MI. Increased risk is related quantitatively to the serum troponin level.

> **Additional Reading:** Diagnosis of acute coronary syndrome. *Am Fam Physician.* 2005;72:119–126.

> Category: Cardiovascular system

339. A 45-year-old carpenter has a history of hepatitis C. He is returning for a check-up and is doing well without complaints. You should make which of the following recommendations?
A) Ibuprofen is considered safe.
B) Even low-dose acetaminophen should be avoided.
C) Vaccination for hepatitis A and B is recommended.
D) Milk thistle should be avoided.
E) Mild-to-moderate alcohol use has little detrimental effect.

Answer and Discussion

The answer is C. HCV infection is the most frequent cause of chronic liver disease and the most common reason for liver transplantation. Chronic liver disease is the tenth leading cause of death in the United States. Preventive care can significantly reduce the progression of liver disease. Because alcohol in the setting of hepatitis C can increase the development of cirrhosis, patients with hepatitis C infection should abstain from alcohol use. Because associated infections with hepatitis A or B virus can lead to liver failure, vaccination of both is recommended. Medications that are potentially hepatotoxic should be avoided or used with caution in patients with chronic liver disease. In general, NSAIDs should be avoided; acetaminophen in a dosage below 2 g per day is a safer alternative. Many herbal remedies are potentially hepatotoxic and should also be avoided. Milk thistle can be used safely in patients who have chronic liver disease and may be beneficial. Weight reduction and exercise can improve liver function in patients with fatty infiltration of the liver. The standard therapy for chronic HCV infection is pegylated interferon and ribavirin (Rebetol).

> **Additional Reading:** Hepatitis C: diagnosis and treatment. *Am Fam Physician.* 2010;81(11):1351–1357.

> Category: Gastroenterology system

340. Which of the following statements concerning the use of metformin is true?
A) The drug is an oral sulfonylurea.
B) Weight gain is common with its use.
C) The most common side effect is headache.
D) Patients using metformin must have periodic liver function tests.
E) The most serious side effect is lactic acidosis.

Answer and Discussion

The answer is E. Metformin belongs to the class of drugs referred to as *biguanides*. Metformin decreases hepatic glucose production by inhibiting gluconeogenesis. The drug also decreases insulin production as a result of decreasing insulin resistance. Metformin decreases plasma triglycerides and LDL cholesterol and increases HDL cholesterol. Hypoglycemia does not occur with metformin monotherapy, and, in contrast to other hypoglycemic agents, weight is not gained and even may be lost with its use. The most common side effects are GI irritation, abdominal cramps, and diarrhea. Patients with inflammatory bowel disease and peptic ulcer disease are not good candidates for metformin therapy. The most severe side effect is lactic acidosis, which can be fatal. Metformin is contraindicated in men with a serum creatine greater than 1.5 mg per dL, or greater than 1.4 mg per dL in women, in patients receiving intravenous radiographic iodinated contrast media, acute MI, CHF, and any ischemic condition.

> **Additional Reading:** Drugs for Type 2 Diabetes. *Treat Guidel Med Lett.* 2011;9(108):47–54.

> Category: Endocrine system

341. A 28-year-old man presents to your office complaining of pain in the perirectal area for the last week. Examination shows an area of tenderness, redness, and induration just superior to the anus in the gluteal cleft. The area is warm and fluctuant, but otherwise unremarkable. The most appropriate management is
A) Warm sitz baths
B) Oral antibiotics and warm sitz baths as an outpatient
C) High-dose, intravenous antibiotics as an inpatient
D) Topical steroids applied to the rectal area
E) Surgical incision and drainage

Answer and Discussion

The answer is E. Pilonidal disease often affects young, white, hirsute men. The disease is related to acute abscesses or chronic draining sinuses that form in the sacrococcygeal region. These sinuses or pits may form a cavity often containing hair. The lesion is often painless unless it becomes infected. Treatment involves incision and drainage and removal of communicating sinus tracts. In many cases, antibiotics are not necessary.

> **Additional Reading:** Pilonidal disease. In: Domino F, ed. *The 5-Minute Clinical Consult.* Philadelphia, PA: Lippincott Williams and Wilkins; 2014.

> Category: Integumentary

342. The drug of choice for treatment of severe coccidioidomycosis ("valley fever") is
A) Ceftriaxone
B) Tetracyline
C) Ciprofloxacin
D) Mefloquin
E) Fluconazole

Answer and Discussion

The answer is E. Coccidioidomycosis ("valley fever") is an infection that is usually asymptomatic. In some cases, nonspecific respiratory symptoms resembling influenza or acute bronchitis occur. Less frequently, acute pneumonia or pleural effusion can develop. Symptoms include fever, cough, chest pain, chills, sputum production, sore throat, and hemoptysis. Physical signs may be absent or limited to scattered rales with or without areas of dullness to percussion over lung fields. Leukocytosis and, in some cases, eosinophilia is seen. Other symptoms include arthritis, conjunctivitis, erythema nodosum, or erythema multiforme. Primary pulmonary lesions sometimes resolve, leaving nodular coin lesions that may be confused with neoplasms and tuberculosis or other granulomatous infections. In some cases, cavitary lesions develop that may vary in size over time and often appear thin-walled. Although dissemination does not occur from these residual areas, a small percentage of these cavities fail to heal. Hemoptysis or the threat of rupture into the pleural space may occasionally require surgery.

Treatment for mild primary coccidioidomycosis may be unnecessary in low-risk patients. Mild-to-moderate nonmeningeal extrapulmonary involvement should be treated with fluconazole or itraconazole. IV fluconazole is preferable for severely ill patients. Amphotericin B is an alternative treatment. As with histoplasmosis, patients with AIDS-associated coccidioidomycosis require maintenance therapy to prevent relapse. Treatment for meningeal coccidioidomycosis must be continued for many months, probably lifelong. Surgical removal of involved bone may be necessary to cure osteomyelitis.

Additional Reading: Antifungal drugs. *Treat Guidel Med Lett.* 2012;10(120):61.

Category: Respiratory system

343. A 65-year-old woman with a seizure disorder controlled with phenytoin presents to your office complaining of muscle cramps, dry skin, and depression. Examination shows carpal-pedal spasms after application of a blood pressure cuff. The most likely diagnosis is
A) Hypothyroidism
B) Hyperventilation with panic attacks
C) Hyperkalemia
D) Hypocalcemia
E) Hyponatremia

Answer and Discussion

The answer is D. Hypocalcemia is defined as a decrease in total plasma calcium concentration <8.8 mg per dL in the presence of normal plasma protein concentration. Causes include hypoparathyroidism, vitamin D deficiency, renal tubular disease, magnesium depletion, acute pancreatitis, hypoproteinemia, septic shock, hyperphosphatemia, and drugs, including phenytoin, phenobarbital, and rifampin. Most patients are asymptomatic. Symptoms, when present, include muscle cramps involving the legs and back, mental status changes, dry skin, depression, and psychosis. Papilledema may occasionally occur, and cataracts may develop after prolonged hypocalcemia. Severe hypocalcemia (<7 mg per dL) may cause tetany, laryngospasm, or generalized seizures. With hypocalcemia giving rise to latent tetany, the patient may exhibit a positive Chvostek's sign (involuntary twitching of the facial muscles caused by a light tapping of the facial nerve just anterior to the exterior auditory meatus) or a positive Trousseau's sign (carpopedal spasm caused by reduction of the blood supply to the hand with a blood pressure cuff inflated to 20 mm Hg above the systolic BP applied to the forearm after 3 minutes). Hypocalcemia can cause heart block and arrhythmias. ECG changes show prolongation of the QTc and ST intervals. T-wave peaking or inversion can also occur. Severe hypocalcemic tetany is treated initially with intravenous infusion of calcium salts (calcium gluconate). In chronic hypocalcemia, oral calcium and vitamin D supplements are usually sufficient. Treatment of hypocalcemia in patients with renal failure must be combined with dietary phosphate restriction and phosphate-binding agents such as calcium carbonate to prevent hyperphosphatemia and metastatic calcification.

Additional Reading: Clinical manifestations of hypocalcemia. In: Basow DS, ed. *UpToDate.* Waltham, MA: UpToDate; 2013.

Category: Neurologic

344. Shy–Drager syndrome is best characterized by
A) Autonomic dysfunction
B) Unilateral foot drop
C) Peripheral neuropathy
D) Proximal muscle weakness
E) Muscle atrophy

Answer and Discussion

The answer is A. Shy–Drager syndrome (now called multiple system atrophy) affects multiple organ systems and causes neurologic damage, including autonomic dysfunction with cerebellar ataxia, parkinsonism, corticospinal, and corticobulbar tract dysfunction. Patients may experience orthostatic hypotension, impotence, urinary retention, fecal incontinence, decreased sweating, iris atrophy, and decreased tearing and salivation. Treatment consists of intravascular volume expansion with the administration of fludrocortisone,

application of constrictive garments to the lower extremities, and the administration of an α-adrenoreceptor stimulator midodrine. Bulbar dysfunction and laryngeal stridor can be fatal if not treated.

Additional Reading: Multiple system atrophy with orthostatic hypotension; 2011. From: http://www.ninds.nih.gov/disorders/msa_orthostatic_hypotension/msa_orthostatic_hypotension.htm

Category: Neurologic

Treatment of Shy–Drager syndrome consists of intravascular volume expansion with the administration of fludrocortisone, application of constrictive garments to the lower extremities, and the administration of an α-adrenoreceptor stimulator midodrine.

345. A 24-year-old yard maintenance worker is bitten by a venomous snake. Which of the following is considered an acceptable treatment?
A) Arterial tourniquet
B) Application of ice
C) Wound incision and forced bleeding
D) Lymphatic tourniquet
E) None of the above

Answer and Discussion

The answer is D. Poisonous snakebites, although rare, are a potentially life-threatening emergency in the United States. Rattlesnakes are responsible for most snakebites and related fatalities. Venomous snakes in the United States can be classified as having hemotoxic or neurotoxic venom. Associated signs and symptoms ranging from fang marks, with or without local pain and swelling, to life-threatening coagulopathy, renal failure, and shock are seen. First-aid techniques such as arterial tourniquets, application of ice, and wound incisions are ineffective and can be harmful. However, suction with a venom extractor within the first 5 minutes after the bite may be useful as are conservative measures, such as immobilization and lymphatic constriction tourniquets until emergency care can be administered. Surgical intervention with fasciotomy is reserved for rare cases. Snakebite prevention should be taught to patients.

Additional Reading: Envenomations: an overview of clinical toxinology for the primary care physician. *Am Fam Physician.* 2009;80(8):793–802.

Category: Nonspecific system

346. Which of the following statements is true regarding low-carbohydrate diets?
A) They may be more effective than low-fat diets in helping patients lose weight in the short term.
B) They cause adverse changes in lipid values.
C) They are often effective years after initiation.
D) They invariably lead to longer healthier lives.

Answer and Discussion

The answer is A. Low-carbohydrate diets restrict caloric intake by reducing the consumption of carbohydrates to 20 to 60 g per day (<20% of caloric intake). The consumption of protein and fat is increased to compensate for the calories that formerly came from carbohydrates. The Atkins Diet is the original low-carbohydrate diet, while others such as the Zone Diet and the South Beach Diet restrict carbohydrates to <40% of calories and focus more on the glycemic index of foods than does the Atkins Diet.

Low-carbohydrate diets are slightly more effective than low-fat diets for initial, short-term weight loss (3 to 6 months), but they are no more effective after 1 year. Low-carbohydrate diets do not adversely affect lipid profiles, but evidence of their effect on long-term cardiovascular health is lacking. Because long-term data on patient-oriented outcomes are lacking for many diets, it is not possible to clearly endorse one diet over another.

Additional Reading: Low-carbohydrate diets. *Am Fam Physician.* 2006;73(11):1942–1948.

Category: Nonspecific system

347. A 42-year-old indigent patient is found to have secondary syphilis and treatment is started. Two hours after his first dose of antibiotics, the patient is noted to have low-grade fever, chills, myalgias, headache, tachypnea, and tachycardia. Appropriate management at this point consists of
A) Stopping all antibiotics
B) Ordering ECG, chest x-ray, blood cultures, and urinalysis
C) Starting intravenous dexamethasone
D) Administering acetaminophen for symptomatic treatment
E) Administering diphenhydramine and epinephrine

Answer and Discussion

The answer is D. The Jarisch–Herxheimer reaction is usually a mild reaction consisting of acute, transient fever (low grade), chills, myalgias, headache, tachycardia, increased respiratory rate, increased circulating neutrophil count (average total WBC count, 12,500 per µL), and vasodilation with mild hypotension that may follow the initiation of treatment for syphilis or other spirochete-related illness. This reaction occurs in approximately 50% of patients with primary syphilis, 90% of those with secondary syphilis, and 25% of those with early latent syphilis. The onset comes within 2 hours of treatment, the temperature peaks at approximately 6 to 8 hours, and defervescence takes place within 12 to 24 hours. The reaction is more delayed in neurosyphilis, with fever peaking after 12 to 14 hours. In patients with secondary syphilis, erythema and edema of the mucocutaneous lesions increase; occasionally, subclinical or early mucocutaneous lesions may first become apparent during the reaction. The pathogenesis of this reaction is undefined, although recent studies have demonstrated the induction of inflammatory mediators such as tumor necrosis factors by treponemal lipoproteins. Patients should be warned to expect such symptoms, which can be managed by symptomatic treatment. Adjunctive steroid and anti-inflammatory therapy has not been shown to prevent the Jarisch–Herxheimer reaction in syphilis and is not recommended for this transient reaction.

Additional Reading: CDC sexually transmitted diseases; 2010. From; http://www.cdc.gov/std/treatment/2010/genital-ulcers.htm

Category: Nonspecific system

The Jarisch–Herxheimer reaction is usually a mild reaction consisting of acute, transient fever (low grade), chills, myalgias, headache, tachycardia, increased respiratory rate, increased circulating neutrophil count (average total WBC count, 12,500 per µL), and vasodilation with mild hypotension that may follow the initiation of treatment for syphilis or other spirochete-related illness.

348. You are covering the local high school football game on Friday night. An 18-year-old star running back goes down on the field after a hard tackle. When you arrive at his side, he is holding his knee. He describes a "pop" followed by severe pain. Which of the following would be most helpful in the initial diagnosis?
A) Ability to walk
B) Lachman's test
C) Anterior drawer test
D) CT of the knee
E) Arthrogram of the knee

Answer and Discussion

The answer is B. ACL (Anterior Cruciate Ligament) injuries typically present after a noncontact deceleration, a "cutting" movement or hyperextension, often accompanied by a "pop," with the inability to continue sports participation and associated knee instability. In all cases of knee injury, it should be determined how quickly swelling occurred after the injury. If an effusion evolved within 4 hours of injury, there is a high likelihood of major osseous, ligamentous, or meniscal injury. The ACL is particularly prone to injury. Physical findings include effusion, positive ACL tests, and chronic quadriceps atrophy. The Lachman's test is performed with the knee in 20 degrees of flexion. The tibia is pulled anteriorly on a secured femur. A positive test result is indicated by increased tibial movement compared with the unaffected knee. The quality of the end point should also be noted; a soft end point indicates an ACL tear. The anterior drawer test (although much less specific) is performed with the knee in 90 degrees of flexion. Similar to the Lachman's test, the tibia is drawn anteriorly, and asymmetric movement is an indicator of ACL injury. The most specific test for ACL disruption is the pivot shift test, but this test is often difficult to perform because of patient guarding and apprehension. Radiographs should be obtained in patients with suspected ACL injuries to rule out associated intra-articular fractures and possibly determine the presence of a marginal avulsion fracture off the lateral tibial plateau (Segond fracture), which helps confirm the diagnosis. MRI is not necessary to diagnose ACL disruption but is often used and may be helpful in diagnosing associated meniscal pathology. Treatment involves rehabilitation with physical therapy and, in some cases, surgical repair.

Additional Reading: Busconi BD, Stevenson JH. Athlete with acute knee injuries. *Sports Medicine Consult: A Problem-Based Approach to Sports Medicine for the Primary Care Physician.* Philadelphia, PA: Lippincott, Williams & Wilkins; 2009.

Category: Musculoskeletal system

349. A 54-year-old nurse presents to your office complaining of gradually increasing right-sided shoulder pain. The patient reports she is unable to sleep on her right side and has a difficult time raising the right arm. Physical examination shows her shoulder's passive range of motion is significantly restricted. X-rays of the shoulder are unremarkable. The most likely diagnosis is
A) Biceps muscle tear
B) Adhesive capsulitis
C) Multiple myeloma
D) Subacromial bursitis
E) Osteoporosis

Answer and Discussion

The answer is B. Adhesive capsulitis, or frozen shoulder, results from thickening and fibrosis of the capsule around the glenohumeral joint and causes loss of motion and pain. Frozen shoulder classically consists of shoulder pain that is slow in onset and presents without any radiographic abnormalities. Usually, the discomfort is localized to the deltoid muscle, and the patient is unable to sleep on the affected side. Loss of passive range of motion (ROM), particularly glenohumeral abduction and external rotation, is hallmark of the disorder. Shoulder impingement and rotator cuff tears may have loss of active ROM but have full passive ROM. An autoimmune cause of frozen shoulder has been proposed, and the condition may be associated with type II diabetes and thyroid disorders. The diagnosis is usually made clinically, and physicians should always be concerned about a possible underlying rotator cuff tear. Radiographs often appear normal but should be obtained to rule out geleno-humeral osteoarthritis, which also is noted to have loss of passive ROM. Arthrography demonstrates generalized constriction of the joint capsule, with loss of the normal axillary and subscapularis spaces. The capsule can be dilated during arthrography, converting the procedure from a diagnostic to a therapeutic one. A carefully designed treatment plan for patients with frozen shoulder may include physical therapy, pain medication such as NSAIDs, and, possibe intra-articular corticosteroid injection. Surgical referral may be indicated after conservative treatment has failed, although the exact timing of surgery should be decided on an individual basis.

Additional Reading: Adhesive capsulitis: a review. *Am Fam Physician*. 2011;83(4):417–422.

Category: Musculoskeletal system

350. During one rescuer cardiopulmonary resuscitation (CPR), the compression/ventilation ratio should be
A) 1:1
B) 5:1
C) 10:1
D) 10:2
E) 30:2

Answer and Discussion

The answer is E. The American Heart Association algorithm for adult basic life support recommends the following sequence when a rescuer finds an unresponsive person: Call for help and an AED (Automated External Defibrillator). The lone rescuer should begin CPR with 30 compressions rather than ventilations to reduce delay to first compression. Compression rate should be at least 100 per minute (rather than "approximately" 100 per minute). Compression depth for adults should range 1½ to 2 inches to at least 2 inches (5 cm). On arrival of a defibrillator or AED, check for a shockable rhythm (ventricular fibrillation or tachycardia). Give one shock (if indicated), then resume CPR, and reshock every 2 minutes.

Additional Reading: Highlights of the 2010 American Heart Association: Guidelines for CPR and ECC. From: http://www.heart.org/idc/groups/heart-public/@wcm/@ecc/documents/downloadable/ucm_317350.pdf.

Category: Cardiovascular system

351. Of the following supplements, which has been associated with an increased risk of lung cancer in smokers?
A) Folic acid
B) β-Carotene
C) Ginseng
D) Vitamin E
E) Saw palmetto

Answer and Discussion

The answer is B. Many carotenoids are known, but their functions are not yet understood. β-Carotene is a vitamin A precursor carried in plasma and LDL. It reduces oxidized LDL uptake but does not prevent LDL oxidation. Sources of dietary carotenoids include fruits, yellow-orange vegetables (e.g., carrots, squash, and sweet potatoes), and deep-green vegetables (e.g., spinach and broccoli). No recommended daily allowance has been established for carotenoids. Research supports the benefit of a carotenoid-rich diet, but not β-carotene supplementation. The β-Carotene and Retinol Efficacy Trial combined β-carotene and retinol supplementation in 18,314 smokers and patients with asbestos exposure. However, the study was terminated prematurely because of a significant increase in lung cancer mortality and a nonsignificant increase in CHD mortality. In 12 years of β-carotene supplementation in 22,071 male physicians, no significant beneficial effects on CHD mortality, nonfatal MI, or stroke were found. In addition, no interactive effect with cigarette smoking (i.e., no harm or benefit) was demonstrated. A nonsignificant reduction in CHD events occurred in the groups who had clinical evidence of atherosclerosis.

Additional Reading: Who should take vitamin supplements? *Med Lett Drugs Ther*. 2011;53(1379–1380):101–103.

Category: Respiratory system

> Research studies suggest that, although once thought to be protective against the development of malignancy, β-carotene actually increased the risk of lung cancer in smokers.

352. A urine culture grows more than 100,000 colony-forming units. The patient is asymptomatic. For which of the following patients is treatment indicated?
A) 94-year-old nursing home resident
B) 72-year-old business executive
C) 68-year-old with a history of breast cancer
D) 78-year-old scheduled for cataract surgery
E) 28-year-old pregnant woman at 38 weeks' gestation

Answer and Discussion

The answer is E. Asymptomatic bacteriuria is defined as the presence of >100,000 colony-forming units per mL of voided urine in persons with no symptoms of UTI. The largest patient population at risk for asymptomatic bacteriuria is the elderly (particularly women). Up to 40% of elderly men and women may have bacteriuria without symptoms. Although early studies noted an association between bacteriuria and excess mortality, more recent studies have failed to demonstrate any such link. Aggressively screening elderly persons for asymptomatic bacteriuria and subsequent treatment of the infection has not been found to reduce infectious complications or mortality. Consequently, this approach is currently not recommended. Three groups of patients with asymptomatic bacteriuria have been shown to benefit from treatment: (1) pregnant women, (2) patients with renal transplants, and (3) patients who are about to undergo GU tract procedures. Between 2% and 10% of pregnancies are complicated by UTIs; if left untreated, 25% to 30% of these women develop pyelonephritis. Pregnancies that are complicated by pyelonephritis have been associated with low-birth-weight infants and prematurity. Thus, pregnant women should be screened for bacteriuria by urine culture at 12 to 16 weeks of gestation. The presence of 100,000 colony-forming units of bacteria per milliliter of urine is considered significant. Pregnant women with asymptomatic bacteriuria should be treated with a 3-to-7-day course of antibiotics, and the urine should subsequently be cultured to ensure cure and the avoidance of relapse.

Additional Reading: Asymptomatic bacteriuria in adults. *Am Fam Physician*. 2006;74(6):985–990.

Category: Nephrologic system

353. Which of the following statements is true regarding orolabial herpes?
A) Highest rate of infection occurs in adolescent children.
B) Lesions are usually painless vesicles that form on the tongue, palate, and gingival area.
C) Topical acyclovir is the drug of choice.
D) Recurrent infections are less severe and shorter in duration.
E) Pain associated with lesions typically lasts 2 to 3 weeks.

Answer and Discussion

The answer is D. Orolabial herpes (gingivostomatitis) is the most prevalent form of mucocutaneous herpes infection. Overall, the highest rate of infection occurs during the preschool years. Female gender, history of sexually transmitted diseases, and multiple sexual partners have also been identified as risk factors for HSV-1 infection. Primary herpetic gingivostomatitis usually affects children below the age of 5 years. It typically takes the form of painful vesicles and ulcerative erosions on the tongue, palate, gingiva, buccal mucosa, and lips. Edema, halitosis, and drooling may be present, and tender submandibular or cervical lymphadenopathy is not uncommon. Hospitalization may be necessary when pain prevents eating or fluid intake. Systemic symptoms are often present, including fever (38.4° to 40°C [101° to 104°F]), malaise, and myalgia. The pharyngitis and flulike symptoms are difficult to distinguish from mononucleosis in older patients. The duration of the illness is 2 to 3 weeks, and oral shedding of the virus may continue for as long as 23 days. Recurrences typically occur two or three times per year. The duration is shorter and the discomfort less severe than in primary infections; the lesions are often single and more localized, and the vesicles heal completely by 8 to 10 days. Pain diminishes quickly in 4 to 5 days. UV radiation predictably triggers recurrence of orolabial HSV-1, an effect that, for unknown reasons, is not fully suppressed by acyclovir. Pharmacologic intervention is therefore more difficult in patients with orolabial infection.

Topical medication for HSV infection is generally not highly effective. In the treatment of primary orolabial herpes, oral acyclovir or valcyclovir can reduce the severity and duration of the outbreak. Standard analgesic therapy with acetaminophen or ibuprofen, careful monitoring of hydration status, and aggressive early rehydration therapy are usually sufficient to avoid hospitalization. Although long-term suppression of orolabial herpes has not been addressed by clinical trials, episodic prophylaxis has been studied because of the predictable trigger effect of UV radiation. Short-term prophylactic therapy with acyclovir may be desirable in some patients who anticipate intense exposure to UV light (e.g., skiers or those who work outdoors), although the clinical effect may vary. Early treatment of recurrent orolabial HSV infection with high doses of antiviral medication has been found to markedly decrease the size and duration of lesions.

Additional Reading: Nongenital herpes simplex virus. *Am Fam Physician*. 2010;82(9):1075–1082.

Category: Integumentary

354. Vegan diets differ from vegetarian diets in that
A) Vegetarian diets can lead to iron deficiency
B) Vegans avoid all animal products in their diets
C) Vegan diets allow for consumption of eggs and their products
D) Vegetarians rarely satisfy nutritional needs

Answer and Discussion

The answer is B. Vegetarian diets differ according to the degree of avoidance of foods of animal origin. According to the traditional definition, a vegetarian diet consists primarily of cereals, fruits, vegetables, legumes, and nuts; animal foods, including milk, dairy products, and eggs are generally excluded. However less restrictive vegetarian diets may include animal foods, such as eggs, milk and dairy products. Vegan diets are more rigid in that all animal products, including eggs, milk, and milk products, are excluded from the diet. Some vegans do not use honey, and may refrain from using animal products such as leather or wool. They also may avoid foods that are processed or not organically grown. Vegetarian diets usually satisfy nutritional needs for growth and development if they are carefully planned with attention to the following possible limiting nutrients: energy, protein, iron, zinc, calcium, vitamin D, vitamin B_{12} (cyanocobalamin), and dietary fiber.

Additional Reading: National Library of Medicine: vegetarian diet. From: http://www.nlm.nih.gov/medlineplus/vegetariandiet.html.

Category: Nonspecific system

> Vegan diets are more rigid than many vegetarian diets in that all animal products, including eggs, milk, and milk products, are excluded from the diet.

355. In assessing the risk of CAD, a diet with high levels of _____ would increase the patient's risk.
A) Trans-fatty acids
B) Polyunsaturated fatty acids
C) Monounsaturated fatty acids
D) Polysaccharides

Answer and Discussion

The answer is A. Diet plays an important role in the risk of CHD. Higher cholesterol levels show a consistent relationship with the incidence of CHD. The type of fat consumed appears to be more important than the amount of total fat. Fatty acids can be divided into 4 categories: saturated, monounsaturated, polyunsaturated, and trans-fats. Saturated fatty acids and trans-fats are associated with an increased risk of CHD. Monounsaturated fatty acids and polyunsaturated fatty acids are associated with a decreased risk of CHD. Additionally, an increase in carbohydrates tends to reduce the serum level of HDL cholesterol in addition to total and LDL cholesterol. Thus, the reduction in CHD risk may be less than predicted by the effect of saturated fat alone on cholesterol levels. Diets with a high glycemic load also decrease the serum HDL concentration. The major sources of trans-fats include margarines and partially hydrogenated vegetable fats. These fats are present in many manufactured foods (e.g., store-bought bread and cookies). Another major source is oils that are maintained at high temperatures for a sustained period of time, such as in fast food restaurants where oils are used to fry meat and potatoes.

Additional Reading: Dietary fatty acids. *Am Fam Physician*. 2009;80(4):345–350.

Category: Cardiovascular system

356. A 40-year-old woman who is otherwise healthy presents to your office complaining of a lump in her neck. On examination, she is found to have a firm 2-cm nodule associated with the left lobe of the thyroid gland. Appropriate management at this time includes
A) Ultrasound of the thyroid
B) Thyroid uptake scan
C) Fine-needle aspiration
D) Radiation ablation
E) Surgical excision

Answer and Discussion

The answer is C. Thyroid nodules are frequently encountered by family physicians. The majority of these are benign; however, children and the elderly have a higher incidence of malignancy. Previous studies have found that the prevalence of thyroid carcinoma was similar (i.e., approximately 5%) in palpable and nonpalpable nodules. Thyroid ultrasonography should be performed in patients with known or suspected thyroid nodules and nearly all single thyroid nodules should be evaluated with needle aspiration biopsy. Hyperfunctioning nodules do not require biopsy. Ultrasonographically guided fine-needle aspiration biopsy of thyroid nodules should be performed if the patient has a history of radiation to the head, neck, or upper chest or a family history of thyroid carcinoma; the diameter of the nodule is 1.0 cm or greater (as in this patient); or suspicious ultrasonographic characteristics are present. In the absence of these findings, follow-up every 6 to 12 months is appropriate because most occult carcinomas are papillary and rarely aggressive. Calcifications associated with thyroid nodules suggest the presence of psammoma bodies, which are associated with papillary carcinoma.

Serum TSH level should be measured during the initial evaluation of a patient with a thyroid nodule. If it is low, radionuclide scintigraphy should be performed.

Additional Reading: Thyroid nodules. *Am Fam Physician.* 2013;88(3):193–196.

Category: Endocrine system

357. Which of the following effects is associated with selective estrogen receptor modulators?
A) Estrogen-like effects on endometrium
B) Estrogen-like effects on lipids
C) Estrogen-antagonistic effects on bone
D) Estrogen-like effects on the breast
E) Decreased risk of thromboembolic events

Answer and Discussion

The answer is B. Raloxifene (Evista) is a selective estrogen receptor modulator that produces estrogen-agonistic effects on bone and lipid metabolism and estrogen-antagonistic effects on uterine endometrium and breast tissue. Because of its tissue selectivity, raloxifene may have fewer side effects than are typically observed with estrogen therapy. The most common adverse effects of raloxifene are hot flushes and leg cramps. The drug is also associated with an increased risk of thromboembolic events. The beneficial estrogenic activities of raloxifene include a lowering of total and LDL cholesterol levels and an augmentation of bone mineral density. Raloxifene has been approved by the FDA for both prevention and treatment of postmenopausal osteoporosis, and it has reduced the risk of vertebral fractures but not nonvertebral fractures.

Additional Reading: Drugs for postmenopausal psteoporosis. *Treat Guidel Med Lett.* 2011;9(111):67–74.

Category: Endocrine system

358. A 68-year-old retired fisherman presents to your office complaining of a lesion that developed on the dorsal aspect of his hand over the last few months. Inspection of the lesion shows a dome-shaped lesion measuring 2 cm in diameter. The volcano-shaped lesion has a protruding mass of keratin. The most likely diagnosis is
A) Basal cell carcinoma
B) Keratoacanthoma
C) Sebaceous cyst
D) Malignant melanoma
E) Dermatofibroma

Answer and Discussion

The answer is B. Keratoacanthoma appears as a skin-colored or pink smooth lesion that becomes dome-shaped during a period of very rapid growth. Onset is rapid; usually within 1 to 2 months the lesion reaches its full size. Common sites include the face, dorsum of the hands, and forearms. When mature, it is volcano-shaped, with protruding masses of keratin resembling lava. Classic keratoacanthoma is not malignant and regresses spontaneously, but atypical lesions may actually be squamous cell carcinoma. Many dermatopathologists include keratoacanthoma in the spectrum of squamous cell carcinoma. Total excision is the preferred treatment for most solitary keratoacanthomas. For smaller lesions, electrodesiccation and curettage or blunt dissection is sufficient. Mohs' surgery can be used in difficult areas, especially around the nose and ears. Alternative therapies include oral isotretinoin, topical (Effudex) and intralesional (Adrucil) fluorouracil, intralesional methotrexate (Rheumatrex), and intralesional 5-interferon alfa-2a (Roferon-A). Radiotherapy is an option for patients with recurrence or larger lesions.

Basal cell carcinoma develops slowly and is seen as a nodule with an eroded center and a "rolled border." The center appears as if gnawed, hence the name "rodent ulcer."

Sebaceous cysts are subcutaneous and may erode though the skin surface. They possess a soft cheesy material, not scaly keratin.

Malignant melanoma are evaluated by the "ABCD" nuemonic. A stands for asymmetry, B is for an irregular border, C is for variations of color (from black to red, white and blue hues), and D is for diameter greater than 1 cm.

Dermatofibroma are firm nodules, the overlying skin is slightly thickened and they may be black, red, or brown colored. Their diameter is generally about a centimeter and there can be multiple lesions. Dermatofibroma are benign focal proliferation of fibroblasts in the skin.

Additional Reading: Common benign skin tumors. *Am Fam Physician.* 2003;67:729–738.

Category: Integumentary

359. In a placebo-controlled trial involving 100 patients, 30 died during the study period (10 receiving active drug and 20 receiving placebo), giving a mortality of 20% with active drug versus 40% with placebo. The number needed to treat (NNT) is
A) 5
B) 10
C) 25
D) 50
E) 100

Answer and Discussion

The answer is A. The benefit of an intervention can be expressed by NNT. NNT is the reciprocal of the absolute risk reduction (the absolute adverse event rate for placebo minus the absolute adverse event rate for treated patients). From a practical standpoint, an NNT interpretation can be shown by the following statement: "This study suggests that I would have to treat five patients with a drug to prevent one death." As an example, consider a placebo-controlled trial involving 100 patients. Thirty patients died during the study period (10 receiving active drug and 20 receiving placebo), giving a mortality rate of 20% with active drug (10 divided by [10 + 40]), versus 40% (20 divided by [20 + 30]) with placebo. The difference between these two rates, the "risk difference," is used to calculate NNT.

40% minus 20% = 20% = 0.2

1 divided by 0.2 = 5

Thus, this study suggests that only five patients need to be treated with the drug (compared with placebo) to prevent one death.

Additional Reading: EBM Glossary. *Am Fam Physician*. From: http://www.aafp.org/journals/afp/authors/ebm-toolkit/glossary.html.

Category: Patient/population-based care

360. The test of choice for screening for hereditary hemochromatosis is
A) Aspartate aminotransferase (AST)
B) Serum ferritin
C) Transferrin saturation
D) Total iron
E) TIBC

Answer and Discussion

The answer is C. Hereditary hemochromatosis is an autosomal-recessive disorder that disrupts the body's regulation of iron. It is the most common genetic disease in whites. Men are more often affected than women. Persons who are homozygous for the HFE gene mutation C282Y comprise 85% to 90% of phenotypically affected persons. End-organ damage or clinical manifestations of hereditary hemochromatosis occur in approximately 10% of persons homozygous for C282Y. Symptoms of hereditary hemochromatosis are nonspecific (e.g., weakness, lethargy, arthralgias, and impotence) and typically absent in the early stages. Late manifestations include arthralgias, osteoporosis, cirrhosis, hepatocellular cancer, cardiomyopathy, dysrhythmia, diabetes mellitus, and hypogonadism. Initial screening of individuals with suspected iron overload and those above the age of 20 years who are first-degree relatives of known cases of hereditary hemochromatosis should be done by measurement of transferrin saturation after an overnight fast. Simultaneous serum ferritin determination increases the predictive accuracy for diagnosis of iron overload. Transferrin saturation is also the test of choice for screening the general adult population for iron overload states.

Treatment of hereditary hemochromatosis includes phlebotomy to reduce total iron levels and achieve normal ferritin levels.

Additional Reading: Hereditary hemochromatosis. *Am Fam Physician*. 2013;87(3):183–190.

Category: Hematologic system

361. Mad cow disease (bovine spongiform encephalopathy [BSE]) has symptoms similar to which of the following conditions?
A) Lyme disease
B) Syphilis
C) Chronic fatigue syndrome
D) Malaria
E) Creutzfeldt–Jakob disease

Answer and Discussion

The answer is E. The FDA Center for Veterinary Medicine is responsible for protection against animal feed that can affect the safety of derived human food. In recent years, the spread of BSE, the so-called mad cow disease, in foreign countries has prompted the Center for Veterinary Medicine to place restrictions on the production of several types of feed. The action was based on research indicating that BSE is transferred among cows through feed made from the rendered carcasses of cattle that contain a prion that has been linked to BSE. The seriousness of the problem was magnified by the emergence in the United Kingdom of the human illness "new-variant Creutzfeldt–Jakob disease," which gave rise to a theory that BSE can be transferred to humans. Because of the potential risk of transmission, the Center for Veterinary Medicine has banned the use of mammalian tissues such as meat, bone meal, meat by-products, and cooked bone marrow in feed for cattle and other ruminant animals. The implementation of the ban is verified through intensive inspection of rendering plants and feed manufacturers.

Additional Reading: Center for Disease Control and Prevention: BSE (Bovine Spongiform Encephalopathy, or Mad Cow Disease). From: http://www.cdc.gov/ncidod/dvrd/bse/.

Category: Neurologic

362. Charcot foot is most commonly seen in patients with
A) Gonorrhea
B) Primary syphilis
C) Rheumatoid arthritis
D) Diabetes mellitus
E) Neurofibromatosis

Answer and Discussion

The answer is D. First described in patients with tertiary syphilis, Charcot foot is now seen mostly in patients with diabetes mellitus. It is a condition of acute or gradual onset and, in its most severe form, causes significant disruption of the bony architecture of the foot. It often results in foot deformities and causes abnormal pressure distribution on the plantar surface, foot ulcers, and, in some cases, requires amputation. The exact pathogenesis is unknown, but underlying sensory neuropathy is nearly universal. Arteriovenous shunting due to autonomic neuropathy is also thought to play a role. Repeated unrecognized microtrauma or an identifiable injury may be the inciting factors of Charcot foot. Approximately 50% of patients with Charcot foot remember a precipitating event such as a slip or a trip, or they may have had unrelated surgery on the foot as an antecedent event. In approximately 25% of patients, a similar problem ultimately develops on the other foot. Clinical findings in patients with an acute Charcot process include warmth, erythema, and swelling, and the disease is often thought to be cellulitis. Pain and tenderness are usually absent because of sensory neuropathy, which is universal and is probably a component of the basic pathogenesis of the Charcot foot. However, because patients with Charcot foot may have some pain if the sensory loss is not complete, the presence of pain does not totally exclude the diagnosis. Such pain is always much less than would be expected for the severity of the clinical and/or radiographic findings. Although cellulitis should be considered in any patient with diabetes, missing the diagnosis of Charcot foot can be serious because failure to initiate proper treatment of the Charcot foot can lead to a total loss of function. Inappropriate treatment with antimicrobial therapy and even incision and drainage can lead to unnecessary complications. Minimal pain or the absence of pain (characteristic of a Charcot fracture) can lead patients and physicians to ignore this serious disease. The initial radiographic findings can be normal, making the diagnosis difficult, but if a Charcot foot is strongly suspected from the clinical presentation, treatment should be initiated and serial radiographs should be taken. The proper treatment for a hot, swollen foot in a patient with sensory neuropathy is immobilization. Most cases of Charcot foot can be treated nonsurgically with pressure-relieving methods such as total contact casting (TCC), which is considered to be the gold standard of treatment.

Additional Reading: Charcot foot: the diagnostic dilemma. *Am Fam Physician.* 2001;64:1591–1598.

Category: Endocrine system

> While cellulitis should be considered in any patient with diabetes, missing the diagnosis of Charcot foot can be serious because failure to initiate proper treatment of the Charcot foot can lead to a total loss of function.

363. A 38-year-old describes severe rectal pain associated with pallor, diaphoresis, and tachycardia that lasts for only a few minutes. The pains occur mostly at night and are described as spasms. The most likely diagnosis is
A) Thrombosed hemorrhoids
B) Irritable bowel syndrome
C) Ulcerative colitis
D) Obstipation
E) Proctalgia fugax

Answer and Discussion

The answer is E. Proctalgia fugax is a unique anal pain. Patients with proctalgia fugax experience severe episodes of spasm-like pain that often occur at night. Proctalgia fugax may only occur once a year, or may be sporadic in waves of three or four times per week. Each episode lasts only minutes, but the pain is severe and may be accompanied by sweating, pallor, and tachycardia. Patients experience urgency to defecate, yet pass no stool. No specific etiology has been found, but proctalgia fugax may be associated with spastic contractions of the rectum or the muscular pelvic floor in irritable bowel syndrome. Other unproven associations are food allergies, especially to artificial sweeteners or caffeine. Reassurance that the condition is benign may be helpful, but little can be done to treat proctalgia fugax. Medications are not helpful, because the episode is likely to be over before the drugs become active. Sitting in a tub of hot water or, alternatively, applying ice may provide symptomatic relief. A low dose of diazepam at bedtime may be beneficial in cases of frequent and disabling proctalgia fugax.

Additional Reading: Evaluation and management of common anorectal conditions. *Am Fam Physician.* 2012;85(6):624–630.

Category: Gastroenterology system

364. The procedure of choice for detecting osteomyelitis in diabetic foot ulcers is
A) Plain films
B) CT scan
C) MRI
D) Technetium bone scan
E) Indium scan

Answer and Discussion

The answer is C. Diabetic foot infection is defined as soft tissue or bone infection below the malleoli and is the most frequent cause of nontraumatic lower-extremity amputation. Diabetic foot infections are diagnosed clinically on the basis of the presence of at least two classic findings of inflammation or purulence. Most infections are polymicrobial. The most common pathogens are aerobic gram-positive cocci, mainly *Staphylococcus* species. Osteomyelitis is a serious complication of diabetic foot infection that increases the likelihood of surgical intervention. Although plain films of the feet are often ordered initially, MRI is the imaging procedure of choice for osteomyelitis in diabetic foot ulcers. MRI can show abnormal bone marrow signal, soft tissue masses, and cortical destruction characteristic of osteomyelitis. Unlike plain films, MRI can detect these changes early (within days) in infection. MRI also provides the anatomic detail, necessary when surgical debridement is required. Treatment is based on the extent and severity of the infection and comorbid conditions. Mild infections are treated with oral antibiotics, wound care, and pressure off-loading in the outpatient setting. Surgical debridement and drainage of deep tissue abscesses and infections should be performed in a timely manner.

Additional Reading: Diabetic foot infections. *Am Fam Physician.* 2013;88(3):177–184.

Category: Endocrine system

365. The *BRCA* genetic locus has been linked with all of the following cancers *except*
A) Breast cancer
B) Ovarian cancer
C) Prostate cancer
D) Colon cancer
E) Gastric cancer

Answer and Discussion

The answer is E. Discovered in the 1980s, *BRCA1* is a gene on chromosome 17 that is known to be involved in tumor suppression. A woman with certain known mutations in *BRCA1* has an increased risk for breast cancer and ovarian cancer. There is a higher risk in Ashkenazi Jewish women (most Jewish people in the United States are of this Eastern European origin). *BRCA2* is another susceptibility gene for breast cancer and is found on chromosome 13. Mutations in *BRCA2* confer an elevated breast cancer risk similar to that occurring with *BRCA1* mutations.

In a family with a history of breast and/or ovarian cancer, the family member who has breast or ovarian cancer should be tested first; if found to have a harmful *BRCA1* or *BRCA2* mutation, then other family members can be tested to see if they also have the mutation.

Additionally, those at higher risk include the following:

- Women of Ashkenazi Jewish descent with any first-degree relative (mother, daughter, or sister) diagnosed with breast or ovarian cancer and 2 second-degree relatives on the same side of the family diagnosed with breast or ovarian cancer.

For women who are not of Ashkenazi Jewish descent

- 2 first-degree relatives diagnosed with breast cancer, 1 of whom was diagnosed at age 50 or younger;
- 3 or more first-degree or second-degree (grandmother or aunt) relatives diagnosed with breast cancer regardless of their age at diagnosis;
- a combination of first- and second-degree relatives diagnosed with breast cancer and ovarian cancer (one cancer type per person);
- a first-degree relative with cancer diagnosed in both breasts (bilateral breast cancer);
- a combination of 2 or more first- or second-degree relatives diagnosed with ovarian cancer regardless of age at diagnosis;
- a first- or second-degree relative diagnosed with both breast and ovarian cancer regardless of age at diagnosis; and
- breast cancer diagnosed in a male relative.

As many as one-third of women below age 29 years with breast cancer carry a *BRCA1* or *-2* mutation, but only 2% of women ages 70 to 79 years with breast cancer carry such a mutation. Genetic studies in high-risk families suggest that *BRCA1* and *-2* mutations may account for 50% of inherited breast and ovarian cancers and are also associated with an increase in prostate and colon cancers.

Known carriers should begin performing monthly breast self-examinations at age 18 years and should begin having annual clinical examinations at age 25 years. Annual mammography is also recommended beginning at age 25 years. Insufficient evidence exists to recommend for or against prophylactic mastectomy. Even this invasive procedure does not appear to provide definitive treatment, as cases have been reported of breast cancer occurring after bilateral mastectomies.

Currently, the USPSTF recommends against routine referral for genetic counseling or routine breast cancer susceptibility gene (*BRCA*) testing for women whose family history is *not* associated with an increased risk for deleterious mutations in breast cancer susceptibility gene 1 (*BRCA1*) or breast cancer susceptibility gene 2 (*BRCA2*). Additionally, the USPSTF recommends that women whose family history is associated with an increased risk for deleterious mutations in *BRCA1* or *BRCA2* genes be referred for genetic counseling and evaluation for *BRCA* testing.

Additional Reading: U.S. Preventive Services Task Force (USPSTF): genetic risk assessment and *BRCA* mutation testing for breast and ovarian cancer susceptibility. *Ann Intern Med.* 2005;143:355–361.

National Cancer Institute; BRCA1 and BRCA2: Cancer Risk and Genetic Testing. From: http://www.cancer.gov/cancertopics/factsheet/Risk/BRCA.

Category: Reproductive system

366. Which of the following statements regarding hepatitis C is correct?
A) Most patients are symptomatic with development of the disease.
B) The course of the disease shows no variability and is progressive.
C) Most patients develop chronic hepatitis.
D) The disease is not transferred through sexual contact.
E) Immune globulin is effective for postexposure prophylaxis.

Answer and Discussion
The answer is C. HCV is the most common chronic blood-borne infection in the United States. Identified in 1988 through molecular biologic techniques, HCV is an enveloped RNA virus that is classified as a separate genus in the Flaviviridae family. HCV is most efficiently transmitted through large or repeated percutaneous exposures to blood, such as transfusions or transplants from infected donors (although the blood supply has been screened for HCV since 1992), inadvertent contamination of supplies shared among patients undergoing chronic hemodialysis, or sharing of equipment among injection drug users. Transmission of HCV may also occur through high-risk (particularly anal) sex, perinatal exposure, percutaneous exposures in the health care setting, or exposure to the blood of an infected household contact. There is no anti-HCV vaccine, and immune globulin does not prevent infection. There is no means to prevent mother-to-child transmission (estimated to occur 5% of the time), and breast-feeding is allowed for mothers with chronic HCV.

The incubation period for newly acquired (acute) HCV infection ranges from 2 weeks to 6 months, averaging 6 to 7 weeks. The course of acute HCV is variable: 60% to 70% are asymptomatic, 20% to 30% have jaundice, and 10% to 20% have nonspecific symptoms such as loss of appetite, fatigue, and abdominal pain; ALT elevations are typically <800 IU per L and rarely exceed 1,000 IU per L. Most patients (80%) develop chronic HCV infection, with a typical, chronic polyphasic fluctuation in ALT between normal and 300 IU per L. No clinical features of the acute disease or risk factors for infection, including a history of percutaneous exposures, have been found to be predictive of chronicity. Since viral replication can be detected as early as 1 to 2 weeks after exposure, acute HCV is best diagnosed with a HCV RNA polymerase chain reaction assay. Emergence of the anti-HCV antibody is expected in 80% of patients by 3 months and 97% by 6 months and is the recommended test to screen for chronic HCV, which is currently recommended by the USPSTF for all patients born between 1945 and 1965, as well as for those with risk factors for infection. The persistence of HCV viremia beyond 6 months defines chronic infection, whereas clearance of detectable virus indicates either self-eradication or treatment success when measured 12 weeks after the end of treatment.

The current standard for combination treatment for chronic HCV (pegylated inferferon plus ribavirin for genotype 2, 3, or 4, plus either protease inhibitor telaprevir or boceprevir for genotype 1 infection) is evolving rapidly at the time of this writing (July 2013). New HCV polymerase inhibitors and nucleoside + nucleotide reverse transcriptase inhibitors are expected by 2014 that have the potential to offer all-oral (i.e., interferon-sparing) treatment for at least genotype 2 and 3 infections, and most likely genotype 1 and 4 infections as well by 2015, with shorter treatment intervals and considerably fewer side effects and toxicities. Recommendations on who to treat are similarly evolving rapidly on the basis of the patient's HCV genotype, stage of liver disease, and preference for treatment versus deferral until newer treatments are available. Although several noninvasive tests are currently available to estimate liver disease stage (such as Fibrosure, Hepascore, and ultrasound elastography and others), a liver biopsy remains the gold standard to stage liver disease.

Additional Reading: *Diagnosis, Management and Treatment of Hepatitis C: an update.* American Association for the Study of Liver Diseases. 2009; 1–6.

Current and future therapies for hepatitis C virus infection. *N Engl J Med.* 2013;368:1907–1917.

Category: Gastroenterology system

367. The most common cause of bacterial conjunctivitis in American adults is
A) *Streptococcus pneumoniae*
B) *Haemophilus influenzae*
C) *Chlamydia trachomatis*
D) *Staphylococcus aureus*
E) *Klebsiella*

Answer and Discussion
The answer is D. The conjunctiva is a thin, translucent, relatively elastic tissue layer with bulbar (outer aspect of the globe) and palpebral (inside of the eyelid) portions. Underneath the conjunctiva lie the episclera, sclera, and uveal tissue layers. Conjunctivitis is the most common cause of red eye. Most frequently, acute conjunctivitis is caused by a bacterial or viral infection. Sexually transmitted diseases such as chlamydia and gonorrhea are less common causes of conjunctivitis. Ocular allergy is one of the major causes of chronic conjunctivitis. Blepharitis (inflammation of the eyelid margin), dry eye, and the prolonged use of ophthalmic medications, contact

lenses, and ophthalmic solutions are also frequent causes of chronic conjunctival inflammation. Adenovirus is by far the most common cause of viral conjunctivitis, although other viruses can also cause the condition. Viral conjunctivitis often occurs in community epidemics, with the virus transmitted in schools, workplaces, and physicians' offices. The usual modes of transmission are contaminated fingers, medical instruments, and swimming pool water. Patients with viral conjunctivitis typically present with an acutely red eye, watery discharge, conjunctival swelling, a tender preauricular node, and, in some cases, photophobia and a foreign-body sensation. Both eyes may be affected simultaneously, or the second eye may become involved a few days after the first eye. Some patients have an associated upper respiratory tract infection. Patients should be instructed to avoid direct contact with other persons for at least 1 week after the onset of symptoms. Treatment is supportive. Cold compresses and topical vasoconstrictors may provide symptomatic relief. Topical antibiotics are rarely necessary, because secondary bacterial infection is uncommon. The three most common pathogens in bacterial conjunctivitis are *S. pneumoniae*, *H. influenzae*, and *S. aureus*. Infections with *S. pneumoniae* and *H. influenzae* are more common in children, whereas *S. aureus* most frequently affects adults. Childhood immunizations for *H. influenzae* and *S. pneumoniae* further decrease the incidence of these causative organisms.

In persons with suspected, but not confirmed, bacterial conjunctivitis, empiric treatment with topical antibiotics may be beneficial. However, this benefit is marginal, so it is advisable to recommend good eyelid hygiene and suggest that patients take antibiotics only if symptoms do not resolve after 1 to 2 days.

Allergic conjunctivitis is distinguished by severe itching and allergen exposure. This condition is generally treated with topical antihistamines, mast-cell stabilizers, or anti-inflammatory agents. Pain and photophobia are not typical features of a primary conjunctival inflammatory process. If these features are present, the physician should consider more serious underlying ocular or orbital disease processes, including uveitis, keratitis, acute glaucoma, and orbital cellulitis. Similarly, blurred vision that fails to clear with a blink is rarely associated with conjunctivitis. Patients with pain, photophobia, or blurred vision should be referred to an ophthalmologist.

Additional Reading: Bacterial conjunctivitis. *Am Fam Physician.* 2010;82(6):665–666.

Category: Special sensory

368. A 33-year-old woman presents with a cold. She also mentions that she started taking omeprazole (Prilosec) over the counter as an antacid as she has been having episodes of indigestion after meals. She finds that it helps but asks about any long-term side effects from taking this regularly. You tell her that evidence has shown that continuing to take this medication will increase her risk for which one of the following?
A) Hypocalcemia
B) Vitamin B_{12} deficiency
C) Clostridium difficile colitis
D) Having a child with birth defects (if taken in the first trimester)
E) Colon cancer

Answer and Discussion

The answer is C. PPIs such as omeprazole (Prilosec) effectively inhibit acid production in the stomach. This reduces symptoms of acid-mediated gastritis, peptic ulcer disease, and gastroesophageal reflux. However, this reduction in stomach acidity can cause unintended consequences involving processes that are physiologically dependent on low pH in the gastrointestinal tract. Theoretical risks include decreased levels of vitamin B_{12}, iron, and/or magnesium; decreased bone density; an increase in gut infections or pneumonia; an increase in gastrointestinal neoplasms; and changes in absorption of other medications.

The evidence is conflicting on some of these risks, but consensus is emerging that chronic use of PPIs increases the risk for pneumonia and gut infections, primarily *Clostridium difficile* colitis. PPIs may also decrease bone density in subsets of patients. These risks need to be weighed against the benefits that these medicines provide before prescribing them on a long-term basis.

Additional Reading: Use of acid-suppressive drugs and risk of pneumonia: a systematic review and meta-analysis. *CMAJ* 2011;183(3):310–319; and Risk of *Clostridium difficile* infection with acid suppressing drugs and antibiotics: meta-analysis. *Am J Gastroenterol.* 2012;107(7):1011–1019.

Category: Gastroenterology system

369. Which of the following drugs is a leukotriene antagonist/inhibitor?
A) Theophylline
B) Prednisone
C) Salmeterol
D) Terbutaline
E) Zafirlukast

Answer and Discussion

The answer is E. Medications used in the treatment of asthma are divided into long-term control medications that are taken regularly and quick-relief (rescue) medications that are taken as needed to relieve bronchoconstriction rapidly. Long-term control medications include anti-inflammatory agents (corticosteroids and leukotriene modifiers) and long-acting bronchodilators. Quick-relief medications include short-acting $\beta2$ agonists, anticholinergics, and systemic corticosteroids.

Patients whose symptoms are mild and infrequent can use a short-acting bronchodilator as needed for relief of symptoms. Patients with more frequent cough, wheeze, chest tightness or shortness of breath should begin treatment with a long-term controller medication. Low daily doses of an inhaled corticosteroid suppress airway inflammation and reduce the risk of exacerbations. For patients who remain symptomatic despite compliance with inhaled corticosteroid treatment and good inhalational technique, addition of a long-acting $\beta2$-agonist is recommended. Patients with more severe disease may need higher doses of inhaled corticosteroids.

Corticosteroids remain the most potent and effective anti-inflammatory agents available for the management of asthma. An inhaled corticosteroid is the most effective long-term treatment for control of the disease in treating all types of persistent asthma in patients of all ages. For long-term use, inhaled steroids are preferred over oral steroids because the inhaled agents have fewer systemic side effects. However, oral steroids are the most effective drugs available for exacerbations of asthma incompletely responsive to bronchodilators. Even when an acute exacerbation responds to bronchodilators, addition of a short course of an oral steroid can decrease symptoms and may prevent a relapse. For asthma exacerbations, daily systemic steroids are generally required for only a few days, without a taper.

Leukotriene modifiers (montelukast and zafirlukast) are less effective alternatives for those who cannot tolerate low-dose inhaled steroids. Leukotriene modifiers are also generally less effective than an inhaled long-acting β agonist. Both of these classes are not recommended for treatment of acute asthma symptoms.

Salmeterol (Serevent) is a long-acting β2 agonist. Its mechanism of action and side effect profile are similar to those of other β2 agonists. Unlike the short-acting agents, salmeterol is not intended for use as a quick-relief agent.

Theophylline, once the mainstay of asthma treatment, is now considered a second- or third-line agent because of its adverse effect profile and potential interactions with many drugs. Furthermore, serum theophylline levels have to be monitored during treatment. In addition to its well-known bronchodilator effects, theophylline has anti-inflammatory activity. Currently, theophylline therapy is generally reserved for use in patients who exhibit nocturnal asthma symptoms that are not controlled with high-dose anti-inflammatory medications.

Zafirlukast (Accolate) and zileuton (Zyflo) antagonize the action of leukotrienes at their receptor (zafirlukast) or inhibit the lipoxygenase pathway (zileuton). Both drugs are approved for the management of chronic asthma in adults and in children older than 12 years. Zafirlukast and zileuton have numerous drug interactions.

Short-acting inhaled β2 agonists are the agents of choice for relieving bronchospasms and preventing exercise-induced bronchospasms. Selective β2 agonists, including albuterol, bitolterol (Tornalate), metaproterenol (Alupent), pirbuterol (Maxair), and terbutaline (Brethaire), are preferred to nonselective β agonists such as epinephrine, ephedrine, and isoproterenol (Isuprel) because the selective agents have fewer cardiovascular side effects and a longer duration of action. Inhaled β2 agonists have a rapid onset of action. Short-term systemic corticosteroid therapy is useful for gaining initial control of asthma and for treating moderate-to-severe asthma exacerbations. The intravenous administration of systemic corticosteroids offers no advantage over oral administration when GI absorption is not impaired. Ipratropium is a quaternary atropine derivative that inhibits vagal-mediated bronchoconstriction. It may be useful as an adjunct to inhaled β2 agonists in patients who have severe asthma exacerbations or who cannot tolerate β2 agonists.

Additional Reading: Drugs for asthma and COPD. *Treat Guidel Med Lett.* 2013;11(132):75–86.

Category: Respiratory system

370. The most common primary cancer of the bone in adults is
A) Multiple myeloma
B) Osteosarcoma
C) Osteoid osteoma
D) Osteitis fibrosa cystica
E) Metastatic prostate cancer

Answer and Discussion

The answer is A. Multiple myeloma is the malignant proliferation of plasma cells involving more than 10% of the bone marrow. Multiple myeloma is the most common primary cancer of the bones in adults. The median age at diagnosis of multiple myeloma is 62 years. Only 2% to 3% of cases are reported in patients younger than 30 years. African Americans in the United States are twice as likely to develop multiple myeloma as whites.

The multiple myeloma cell produces monoclonal immunoglobulins that may be identified on serum or urine protein electrophoresis. Bone pain related to multiple lytic lesions is the most common clinical presentation. However, up to 30% of patients are diagnosed incidentally while being evaluated for unrelated problems, and one-third of patients are diagnosed after a pathologic fracture, commonly of the axial skeleton. Multiple myeloma must be differentiated from other causes of monoclonal gammopathy, including monoclonal gammopathy of undetermined significance,

heavy chain disease, plasmacytoma, and Waldenstrom macroglobulinemia. Routine laboratory workup may show pancytopenia, abnormal coagulation, hypercalcemia, azotemia, elevated alkaline phosphatase and ESR, and hypoalbuminemia. Examination may reveal proteinuria, hypercalciuria, or both. Urine dipstick tests may not indicate the presence of Bence Jones proteinuria. All patients with suspected multiple myeloma require a 24-hour urinalysis by protein electrophoresis to determine the presence of Bence Jones proteinuria and kappa or lambda light chains. Serum protein electrophoresis identifies an M protein as a narrow peak or "spike" in the γ, β, or α2 regions of the densitometer tracing. Chemotherapy with melphalan and prednisone is the standard treatment for multiple myeloma. Other treatment modalities include polychemotherapy (thalidomide, immunomodulatory drugs, proteasome inhibitors) and bone marrow transplantation. Only 50% to 60% of patients respond to therapy. The aggregate median survival for all stages of multiple myeloma is 3 to 5 years.

Additional Reading: Multiple myeloma: diagnosis and treatment. *Am Fam Physician.* 2008;78(7):853–859.

Category: Hematologic system

371. A 21-year-old returns from a camping trip early complaining of a dull numbness affecting his upper left extremity. He recalls a sharp pinprick sensation before the development of symptoms. The patient now describes a cramping pain and muscle rigidity of the back and chest area. A red, indurated area is found on the distal left arm. The patient has profuse sweating, nausea, vomiting, and shortness of breath. The likely diagnosis is
A) Lyme disease
B) Tick paralysis
C) Malaria
D) Black widow spider envenomation
E) Rocky Mountain spotted fever

Answer and Discussion

The answer is D. Black widow spider bites are associated with a sharp, pinprick-like pain, followed by a dull, sometimes numbing pain in the affected extremity and by cramping pain and muscular rigidity in the abdomen or the shoulders, back, and chest. Associated manifestations may include severe abdominal pain, restlessness, anxiety, sweating, headache, dizziness, ptosis, eyelid edema, rash and pruritus, respiratory distress, nausea, vomiting, salivation, weakness, and increased skin temperature over the affected area. Blood pressure and CSF pressure are usually elevated in more severe cases in adults. An ice cube may be placed over a black widow spider bite to reduce pain. Patients younger than 16 years or older than 60 years, those with hypertensive CVD, or those with symptoms and signs of severe envenomation should be hospitalized and, when symptomatic treatment is unsuccessful, should be given antivenin. Antivenin must be given within 30 minutes and the manufacturer recommends skin testing prior to administration (however, skin testing does not always predict anaphylaxis). Children may require respiratory assistance. Vital signs should be checked frequently during the 12 hours after the bite. In the elderly, acute hypertension may require treatment. For muscle pain and spasms, intravenous calcium gluconate may be given slowly and requires cardiac monitoring. Several doses at 4-hour intervals may be necessary.

Additional Reading: Common spider bites. *Am Fam Physician.* 2007;75(6):869–873.

Category: Nonspecific system

372. A 75-year-old man presents to your office complaining of flashes of light and blurred vision. He reports no pain. In-office examination reveals no findings other than decreased visual acuity. Appropriate management consists of
A) Patching of the affected eye
B) Course of oral steroids
C) Ultrasound of the carotids
D) Initiation of aspirin therapy
E) Immediate ophthalmology referral

Answer and Discussion

The answer is E. Retinal detachment can occur as the result of a retinal tear (occurs more frequently in myopia, after cataract surgery, or after ocular trauma) by detachment without a tear as a result of vitreal traction (seen in proliferative retinopathy of diabetes or sickle cell disease) or by transudation of fluid into the subretinal space (e.g., severe uveitis or primary or metastatic choroidal tumors). Retinal detachment is painless. Early symptoms may include dark or irregular vitreous floaters, flashes of light, or blurred vision. As the detachment progresses, the patient notices a curtain or veil in the field of vision. If the macula is involved, central visual acuity is significantly affected. Direct ophthalmoscopy may show retinal irregularities and a retinal elevation with darkened blood vessels. Indirect ophthalmoscopy, including scleral depression, is necessary for detecting peripheral breaks and detachment. If a vitreous hemorrhage obscures the retina, especially in myopia, postcataract extraction, or eye injury, retinal detachment should be suspected and B-scan ultrasonography performed. Although often localized, retinal detachments due to retinal tears can expand to involve the entire retina if not treated promptly. Any patient with a suspected or established retinal detachment should be seen urgently by an ophthalmologist.

Additional Reading: Ocular emergencies. *Am Fam Physician.* 2007;76(6):829–836.

Category: Special sensory

> Retinal detachment is painless. Early symptoms may include dark or irregular vitreous floaters, flashes of light, or blurred vision. As the detachment progresses, the patient notices a curtain or veil in the field of vision.

373. Which of the following statements concerning diarrhea in the United States is true?
A) Resistance to antimicrobial agents is not a concern with treatment of diarrhea.
B) Traveler's diarrhea is caused by a virus in most cases.
C) Pathogens are not identifiable in more than 50% of cases of diarrhea.
D) The goal of treatment is eradication of the causative agent.

Answer and Discussion

The answer is C. Diarrhea is defined as watery or liquid stools, usually with increases in daily frequency and in total stool weight (>200 g per day). The pathogens that commonly cause sporadic diarrhea in adults in developed countries are *Campylobacter, Salmonella,* and *Shigella* species; *E. coli; Yersinia* species; protozoa; and viruses. However, pathogens are not identifiable in more than one-half of cases. Traveler's diarrhea is caused by bacteria in approximately 80% of patients. Common pathogens are enterogenic *E. coli, Salmonella, Shigella, Campylobacter, Vibrio, Yersinia,* and *Aeromonas* species. Death from diarrhea is rare, but infants, elderly patients, and those in long-term care facilities are at greater risk. The goals of treatment include reducing the infectious period, length of illness, risk of transmission to others, risk of dehydration, and rates of severe illness.

Antimotility and antisecretory agents (bismuth subsalicylate reduces duration of diarrhea compared with placebo, but less effective than loperamide) are likely to be beneficial in the treatments of acute diarrhea in adults.

Empiric treatment of traveler's diarrhea shortened the length of illness, although it was occasionally associated with prolonged presence of the causative pathogen in the stool and the development of resistant strains. Empiric treatment of community-acquired diarrhea with ciprofloxacin shortened the length of illness by 1 to 2 days. Development of resistant strains occurred with the use of some antibiotics but not with others. Adverse effects were similar to those noted for traveler's diarrhea. One must balance the trade-off between the benefits and harms of using empiric antibiotics for mild-to-moderate diarrhea. However in treating traveler's diarrhea in adults, the empiric use of antibiotics is likely to be beneficial.

Additional Reading: Diarrhea in adults (acute). *Am Fam Physician.* 2008;78(4):503–504.

Category: Gastroenterology system

374. A 25-year-old HIV patient presents with pain associated with his gums. He has also noted bleeding of his gums when he brushes his teeth. The most likely severe complication of this condition is
A) Necrotizing ulcerative gingivitis
B) Plaque deposition
C) Dental caries
D) Glossitis
E) Bacterial endocarditis

Answer and Discussion

The answer is A. HIV-infected persons may present with various periodontal diseases, from mild inflammation (HIV gingivitis) to localized acute necrotizing ulcerative gingivitis and from localized periodontitis to necrotizing stomatitis. Patients with HIV gingivitis present with a bright erythematous line along the gingival margin and complain of spontaneous bleeding. In acute necrotizing ulcerative gingivitis, the gingiva appears erythematous, with ulcerations of the papillae that become tender and bleed when teeth are brushed. Rapid bone and soft tissue loss and loosening teeth are characteristic of HIV periodontitis. Patients complain of "deep" pain, and the condition can rapidly progress to large areas of necrotizing stomatitis. Patients affected with HIV gingivitis should be referred to an oral surgeon for debridement, scaling, and curettage of the involved areas. This treatment is followed by administration of metronidazole (Flagyl), irrigation with povidone iodine, and daily mouth rinsing with chlorhexidine gluconate (Peridex). Because it may potentiate peripheral neuropathy, metronidazole should not be given to patients taking didanosine (Videx) or zalcitabine (Hivid). In these patients, clindamycin or amoxicillin may be used.

Additional Reading: Oral manifestations of systemic disease. *Am Fam Physician.* 2010;82(11):1381–1388.

Category: Integumentary

375. Which of the following medications would be most effective to treat postmenopausal flushing?

A) Venlafaxine
B) Amitryptyline
C) Green tea
D) Trazadone
E) Propanolol

Answer and Discussion

The answer is A. The SSRIs including paroxetine and venlafaxine have been used to relieve the symptoms of vasomotor instability (hot flushes) associated with menopause and are considered first-line therapy in women who are not taking estrogen. Their efficacy has been demonstrated in a number of randomized trials.

> **Additional Reading:** Counseling patients about hormone therapy and alternatives for menopausal symptoms. *Am Fam Physician.* 2010;82(7):801–807.

> **Category:** Reproductive system

376. Patients with antithrombin deficiency are at increased risk for

A) Myelodysplasia
B) Thrombosis
C) Multiple myeloma
D) Vitamin K deficiency
E) Bleeding complications while taking warfarin

Answer and Discussion

The answer is B. Antithrombin is a protein that inhibits thrombin and factors Xa, IXa, and XIa. Deficiency of plasma antithrombin is inherited in an autosomal-dominant fashion with a prevalence of approximately 0.2% to 0.4%; approximately one-half of these persons experience venous thrombotic episodes. Acquired deficiencies in antithrombin levels are observed in patients with acute thrombosis, disseminated intravascular coagulation, liver disease, or nephrotic syndrome and during heparin therapy, estrogen therapy (including contraceptive use), or L-asparaginase therapy. Homozygous deficiency is usually lethal to the fetus in utero. Laboratory screening involves quantification of plasma inhibition of thrombin in the presence of heparin. Oral anticoagulation with warfarin is highly effective prophylaxis for patients who have experienced or are at risk of thrombosis.

> **Additional Reading:** Recurrent venous thromboembolism. *Am Fam Physician.* 2011;83(3):293–300.

> **Category:** Cardiovascular system

377. An essential tremor most commonly affects the

A) Head
B) Voice
C) Tongue
D) Legs
E) Hands

Answer and Discussion

The answer is E. Tremor is a symptom of many disorders, including Parkinson's disease, essential tremor, orthostatic tremor, cerebellar disease, peripheral neuropathy, and alcohol withdrawal. Tremors may be classified as postural, rest, or action tremors. Symptomatic treatment is directed to the tremor type:

- *Parkinson's tremor.* The tremor in Parkinson's disease occurs at rest and is characterized by a frequency of 4 to 6 Hz and medium amplitude. It is classically referred to as a *pill-rolling* tremor of the hands, but can also affect the head, trunk, jaw, and lips. Combination therapy with carbidopa and levodopa is commonly used for parkinsonian tremor.
- *Essential tremor.* Essential tremor is the most common movement disorder. Its onset occurs anywhere between the second and sixth decades of life and its prevalence increases with age. The tremor is usually bilateral. The tremor is minimal or absent at rest. The tremor is slowly progressive over a period of years, and the specific pathophysiology of essential tremor remains unknown. Essential tremor occurs sporadically or can be inherited (in 50% of patients, inheritance is autosomal dominant). It most commonly affects the hands, but can also affect the head, voice, tongue, and legs. In many cases, essential tremor is alleviated by small amounts of alcohol, an effect not found in Parkinson's disease. Essential tremor may be amenable to propranolol or primidone.
- *Other tremors.* Propranolol may be useful in treating alcohol withdrawal tremor, and INH may control the cerebellar tremor associated with multiple sclerosis. Clonazepam may relieve orthostatic tremor. Other agents are also available for the treatment of tremor. When medical therapy fails to control the tremor, surgical options such as thalamotomy, pallidotomy, and thalamic stimulation should be considered in severe cases. Thalamic stimulation, the most recent of these surgical approaches, offers the advantage over ablative procedures of alleviating tremor without the creation of a permanent lesion.

> **Additional Reading:** Differentiation and diagnosis of tremor. *Am Fam Physician.* 2011;83(6):697–702.

> **Category:** Neurologic

378. Which of the following statements is true regarding firearm-related injuries?

A) The incidence has risen significantly over the last few years.
B) Most of the nonfatal injuries occurring in adult men ages 15 to 44 years were inflicted by others.
C) The rates for African American and Hispanic individuals have decreased.
D) Law-enforcement practices have not affected the incidence.
E) Increases in the cocaine market have attributed to increases in firearm injuries.

Answer and Discussion

The answer is C. The overall annual rates of nonfatal and fatal firearm-related injuries in the United States declined consistently from 1993 to 1997. The annual nonfatal rate decreased by 40.8%. The annual mortality rate also declined by 21.1%. The declines in the rates of nonfatal and fatal firearm-related injury were generally consistent across all population subgroups. The decreases in the rates of nonfatal and fatal injuries were similar in men and women. Declines in fatality rates in African Americans and Hispanics were similar and were both greater than the decline in non-Hispanic whites. In the rates of nonfatal injury, no consistent pattern was seen in the estimated decline across age groups, but, in the rates of fatal injury, age and percentage change were inversely related. Most of the nonfatal injuries occurred among men 15 to 44 years of age were self-inflicted and were associated with hunting, target shooting, and routine gun handling.

Numerous factors may have contributed to the decline in the rates of nonfatal and fatal assaultive firearm-related injury. These factors include improvements in economic conditions; the aging of the population; the decline in the "crack" cocaine market; changes in legislation, sentencing guidelines, and law-enforcement practices; and improvements associated with violence-prevention programs.

> Additional Reading: Center for Disease Control and Prevention: Firearms. From: http://www.cdc.gov/search.do?action=search&subset=mmwr&queryText=firearms.

Category: Patient/population-based care

379. The HIPAA has recently been updated and calls for
A) Mandatory health insurance for all people who earn less than $12,000 per year
B) Stringent codes for the uniform transfer of medically related data
C) Health maintenance organizations to allow more diagnostic testing of patients and less scrutiny of physicians
D) All Americans to invest in a medical savings account
E) Improved access of third parties to patients' medical records

Answer and Discussion

The answer is B. The HIPAA, also known as the *Kassenbaum–Kennedy legislation*, was signed into law in 1996 and includes the "portability" aspect of the law (which protects the ability of people with current or preexisting medical conditions to get health insurance) and the "accountability" aspects of the law (which include enforcement). Its multiple provisions include strict codes for the uniform transfer of electronic data, including billing and other routine exchanges, and new patient rights regarding personal health information, including the right to access this information and to limit its disclosure. Also outlined are specific physical, procedural, and technological security protections all health care organizations must take to ensure the confidentiality of patients' medical information. The purpose of HIPAA is to improve the portability of health insurance coverage in the group and individual markets, focus on health care fraud and abuse, promote the use of medical savings accounts, improve access to long-term care services and coverage, and simplify the administration of health insurance. Every medical practice in the United States must comply with these regulations, including transaction standards (i.e., the rules standardizing electronic data exchange of health-related information).

> Additional Reading: HIPAA again: confronting the updated privacy and security rules. *Fam Pract Manag.* 2013;20(3):18–22.

Category: Patient/population-based care

> The purpose of HIPAA is to improve the portability of health insurance coverage in the group and individual markets, focus on health care fraud and abuse, promote the use of medical savings accounts, improve access to long-term care services and coverage, and simplify the administration of health insurance.

---

380. The drug of choice for the treatment of chronic opioid dependence is
A) Naloxone
B) Bupropion
C) Disulfiram
D) Methadone
E) Diazepam

Answer and Discussion

The answer is D. Opioid dependence is a chronic, often relapsing, disorder that can be very challenging to treat. Between 500,000 and 1,000,000 Americans are believed to be opioid dependent at any point in time. Opioid-related disorders are more prevalent in men than in women by a ratio of up to 4:1. Opioid dependency is often linked to a history of drug-related criminal activity, antisocial personality disorder, and coexisting mood disorders, especially depression. Methadone and buprenorphine seem equally effective at stabilizing opioid use. Methadone has the longest track record and is effective in reducing illicit narcotic use, retaining patients in treatment, and decreasing illegal drug use. Ongoing methadone maintenance decreases the risk of contracting and transmitting HIV, HBV, and HCV and is considered a cost-effective intervention. Long-term maintenance is more successful in averting relapse than shorter-term treatment. The goals of early treatment are to decrease withdrawal symptoms, diminish opioid craving, and arrive at a tolerance threshold, while preventing euphoria and sedation from overmedication. Detoxification is indicated when a patient demonstrates consistent, long-term abstinence and possesses adequate supportive resources (e.g., productive use of time, a stable home life). Patient acceptance of community resources for opiate addicts such as Narcotics Anonymous is a good prognostic sign. Narcotics Anonymous is also a useful tool in relapse prevention.

> Additional Reading: Opioid dependence. *Am Fam Physician.* 2012;86(6):565–566.

Category: Psychogenic

381. The use of antiobesity medication is acceptable when the BMI is
A) >10 kg per m^2
B) >20 kg per m^2
C) >30 kg per m^2
D) Greater than the normal weight of the individual
E) More than the calculated fat percentage of the patient

Answer and Discussion

The answer is C. Obesity is epidemic in the United States and other industrialized nations. Obesity is defined as a BMI (= weight in kg divided by height in m^2) of 30 kg per m^2 or more. There are three classes of severity:

- Class I (BMI of 30.0 to 34.9 kg per m^2)
- Class II (BMI of 35.0 to 39.9 kg per m^2)
- Class III (BMI of 40.0 kg per m^2 or higher).

The age-adjusted prevalence rates of classes I, II, and III obesity in American adults are estimated to be 14.4%, 5.2%, and 2.9%, respectively. These estimates represent a substantial increase in the prevalence of all three obesity classes since the mid-1990s. Although behavior modification strategies are helpful for most obese patients, they do not guarantee long-term weight-loss maintenance. Without ongoing management, most or all of the weight patients lose can be regained within 3 to 5 years. This limitation contributes to the active development of pharmacologic approaches to obesity. Current guidelines consider pharmacotherapy to be an adjunct to lifestyle modification programs and are targeted toward at-risk patients (patients with a BMI of 30 or greater or a BMI of 27 or greater combined with medical comorbidities such as hypertension or insulin resistance).

- *Noradrenergic drugs.* One class of weight-loss medications is the noradrenergic drugs that affect weight loss by suppressing one's appetite. Some noradrenergic agents include phentermine resin

(Ionamin), mazindol (Sanorex), phenylpropanolamine (Dexatrim, recently removed from the market), phendimetrazine (Plegine), and diethylpropion (Tenuate). When combined with dietary programs, these drugs produced modest short-term net weight losses compared with dietary changes and placebo. The FDA has not labeled any of these drugs for long-term treatment of obesity.

- *Orlistat.* Orlistat (Xenical) is an intestinal lipase inhibitor that has been approved by the FDA for long-term use. After 12 weeks of treatment with orlistat (360 mg per day), patients showed weight losses of up to 5 kg (11 lb), compared with 2- to 3-kg losses (4.4 to 6.6 lb) among patients in the placebo group. Weight losses appear to be dosage dependent, with lower dosages producing smaller weight losses. Flatus, oily stools, and diarrhea are common but usually resolve during the second year of treatment. Vitamin deficiencies can occur with its use, and a vitamin supplement is recommended.

- *Sibutramine.* Sibutramine (Meridia), which has been approved by the FDA for long-term treatment of obesity, is a centrally acting, specific reuptake inhibitor of norepinephrine and serotonin, thus having satiating and potential thermogenic effects. Several clinical studies of 12 to 52 weeks' duration showed weight losses of 4.7 to 7.6 kg (10.3 to 16.7 lb) in patients receiving sibutramine. Weight losses were dosage dependent and tended to plateau by the 24th week. Efficacy of sibutramine at 1 year has also been established. Patients taking 5-, 10-, and 15-mg daily dosages experienced dosage-related weight loss for up to 12 weeks, and all dosages were well tolerated. Common adverse effects are headache, dry mouth, insomnia, and constipation. The most common serious side effect is hypertension. Sibutramine should not be used with SSRIs and in patients with cardiovascular disorders, particularly poorly controlled hypertension.

Because of the inherent difficulties in treating obesity, physicians should attempt to develop continuous care programs emphasizing lifestyle modifications such as enduring changes in dietary and activity habits. Patients using behavior modification strategies to make these changes are more likely to succeed in long-term weight maintenance. Weight loss related to drug treatment is modest (5% to 10%) and occurs in the first 6 months. Medication appears to be more effective at maintaining weight loss.

Additional Reading: Two new drugs for weight loss. *Med Lett Drugs Ther.* 2012;54(1398):69–71.

Category: Endocrine system

382. Which of the following statements regarding onychomycosis is true?
A) The infection is caused by *Trichophyton rubrum*.
B) Fungi are responsible for 90% of nail dystrophies.
C) Ciclopirox (Penlac) is very effective for the treatment of onychomycosis.
D) Griseofulvin and ketoconazole are first-line medications for the treatment of onychomycosis.
E) Periodic testing of renal function is indicated with the use of antifungal medication.

Answer and Discussion

The answer is A. Onychomycosis (tinea unguium) is a fungal infection of the nail bed, matrix, or plate. Toenails are affected more often than fingernails. The infection is usually caused by *T. rubrum*, which invades the nail bed and the underside of the nail plate

beginning at the hyponychium and then migrating proximally through the underlying nail matrix. Because fungi are responsible for only approximately one-half of nail dystrophies, the diagnosis of onychomycosis may need to be confirmed by potassium hydroxide preparation, culture, or histology. Psoriasis, lichen planus, contact dermatitis, trauma, nail-bed tumor, and yellow nail syndrome may be mistakenly diagnosed as onychomycosis. The FDA has approved ciclopirox nail lacquer for the treatment of mild-to-moderate onychomycosis caused by *T. rubrum* without involvement of the lunula. Although safe and relatively inexpensive, ciclopirox therapy is seldom effective. Triazole and allylamine antifungal drugs have largely replaced griseofulvin and ketoconazole as first-line medications in the treatment of onychomycosis. These agents offer shorter treatment courses, higher cure rates, and fewer relapses. Of the drugs available, terbinafine (Lamisil) and itraconazole (Sporanox) are considered first line and fluconazole (Diflucan) is an alternative for those who cannot tolerate the first-line agents. Liver enzyme monitoring is recommended before continuous medication therapy is initiated and every 4 to 6 weeks during treatment. Onychomycosis is expensive to treat. Costs include medications, procedures, laboratory tests, and health care providers' time, as well as expenses associated with the management of adverse drug effects and treatment failures.

Additional Reading: Antifungal drugs. *Treat Guidel Med Lett.* 2012;10(120):61.

Category: Integumentary

383. A 31-year-old man who enjoys scuba diving presents to your office after a dive complaining of severe back pain, loss of sensation around the trunk, and numbness of the legs. Appropriate management consists of
A) Administration of acetazolamide
B) Furosemide (Lasix) and fluid restriction
C) NSAIDs and narcotic pain medication
D) Intravenous steroids
E) Transfer to a facility with a recompression chamber

Answer and Discussion

The answer is E. Recreational scuba diving, which is defined as pleasure diving without mandatory decompression to a maximum depth of 130 ft, has become a popular activity since the mid-1980s. Although divers are concentrated along coastal regions, many others dive in inland lakes, streams, quarries, and reservoirs, or fly to distant dive sites. Physicians practicing almost anywhere in the United States may see a patient with a dive-related injury or complaint. Injuries related to diving are usually mild and include ear-related complaints. Barotrauma to the middle or inner ear can occur during the descent or ascent phases of the dive and may cause vertigo and other neurologic symptoms. Middle-ear barotrauma of descent is the most common type of diving injury and may involve hemorrhage and rupture of the tympanic membrane. Symptoms include the acute onset of pain, vertigo, and conductive hearing loss. In severe cases (usually during ascent), increased pressure in the middle ear can cause reversible weakness of the facial nerve and Bell's palsy (facial baroparesis). The most severe illness related to diving is decompression illness (the "bends"). Neurologic decompression sickness can present with a wide spectrum of symptoms. A prodrome of malaise, fatigue, anorexia, and headache is common. The most severe presentation is partial myelopathy referable to the thoracic spinal cord. Patients complain of paresthesias and sensory loss in the trunk and extremities, a tingling or constricting sensation around the thorax, ascending leg weakness ranging from mild to severe pain in the lower back or pelvis, and loss of bowel and/or bladder control. The neurologic examination often reveals monoparesis or paraparesis, a sensory level, and sphincter disturbances. However, neurologic examination may also be normal. The diagnosis of neurologic decompression sickness is clinical and should be suspected in any patient with a recent history of diving who has a consistent presentation. Flying shortly after a dive can precipitate symptoms. The initial management of neurologic decompression sickness requires transport to a recompression facility. The majority of recreational divers with neurologic decompression sickness have an excellent recovery after prompt recompression therapy.

> **Additional Reading:** Decompression sickness. In: Domino F, ed. *The 5-Minute Clinical Consult*. Philadelphia, PA: Lippincott Williams and Wilkins; 2014.

Category: Nonspecific system

384. A 41-year-old woman presents with complaining of recurring headaches. They are typically unilateral, have a pulsatile quality, and are associated with nausea, and occasionally she experiences photophobia as well. The patient describes the headaches as intense, usually requiring her to limit her activities and can last for 1 to 2 days. She has tried several over-the-counter migraine medications that help a little, but asks you to prescribe something "stronger." Which one of the following would be the best choice for you to prescribe as first-line abortive therapy?
A) Acetaminophen
B) Acetaminophen/oxycodone (Percocet)
C) Butalbital/aspirin/caffeine (Fiorinal)
D) Prednisone
E) Sumatriptan (Imitrex)

Answer and Discussion

The answer is E. Several different medications are recommended as first-line abortive therapies to treat acute migraine. But there are only a few trials directly comparing different medication classes and no definitive algorithms as to which class works best. NSAIDs and acetaminophen/aspirin/caffeine compounds are recommended as first-line therapies and can be obtained over the counter. Triptans are effective and safe for treatment of acute migraine and are recommended as first-line therapy but require a prescription. Opiates and barbiturates are not recommended because of their potential for abuse. Acetaminophen and oral corticosteroids alone are not effective.

> **Additional Reading:** Drugs for migraine. *Treat Guidel Med Lett.* 2011;9(102):7–12.

Category: Neurologic

385. Which of the following should be used in the management of those taking chronic opioids for non–cancer-related pain?
A) Urine drug screens
B) Random pill counts
C) State-sponsored physician prescribing records
D) Opioid contracts
E) All of the above

Answer and Discussion

The answer is E. The management of those taking chronic narcotics can be challenging. The physician should explain the process of monitoring those taking chronic opioids for non–cancer-related pain and should have the patient sign an opioid contract that outlines the process. Various methods should be used in the monitoring process on the basis of the level of risk associated with abuse. Methods include urine drug screens, random pill counts, and state-sponsored physician prescribing records that are available in some states.

> **Additional Reading:** Opioid treatment guidelines: clinical guidelines for the use of chronic opioid therapy in chronic noncancer pain. *J Pain.* 2009;10(2):113–130.

Category: Psychogenic

386. All the following about DM II medications is correct except
A) Sulfonuylurea increase insulin secretion by closing potassium channels on the surface of pancreatic β cells.
B) Metformin decreases hepatic glucose output and, to a lesser extent, sensitizes peripheral tissue.
C) Thiazolidinediones will cause hypoglycemia when used as monotherapy.
D) α-Glucosidase inhibitors act at the brush border in the small intestine, inactivating the enzyme that breaks down complex carbohydrates, slowing absorption, and flattening the postprandial glycemic curve.

Answer and Discussion

The answer is C. Sulfonuylurea insulin secretagogues (e.g., glipizide [Glucotrol], glimepiride [Amaryl]) and nonsulfonylurea insulin secretagogues (e.g., nateglinide [Starlix]) increase insulin secretion by closing potassium channels on the surface of pancreatic β cells. Hypoglycemia can occur with any insulin secretagogue. While sulfonylureas can cause weight gain, this effect is less common with nonsulfonylurea secretagogues. A recent review concluded that CVD events were unchanged with the use of sulfonylureas, but there was insufficient evidence to make any conclusions about the effects of nonsulfonylurea secretagogues on cardiovascular outcomes.

Biguanides (metformin) decrease hepatic glucose output and, to a lesser extent, sensitizes peripheral tissues to insulin. A review found no increase in fatal or nonfatal lactic acidosis with metformin use. However, current guidelines recommend that metformin should not be used in patients with chronic or acute renal insufficiency and should be discontinued when creatinine levels reach 1.4 mg per dL (120 μmol per L) in women or 1.5 mg per dL (130 μmol per L) in men. Metformin has been shown to decrease progression from impaired glucose tolerance to type 2 diabetes, and it is the only hypoglycemic agent shown to reduce mortality rates in patients with type 2 diabetes.

Thiazolidinediones (rosiglitazone [Avandia], pioglitazone [Actos]) increase insulin sensitivity in peripheral tissues and also decrease glucose production by the liver. These agents are not associated with hypoglycemia when used as monotherapy. However, a review concluded that rosiglitazone (Avandia) was associated with an increased risk of MI and death from cardiovascular causes, although another review concluded that although the risk of MI and heart failure are significantly increased, overall cardiovascular mortality rates were unaffected. In a meta-analysis, pioglitazone (Actos) was associated with a reduction in deaths, MI, and stroke. The incidence of serious heart failure was increased by 40%, but there was no change in CVD mortality rates.

α-Glucosidase inhibitors (acarbose [Precose]) act in the small intestine, inactivating the enzyme that breaks down complex carbohydrates, slowing absorption, and flattening the postprandial glycemic curve.

> **Additional Reading:** Management of blood glucose in type 2 diabetes mellitus. *Am Fam Physician.* 2009;79(1):29–36.

Category: Endocrine system

387. Clinical findings associated with Cushing disease include all of the following, except
A) Weight gain
B) Menstrual irregularity
C) Depression/emotional lability
D) Excessive thirst
E) Glucose intolerance

Answer and Discussion

The correct answer is D. Cushing disease is defined as glucocorticoid excess due to excessive ACTH secretion from a pituitary tumor, the most common cause of primary Cushing syndrome. Cushing syndrome is defined as excessive corticosteroid exposure from exogenous sources (medications) or endogenous sources (pituitary, adrenal, pulmonary, etc. or tumor). Exogenous intake of steroids is the primary cause of secondary Cushing syndrome.

In addition to the above common signs, physical findings include the following:

- Obesity (usually central)
- Facial plethora
- Moon face (facial adiposity)
- Thin skin
- Hypertension
- Hirsutism
- Proximal muscle weakness
- Purple striae on the skin
- Acne
- Easy bruisability

Additional Reading: Cushing disease and Cushing syndrome. In: Domino F, ed. *The 5-Minute Clinical Consult*. Philadelphia, PA: Lippincott Williams and Wilkins; 2014.

Category: Endocrine system

QUESTIONS

Each of the following questions or incomplete statements is followed by suggested answers or completions. Select the ONE BEST ANSWER in each case.

1. A 14-year-old boy presents to your office with a mildly pruritic rash that involves his chest and back. He reports it began with a single lesion on his back, but now has spread to involve his entire back and chest. You note on your examination the presence of multiple secondary lesions that appear to follow cleavage lines. The most likely diagnosis is
A) Herpes zoster
B) Pityriasis rosea
C) Tinea versicolor
D) Varicella
E) Rhus dermatitis

Answer and Discussion

The answer is B. Pityriasis rosea typically occurs in children and young adults. It is characterized by an initial herald patch, followed by the development of a diffuse papulosquamous rash. Pityriasis rosea is easier to identify when the general eruption appears with smaller secondary lesions that follow Langer's lines (cleavage lines) in a "Christmas treelike pattern." Many diseases can mimic pityriasis rosea including drug exanthems, but the most worrisome condition to be ruled out is secondary syphilis. Topical or systemic steroids and antihistamines are often used to relieve itching. Asymptomatic lesions do not require treatment.

> Additional Reading: Pityriasis rosea. *Nelson Textbook of Pediatrics,* 19th ed. Philadelphia, PA: Elsevier/Saunders; 2011.

> Category: Integumentary

Pityriasis rosea is characterized by an initial herald patch, followed by the development of a diffuse papulosquamous rash.

---

2. What is the most common cause of nephritic syndrome in a 4-year-old?
A) Trauma
B) Recent strep infection
C) Dehydration
D) Nonsteroidal anti-inflammatory drugs (NSAIDs)
E) *Varicella* infection

Answer and Discussion

The answer is B. Poststreptococcal glomerulonephritis is the leading cause of acute nephritic syndrome. The condition is most frequently encountered in children between 2 and 6 years of age with a recent history of pharyngitis. It is rare in children younger than 2 and adults older than 40. The incidence of poststreptococcal glomerulonephritis appears to be decreasing. The condition typically develops approximately 10 days after pharyngitis or 2 weeks after a skin infection with a nephritogenic strain of group A hemolytic *Streptococcus.* It has not been determined whether antibiotic treatment of the primary skin infection affords protection from the development of poststreptococcal glomerulonephritis. The classic presentation of poststreptococcal glomerulonephritis is a nephritic syndrome with oliguric acute renal failure. Most patients have milder disease, and subclinical cases are common. Patients with severe disease experience gross hematuria characterized by red or smoky urine, headache, and generalized symptoms such as anorexia, nausea, vomiting, and malaise. Inflammation of the renal capsule can lead to flank or back pain. Physical examination may show hypervolemia, edema, or hypertension. Acute poststreptococcal glomerulonephritis is usually diagnosed on clinical and serologic grounds without the need for biopsy, especially in children with a typical history. The overall prognosis in classic poststreptococcal acute proliferative glomerulonephritis is good. Most patients recover spontaneously and return to baseline renal function within 3 to 4 weeks with no long-term complications.

> Additional Reading: Evaluation of poststreptococcal illness. *Am Fam Physician.* 2005;71:1949–1954.

> Category: Nephrologic system

3. At what age do children normally articulate most words and know basic colors?
A) 3 years
B) 4 years
C) 5 years
D) 6 years
E) 7 years

Answer and Discussion

The answer is B. Motor development during the preschool years results in children running, jumping, and climbing. Children learn to balance on one foot and hop. Vocabulary continues to develop rapidly with the mastery of hundreds of words. Language development proceeds with multiword sentences, the use of pronouns, and the gradual improvement in articulation skills. Children normally master the concept of numbers 1, 2, and 3 by 3.5 years. Four-year-old children should know basic colors and clearly articulate most words.

> **Additional Reading:** Screening for developmental delay. *Am Fam Physician.* 2011;84(5):544–549.

> **Category:** Psychogenic

4. At what age is it necessary to perform orchiopexy in a child affected with cryptorchism?
A) 12–24 months
B) 36–48 months
C) 5 years
D) 7 years
E) Orchiopexy is not necessary.

Answer and Discussion

The answer is A. Either one or both testes may be absent from the scrotum at birth in about one in five premature or low-birth-weight male infants and in 3% to 6% at full-term infants. Cryptorchism is found in 1% to 2% of male children after 1 year of age but can be confused with retractile testes that is associated with a strong cremasteric reflex, which requires no treatment. Cryptorchism should be corrected before age 12 to 24 months in an attempt to reduce the risk of infertility, which occurs in up to 75% of male children with bilateral cryptorchism and in 50% of male children with unilateral cryptorchism. It is not clear, however, whether such early orchiopexy improves ultimate fertility. Some patients have underlying hypogonadism. Cryptorchism is also associated with testicular carcinoma mainly in the undescended testicle and particularly with intra-abdominal malposition; however, up to 10% of cancers can occur on the unaffected side.

> **Additional Reading:** Undescended testis (cryptorchidism). *Nelson Textbook of Pediatrics,* 19th ed. Philadelphia, PA: Elsevier/Saunders; 2011.

> **Category:** Reproductive system

5. A 5-year-old presents to your office complaining of scrotal pain and you note swelling of the left testis. Appropriate management at this time includes
A) Continued observation
B) Elevation of the scrotum and ice therapy
C) Ultrasound evaluation with Doppler color flow
D) Doppler stethoscope evaluation
E) Computed tomography (CT) scan of the pelvis

Answer and Discussion

The answer is C. Testicular torsion should be suspected in patients who complain of acute scrotal pain and swelling. Testicular viability is in jeopardy with delay in diagnosis, ultimately impacting the patient fertility. Associated conditions that may resemble testicular torsion not warranting surgery are torsion of a testicular appendage, epididymitis/orchitis, trauma, incarcerated hernia, varicocele, and idiopathic scrotal edema. Testicular torsion is most common in men younger than 25 years old, although it can occur in men of any age. A prepubertal or young male adult with acute scrotal pain should be diagnosed as testicular torsion until proven otherwise. Physical exam finding of higher testicular lie and absent cremasteric reflex are supportive evidence for this condition. Scrotal imaging with Doppler color flow ultrasound is necessary when the diagnosis remains unclear. Once the correct diagnosis is established, prompt surgical evaluation should be performed. It is reasonable to perform manual detorsion for immediate noninvasive treatment followed by elective orchiopexy.

> **Additional Reading:** Testicular torsion. *Am Fam Physician.* 2006;74(10):1739–1743.

> **Category:** Reproductive system

6. Which of the following statements is true regarding head lice infestations?
A) African Americans are less likely affected.
B) Retreatment with pyrethrin is rarely needed.
C) Head lice can live off the body up to 1 week.
D) Dogs are common vectors for head lice.
E) Hallmark of pediculosis are erythematous patches and plaques.

Answer and Discussion

The answer is A. Pediculosis capitis or head lice is an infestation of lice in the scalp hair as it feeds on human blood. Modes of transmission are through fomites and head-to-head contact. For some unknown reason, head lice rarely affects African Americans. Head lice can live off the body up to 1 month. The hallmark of all types of pediculosis is pruritus.

There is known resistance of head lice to pyrethroids. Malathion 0.5% in isopropanol is the treatment of choice for head lice. This medication is applied to dry hair and scalp until wet and washed 12 hours after initial application. A reapplication 7 to 9 days after initial treatment may be necessary. Household members should be treated at the same time. Fine-toothed combs are used after application of a damp towel to the scalp for 30 minutes. Washing or dry-cleaning clothing and bed linens is advised. Brushes and combs used should be disposed of by coating with a pediculicide for 15 minutes followed by rinsing in boiling water. Children are cleared to go back to school after the initial treatment. Spinosad (Natroba) is safe and effective for the treatment of head lice for ages 4 years and above; nit combing following treatment is not necessary.

> **Additional Reading:** Pediculosis. *Nelson Textbook of Pediatrics,* 19th ed. Philadelphia, PA: Elsevier/Saunders; 2011; and Spinosad (Natroba) for head lice. *Am Fam Physician.* 2013;87(12): 874–876.

> **Category:** Integumentary

7. A 4-year-old presents with short stature. Further evaluation confirms a delayed bone age. The most likely diagnosis is
A) Hormonal disorder
B) Cartilage defects
C) Growth plate disorder
D) Genetic influence of the parents

Answer and Discussion

The answer is A. Short stature may affect children as a result of intrinsic growth defects or because of acquired extrinsic factors that impair growth. In general, delayed bone age in a child with short stature is suggestive of an endocrinologic or systemic disorder, constitutional delay, and undernutrition. Normal bone age in a short child is more likely to be caused by familial short stature.

> Additional Reading: Analysis of growth patterns. *Nelson Textbook of Pediatrics,* 19th ed. Philadelphia, PA: Elsevier/Saunders; 2011.

> Category: Endocrine system

8. An 8-year-old is seen in the emergency room secondary to abdominal pain. Further evaluation confirms the presence of intussusception. The most likely precipitating cause is
A) Colon polyp
B) Meckel's diverticulum
C) Lymphoma
D) Parasite infection
E) Foreign body

Answer and Discussion

The answer is C. In children older than 6 years, lymphoma is the most common cause. Intussusception is the most common cause of intestinal obstruction in the first 2 years of life. It is more common in boys than in girls. In most cases (85%), the cause is not apparent. Associated conditions that can result in intussusception include polyps, Meckel's diverticulum, Henoch–Schonlein purpura, lymphoma, lipoma, parasites, foreign bodies, and viral enteritis with hypertrophy of Peyer patches. Intussusception of the small intestine occurs in patients with celiac disease and cystic fibrosis related to the bulk of stool in the terminal ileum. Henoch–Schonlein purpura may also cause isolated small-bowel intussusception. Intermittent small-bowel intussusception is a rare cause of recurrent abdominal pain.

> Additional Reading: Gastrointestinal emergencies. *The Harriet Lane Handbook: A Manual for Pediatric House Officers,* 19th ed. Philadelphia, PA: Elsevier/Mosby; 2012.

> Category: Gastroenterology system

9. The initial treatment of choice for symptomatic labial adhesions is
A) Testosterone cream
B) Estrogen cream
C) GnRH antagonist
D) Hydrocortisone cream
E) Surgical separation

Answer and Discussion

The answer is B. Labial adhesions are common in prepubertal girls. The cause is thought related to low levels of circulating estrogen. Most women with small areas of labial adhesions are asymptomatic. However, interference with urination or accumulation of urine behind the adhesion can lead to discomfort and symptoms. Dysuria and recurrent vulvar and vaginal infections are associated symptoms. In rare situations, urinary retention may occur. Asymptomatic labial fusion usually does not require treatment. Symptomatic adhesions may be treated with a short course of estrogen cream applied twice daily for 7 to 10 days; this may separate the labia. A new alternative treatment is to use estrogen transdermal patches in close proximity to the labia. When medical treatment fails or if severe urinary symptoms exist, surgical separation of the labia is indicated. This can be done as an office procedure using 1% to 2% topical xylocaine gel.

Because of inadequate levels of estrogen, recurrences of labial adhesion are common until puberty. Following puberty, the condition usually resolves spontaneously. Improved hygiene and removal of vulvar irritants may help prevent recurrences.

> Additional Reading: Labial adhesions. *Textbook of Family Medicine,* 8th ed. Philadelphia, PA: Saunders/Elsevier; 2011.

> Category: Reproductive system

10. Which of the following statements is true regarding iron deficiency in childhood?
A) Iron deficiency commonly occurs in term infants during the first 3 months.
B) Ingestion of cow's milk can result in iron overload.
C) Iron deficiency rarely leads to complications.
D) Pica is associated with iron deficiency.
E) Mild iron deficiency typically leads to symptoms of pallor, fatigue, and delayed motor development.

Answer and Discussion

The answer is D. The incidence of iron deficiency in children has decreased substantially due to improved nutrition and the increased availability of iron-fortified infant formulas and cereals. Normal-term infants are born with sufficient iron stores to prevent iron deficiency for the first 4 to 5 months of life. Thereafter, sufficient iron needs to be absorbed to maintain the needs of rapid growth. For this reason, nutritional iron deficiency is most common between 6 and 24 months of life. A deficiency earlier than age 6 months may occur if iron stores at birth are reduced by prematurity, small birth weight, neonatal anemia, or perinatal blood loss or if there is subsequent iron loss due to hemorrhage. Iron-deficient children older than 24 months should be evaluated for blood loss. Iron deficiency, in addition to causing anemia, has adverse effects on multiple organ systems. Symptoms and signs vary with the severity of the deficiency. Mild iron deficiency is usually asymptomatic. In infants with more severe iron deficiency, pallor, fatigue, irritability, and delayed motor development are common. Children whose iron deficiency is due in part to ingestion of unfortified cow's milk may be fat and flabby, with poor muscle tone. A history of pica is common.

> Additional Reading: Anemia. *The Harriet Lane Handbook: A Manual for Pediatric House Officers,* 19th ed. Philadelphia, PA: Elsevier/Mosby; 2012.

> Category: Hematologic system

A history of pica is common in iron-deficiency anemia.

11. In treating acute sinusitis in children, which of the following sinuses is unlikely to be infected in a 6-year-old?
A) Frontal
B) Maxillary
C) Ethmoidal
D) Sphenoidal

Answer and Discussion

The answer is A. Acute bacterial infection of the sinuses that lasts <30 days and completely resolves is called acute bacterial sinusitis. The maxillary and ethmoidal sinuses most commonly involved when mucociliary function and drainage are impaired by an upper respiratory infection (URI) or allergic rhinitis. Both the ethmoid and maxillary sinuses are present at birth, forming in the third to fourth gestational month. The sphenoid sinuses pneumatize as an extension of a posterior ethmoid cell by age 5 years, and the frontal sinuses form from an anterior ethmoid cell appearing at about age 7 to 8 years. Frontal sinusitis is unusual before age 10 years.

Additional Reading: Sinusitis. *Nelson Textbook of Pediatrics,* 19th ed. Philadelphia, PA: Elsevier/Saunders; 2011.

Category: Respiratory system

12. Which of the following statements regarding attention-deficit/hyperactivity disorder (ADHD) is true?
A) Specific biologic markers are used in the diagnosis.
B) The Conner's ADHD Index is a checklist that helps identify children affected with ADHD.
C) Stimulant medications rarely benefit children with ADHD.
D) Symptoms of ADHD typically progress over time.
E) Drug therapy combined with psychosocial therapy is universally better than medication alone.

Answer and Discussion

The answer is B. ADHD is manifest by inappropriate-for-age hyperactivity, impulsivity, and lack of attention. ADHD cannot be easily diagnosed by a specific test or biologic marker, and some are unclear if the disorder is a truly pathologic condition or just one end of the behavioral spectrum. ADHD is more frequently diagnosed in children with behavioral difficulties and academic underachievement. The prevalence of ADHD is between 6.8% and 10.3%, with boys affected threefold more often than girls. Associated psychiatric conditions, including oppositional–defiant disorder, conduct disorder, depressive disorder, and anxiety disorders, are common. The Conners' ADHD Index and symptom scales from the *Diagnostic and Statistical Manual of Mental Disorders*, 4th ed. (DSM-IV) are ADHD-specific checklists and have a high sensitivity for identification of children with the disorder. Reviews of the pharmacologic management of ADHD with methylphenidate hydrochloride (Ritalin, Concerta), dextroamphetamine sulfate (Adderall, Dexedrine), and pemoline (Cylert) show these drugs to be generally effective for most children affected. Nonpharmacologic treatments that may have some beneficial effect on behavior and academic performance are behavioral modification and intensive contingency-management therapy. Combining drug therapy with psychosocial therapy shows no clear advantage when compared with drug therapy alone. However, the addition of behavioral therapies to medication may have some benefit, including reduction of anxiety and improvement in social skills. The symptoms of ADHD tend to decrease over the long term, but may continue into adolescence and adulthood. The most common treatment is stimulant medication.

Additional Reading: Current strategies in the diagnosis and treatment of childhood attention-deficit/hyperactivity disorder. *Am Fam Physician.* 2009;79(8):657–665.

Category: Psychogenic

13. A 12-year-old obese boy presents to your office complaining of bilateral leg pain that occurs only at night. His mother denies any pain during the day and reports he has not had a limp. The most likely diagnosis is
A) Slipped capital femoral epiphysis
B) Legg–Calve–Perthes disease
C) Osgood–Schlatter's disease
D) Patellofemoral syndrome
E) "Growing pains"

Answer and Discussion

The answer is E. A diagnosis of "growing pains" must meet three criteria: (1) the leg pain is bilateral; (2) the pain occurs only at night; and (3) the patient has no limp, pain, or symptoms during the day. To inaccurately diagnose a limping child with growing pains can be dangerous, as the physician risks missing the underlying pathology. However, if a child does fit the criteria for growing pains, the parents should be reassured that this is a benign, self-limited process that occurs for unknown reasons.

Additional Reading: Growing pains. *Nelson Textbook of Pediatrics,* 19th ed. Philadelphia, PA: Elsevier/Saunders; 2011.

Category: Musculoskeletal system

14. The gold standard for diagnosing peritonsillar abscess is
A) Lateral plain films
B) Ultrasound
C) CT scan
D) MRI evaluation
E) Needle aspiration

Answer and Discussion

The answer is E. Peritonsillar abscess is most common in persons 20 to 40 years of age. Young children are seldom affected unless they are immunocompromised, but the infection can cause significant airway obstruction in children. The infection affects men and women equally. Chronic tonsillitis or multiple trials of oral antibiotics for acute tonsillitis may predispose persons to the development of a peritonsillar abscess. The presenting symptoms include fever, throat pain, and trismus. Ultrasonography and CT scanning are useful in confirming a diagnosis. Needle aspiration remains the gold standard for diagnosis and treatment of peritonsillar abscess. After performing aspiration, appropriate antibiotic therapy (including penicillin, clindamycin, cephalosporins, or metronidazole) must be initiated. In advanced cases, incision and drainage or immediate tonsillectomy may be required. *Streptococcus pyogenes* (group A β-hemolytic *Streptococcus*) is the most common aerobic organism associated with peritonsillar abscess. The most common anaerobic organism is *Fusobacterium.* For most abscesses, a mixed group of both aerobic and anaerobic organisms cause the infection.

Additional Reading: Peritonsillar abscess. *Am Fam Physician.* 2008;77(2):199–202.

Category: Respiratory system

15. A 12-year-old boy is brought in to your office by his mother and father. The child has been experiencing swelling of his joints, fevers, and a rash. An examination reveals hepatosplenomegaly and lymphadenopathy. Laboratory evaluation shows anemia, leukocytosis, and thrombocytosis. You suspect juvenile rheumatoid arthritis (JRA). Which of the following medications would be first-line treatment?
A) Acetaminophen
B) Ibuprofen
C) Codeine
D) Methotrexate
E) Prednisone

Answer and Discussion

The answer is B. JRA, formerly known as Still's disease, is a diverse group of diseases that is clinically distinct from adult rheumatoid arthritis. Most children with JRA have long remissions without loss of function or significant residual deformity. There are no specific laboratory tests to diagnose JRA. One must exclude other causes for arthritis, including reactive arthritis from extra-articular infection, septic arthritis, neoplastic disorders, endocrine disorders (e.g., thyroid disease, type 1 diabetes mellitus), degenerative or mechanical disorders, or idiopathic pediatric joint pain. Diagnosis of JRA requires signs of inflammation rather than simply arthralgias persisting for more than 6 weeks, with onset before age 16 years. JRA has three major subtypes: pauciarticular (40% to 50%), polyarticular (25% to 40%), and systemic (10% to 20%). Each type has different clinical presentations and courses, and treatment is determined by differentiating among the various types. Pauciarticular JRA involves four or fewer joints, usually large joints asymmetrically. Early-onset pauciarticular JRA affects mostly girls younger than 4 years and has a 30% risk of chronic iridocyclitis and a 10% risk of ocular damage. Late-onset pauciarticular JRA affects mostly boys older than 8 years; many of whom later develop spondyloarthropathies; 10% develop iridocyclitis. Slit-lamp ophthalmic examinations are recommended. Polyarticular JRA is defined as arthritis in five or more joints; patients are either RF positive or RF negative. RF-positive patients usually are girls aged 8 years or older, have symmetric small-joint arthritis, and have a worse prognosis than do RF-negative patients. Systemic-onset JRA is characterized by high intermittent fevers (>102°F), rash, hepatosplenomegaly, lymphadenopathy, arthralgias, pericarditis, pleuritis, and growth delay. Anemia, leukocytosis, and thrombocytosis are common laboratory findings. Extra-articular symptoms are usually mild and self-limited. Boys and girls are equally affected. NSAIDs are the first-line treatment for JRA. Clinical improvement may not be seen for up to 1 month. Methotrexate is often used with NSAIDs, particularly for systemic and polyarticular JRA. Corticosteroids are used orally for severe, life-threatening, systemic JRA and intra-articularly for pauciarticular JRA. Most children with JRA require a great deal of physical as well as psychological support. Physical and occupational therapy is important because children often stop using painful joints, adding to disability.

Additional Reading: Rakel R. Juvenile rheumatoid arthritis. *Textbook of Family Medicine*, 8th ed. Philadelphia, PA: Saunders/Elsevier; 2011.

Category: Musculoskeletal system

16. An asthmatic 8-year-old is complaining of wheezing and shortness of breath in your office. An albuterol nebulizer treatment is given, and the child's peak expiratory flow rate (PEFR) is measured at 75%. The appropriate next step would be
A) Add an oral steroid
B) Add theophylline
C) Add ipratropium
D) Administer epinephrine
E) Intubate the child

Answer and Discussion
The answer is A. Early treatment of asthma exacerbations is important to prevent progression to severe disease. First-line treatment should be with a short-acting inhaled β2-agonist such as albuterol; two to four puffs from a metered-dose inhaler can be given every 20 minutes up to three times, or a single treatment can be given by nebulizer. If the response is acceptable as assessed by sustained symptom relief or improvement in PEFR to more than 80% of the child's best, the short-acting β2-agonist can be continued every 3 to 4 hours for 24 to 48 hours. For patients taking inhaled corticosteroids, the dose may be doubled for 7 to 10 days. If the child does not completely improve from the initial therapy, with PEFR between 50% and 80%, the β2-agonist should be continued, and an oral corticosteroid

should be added. If the child experiences marked distress or if PEFR persists below 50%, the patient should repeat the β2-agonist immediately. Further emergent treatment may be necessary.

Additional Reading: Rakel R. Asthma. *Textbook of Family Medicine,* 8th ed. Philadelphia, PA: Saunders/Elsevier; 2011.

Category: Respiratory system

17. An 18-month-old female child presents to your office with her mother. A urinary tract infection (UTI) is discovered. Appropriate treatment at this time including antibiotic coverage includes
A) Intravenous pyelogram
B) Cystoscopy
C) Renal ultrasound and voiding cysturethrography (VCUG)
D) Observation with no further testing

Answer and Discussion
The answer is C. Practice guidelines from the American Academy of Pediatrics (AAP) recommend renal ultrasonography in all children 2 months to 2 years of age with a documented first UTI. VCUG is no longer routinely recommended. VCUG is warranted if renal and bladder sonogram reveal hydronephrosis, scarring, presence of findings suggestive of high-grade vesicoureteral reflux (VUR) or obstructive uropathy, or clinical scenarios considered to be complex or atypical. After the age of 2 years, some controversy exists. Some authorities recommend postponing workup for the first UTI in girls.

Additional Reading: Urinary tract infection: clinical practice guideline for the diagnosis and management of the initial UTI in febrile infants and children 2 to 24 months. *Pediatrics.* 2011;128(3):595–610.

Category: Nephrologic system

Practice guidelines from the AAP recommend renal ultrasonography to screen for anatoming abnormalities in all children 2 months to 2 years of age with a documented first UTI.

18. Which of the following statements is true regarding child safety seats?
A) Newborn infants should face forward in the backseat of cars.
B) A child outgrows a forward-facing seat when their shoulders extend beyond the back of the seat.
C) Once a child is >40 lbs, it is important to make sure the harness of the child seat is used.
D) Low-back booster seats are safe to use in children >40 lbs.
E) To sit with a standard seatbelt, the child's weight should be at least 81 lbs.

Answer and Discussion
The answer is E. Motor vehicle crashes continue to be the leading cause of death in children 1 to 14 years of age. Properly used child safety seats significantly reduce child morbidity and mortality. Although many parents know child safety seats are important, >80% of seats are misused. Children should sit in the backseat. The rear-facing position should be used until the child is 1 year of age and weighs 20 lbs (9 kg). Forward-facing child seats face forward and are for children heavier than 20 lbs and older than 1 year. A child outgrows this seat when the ears are above the back of the seat or when the child passes the height or weight limit of the seat (usually 40 lbs). High-back booster seats face forward and have removable harnesses.

They are meant for use with children heavier than 20 to 30 lbs (9 to 13.5 kg), depending on the manufacturer, and older than 1 year. The high back protects the head and neck in a rear-end collision. The harness should be used until the child exceeds the weight limit of the harness system (usually 40 lbs). Once the child is heavier than 40 lbs, the harness is removed, and the seat is used to position the vehicle seatbelt correctly (over the midclavicle and midchest, and tight over the upper thighs). High-back belt-positioning booster seats boost the child up so that the vehicle seatbelt fits correctly. They can only be used with a shoulder–lap belt system. High-back booster seats are for use with children heavier than 40 lbs and can be used until the child fits properly in the vehicle seatbelt system. Because safer restraint systems are available for children weighing more than 40 lbs, the use of low-back booster seats is not recommended. To properly fit a child in a standard car seatbelt, three elements must be present: (1) the child's legs should bend over the edge of the auto seat with the buttocks against the seat back; (2) the shoulder portion of the belt should be over the midclavicle and center of the chest; and (3) the lap belt should be tight over the upper thighs or the pelvis. A child should have a sitting height of 29 in. (74 cm) to have a proper seatbelt fit. This sitting height roughly correlates to a standing height of 58 in. (147 cm) and a weight of 81 lbs (36.5 kg). Increased education of parents regarding proper use of child safety seats can protect children from potentially fatal crash forces. Parents may also be educated about community resources and the several types of child safety seats.

> **Additional Reading:** New recommendations on motor vehicle safety for child passengers. *Am Fam Physician.* 2013;87(7): 472–474.

> **Category:** Patient/population-based care

19. Which of the following findings is *not* associated with rotavirus infections?
A) Metabolic acidosis
B) Hypernatremia
C) White blood cells (WBCs) noted in the stool
D) Normal WBC count
E) Lactic acidosis

Answer and Discussion

The answer is C. Vomiting is the first manifestation of rotavirus in the majority of patients, followed within 24 hours by low-grade fever and repeated bouts of watery diarrhea. Diarrhea usually lasts 4 to 8 days but can last longer in young infants or immunocompromised patients. The WBC count is rarely elevated. As patients become dehydrated from unreplaced fecal water loss, they may become hypernatremic. The stool does not contain blood or white cells. Metabolic acidosis results from bicarbonate loss in the stool, ketosis from poor intake, and lactic acidemia from hypotension and hypoperfusion. Replacement of fluid and electrolyte deficits and ongoing losses is critical, especially in small infants. The use of oral rehydration fluid is appropriate in most cases. The use of clear liquids or hypocaloric (dilute formula) diets for more than 48 hours is not advisable in uncomplicated viral gastroenteritis because starvation depresses digestive function and prolongs diarrhea. Intestinal lactase levels are reduced during rotavirus infection. Brief use of a lactose-free diet is associated with a shorter period of diarrhea but is not critical to successful recovery in most healthy infants. Reduced fat intake during recovery may reduce nausea and vomiting. Antidiarrheal medications are not effective and can be dangerous (loperamide, tincture of opium, diphenoxylate with atropine). Bismuth subsalicylate preparations may reduce stool volume but are not necessary for recovery. Specific identification of rotavirus is not required in every case, especially in outbreaks. Rotavirus antigens can be identified in stool. False positives (which may actually be nonpathogenic rotavirus) are seen in neonates. Some immunity is imparted by the first episode of rotavirus infection. Repeat infections occur but are usually less severe. Prevention of rotavirus is mainly by good hygiene and prevention of fecal–oral contamination. In July 1999, the AAP recommended suspending the use of oral rotavirus vaccine in the United States because of its association with intussusception in the first 3 weeks following vaccine administration. Recently, newer vaccines have been developed with an improved safety record.

> **Additional Reading:** Rotavirus. From: http://www.cdc.gov/rotavirus/

> **Category:** Gastroenterology system

20. Which of the following is *not* associated with early sexual activity?
A) Academic deficiencies
B) Repeat pregnancies
C) Sex education classes
D) Increased sexually transmitted diseases (STDs)
E) Low socioeconomic status

Answer and Discussion

The answer is C. Early sexual activity can have a substantial negative impact on adolescents. Currently in the United States, more than 900,000 teenagers become pregnant each year. Those who give birth tend to have more academic deficiencies, poorer socioeconomic outcomes, and repeat pregnancies, and they are more likely to be single parents. In addition, adolescents who engage in early sexual activity expose themselves to STDs. Of all STD cases reported in the United States, more than two-thirds occur in adolescents and young adults. Prevention strategies should be established to reduce early sexual activity in adolescents.

> **Additional Reading:** Sexual activity. *Nelson Textbook of Pediatrics,* 19th ed. Philadelphia, PA: Elsevier/Saunders; 2011.

> **Category:** Patient/population -based care

21. When evaluating febrile seizures, when is a lumbar puncture indicated?
A) If the seizure is generalized
B) If the seizure lasts 10 minutes
C) If there is a second seizure within 24 hours
D) If the seizure is associated with a recent vaccination
E) All children affected with a febrile seizure should have a lumbar puncture.

Answer and Discussion

The answer is C. The majority of seizures in children <5 years are febrile type seizures, and children with a positive family history have a higher incidence. A febrile seizure is defined as any seizure occurring in a child who is 6 months to 5 years of age accompanied by a current or recent fever (at least 38°C [100.4°F]) and without previous seizure or neurologic events. Febrile seizures are typically categorized as simple or complex. Simple febrile seizures are characteristically generalized, usually last <15 minutes, and occur only once in a 24-hour period. Complex febrile seizures may have focal features, last >15 minutes, and recur within a 24-hour period. Viral infections are often present with febrile seizures, with human herpes virus 6 and 7 and influenza A and B being important causes. There is also a significant increased risk of febrile seizures within 24 hours of receiving vaccination for diphtheria and tetanus toxoids and whole-cell pertussis, and within 8 to 14 days of receiving a measles, mumps, and rubella (MMR) vaccination. The risk of recurrent febrile seizures is increased in patients whose initial febrile seizure occurred at <12 months of age, patients with a lower rectal temperature at first seizure (<40°C [104°F]), patients with shorter duration of fever before their first seizure (<24 hours), patients with a family history of febrile seizures, and patients with complex features with the first febrile seizure. The risk of development of epilepsy is slightly higher among persons having simple febrile seizures but is significantly increased among those who have one or more complex febrile seizures. Initial evaluation of children with febrile seizure includes airway and circulatory support, ideally with noninvasive measures until the postictal state resolves. A thorough medical history that includes past seizures and other neurologic conditions, exposure to medications or toxins, allergies, or trauma may point to a specific seizure cause. Treatment with antipyretics is rarely necessary in the typical seizure case. Patients with seizures that last longer than 5 minutes should receive benzodiazepines to control the seizure. After the seizure ends, the physician should conduct a mental status examination and a physical evaluation. Routine laboratory studies include only a blood glucose test; an electrolyte test may be appropriate if a metabolic abnormality is being considered.

In most cases no further workup is necessary, but lumbar puncture is indicated in patients with suspected meningitis. A lumbar puncture should be considered in children younger than 12 months who have a febrile seizure as other signs of infection may not be evident. For children 12 to 18 months of age, clinical signs and symptoms of meningitis may be subtle, necessitating a lumbar puncture. Lumbar puncture is similarly indicated when a child greater than 18 months with neck stiffness, Kernig, or Brudzinski signs or a clinical picture pointing to an intracranial infection.

Neuroimaging only is appropriate in patients at risk of cerebral abscess, in those who have clinical evidence of increased intracranial pressure, in patients who have evidence of trauma, or in patients who have status epilepticus or have had a complex seizure. Children with simple febrile seizures can be cared for at home after providing parental education and making plans to follow up with the family. Routine prophylaxis using phenobarbital, valproic acid, oral diazepam, or antipyretics is controversial and usually not indicated.

Additional Reading: Febrile seizures. *Nelson Textbook of Pediatrics,* 19th ed. Philadelphia, PA: Elsevier/Saunders; 2011; and

Evaluation and management of febrile seizures in the out-of-hospital and emergency department settings. *Ann Emerg Med.* 2003;41:215–222.

Category: Neurologic

22. Which of the following statements is true regarding sexual development in girls?
A) The average age of menarche is earlier than it was 75 years ago.
B) African American girls usually experience menarche at an older age.
C) Breast development is usually the last physical characteristic to develop.
D) Girls who mature earlier are typically taller than girls who develop late.
E) The height spurt correlates more with pubic hair development than with breast development.

Answer and Discussion

The answer is A. Teenagers are now entering puberty earlier because of various factors, including better nutrition and improved socioeconomic conditions. In the United States, the average age at menarche is 12.16 years in African American girls and 12.88 in White girls. However, menarche may be delayed until age 16 years or may begin as early as age 10. The first objective sign of puberty in girls is the beginning of the height spurt. This is followed by development of breast buds between ages 8 and 11 years. Although breast development usually precedes the growth of pubic hair, in some girls the sequence may be reversed. Among girls, the growth spurt starts at about age 9 years and reaches a peak at age 11.5 years. The spurt usually ends by age 14 years. Girls who mature early reach their peak height velocity sooner and attain their final height earlier. Girls who mature late attain a greater ultimate height because of the longer period of growth before the growth spurt. Final height is related to skeletal age at onset of puberty as well as genetic factors. The height spurt correlates more closely with breast developmental stages than with pubic hair stages.

Additional Reading: Physiology of puberty. *Nelson Textbook of Pediatrics,* 19th ed. Philadelphia, PA: Elsevier/Saunders; 2011.

Category: Reproductive system

23. Which of the following blood tests may be helpful in determining a recent strep infection in a patient that has a possible poststreptococcal complication?
A) Erythrocyte sedimentation rate
B) C-reactive protein
C) Complete blood count (CBC)
D) Antistreptolysin O titer

Answer and Discussion

The answer is D. Group A beta-hemolytic streptococcal pharyngitis, scarlet fever, and in rare cases asymptomatic carrier states are associated with poststreptococcal complications. Children are most commonly affected in streptococcal pharyngitis, acute rheumatic fever, pediatric autoimmune neuropsychiatric disorders associated with streptococcal infection, and poststreptococcal glomerulonephritis. The hallmarks of rheumatic fever include arthritis, carditis, cutaneous disease, chorea, and subsequent acquired valvular disease. Pediatric autoimmune neuropsychiatric disorders include a subgroup of illnesses involving the basal ganglia in children with obsessive–compulsive disorders, tic disorders, dystonia, chorea encephalitis, and dystonic choreoathetosis. Poststreptococcal glomerulonephritis occurs most frequently in children between 2 and 6 years of age with a recent history of pharyngitis and a rash during the winter months.

The clinical examination of a patient with possible poststreptococcal complications should include an evaluation for signs of inflammation (i.e., CBC, erythrocyte sedimentation rate, C-reactive protein) and evidence of a preceding streptococcal infection. Antistreptolysin O titers should be obtained to confirm a recent invasive streptococcal infection. Other important antibody markers include antihyaluronidase, antideoxyribonuclease B, and antistreptokinase antibodies.

Additional Reading: Evaluation of poststreptococcal illness. *Am Fam Physician.* 2005;71:1949–1954.

Category: Nonspecific system

24. A 13-year-old girl is brought to your office by her mother. The child has experienced a recent sore throat with fevers and is now complaining of bilateral knee pain. Laboratory evaluation shows an elevated sedimentation rate. The most likely diagnosis is
A) JRA
B) Acute rheumatic fever
C) Lyme's disease
D) Osgood–Schlatter disease
E) Patellofemoral syndrome

Answer and Discussion

The answer is B. Rheumatic fever is complication of acute group A streptococcal pharyngitis that presents as an acute systemic febrile illness. Associated findings include a migratory arthritis involving the large joints, signs and symptoms of carditis and valvulitis, the erythema marginatum rash, subcutaneous nodules, and choreoathetotic movements of Sydenham's chorea. Damage to the cardiac valves may be chronic and progressive, resulting in significant cardiac dysfunction. Although the Modified Jones Criteria help with the clinical diagnosis, no specific symptoms, clinical signs, or laboratory tests are pathognomonic for rheumatic fever. Additionally, not all patients with rheumatic fever fulfill the Modified Jones Criteria. The criteria consist of major manifestations that include carditis, erythema marginatum, polyarthritis, subcutaneous nodules, and Sydenham's chorea. Minor manifestations include clinical (e.g., arthralgia, fever) and laboratory (e.g., elevated C-reactive protein and erythrocyte sedimentation rate, prolonged PR interval on electrocardiograph) findings. A diagnosis of rheumatic fever is supported by evidence of preceding group A streptococcal infection (i.e., positive throat culture or rapid streptococcal antigen test, elevated or rising antistreptolysin titer), and the presence of two major manifestations or of one major and two minor manifestations. Arthritis is the most frequent and least specific manifestation of rheumatic fever. It usually affects the large joints and may be the first sign of illness. The lower extremities generally are affected first, followed by the upper extremities. Joint involvement occurs early in the illness and is more common and severe in younger patients. The arthritis may be painful, but it is transient; the inflammation lasts about 2 to 3 days in each joint and 2 to 3 weeks in total. Radiographic evaluation can show slight joint effusions but usually the results are normal. The arthritis is self-limited, resolves without complications, and is treated with salicylates and NSAIDs. Carditis associated with rheumatic fever presents as pericarditis, myocarditis, and, most commonly, endocarditis. Pericarditis can present with chest discomfort, pleuritic chest pain, pericardial friction rubs, and distant heart sounds. Myocarditis is rare in isolation and can present with signs and symptoms of heart failure. Endocarditis may be asymptomatic or present with a new heart murmur. Cardiac murmurs do not always indicate valvular involvement, and they may be transient. If valvular disease occurs, it is most likely in the mitral, aortic, tricuspid, or pulmonary valve, in that order. Electrocardiograph and echocardiogam abnormalities may be present in about one-third of patients with carditis. Rheumatic heart disease is an important long-term consequence of rheumatic fever and is the major cause of acquired valvular disease internationally. Rheumatic heart disease typically occurs 10 to 20 years after the original rheumatic fever episode. Significant mitral stenosis can occur and require surgery. Sydenham's chorea is characterized by involuntary movements, muscular weakness, and emotional disturbances. It is usually more marked on one side of the body than the other and may be completely unilateral. Atypical behavior such as crying and restlessness are seen and, in rare cases, features of a psychosis may

be noted. There is no sensory loss or involvement of the pyramidal tracts. Sydenham's chorea is typically self-limited and occurs in <5% of those affected. The condition typically lasts 2 to 3 months. Antistreptococcal prophylaxis should be maintained continuously after an attack of acute rheumatic fever or chorea to prevent recurrences.

Additional Reading: Evaluation of poststreptococcal illness. *Am Fam Physician.* 2005;71:1949–1954.

Category: Cardiovascular system

25. A child presents to the emergency room with abdominal pain. An abdominal series shows a "bird's beak" sign. The most likely diagnosis is
A) Intussusception
B) Volvulus
C) Pyloric stenosis
D) Malrotation
E) Acute appendicitis

Answer and Discussion

The answer is B. Sigmoid volvulus is a rare problem seen in children and adolescents. Volvulus occurs when a floppy sigmoid loop rotates around its base, producing arterial and venous obstruction of the affected segment, followed by rapid distention of the closed loop. Because the consequences can be life-threatening, sigmoid volvulus should be included in the differential diagnosis of acute and recurrent episodes of abdominal pain or bowel obstruction in children, especially if colonic dilation is seen on radiographs. Boys are more commonly affected than girls. Symptoms can be either acute or recurrent. The most common symptoms are abdominal pain that is relieved by passage of stool or flatus, abdominal distention, and vomiting. Radiographic evaluation often reveals colonic dilation. Barium enema often confirms or suggests the diagnosis and should be performed under fluoroscopic control; a "twisted-taper" or "bird's-beak" appearance of the affected colon is characteristic. The most common associated conditions include Hirschsprung's disease and imperforate anus. Although sigmoid volvulus can resolve spontaneously, nonoperative management begins with fluid resuscitation and antibiotics, followed by barium enema detorsion of the sigmoid. Other nonoperative modalities include proctosigmoidoscopy and decompression by rectal tube. Operative management most commonly consists of sigmoidectomy.

Additional Reading: Vomiting. *Nelson Textbook of Pediatrics,* 19th ed. Philadelphia, PA: Elsevier/Saunders; 2011.

Category: Gastroenterology system

> Barium enema often confirms or suggests the diagnosis of a sigmoid volvulus, and should be performed under fluoroscopic control; a "twisted-taper" or "bird's-beak" appearance of the affected colon is characteristic.

26. The drug of choice for otitis media is
A) Azithromycin
B) Amoxicillin
C) Cefuroxime
D) Amoxicillin–clavulanate
E) Ceftriaxone

Answer and Discussion

The answer is B. The 2004 acute otitis media (AOM) guideline published by the AAP and the American Academy of Family Physicians suggested an "observation option" for selected children and proposed that the initial antibiotic therapy be prioritized according to diagnostic certainty. The recommendation was to prescribe amoxicillin (assuming no penicillin allergy) when a decision to treat with an antibiotic had been made if the child had not been administered amoxiccilin in the previous month *or* there was no concurrent purulent conjunctivitis.

Antibiotic resistance is growing among the organisms that commonly cause AOM. Associated risk factors for resistant pathogens include recent antibiotic treatment, children in day care facilities, infections occurring in the winter, and AOM in children <2 years of age. Amoxicillin remains the antibiotic of first choice, although a higher dosage (80 mg/kg/day) is recommended to ensure adequate eradication of resistant *Streptococcus pneumoniae*. Oral cefuroxime (Ceftin) or amoxicillin–clavulanate (Augmentin) and intramuscular ceftriaxone (Rocephin) are suggested second-line choices for treatment failure. Compliance with antibiotic regimens is enhanced by selecting medications that require less frequent dosing (such as one or two times a day) and by prescribing shorter (5 days or less) treatment courses. Selective use of tympanocentesis if the patient does not respond to empiric therapy can help confirm the diagnosis and guide effective therapy.

> **Additional Reading:** The diagnosis and management of acute otitis. *Pediatrics.* 2013;131(3):e964–e999.

> **Category:** Special sensory

27. Which of the following is a contraindication to influenza vaccine?
A) Allergy to eggs
B) Recent strep infection
C) Allergy to aluminum
D) Age <6 years

Answer and Discussion

The answer is A. Influenza vaccine (Fluzone, Fluvirin) should optimally be given in October and November, but can be given throughout the influenza season. Unvaccinated children younger than 9 years should be given two doses at least 1 month apart. Children aged 6 to 35 months are given 0.25 mL IM, whereas children aged 3 years and older are given 0.5 mL IM. (Fluvirin is indicated for use in only children aged 4 years and older.) Because vaccine viruses are first grown in eggs, the vaccine is contraindicated in persons with a history of allergy to eggs or egg products. It is also contraindicated in persons known to be sensitive to thimerosal. The Food and Drug Administration has approved a live attenuated influenza vaccine that is administered nasally (FluMist). It is to be used in healthy children aged 5 to 17 years and adults aged 18 to 49 years. Its safety in asthmatic individuals has not been established, and it is not currently recommended for use in patients with high-risk conditions, such as chronic cardiovascular, pulmonary, renal, or metabolic disorders, and in pregnant women. It is contraindicated in persons with a history of allergic reactions to any vaccine component, including eggs and children receiving chronic aspirin therapy or who are immunosuppressed.

> **Additional Reading:** Seasonal influenza vaccination resources for health professionals. From: http://www.cdc.gov/flu/professionals/vaccination/

> **Category:** Patient/population-based care

28. Which of the following statements regarding immunizations is true?
A) MMR vaccine can cause autism.
B) Hepatitis B vaccine can lead to multiple sclerosis.
C) Children with egg allergies may be given MMR vaccine.
D) Children with a prior local reaction to neomycin should avoid the varicella vaccine.

Answer and Discussion

The answer is C. Controversy has risen about the safety of some vaccines because of rare but serious adverse effects that have been attributed to them. Pain, swelling, and redness at the injection site are common local reactions to vaccines. Fever and irritability may occur after some immunizations. Currently, no substantial evidence links MMR vaccine to autism or hepatitis B vaccine to multiple sclerosis. Thimerosal is being eliminated from routine childhood vaccines because of concerns that multiple immunizations with vaccines containing this preservative could exceed recommended mercury exposures. Children with a history of egg allergy may be given MMR vaccine, even though it is derived from chick embryo fibroblast tissue culture. However, influenza vaccine should not be given to a person with a history of egg allergy. Traces of antibiotics such as neomycin, which is present in varicella (chickenpox), trivalent inactivated poliovirus (IPV), and MMR vaccines, have been considered possible causes of adverse reactions. A history of anaphylactic reaction to neomycin is a contraindication to future immunization, whereas a local reaction is not.

> **Additional Reading:** Vaccine adverse events: separating myth from reality. *Am Fam Physician.* 2002;66:2113–2120.

> **Category:** Patient/population-based care

29. Which of the following statements regarding pertussis is true?
A) Whole-cell vaccine has been shown to be safer than acellular vaccine.
B) The incidence of pertussis is decreasing.
C) Those vaccinated against pertussis have no risk of contracting the disease.
D) Use of diphtheria and tetanus toxoids and acellular pertussis (DTaP) in adolescents is contraindicated.
E) Acellular pertussis vaccine is indicated throughout the primary vaccination series.

Answer and Discussion

The answer is E. Fifty million cases of pertussis are seen each year, leading to about 400,000 deaths. In recent years, high-income countries see large increases in adolescent pertussis rates; the incidence of pertussis in U.S. teens has risen 19-fold since 1996. Whole-cell vaccines have been available for 70 years. Concerns about adverse effects (e.g., convulsions, encephalopathy, hypotonic episodes, fever, vomiting) paved the way for the development of acellular recombinant vaccines in the 1970s and 1980s.

The Centers for Disease Control and Prevention (CDC) recommend DTaP vaccine at 2, 4, 6, and 15 to 18 months of age, with a booster of the tetanus toxoid, reduced diphtheria toxoid, and acellular pertussis (Tdap) vaccine between 11 and 18 years of age, and a one-time Tdap booster as an adult.

Cochrane review included 52 safety studies and 6 effectiveness trials. In general, acellular and whole-cell vaccines had a low incidence of adverse effects; however, in patient receiving acellular vaccines, there was better compliance to the full series and fewer patients had adverse effects such as febrile convulsions and hypotonic-hyporesponsive episodes. Although not statistically significant compared with whole-cell vaccines, adverse effects from acellular vaccines increased as the series progressed, including fever (60 to 162 per 1,000 persons), local redness (96 to 162 per 1,000 persons), and swelling (117 to 275 per 1,000 persons). There was no difference seen between vaccines when compared as a cause of death from infection, with such events being rare.

Additional Reading: Cochrane briefs acellular vaccines for preventing pertussis in children. *Am Fam Physician.* 2011;84(5):504.

Category: Patient/population-based care

30. You are called to see an infant in the newborn nursery. The child was delivered 60 hours prior to your visit. The child appears jaundiced but otherwise healthy. A total serum bilirubin level is measured at 18 mg/dL. Appropriate treatment includes
A) Observation
B) Stop breast-feeding and switch to formula feedings
C) Begin phototherapy
D) Perform a septic workup
E) Start IV hydration

Answer and Discussion

The answer is C. Hyperbilirubinemia is very common in term newborns. Current recommendations include the following: phototherapy should be instituted when the total serum bilirubin level is ≥15 mg/dL (257 µmol/L) in infants 25 to 48 hours old, 18 mg/dL (308 µmol/L) in infants 49 to 72 hours old, and 20 mg/dL (342 µmol/L) in infants older than 72 hours. It is unlikely that term newborns with hyperbilirubinemia have serious underlying pathology. Physiologic jaundice peaks on the third or fourth day and declines over the first week following birth. Infants who are breast-fed are more likely to develop physiologic jaundice because of relative caloric deprivation in the first few days of life. If jaundice occurs in breast-fed infants, feedings should be increased to more than 10 times per day. In some cases formula supplementation may be necessary. Pathologic jaundice occurs if it presents within the first 24 hours after birth, the total serum bilirubin level rises by >5 mg/dL (86 µmol/L) per day or is >17 mg/dL (290 µmol/L), or an infant has signs and symptoms suggestive of serious illness. The management consists of excluding pathologic causes of hyperbilirubinemia and initiating treatment to prevent harmful neurotoxicity.

Additional Reading: A practical approach to neonatal jaundice. *Am Fam Physician.* 2008;77(9):1255–1262.

Category: Hematologic system

31. Bottle-feeding at bedtime can result in
A) Increased risk for aspiration
B) Dental caries
C) Oral candidiasis
D) Nasal polyps
E) Development of hiatal hernia

Answer and Discussion

The answer is B. Baby-bottle tooth decay can occur after a child repeatedly falls asleep with a bottle in his or her mouth. It is more commonly seen in lower socioeconomic groups and can lead to major dental problems with the development of caries. Prevention should be aimed at educating the parents about this problem so that they can avoid bottle-feeding at bedtime.

Additional Reading: A practical guide to infant oral health. *Am Fam Physician.* 2004;70(11):2113–2120.

Category: Special sensory

32. Which of the following is true concerning DTaP vaccination?
A) The vaccine is routinely administered at 4, 6, and 12 months and again at 5 years of age.
B) The whole-cell form is indicated for those who are immunocompromised.
C) The oral form is an inactivated vaccine.
D) Development of pertussis has been linked to the whole-cell form.
E) The acellular form is recommended for routine vaccination of all infants.

Answer and Discussion

The answer is E. Current recommendations for the diphtheria, pertussis, and tetanus immunization of young children state that DTaP is usually given at 2, 4, 6, and 12 to 15 months, with an additional dose at 4 to 6 years. The acellular pertussis form is preferred for all doses to help reduce the occurrence of side effects. Tetanus toxoid, reduced diphtheria toxoid, and acellular pertussis vaccine (Tdap adolescent preparation) is recommended at age 11 to 12 years for those who have completed the recommended childhood DPT/DTaP vaccination series and have not received a tetanus and diphtheria toxoid (Td) booster dose. Adolescents aged 13 to 18 years who missed the 11-to-12-year Td/Tdap booster dose should also receive a single dose of Tdap if they completed the recommended childhood DPT/DTaP vaccination series. Subsequent boosters are recommended every 10 years. Contraindications to the DPT vaccine include the following:

1. Previous anaphylaxis to the vaccine
2. Moderate or severe illness
3. Previous encephalopathy within 7 days after DPT injection
4. Progressive neurologic problem that is undiagnosed
5. Fever higher than 105°F after previous DPT injection
6. Continuous crying lasting 3 hours or more after previous DPT injection
7. Seizure within 3 days after previous DPT injection
8. Previous collapse, limp, or pale episode with previous DPT injection

Items 5 through 8 are relative contraindications and should be evaluated individually. The DTaP immunization should be given intramuscularly. A combined vaccine with DPT and Hib (Tetramune), which can be given at 2, 4, 6, and 12 to 15 months, is available.

Additional Reading: DTaP ACIP vaccine recommendations. From: http://www.cdc.gov/vaccines/hcp/acip-recs/vacc-specific/dtap.html

Category: Patient/population-based care

33. Which of the following vaccines is no longer recommended for routine vaccination in children?
A) Live oral polio vaccine
B) Inactivated injectable polio vaccine
C) DTaP
D) Haemophilus influenzae type b
E) Hepatitis B

Answer and Discussion

The answer is A. Sabin's vaccine (oral poliovirus vaccine [OPV]) for poliomyelitis prevention is an oral, live, attenuated, trivalent vaccine that was given at 2, 4, and 18 months, and 5 years. Because of cases of the risk associated with the live vaccine, it is no longer used. In its place, the injectable (Salk) vaccine, referred to as *IPV vaccine,* should be administered. The IPV vaccine has now been recommended for routine immunization in all infants because of the risk of developing polio from the live attenuated Sabin's vaccine. The schedule is the same for IPV vaccine.

Additional Reading: Polio vaccine. From: http://www.cdc.gov/vaccines/vpd-vac/polio/default.htm

Category: Patient/population-based care

34. Infant formula typically contains
A) 1 calorie/ounce
B) 10 calories/ounce
C) 20 calories/ounce
D) 50 calories/ounce
E) 100 calories/ounce

Answer and Discussion

The answer is C. Commonly, formula preparations provide 20 calories/ounce. Formulas exist as cow's milk–based, soy-based, and casein-based preparations. Cow's milk–based formula is the preferred, non–breast milk preparation for otherwise healthy term infants who do not breast-feed or for whom breast-feeding has been terminated prior to 1 year of age. Cow's milk–based formula closely resembles human breast milk and is composed of 20% whey and 80% casein with 50% more protein/dL than breast milk, as well as iron, linoleic acid, carnitine, taurine, and nucleotides. Approximately 32 ounces meets 100% of the recommended daily allowance (RDA) for calories, vitamins, and minerals. These formula preparations are diluted to a standard 20 calories/ounce and are typically whey-dominant protein preparations with vegetable oils and lactose. There are also multiple lactose-free preparations. Most standard formula preparations do not meet the recommended daily allowance for fluoride, and exclusively formula-fed infants may require 0.25 mg/day of supplemental fluoride.

Additional Reading: Nutrition and growth. *The Harriet Lane Handbook: A Manual for Pediatric House Officers,* 19th ed. Philadelphia, PA: Elsevier/Mosby; 2012.

Category: Nonspecific system

35. Which of the following is a risk factor for the development of otitis media in children?
A) Low birth weight
B) Premature birth
C) Family history of allergies/asthma
D) Low socioeconomic class
E) Pacifier use

Answer and Discussion

The answer is E. Otitis media usually results as a complication of an URI (viral). It is particularly common in children between 6 months and 3 years of age. The most common etiologic agents include *Streptococcus pneumoniae, Haemophilus influenzae,* and *Moraxella (Branhamella) catarrhalis.* In newborns, *Escherichia coli* and *Staphylococcus aureus* are major causes. Viral causes include respiratory syncitial virus (RSV), parainfluenza virus, influenza virus, enteroviruses, and adenoviruses. Risk factors include attending day care at or before 2 months of age, in day care >30 hours/week, bottle-feeding, exposure to cigarette smoke, pacifier use, and Polynesian, Native American, or Alaskan/Canadian Eskimo descent. Low birth weight, young gestational age, and a family history of allergies or asthma are not significantly associated with an increased risk of AOM.

Symptoms include earache, nausea, vomiting, diarrhea, hearing loss, and otorrhea. Fever may be present, but it may be absent in as many as 33% of those affected. Signs include bulging of the tympanic membrane with loss of the light reflex and normal landmarks as well as tympanic membrane immobility. Perforation and vestibular dysfunction may also occur. Diagnosis is based on clinical findings and requires the presence of fluid under pressure in the middle ear plus one sign of acute local or systemic illness. Eardrum motion is best assessed by looking at the pars flaccida in the superior part of the drum. A red drum with normal mobility is common in crying children and is not diagnostic of acute bacterial infection. The drug of choice for treatment is amoxicillin in patients who are not at increased risk of being infected with a drug-resistant organism. Complications include mastoiditis, labyrinthitis, conductive and sensory neural hearing loss, and meningitis.

Additional Reading: The diagnosis and management of acute otitis. *Pediatrics.* 2013;131(3): e964–e999.

Category: Special sensory

Risk factors for otitis media include attending day care at or before 2 months of age, in day care for more than 30 hours/week, bottle-feeding, exposure to cigarette smoke, pacifier use, Polynesian descent, Native American descent, and Alaskan and Canadian Eskimo descent.

36. Elevations in blood lead levels (BLLs) can result in
A) Decline in intelligence quotients (IQs)
B) Development of personality disorders
C) Hyperactivity disorder
D) Clear cell carcinoma of the vagina
E) Visual deficits

Answer and Discussion

The answer is A. A significant number of preschool-age children in the United States have BLLs >10 μg/dL (0.50 μmol/L), and these levels have been associated with a decline in IQ. The CDC advocates the use of a screening questionnaire to identify lead exposure or toxicity in all children. Efforts to remove lead from gasoline and paint have led to a reduction of BLLs in children. Secondary prevention through lead paint removal is effective in homes that have a high lead burden. Children with lead levels of 45 to 69 μg/dL (2.15 to 3.35 μmol/L) should receive chelation therapy using succimer (DMSA) or edetate calcium disodium (CaNa2EDTA). Use of both CaNa2EDTA and dimercaprol (BAL in oil) is indicated in children with BLLs higher than 70 μg/dL (3.40 μmol/L).

Additional Reading: Lead poisoning in children. *Am Fam Physician.* 2010;81(6):751–757.

Category: Patient/population-based care

37. A 14-year-old boy presents to your office complaining of pain in his left leg. Radiographs of the area show an aneurysmal bone cyst associated with the metaphysis and periosteal elevation of the mid tibia. The most appropriate management includes
A) Leg casting for 6 to 8 weeks
B) NSAIDs and reassurance
C) Administration of growth hormone
D) Technetium bone scan
E) Orthopaedic surgery referral

Answer and Discussion

The answer is E. Unicameral bone cysts (simple bone cysts) usually affect the metaphysis in long bones of pediatric patients (predominantly the femur, humerus). Most are asymptomatic and come to the attention of the patient, parents, and physician when a fracture occurs in the area of the bone cyst. Most small cysts heal without difficulty; a larger cyst may require surgery that involves removal of the cyst and bone grafting. Most patients recover without permanent disability. An aneurysmal bone cyst is a cyst that occasionally grows larger; these cysts usually occur before 20 years of age. Areas of involvement include expansion beyond the metaphyseal cartilage of the long bones. Patients may report pain and swelling in the region of the cyst. Radiographs may show well-circumscribed areas of rarefaction with periosteal elevation. Treatment usually involves surgery to remove the cyst. Occasionally, radiation therapy is used for vertebral lesions that threaten the spinal cord if surgery is contraindicated; however, postradiation sarcomas can occur. The prognosis for unicameral and aneurysmal bone cysts after treatment is excellent.

> **Additional Reading:** Benign tumors and tumor-like processes of bone. *Nelson Textbook of Pediatrics,* 19th ed. Philadelphia, PA: Elsevier/Saunders; 2011.

> **Category:** Musculoskeletal system

38. The definition of *amblyopia* is
A) Congenital cataracts noted at birth
B) Retinal detachment seen in premature children
C) Irregular pupillary size
D) Increased distance between the medial and lateral canthus
E) Subnormal visual acuity in one or both eyes despite correction of refractive error

Answer and Discussion

The answer is E. Amblyopia is subnormal visual acuity in one or both eyes despite correction of a refractive error. It results when the child suppresses the vision in one eye to avoid diplopia. Organic disease may be present but is insufficient to explain the level of vision. Amblyopia is frequently asymptomatic and detected only by screening programs. It is more resistant to treatment at an older age; thus children should be treated early. Other causes (neurologic, psychologic) must be considered if the history and ophthalmologic examination are not suggestive of amblyopia.

Treatment includes correction of refraction error or removal of cataract, as well as forced use of the amblyopic eye by patching the better eye. Some children cannot tolerate the patch, in which case the sound eye is blurred with glasses or drops (penalization therapy) to stimulate proper visual development of the more severely affected eye.

> **Additional Reading:** Amblyopia. *Nelson Textbook of Pediatrics,* 19th ed. Philadelphia, PA: Elsevier/Saunders; 2011.

> **Category:** Special sensory

39. Leukocoria is most likely associated with
A) Pregnancy
B) Infection
C) Retinoblastoma
D) Leukemia
E) Pyuria

Answer and Discussion

The answer is C. An abnormal pupillary light reflex (called *leukocoria* if the pupil appears white) may indicate a disorder anywhere within the eye. Associated disorders include corneal opacity, blood (hyphema) or other material in the anterior chamber, cataract, vitreous opacity, or retinal disease. The most serious diagnosis is retinoblastoma, a malignancy that is thought to arise from retinal germ

cells. Because it may be hereditary, a family history of retinoblastoma or of enucleation is of special concern. Although retinoblastoma is almost uniformly fatal without treatment, the cure rate is better than 90% when the condition is promptly recognized and treated, and many children can be effectively treated without enucleation.

> **Additional Reading:** Abnormalities of pupil and iris. *Nelson Textbook of Pediatrics,* 19th ed. Philadelphia, PA: Elsevier/Saunders; 2011.

> **Category:** Special sensory

40. Which of the following statements is true regarding hyperbilirubinemia?
A) Physiologic jaundice is rare in newborns.
B) Switching from formula feeding to breast-feeding may help decrease bilirubin levels.
C) Coombs' testing offers little information in the workup of hyperbilirubinemia.
D) For the condition of kernicterus to occur in premature infants, the level of bilirubin must be higher than in term newborns.
E) Complications of kernicterus include hearing loss, seizures, and mental retardation.

Answer and Discussion

The answer is E. Kernicterus occurs when the serum unconjugated (indirect) bilirubin becomes dangerously elevated (usually >25 mg/dL) in newborns. Symptoms include poor feeding, flaccidity, apnea, opisthotonos, and seizures; in severe cases, death may occur. Children who do survive may suffer hearing loss, seizures, and mental retardation. Risk factors include prematurity, blood incompatibilities, infection, and acidosis. Physiologic jaundice is the most common form of jaundice and occurs in up to 50% of newborns. The condition is benign and usually resolves in 1 week. Most bilirubin levels peak in 3 to 5 days. The workup of a child with hyperbilirubinemia should include the following:

- Careful history to detect risk factors and physical examination to rule out petechiae, hepatosplenomegaly, bruising, and signs of infection
- Measurement of bilirubin levels
- CBC, reticulocyte count, and peripheral blood smear
- Coombs' test
- Typing of mother's and infant's blood
- Thyroid function tests

Treatment for hyperbilirubinemia of newborns includes the following:

- Increasing formula feedings for the infant will increase gastrointestinal (GI) motility and frequency of stools, thereby minimizing the enterohepatic circulation of bilirubin.
- Increasing frequency of breast-feeding. If bilirubin continues to rise, switch from breast-feeding to formula for a few days until bilirubin is <15 mg/dL (the mother should continue with breast pumping during this time).
- Phototherapy, which helps degrade unconjugated bilirubin
- Exchange transfusion for severe cases of persistent hyperbilirubinemia (usually >20 mg/dL) or hemolysis with anemia
- In premature infants, kernicterus may occur with lower bilirubin levels.

> **Additional Reading:** Kernicterus. *Nelson Textbook of Pediatrics,* 19th ed. Philadelphia, PA: Elsevier/Saunders; 2011.

> **Category:** Neurologic

41. Preterm breast milk
A) Has the same components as breast milk produced at term
B) Persists for 1 week before the composition approaches that of term infant breast milk
C) Contains lower concentrations of important electrolytes and immunoglobulins
D) Typically requires fortification with human milk fortifiers
E) Contains excessive amounts of calcium

Answer and Discussion

The answer is D. The composition of breast milk in mothers of preterm infants is different from that of term infants. This difference persists for approximately 4 weeks before the composition approaches that of term infant breast milk. The difference in preterm milk composition reflects the increased nutrient demands of preterm infants. Preterm breast milk contains higher concentrations of total and bound nitrogen, immunoglobulins, sodium, iron, chloride, and medium-chain fatty acids. However, it may not contain sufficient amounts of phosphorus, calcium, copper, and zinc. Preterm infants are more likely to require fortification with human milk fortifiers (HMF) to correct these deficiencies.

> **Additional Reading:** Enteral nutrition components. *The Harriet Lane Handbook. A Manual for Pediatric House Officers.* Johns Hopkins Hospital; 2012.

> **Category:** Nonspecific system

42. A 12-year-old boy presents to your office complaining of gradually increasing hip pain that radiates to the thigh and knee. Physical examination shows an obese boy with pain associated with hip abduction and adduction. Radiographs show evidence of acetabular dysplasia. The most likely diagnosis is
A) Congenital dislocation of the hip
B) Osgood–Schlatter disease
C) Slipped capital femoral epiphyses
D) Sacral insufficiency fracture
E) Transient synovitis of the hip

Answer and Discussion

The answer is C. Slipped capital femoral epiphyses are usually seen in overweight boys between 11 and 14 years of age. The condition occurs when the femoral head slips posteriorly and inferiorly, exposing the anterior and superior aspects of the metaphysis of the femoral neck. When the condition occurs before puberty, an underlying endocrine disorder (hypothyroidism, growth hormone deficiency) should be suspected. Symptoms, including pain and a limp, are usually gradual in onset and usually involve the hips or are referred to the thigh or knee. The condition is bilateral in 20% of cases. Radiographs should be performed, including frog-leg views. Findings include abnormalities with the femoral head, including acetabular dysplasia. Treatment involves orthopaedic referral with surgical pinning. Complications include avascular necrosis of the hip and erosion of cartilage.

> **Additional Reading:** Slipped capital femoral epiphysis. *Nelson Textbook of Pediatrics,* 19th ed. Philadelphia, PA: Elsevier/Saunders; 2011.

> **Category:** Musculoskeletal

43. A 4-year-old is brought to your office. The parent complains that the child's hair is falling out. Closer inspection shows the hair shafts are broken just above the scalp. There are scaly, pruritic, mildly inflamed gray patches, and scrapings of the area show the presence of hyphae. The treatment of choice is

A) Topical antifungals
B) Oral antifungals
C) Topical hydrocortisone cream
D) Permethrin cream
E) Shave the hair off at the scalp and let it regrow

Answer and Discussion

The answer is B. Tinea capitis is a fungal infection of the scalp that usually affects infants and young children. It is contagious and may become epidemic. It is caused by fungi including *Trichophyton, Microsporum,* and *Epidermophyton.* Lesions of the scalp usually cause scaly, gray patches that are pruritic. Multiple areas of hair loss may occur with hair shafts broken just above the scalp. Microscopic examination of scrapings after treatment with 10% potassium hydroxide reveals fungal hyphae. Hair examined with black light fluorescences show a greenish-yellow color in cases of microsporosis. Treatment for most tinea infections involves the use of topical antifungals but is not sufficient for tinea capitis, which requires oral administration of antifungals, such as griseofulvin. Severely inflamed lesions benefit from systemic or intralesional steroids. Until tinea capitis is cured, an imidazole or ciclopirox cream should be applied to the scalp to prevent spread, especially to other children, and selenium sulfide 2.5% shampoo should be used daily. Children can attend school during treatment, and the risk of transmission is low.

> **Additional Reading:** Tinea capitis. *Nelson Textbook of Pediatrics,* 19th ed. Philadelphia, PA: Elsevier/Saunders; 2011.

> **Category:** Integumentary

44. An 18-year-old high school student presents with a painless mass in his neck. He also reports a slight cough over the last 6 weeks. Additionally, he reports some fatigue and generalized pruritus. The most likely diagnosis is
A) Infectious mononucleosis
B) Brachial cleft cyst
C) *Streptococcus* pharyngitis
D) Lyme's disease
E) Hodgkin's disease

Answer and Discussion

The answer is E. The incidence of Hodgkin's disease increases throughout childhood and peaks in the late teens. The most common presenting complaint is a painless mass in the neck. Other presentations include a persistent cough secondary to a mediastinal mass or, less commonly, splenomegaly or enlarged axillary or inguinal lymph nodes. About one-third of children with Hodgkin's disease present with constitutional symptoms. These symptoms may include intermittent fever, night sweats, and weight loss. These are referred to as "B" symptoms. The "A" designation refers to the absence of these symptoms. Other symptoms include anorexia, fatigue, and pruritus. Any persistent painless mass (especially a neck mass) that does not respond to antibiotics should be evaluated. This investigation should include a lymph node biopsy. Because of sampling errors and difficulties in obtaining an accurate diagnosis, excisional biopsy (rather than needle biopsy) of enlarged lymph nodes should be performed. A persistent cough, especially in the presence of any "B" symptoms, should be investigated. As part of this evaluation, a chest radiograph should be obtained. It is also important to investigate "B" symptoms associated with any lymphadenopathy or splenomegaly. Laboratory tests can often be helpful in confirming the diagnosis. Although nonspecific, elevations in the erythrocyte sedimentation rate, lactate dehydrogenase level, and ferritin level are suspicious findings in children with other signs or symptoms of Hodgkin's disease. Infrequently, the CBC reveals abnormalities, including anemia and eosinophilia.

Additional Reading: Role of the primary care physician in Hodgkin lymphoma. *Am Fam Physician.* 2008;78(5):615–622.

Category: Hematologic system

> The incidence of Hodgkin's disease increases throughout childhood and peaks in the late teens. The most common presenting complaint is a painless mass in the neck.

45. The condition of facial acne is associated with
A) Ingestion of fatty foods
B) Presence of *Propionibacterium acnes*
C) Consumption of chocolate
D) Presence of *Staphylococcus aureus*
E) Poor hygiene

Answer and Discussion

The answer is B. Acne is one of the most common presenting complaints in a family physician's office. Adolescent patients between 12 and 25 years of age are the most commonly affected. The condition results when keratinization blocks follicular canals. Increased sebum production occurs, and bacterial proliferation causes inflammation. Increased androgen production is often related to the development of acne. The plugged pilosebaceous unit is referred to as a "whitehead" if the lesion is a closed comedone, or a "blackhead" if the comedone is open. The most common infecting bacterium is *Propionibacterium acnes,* which proliferates and releases chemotactic factors that attract leukocytes. The diagnosis of acne is made by observing characteristic lesions on the face, back, shoulders, and chest. Treatment involves washing with mild soaps on a regular basis; application of benzoyl peroxide; topical tretinoin (Retin-A); or topical antibiotics such as erythromycin, clindamycin, tetracycline, or meclocycline. Oral antibiotics may be necessary for more severe cases. Severe nodulocystic acne that fails to respond to the previously mentioned measures may be treated with oral isotretinoin (Accutane). Close monitoring of liver function tests, triglyceride levels, and CBCs are required. In addition, the drug has many other side effects (i.e., xerosis, epistaxis, myalgias, and arthralgias) and is highly teratogenic. Patients should be aware that acne is not a disease of hygiene. They should not try to scrub the lesions away, and they should not use alcohol-based astringents that can dry and irritate their skin. Patients should be instructed to wash their face twice a day with a mild soap and water. Patients should also be informed that acne has no relationship to diet (e.g., chocolate, pizza, soda). Many think acne is caused by stress, but no studies support this association. It may be that the acne itself causes stress, not vice versa. Cosmetics have long been blamed for the development of acne lesions. Although the causal relationship between cosmetics and acne may be overstated, patients should be directed to use oil-free, non-comedogenic cosmetics. Oil from hair products and suntan lotions can also exacerbate acne. Female patients should be informed that acne usually worsens during the week before menses. Mechanical trauma can make acne worse. Therefore, patients should be encouraged to avoid picking at lesions because doing so may cause more inflammation.

Additional Reading: Diagnosis and treatment of acne. *Am Fam Physician.* 2012;86(8):734–740.

Category: Integumentary

46. Absence seizures are associated with which of the following features?
A) Subnormal intelligence
B) Three-per-second spike-and-wave electroencephalogram (EEG) pattern
C) Staring episodes that last 30 to 45 minutes
D) March-like progression of tonic–clonic activity
E) No genetic transmission

Answer and Discussion

The answer is B. Absence seizures (formerly called *petit mal seizures*) are characterized by brief, 10- to 30-second staring episodes, followed by a resumption of normal activity. Attacks may occur up to 100 times daily and can be precipitated by hyperventilation. The seizures usually affect children, and there is a genetic predisposition. Affected children usually have normal intelligence, and most cases resolve before 20 years of age. EEG findings show a characteristic 3-per-second bilateral spike-and-wave pattern. Treatment usually involves the use of valproic acid and/or ethosuximide and clonazepam.

Additional Reading: Seizures in childhood. *Nelson Textbook of Pediatrics,* 19th ed. Philadelphia, PA: Elsevier/Saunders; 2011.

Category: Neurology

47. Idiopathic aseptic necrosis of the femoral head is also known as
A) Slipped capital femoral epiphyses
B) Osgood–Schlatter disease
C) Legg–Calvé–Perthes disease
D) Morton's neuroma
E) Transient synovitis of the hip

Answer and Discussion

The answer is C. Idiopathic aseptic necrosis of the femoral head is also known as *Legg–Calvé–Perthes disease.* The disease is usually unilateral and is most common in boys 2 to 12 years of age. Symptoms include hip, groin, or thigh pain and difficulty ambulating, which is usually gradual in onset and progressive. Physical examination may show an abnormal gait (painless limp) and atrophy of the thigh muscles. Lateral radiographs (frog view) are required and show areas of lucency and fragmentation of the femoral head, which may progress to sclerosis and destruction. Radiographs are often normal early in the disease process; however, bone scans may show decreased uptake in the area of the femoral head. Treatment involves expectant observation both clinically and radiographically, abduction casts to contain the femoral head within the acetabulum, and surgery in select cases. It should be remembered that children who present with knee pain may have hip pathology.

Additional Reading: The hip. *Nelson Textbook of Pediatrics,* 19th ed. Philadelphia, PA: Elsevier/Saunders; 2011.

Category: Musculoskeletal

48. Which of the following is associated with infectious mononucleosis?
A) Submental lymphadenopathy
B) Strawberry tongue
C) Cobble-stoned appearance of posterior pharynx
D) Palatal petechiae
E) Negative heterophile antibody test

Answer and Discussion

The answer is D. Infectious mononucleosis is relatively common in patients 10 to 30 years of age who present with sore throat and fatigue, palatal petechiae, posterior cervical or auricular adenopathy, marked adenopathy, or inguinal adenopathy. An atypical lymphocytosis of at least 20% or atypical lymphocytosis of at least 10% plus lymphocytosis of at least 50% strongly supports the diagnosis, as does a positive heterophile antibody test. False-negative results of heterophile antibody tests are relatively common early in the course of infection. Symptomatic treatment, the mainstay of care, includes adequate hydration, analgesics, antipyretics, and adequate rest. Bed rest should not be strictly enforced, and the patient's energy level should guide activity. Corticosteroids, acyclovir, and antihistamines are not recommended for routine treatment of infectious mononucleosis, although corticosteroids may benefit patients with respiratory compromise or severe pharyngeal edema. Patients with infectious mononucleosis should be withdrawn from contact or collision sports for at least 4 weeks after the onset of symptoms. Fatigue, myalgias, and need for sleep may persist for several months after the acute infection has resolved.

> **Additional Reading:** Epstein–Barr virus. *Nelson Textbook of Pediatrics*, 19th ed. Philadelphia, PA: Elsevier/Saunders; 2011.

Category: Nonspecific

49. Which of the following is routinely given at birth to prevent hemorrhagic disease of the newborn?
A) Erythromycin
B) Vitamin C
C) Vitamin K
D) Factor X
E) von Willebrand's factor

Answer and Discussion

The answer is C. Following birth, there is a modest decrease in the vitamin K (phytonadione)–dependent factors II, VII, IX, and X, which gradually return to normal in 7 to 10 days. The cause of this decrease is inadequate free vitamin K available from the mother and the newborn's inability to synthesize vitamin K because of a lack of intestinal flora. Therefore, 1 mg of vitamin K is administered intramuscularly at birth to prevent hemorrhagic disease of the newborn in term infants. Larger doses predispose to the development of hyperbilirubinemia and kernicterus. Breast milk is a poor source of vitamin K. As a result, hemorrhagic complications occur more frequently in breast-fed infants. Mothers taking medications that interfere with vitamin K function (i.e., phenobarbital and phenytoin) may have infants at increased risk for early-onset bleeding.

> **Additional Reading:** Hemorrhage in the newborn infant. *Nelson Textbook of Pediatrics,* 19th ed. Philadelphia, PA: Elsevier/Saunders; 2011.

Category: Hematologic

50. Which of the following statements about Down's syndrome is true?
A) Younger mothers are at increased risk for having a child affected with Down's syndrome.
B) There is an increased risk of leukemia in children affected with Down's syndrome.
C) Most children affected have normal IQs.
D) The condition is not passed on to children of affected mothers.
E) Those affected usually have a normal life expectancy.

Answer and Discussion

The answer is B. Down's syndrome is a condition characterized by an extra chromosome 21. The incidence is reported to be 1 in 700 to 800 births, but it varies depending on maternal age. Older mothers (especially those older than 35) are at increased risk. The disease may result from trisomy 21, translocation, or mosaicism.

Signs and symptoms include a flattened, hypoplastic midface with a depressed nasal bridge, hypotonicity, delayed physical and mental development with decreased IQ, microcephaly with a flattened occiput, slanted eyes with epicanthal folds, Brushfield spots (gray to white spots around the periphery of the iris), single palmar crease, short fingers, and abnormal feet with a wide gap between the first and second toe. Other associated conditions include congenital heart disease (e.g., ventricular septal defects) and GI anomalies (e.g., tracheoesophageal fistula, pyloric stenosis, duodenal atresia, and imperforate anus). The life expectancy of a child affected with Down's syndrome is reduced by the presence of heart disease and an increased risk of acute leukemia. Some affected women are fertile; however, they have a 50% chance that their fetus will also have Down's syndrome. Many of these affected fetuses abort spontaneously. All men with Down's syndrome are infertile.

> **Additional Reading:** Down syndrome and other abnormalities of chromosome number. *Nelson Textbook of Pediatrics,* 19th ed. Philadelphia, PA: Elsevier/Saunders; 2011.

Category: Nonspecific

> **Signs and symptoms of Down's syndrome include a flattened, hypoplastic midface with a depressed nasal bridge, hypotonicity, delayed physical and mental development with decreased IQ, microcephaly with a flattened occiput, slanted eyes with epicanthal folds, Brushfield spots (gray to white spots around the periphery of the iris), single palmar crease, short fingers, and abnormal feet with a wide gap between the first and second toe.**

51. The most common cause of a limp in a 5-year-old boy is
A) Stress fracture
B) Transient synovitis of the hip
C) Legg–Calvé–Perthes disease
D) Slipped capital femoral epiphyses
E) Septic joint

Answer and Discussion

The answer is B. Transient synovitis of the hip is the most common cause of hip pain and limping in U.S. children. The condition usually follows an upper respiratory illness and resolves spontaneously within a few days. Children 3 to 10 years of age, particularly boys, are the most commonly affected. Physical examination shows a limp and limited motion of the hip, especially with internal rotation. The hip is usually kept flexed, abducted, and externally rotated. Radiographs are usually negative but may show soft tissue swelling associated with the hip joint. A CBC and the erythrocyte sedimentation rate are usually normal. Treatment involves rest and anti-inflammatory drugs. Symptoms usually resolve in 7 to 10 days. Traction of the hip in slight flexion may also be used. Follow-up radiographs (at 1 and 3 months from time of presentation or perhaps sooner if the child's limp persists) are recommended because of the risk for development of avascular necrosis of the femoral head. If septic arthritis is suspected, aspiration of the hip may be necessary.

Additional Reading: The hip. *Nelson Textbook of Pediatrics,* 19th ed. Philadelphia, PA: Elsevier/Saunders. 2011.

Category: Musculoskeletal system

52. Which of the following statements concerning circumcision is true?
A) It is medically indicated for all male children.
B) Premature infants should not be circumcised.
C) Male infants with posthitis should not be circumcised.
D) Hypospadias is not a contraindication for circumcision.
E) Circumcision can be performed in the office until 4 months of age.

Answer and Discussion
The answer is B. Controversy surrounds the necessity of circumcision. UTIs are 10 to 15 times more common in uncircumcised infants. Many recommend circumcision in infants who are predisposed to UTI, such as those with congenital hydronephrosis and vesicoureteral reflux. Other indications for circumcision include recurrent balanitis (inflammation of the glans), posthitis (inflammation of the foreskin), or paraphimosis (retraction of the prepuce behind the glans that may interfere with blood flow). Routine circumcision is often more a social issue than a medical indication. Because phimosis (tightness of the foreskin so that it cannot be retracted over the glans penis) cannot usually be detected before puberty, it is not an indication for circumcision. Contraindications for circumcision include prematurity, genital anomalies (including hypospadias or ambiguous genitalia), and bleeding disorders. Circumcision should be performed at least 12 to 24 hours after birth and within 6 weeks of birth, preferably before discharge from the hospital. If delay occurs beyond 6 weeks, circumcision should be postponed until after 1 year of age with general anesthesia. Most recommend using a dorsal penile nerve block with 1% lidocaine without epinephrine for local anesthesia. EMLA cream can also be applied.

Additional Reading: Anomalies of the penis and urethra. *Nelson Textbook of Pediatrics,* 19th ed. Philadelphia, PA: Elsevier/Saunders. 2011.

Category: Reproductive system

53. Which of the following statements is true regarding infectious mononucleosis?
A) Guillain–Barré syndrome is an associated complication.
B) The disease can result in positive rheumatoid factor formation.
C) Heterophil agglutination tests are usually positive at the onset of the disease.
D) Rupture of the aorta can be associated with the disease.
E) Glaucoma is often seen with prolonged cases.

Answer and Discussion
The answer is A. Infectious mononucleosis is caused by the Epstein–Barr virus. It usually affects individuals between 10 and 35 years of age. Symptoms include fever, sore throat, anorexia, generalized fatigue, lymphadenopathy (especially affecting the posterior cervical chain), splenomegaly, and a maculopapular rash. Hepatitis with hepatomegaly is often seen with occasional jaundice. Laboratory findings include leukocytosis with many atypical lymphocytes (i.e., larger with vacuolated cytoplasm) and a positive monospot test (with heterophil agglutination) that becomes positive before the fourth week after the onset of the illness. The results of these tests are usually negative in infants and children younger than 4 years. False-positive rapid plasma reagin and Venereal Disease Research Laboratory

tests may occur, as well as abnormal liver function tests. Treatment involves supportive therapy with saline gargles, anti-inflammatory drugs, and antipyretic medication. In severely ill patients with severe pharyngitis, corticosteroids can be used to help decrease inflammation. Complications include the development of Guillain–Barré syndrome, myocarditis, and encephalitis. Spleen rupture may also occur with trauma; therefore, contact sports should be avoided until the splenomegaly has resolved.

Additional Reading: Epstein–Barr virus. *Nelson Textbook of Pediatrics,* 19th ed. Philadelphia, PA: Elsevier/Saunders; 2011.

Category: Nonspecific system

54. Which of the following is true regarding medications used in the treatment of acne?
A) A low estrogen-containing oral contraceptive can be helpful in the treatment of acne.
B) Doxycycline, tetracycline, and minocycline are contraindicated before the age of 18.
C) Lipid values must be monitored when using isotretinoin.
D) Oral contraceptives are adequate to prevent pregnancy when administering isotretinoin.

Answer and Discussion
The answer is C. Topical retinoids, benzoyl peroxide, sulfacetamide, and azelaic acid are recommended in patients with mild or moderate comedones. Topical erythromycin or clindamycin can be used in addition in patients with mild to moderate inflammatory acne or mixed acne. A 6-month course of oral erythromycin, doxycycline, tetracycline, or minocycline can be prescribed in patients with moderate to severe inflammatory acne. A low-androgen-containing oral contraceptive pill is also effective in women with moderate to severe acne. Isotretinoin is reserved for use in the treatment of the most severe or refractory cases of inflammatory cystic type acne. Because of its poor side-effect profile and teratogenicity, isotretinoin must be prescribed by a physician who is registered with the System to Manage Accutane-Related Teratogenicity (SMART) program. Serious side effects of isotretinoin include hepatitis, hypertriglyceridemia, intracranial hypertension, arthralgia, myalgias, night blindness, and hyperostosis. Serum liver function tests and triglyceride levels must be monitored monthly in patients receiving isotretinoin. Isotretinoin is teratogenic and can result in severe fetal abnormalities involving several systems. As a result, two forms of contraception must be used during isotretinoin therapy and for 1 month after treatment has been discontinued. To ensure that female patients are not pregnant when treatment is initiated, two negative urine pregnancy tests are required before isotretinoin is prescribed. Pregnancy status is rechecked at monthly visits. The link between isotretinoin and depression is controversial.

Additional Reading: Diagnosis and treatment of acne. *Am Fam Physician.* 2012;86(8):734–740.

Category: Integumentary

55. A 2-year-old presents with an erythematous rash on the face (slapped-cheek appearance) that has spread to involve the trunk; the extremities are spared. She also has a low-grade fever and malaise. Which of the following is the most likely diagnosis?
A) Measles
B) Congenital syphilis
C) Erythema infectiosum
D) Meningococcemia
E) Rubeola

Answer and Discussion

The answer is C. Erythema infectiosum is referred to as *fifth disease* because it represents the fifth major viral childhood illness (which also includes measles, mumps, rubella, and rubeola). The disease is caused by parvovirus B19 and is characterized by mild constitutional symptoms, such as low-grade fever, malaise, and joint pain (particularly in adult women). Also, there is a classic indurated, erythematous maculopapular facial rash that may progress to the trunk and extremities (but spares the palms and soles). The rash is often pronounced on extensor surfaces. The rash is often referred to as a "slapped-cheek" appearance and can be exacerbated with exposure to sunlight, heat, emotional stress, or fever. The illness usually lasts 5 to 10 days, and only symptomatic treatment is necessary. Occasionally, complications include arthropathies, myocarditis, and a transient aplastic crisis. Fifth disease may occasionally cause fetal death secondary to fetal hydrops; therefore, pregnant women should avoid contact with affected patients. Children are not infectious once the rash develops because the rash and arthropathy (when present) are immune-mediated, postinfectious reactions. Therefore, isolation from school and/or day care is not necessary.

> **Additional Reading:** Parvovirus B19. *Nelson Textbook of Pediatrics,* 19th ed. Philadelphia, PA: Elsevier/Saunders; 2011.
>
> **Category:** Nonspecific system

56. The treatment of choice for iron poisoning is
A) Pralidoxime chloride
B) Deferoxamine
C) Penicillamine
D) Edetate calcium disodium
E) Plasmapheresis

Answer and Discussion

The answer is B. There are five stages described for iron intoxication:

- Stage 1. Hemorrhagic gastroenteritis, which occurs 30 to 60 minutes after the ingestion. Lasting for 4 to 6 hours, this may result in hematemesis, abdominal pain, irritability, explosive diarrhea, shock, coma, and metabolic acidosis.
- Stage 2. After these findings, there is usually a symptom-free period that lasts up to 24 hours.
- Stage 3. The next 48 hours after ingestion is usually a period of delayed shock with iron levels >500 mg/dL. Cerebral dysfunction, fever, seizures, and coma may occur.
- Stage 4. Two to 5 days after ingestion, liver damage starts to appear and may lead to hepatic failure. Other manifestations include coagulopathies and hypoglycemia.
- Stage 5. GI scarring, bowel obstruction, and pyloric stenosis may develop 2 to 5 weeks after the initial ingestion.

In addition to the previously mentioned symptoms, vomiting, hyperglycemia, leukocytosis, and an abdominal radiograph that shows the iron particles are usually related to a serum iron level >300 mg/dL. Severe cases may cause seizures, coma, pulmonary edema, and vascular collapse. Treatment involves inducing vomiting, as well as gastric lavage, followed by use of the chelating agent deferoxamine. Charcoal does not bind iron. In severe cases, hemodialysis and exchange transfusion may be necessary.

> **Additional Reading:** Poisoning. *Nelson Textbook of Pediatrics,* 19th ed. Philadelphia, PA: Elsevier/Saunders; 2011.
>
> **Category:** Nonspecific system

57. A 1-year-old infant is brought into the office by a concerned mother. The child has an erythematous diaper rash with small satellite lesions that have not improved with application of petroleum jelly. The most appropriate treatment is
A) Zinc oxide
B) Clotrimazole (Lotrimin) ointment
C) Neosporin ointment
D) Mupirocin (Bactroban) ointment
E) Hydrocortisone cream

Answer and Discussion

The answer is B. Diaper dermatitis secondary to Candida albicans is an intensely red and scorched-appearing rash that involves the perineal area. The rash may be well demarcated and possesses vesicles that weep, pustules, papules, and the characteristic satellite lesions. Treatment consists of antifungal ointment (i.e., clotrimazole or nystatin) and, possibly, short-term use of hydrocortisone cream for severe dermatitis. Soothing cream (zinc oxide) should be applied with each diaper change. Also, keeping the area dry can help deter the development of yeast dermatitis.

> **Additional Reading:** Candida. *Nelson Textbook of Pediatrics,* 19th ed. Philadelphia, PA: Elsevier/Saunders; 2011.
>
> **Category:** Nonspecific system

58. Which of the following medications is recommended in the treatment of mild to moderate croup?
A) Acyclovir
B) Dexamethasone
C) Theophylline
D) Atropine
E) No medications have been found to be useful.

Answer and Discussion

The answer is B. Viral croup is the main cause of airway obstruction in children 6 months to 6 years of age. For children with mild croup, symptomatic care and mist therapy may be all that is necessary. Epinephrine has been used in the past to treat more severe cases of croup, but recent studies have found that glucocorticoid use is associated with shorter hospital stays, improvement in croup scores, and less use of epinephrine. Studies have shown that treatment with oral dexamethasone is as effective as intramuscular dexamethasone or nebulized budesonide. While more studies are needed to establish guidelines, oral dexamethasone can be used to treat mild to moderate croup with close follow-up and instructions for further care, if needed.

> **Additional Reading:** Croup: an overview. *Am Fam Physician.* 2011;83(9):1067–1073.
>
> **Category:** Respiratory system

59. Which of the following medications would not be a suitable alternative for second-line treatment of otitis media in a 6-year-old?
A) Azithromycin
B) Cefaclor
C) Cefixime
D) Ciprofloxacin
E) Erythromycin

Answer and Discussion

The answer is D. Ciprofloxacin is generally not indicated for patients below age 18 years because of the risk of damage to cartilage development. Although amoxicillin is considered the drug of choice, the other options can be used as second-line agents.

Additional Reading: The diagnosis and management of acute otitis. *Pediatrics.* 2013;131(3):e964–e999.

Category: Special sensory

60. Immunizations (excluding hepatitis B) for premature infants should be
A) Delayed because of the infant's immaturity
B) Administered at same designated times as normal infants on the basis of their age
C) Withheld for 1 year
D) Given earlier to help prevent diseases to which they are more susceptible
E) Given in reduced amounts on the basis of the infants' weight

Answer and Discussion

The answer is B. Premature infants are predisposed to certain problems, including poor sucking and diminished gag and cough reflexes, which can lead to an increased risk of aspiration and difficulty feeding. Other problems include pulmonary immaturity, decreased ability to maintain body temperature, impaired renal excretion, limited iron stores with a predisposition to develop anemia, metabolic disturbances, and decreased ability to fight infection. Immunizations should take place at the same designated times as for term infants with no adjustments made for premature age. One exception to this recommendation is that hepatitis B vaccination should be delayed for 1 month if mothers are negative for hepatitis B surface antigen.

Additional Reading: General immunization practices. *Nelson Textbook of Pediatrics,* 19th ed. Philadelphia, PA: Elsevier/Saunders; 2011.

Category: Patient/population-based care

> Premature infants are predisposed to certain problems, including poor sucking and diminished gag and cough reflexes, which can lead to an increased risk of aspiration and difficulty feeding.

61. Which of the following conditions is associated with children of teenage mothers?
A) Cognitive delays in IQ
B) Schizophrenia
C) Major depression
D) Manic–depressive disorder
E) Suicide

Answer and Discussion

The answer is A. The children of teenage mothers have been shown to have cognitive delays on IQ and vocabulary tests. They may also show problems of emotion, including rebelliousness, aggressiveness, uncontrollable anger, and impulsiveness. They are at greater risk for low birth weight and they have an increased risk of experiencing an accident within the home and of being hospitalized before the age of 5 years. There appears to be no link with major affective disorders.

Additional Reading: Adolescent pregnancies. *Nelson Textbook of Pediatrics,* 19th ed. Philadelphia, PA: Elsevier/Saunders; 2011.

Category: Patient/population-based care

62. A 3-year-old boy presents with a bilateral conjunctivitis, cracking of his lips, cervical lymphadenopathy, and swelling of his hands. The most likely diagnosis is
A) Kawasaki's disease
B) Infectious mononucleosis
C) Scarlet fever
D) Rocky Mountain fever
E) Lyme's disease

Answer and Discussion

The answer is A. Kawasaki's disease was previously referred to as mucocutaneous lymph node syndrome. The cause of Kawasaki's disease is unclear, and unfortunately a specific diagnostic test for its detection does not exist. The majority of affected patients are younger than age 5 years, and boys are more frequently affected. Diagnosis is based on the following criteria and include fever for more than 5 days and at least four of the following features: (1) bilateral, painless, nonexudative conjunctivitis, (2) lip cracking and fissuring, strawberry tongue, inflammation of the oral mucosa, (3) cervical lymphadenopathy ($\geq$1.5 cm in diameter and usually unilateral), (4) exanthema, and (5) redness and swelling of the hands and feet with subsequent desquamation. Adverse cardiovascular effects are the most serious component of Kawasaki's disease. Cardiovascular complications include myocarditis, pericarditis, valvular heart disease (usually mitral or aortic regurgitation), and coronary arteritis. Coronary artery lesions range from mild transient dilation of a coronary artery to large aneurysm formation. Those at greatest risk of aneurysm formation are boys, children under the age of 6 months, and those not treated with intravenous immunoglobulin (IVIG). The gold standard for diagnosing coronary artery aneurysms is angiography; however, two-dimensional echocardiography is highly sensitive and is the current standard screening test in children with Kawasaki's disease. Fortunately, most coronary artery aneurysms resolve within 5 years of diagnosis. Giant aneurysms (>8 mm) are much less likely to resolve, and about half become stenotic. Of additional concern, acute thrombosis of an aneurysm can occur, resulting in a myocardial infarction, and can be fatal. The treatment of Kawasaki's disease consists of therapy with intravenous immunoglobulin and high-dose aspirin. This therapy is effective in decreasing the incidence of coronary artery dilation and aneurysm formation. Currently, corticosteroids are not felt to be effective in Kawasaki's disease.

During the acute and subacute phases of the illness, patients should be monitored closely by serial electrocardiography, chest radiograph, and echocardiography. Selective coronary angiography is recommended in patients with evidence of myocardial ischemia.

Additional Reading: Kawasaki disease. *Nelson Textbook of Pediatrics,* 19th ed. Philadelphia, PA: Elsevier/Saunders; 2011.

Category: Cardiovascular system

63. The major difference between stuttering and developmental dysfluency is
A) Stuttering involves repetition of word parts and prolongation of sounds
B) Stuttering involves repetition of whole words and phrases
C) Stutterers tend to speak more slowly than those with developmental dysfluency
D) Those affected with developmental dysfluency are more easily frustrated
E) Those with developmental dysfluency may display inappropriate articulating postures

Answer and Discussion

The answer is A. The etiology of stuttering is controversial. Majority of stuttering cases are classified as developmental problems, although stuttering can also be classified as a neurologic or, less commonly, psychogenic problem. Stutterers also have difficulty coordinating airflow, articulation, and resonance. In addition, small asynchronies have also been found in the fluent speech of stutterers. Stuttering is a common disorder that usually resolves by adulthood. Boys are more frequently affected, and there appears to be an increased genetic risk. Generally, there is cause for concern if a patient's speech has five or more breaks per 100 words. Almost 80% of children who stutter recover fluency by the age of 16 years. Mild stuttering is self-limited, but more severe stuttering requires speech therapy, which is the mainstay of treatment. Delayed auditory feedback and computer-assisted training are currently used to help slow down speech and control other speech mechanisms. Pharmacologic therapy is seldom used, although haloperidol has been somewhat effective. Differentiating between normal developmental dysfluency and stuttering is important. In general, developmental dysfluency involves the repetition of whole words and phrases, whereas stuttering involves the repetition of word parts and the prolongation of sounds. In addition, stutterers frequently speak at a faster tempo, display silent pauses, have inappropriate articulating postures, become more dysfluent in response to stress, and are more easily frustrated.

Additional Reading: Stuttering: an overview. *Am Fam Physician.* 2008;77(9):1271–1276.

Category: Special sensory

64. Bites from which of the following animals require rabies postexposure prophylaxis?
A) Fox
B) Squirrel
C) Hamster
D) Gerbil
E) Rat

Answer and Discussion

The answer is A. Rabies in humans is rare in the United States, but the CDC estimates that as many as 39,000 persons receive postexposure prophylaxis annually. The risk of infection must be carefully evaluated by the clinician in the management of potential human rabies exposures. Bats, skunks, raccoons, foxes, and most other carnivores should receive postexposure prophylaxis. Bites of squirrels, hamsters, guinea pigs, gerbils, chipmunks, rats, mice, other small rodents, rabbits, and hares almost never require antirabies postexposure prophylaxis. The CDC considers administration of postexposure prophylaxis to be a medical urgency, not a medical emergency, although Advisory Committee on Immunization Practices (ACIP) emphasizes that decisions about using prophylaxis should not be put off.

Additional Reading: Human rabies prevention—United States, 2008 Recommendations of the Advisory Committee on Immunization Practices (ACIP). *MMWR.* 2008;57(RR-3):1–28.

Category: Nonspecific system

65. Which of the following is a clinical finding of coarctation of the aorta?
A) Bounding femoral pulses
B) Blood pressure higher in the legs than in the arms in infants older than 1 year of age
C) Rib notching on chest radiograph
D) Diastolic murmur heard at the apex, radiating to the axilla
E) Dilation of the thoracic aorta near the ligamentum arteriosus

Answer and Discussion

The answer is C. Coarctation of the aorta is one of the more common congenital heart defects (CHDs). Boys are more commonly affected than girls. The condition occurs when there is discrete narrowing of the thoracic aorta near the ligamentum arteriosus, leading to proximal hypertension and left ventricular overload. Other findings include a ventricular septal defect, patent ductus arteriosus, and bicuspid aortic valve. In most cases, those affected are asymptomatic during infancy. However, congestive heart failure can occur and may require immediate surgical intervention. Signs associated with coarctation of the aorta include diminished or absent femoral pulses, blood pressure higher in the arms than in the legs in infants older than 1 year, 2/6 to 3/6 systolic ejection murmur heard over the apex and upper left sternal border, rib notching on chest radiograph (which is a result of enlargement of the intercostal arteries), and left ventricular hypertrophy. Diagnosis is based on physical findings and echocardiography or with CT or MRI angiography. Treatment depends on the severity of coarctation and the heart's ability to maintain perfusion. In severe cases, prostaglandin E_1 may be used to keep a patent ductus arteriosus dilated until surgery or balloon angioplasty can be performed. In more stable patients, β-blockers and afterload-reducing agents can be used to postpone definitive treatment until the child is 3 to 5 years of age, when the treatment can be performed electively. Those patients who do well initially without evidence of congestive heart failure and requiring no surgery usually do quite well regarding further complications in childhood and adolescence. Those affected are at risk for hypertension and cardiac dysfunction as well as subacute infective endocarditis.

Additional Reading: Coarctation of the aorta. *Nelson Textbook of Pediatrics,* 19th ed. Philadelphia, PA: Elsevier/Saunders; 2011.

Category: Cardiovascular system

66. Which of the following statements about cystic fibrosis is true?
A) It is an autosomal-dominant transmitted disease.
B) The condition is associated with pancreatic insufficiency.
C) It is commonly diagnosed with a pulmonary function test.
D) Those affected do not live beyond 20 years of age.
E) Fertility is not affected in those with cystic fibrosis.

Answer and Discussion

The answer is B. Cystic fibrosis is the most common fatal genetic disease in the United States. It is transmitted as an autosomal-recessive trait. The incidence in the United States is reported to be approximately 1:3,500 in whites and 1:17,000 in African Americans. Those who are heterozygous are unaffected. The disorder involves exocrine glands and affects predominantly the GI and respiratory systems. Complications include meconium ileus present at birth, chronic cough and wheezing with copious mucous production, pancreatic insufficiency with possible development of insulin-dependent diabetes (up to 8%), retarded growth, infertility, and chronic obstructive pulmonary disease. The diagnosis is made by the pilocarpine iontophoresis sweat test. Levels of sodium and chloride >60 mEq/L are usually diagnostic. Survival beyond 30 years of age is occurring more frequently. Death usually results from pulmonary complications such as infections with *S. aureus, Pseudomonas aeruginosa,* and *H. influenzae.*

Additional Reading: Cystic fibrosis. *Nelson Textbook of Pediatrics,* 19th ed. Philadelphia, PA: Elsevier/Saunders; 2011.

Category: Nonspecific system

67. Of the following antibiotics, which one would be acceptable to use when treating penicillin-resistant *S. pneumoniae* otitis media?
A) Azithromycin
B) Clarithromycin
C) Cefuroxime
D) Cefaclor
E) Cephalexin

Answer and Discussion

The answer is C. Only five antibiotics—high-dose amoxicillin (80 mg/kg/day), amoxicillin-clavulanate, cefuroxime, cefprozil (Cefzil), and ceftriaxone—have demonstrated a modest degree (60% to 80%) of clinical efficacy in the treatment of AOM caused by penicillin-resistant *S. pneumoniae*.

Additional Reading: The diagnosis and management of acute otitis. *Pediatrics.* 2013;131(3):e964–e999.

Category: Special sensory system

68. A 3-year-old boy presents to your office with a history of seven ear infections over the last year. Appropriate management of this child consists of
A) Tonsillectomy and adenoidectomy
B) Single-dose prophylactic antibiotics given at night
C) Tympanostomy tube placement
D) Long-term use of antihistamine-decongestant preparations
E) Continued observation

Answer and Discussion

The answer is B. Chronic otitis media usually results from AOM and eustachian tube dysfunction. Despite short courses of antibiotics, affected children have recurrent infections that appear to be more prevalent in the winter months. Persistent chronic otitis media may lead to hearing deficits and subsequent language delays. Prophylaxis should be attempted if the child experiences more than four infections in 1 year or three or more infections within 6 months. Treatment for this difficult problem consists of prophylactic antibiotics given in a single dose at bedtime. Medications for chronic suppression therapy include amoxicillin, sulfisoxazole, or trimethoprim–sulfamethoxazole. If a sulfonamide is used, the child should have a CBC periodically, and parents or guardians should be instructed to discontinue the medication immediately if a rash or mouth sore develops. Steroid use has not been advocated, and myringotomy tube placement should be reserved for children in whom prophylactic therapy fails.

Additional Reading: The diagnosis and management of acute otitis. *Pediatrics.* 2013;131(3):e964–e999.

Category: Special sensory

69. Which of the following statements about breast-feeding is true?
A) The infant should feed on each side for 8 to 15 minutes every 2 to 3 hours after birth.
B) Colostrum is excreted 7 to 10 days after delivery and contains important antibodies, high calories, and other nutrients.
C) The mother should weigh infants before and after feeding to quantify the amount consumed.
D) Breast-feeding usually provides adequate nutrition for 2 to 4 months; supplementation should begin at that point.
E) Breast-feeding should be based on timed intervals rather than on demand.

Answer and Discussion

The answer is A. Breast-feeding is encouraged for all mothers. Currently, as many as 50% of mothers (especially those in higher socioeconomic groups) breast-feed. In most cases, the infant should feed at each breast for 8 to 15 minutes every 2 to 3 hours after birth and can be started immediately after delivery. *Colostrum,* a yellowish fluid excreted from the breast immediately after delivery, contains important antibodies, high calories, and high proteins, as well as other nutrients and helps stimulate the passage of meconium. Some studies have shown that delaying breast-feeding, trying to quantify amounts of feeding with prefeed and postfeed weights, and providing infant formula decrease the percentage of women who breast-feed by discouraging the practice. Breast-feeding is usually adequate nutrition for 6 to 9 months. If mothers develop sore nipples, they should be counseled with regard to proper positioning of the baby's mouth on the breast. The production of a lubricant from Montgomery's glands occurs and helps protect the breast from excessive drying. Typically, breast-fed infants require more frequent feedings than bottle-fed infants. Breast-feeding should occur based on demand rather than by the clock. Breast engorgement can be avoided with more frequent feedings or manual expression of excessive milk production with breast pumps. New mothers should initiate breast-feeding as soon as possible after giving birth. When mothers initiate breast-feeding within one-half hour of birth, the baby's suckling reflex is strongest, and the baby is more alert. Early breast-feeding is associated with fewer nighttime feeding problems and better mother–infant communication. Babies who are put to breast earlier have been shown to have higher core temperatures and less temperature instability.

Additional Reading: Strategies of breastfeeding success. *Am Fam Physician.* 2008;78(2):225–232.

Category: Patient/population-based care

70. The most common bacterial pathogen associated with lung infections in adolescents is
A) Adenovirus
B) *Streptococcus pneumoniae*
C) *H. influenzae*
D) *Mycoplasma pneumoniae*
E) *Chlamydia*

Answer and Discussion

The answer is D. *Mycoplasma* is the most common pathogen responsible for lung infections in patients between 5 and 35 years of age. It may involve close contacts, school children, military recruits, and family members and is spread via respiratory droplets. Symptoms include malaise, sore throat, coryza, myalgias, and an increasing productive cough of mucopurulent or blood-streaked sputum. A maculopapular rash occurs in 10% to 20%. Unlike Pneumococcal pneumonia, the course is less severe. Bullous myringitis has also been associated with *Mycoplasma* infections. Chest radiographs of those affected with *Mycoplasma* pneumonia show patchy infiltrates in the lower lobes and, rarely, lobar consolidation. The WBC count may be normal or mildly elevated. Diagnosis can be made with acute and convalescent titers but is unnecessary. The drug of choice for treatment is a macrolide antibiotic. Alternative medications include fluoroquinolones and tetracyclines. Because the *Mycoplasma* organism does not have a cell wall, the β-lactam antibiotics are ineffective.

Additional Reading: Community-acquired pneumonia. *Nelson Textbook of Pediatrics,* 19th ed. Philadelphia, PA: Elsevier/Saunders; 2011.

Category: Respiratory system

> *Mycoplasma* is the most common pathogen responsible for lung infections in patients between 5 and 35 years of age.

71. The major complication of slipped capital femoral epiphysis is
A) Avascular necrosis of the hip
B) Osteochondritis dissecans
C) Leg-length discrepancy
D) Transient synovitis of the hip
E) Intoeing

Answer and Discussion

The answer is A. Slipped capital femoral epiphysis typically occurs during the adolescent growth spurt and is most frequent in obese children. In many cases, both hips are affected. Most cases of slipped capital femoral epiphyses are stable and have a good prognosis if diagnosed early in their course. Unstable slipped capital femoral epiphysis has a worse prognosis because of the high risk of avascular necrosis. Early radiographic clues are the metaphyseal blanch sign and Klein's line. Once diagnosed, treatment in most cases includes surgical pinning.

> **Additional Reading:** The hip. *Nelson Textbook of Pediatrics,* 19th ed. Philadelphia, PA: Elsevier/Saunders; 2011.

> **Category:** Musculoskeletal system

72. In December, a 4-month-old infant is brought to the emergency room. The parents report the child has had a runny nose, fever, cough, and audible wheezing. The child is attending a day care center, and other children have had similar symptoms. On examination, the child has some rales, wheezing, and intercostal retractions with grunting. The most likely infecting organism is
A) *S. pneumoniae*
B) *H. influenzae*
C) Adenovirus
D) RSV
E) Coxsackievirus

Answer and Discussion

The answer is D. RSV is a pneumovirus that usually affects children between 1 and 6 months of age, with a peak incidence at 2 to 3 months of age. The commonly encountered virus gives rise to bronchiolitis and pneumonia. The virus occurs during the winter months and is characterized by rhinorrhea, fever, cough, and wheezing; in more severe cases, tachypnea, dyspnea, and hypoxia are present. The virus is spread by close contacts via fomites and respiratory secretions and tends to occur in outbreaks in places such as day care centers. Physical examination shows nasal flaring, rales, and wheezing as well as intercostal retractions with grunting in infants. Laboratory evaluation usually shows a normal leukocyte count with elevated granulocytes. Chest radiographs may show hyperexpansion, areas of atelectasis, and/or bronchopneumonia. The virus may be quickly detected by immunofluorescence microscopy of nasal swabs or enzyme-linked immunoassay antigen detection tests. Treatment of URIs is usually symptomatic. Lower respiratory infections may be treated with supplemental oxygen and hydration. Bronchodilators and corticosteroids are not generally helpful. Aerosolized ribavirin (an antiviral agent) is no longer recommended except in severely immunocompromised patients. Respiratory support may be necessary in severe cases.

> **Additional Reading:** Respiratory syncytial virus. *Nelson Textbook of Pediatrics,* 19th ed. Philadelphia, PA: Elsevier/Saunders; 2011.

> **Category:** Respiratory system

73. Of the following, which is the first sign of sexual development in girls?
A) The presence of axillary hair
B) The development of pubic hair
C) Menstruation
D) Development of breast buds
E) Closure of the epiphyseal growth plate

Answer and Discussion

The answer is D. The development of breast buds (subareolar tissue) is usually the first sign of puberty (8 to 13 years of age). This is followed closely by the development of pubic hair (6 to 12 months later) and then axillary hair. The growth spurt often begins even before the development of breast buds. Menarche usually occurs 2.0 to 2.5 years after the development of the breast buds. Growth in height occurs predominantly before menarche and then slows thereafter. As the young girl's body changes, the percentage of body fat increases and redistributes, giving rise to adult contours. *Precocious puberty* is defined as the presence of breast development or pubic hair before 8 years of age. *Pubertal delay* is defined as absence of breast development before the age of 13 years or the lack of menstruation 5 years after breast growth.

> **Additional Reading:** Physiology of puberty. *Nelson Textbook of Pediatrics,* 19th ed. Philadelphia, PA: Elsevier/Saunders; 2011.

> **Category:** Reproductive system

74. Which of the following patient group-treatment scenarios is appropriate for the treatment/exposure of bacterial meningitis?
A) Neonates—ampicillin and cefotaxime
B) 1 month to 10 years of age—ampicillin and gentamicin
C) 10 to 18 years old—cefuroxime and erythromycin
D) Adults—ampicillin and metronidazole
E) Isoniazid for individuals exposed to meningococcal meningitis

Answer and Discussion

The answer is A. The treatment of bacterial meningitis depends on the age of the patient. In neonates, the common infecting organisms include group B or D streptococci, *Listeria,* and gram-negative organisms such as *E. coli.* Recommended treatment includes ampicillin and cefotaxime until susceptibilities are known. In infants and children 1 month to 10 years of age, the common infecting organisms include pneumococci and meningococci. Combination therapy is recommended and includes ampicillin, vancomycin, and cefotaxime or ceftriaxone. Various combinations should be confirmed on the basis of local sensitivities and most recent recommendations. For patients allergic to penicillin, vancomycin and rifampin may be considered. In addition to intravenous antibiotics, dexamethasone may decrease the incidence of permanent neurologic and audiologic complications and should be administered.

Family members, nursery school children, and other close contacts of those affected by meningococcal or *H. influenzae* meningitis should also receive rifampin as a prophylactic measure.

> **Additional Reading:** The inner ear and diseases of the bony labyrinth. *Nelson Textbook of Pediatrics,* 19th ed. Philadelphia, PA: Elsevier/Saunders; 2011.

> **Category:** Neurologic system

75. Conductive hearing loss noted in children may be caused by
A) Meningitis
B) Medications
C) Chronic eustachian tube dysfunction
D) Intracranial hemorrhage
E) Chronic exposure to loud noises

Answer and Discussion

The answer is C. Signs of hearing loss may include delayed speech development, behavioral problems, and impaired comprehension. Hearing loss can be categorized as conductive or sensorineural. Conductive hearing loss is usually caused by otitis media with effusion. Other causes include foreign bodies in the ear, allergies, or chronic eustachian tube dysfunction. Sensorineural hearing loss can be caused by meningitis and other congenital infections, intracranial hemorrhage, chronic noise exposure, congenital defects, medications that are ototoxic, and trauma. Although hearing screening has been mandated in 34 states for all children, absolute indications for audiologic evaluation include premature birth (birth weight <2,500 g or birth weight >2,500 g with complications including asphyxia, seizures, intracranial hemorrhage, hyperbilirubinemia, persistent fetal circulation, and assisted ventilation), intrauterine infection, bacterial meningitis, anomalies of the first or second branchial arch, anomalies of the neural crest or ectoderm, family history of hereditary or unexplained deafness, parental concern, and delayed speech or language development or other disabilities (including mental retardation, autism, cerebral palsy, and blindness). Infants are tested using either otoacoustic emissions (OAE) or auditory brain stem–evoked responses (ABR). The auditory brain stem–evoked response uses external scalp electrodes to detect waveforms that occur in predictable patterns after an auditory stimulus. The prompt recognition of hearing problems in children can help prevent delays in language development.

> **Additional Reading:** Hearing loss. *Nelson Textbook of Pediatrics*, 19th ed. Philadelphia, PA: Elsevier/Saunders; 2011.

> **Category:** Special sensory

76. In boys, the first sign of puberty is
A) Development of pubic hair
B) Testicular enlargement
C) Spermarche
D) Enlargement of the penis
E) Skeletal growth spurt

Answer and Discussion

The answer is B. At the onset of puberty, boys have testicular enlargement followed by the appearance of pubic hair, enlargement of the penis, and spermarche. Skeletal and muscle growth are late events in male puberty. The age at which pubertal milestones are attained varies among the population studied and is influenced by activity level and nutritional status.

> **Additional Reading:** Physiology of puberty. *Nelson Textbook of Pediatrics*, 19th ed. Philadelphia, PA: Elsevier/Saunders; 2011.

> **Category:** Reproductive system

77. Which of the following conditions is associated with giving whole milk to infants younger than 1 year?
A) Iron-deficiency anemia
B) Inflammatory bowel disease
C) Mental retardation
D) Hirschsprung's disease
E) None of the above

Answer and Discussion

The answer is A. This condition has a variety of causes, including inadequate iron stores at birth because of prematurity, fetal–maternal blood loss, iron-deficient mother, or lack of iron ingestion by the child that fails to keep up with expanding blood volume as the child grows (especially between 9 and 18 months of age); in older adolescent patients, it may be caused by menstrual blood loss. Whole milk given to infants younger than 1 year may also cause chronic irritation of the colon, resulting in blood loss and development of iron-deficiency anemia. The U.S. Preventive Services Task Force recommends that high-risk infants be screened for iron-deficiency anemia between 6 and 12 months of age. Screening for iron-deficiency anemia is not recommended in the general infant population because of low overall prevalence. The CDC has developed specific criteria for anemia: hemoglobin levels <11.0 g/dL (110 g/L) for children between 6 months and 5 years of age. In 1993, it was estimated that the prevalence of iron-deficiency anemia among children younger than 5 years was <3%, and most cases were mild; however, among high-risk groups, the prevalence may be up to 30%. Increased prevalence of iron-deficiency anemia occurs among African Americans, Native Americans, Alaska Natives, persons of low socioeconomic status, preterm and low-birth-weight infants, immigrants from developing countries, and infants whose primary nutritional source is unfortified cow's milk.

Strategies to prevent iron-deficiency anemia among infants are recommended. Family physicians should discuss issues of infant nutrition with expectant and new parents and encourage the consumption of iron-fortified formulas and cereals or encourage breast-feeding supplemented with iron-fortified cereals between the ages of 4 and 6 months.

> **Additional Reading:** Iron deficiency anemia: evaluation and management. *Am Fam Physician.* 2013;87(2):98–104.

> **Category:** Hematologic system

78. A 14-year-old boy presents with tenderness associated with the right breast. There are no other findings. Testicular examination is unremarkable. Appropriate management of this patient includes
A) Mammogram
B) Ultrasound of the breast
C) Genetic typing
D) Biopsy
E) Reassurance and continued observation

Answer and Discussion

The answer is E. Benign gynecomastia of adolescence is a very common finding among boys in middle to late puberty. The breast tissue is usually asymmetric and often tender to palpation. Provided the history and physical examination, including palpation of the testicles, are unremarkable, reassurance and periodic reevaluation are all that is necessary. Most cases resolve in 1 to 2 years. Familial gynecomastia is a common genetic disorder transmitted as a X-linked recessive trait or a sex-limited dominant trait causing limited breast development around the time of puberty. It requires no further evaluation in an otherwise normal boy unless there is evidence of hypogonadism. In rare cases, those with severe gynecomastia may require cosmetic surgery. Pathologic gynecomastia occurs in cases of Klinefelter's syndrome and prolactin-secreting adenomas and with a wide variety of drug use including marijuana and phenothiazines.

> **Additional Reading:** Gynecomastia. *Nelson Textbook of Pediatrics*, 19th ed. Philadelphia, PA: Elsevier/Saunders; 2011.

> **Category:** Integumentary

79. Which of the following is the medication of choice for the treatment of pinworms (*Enterobius vermicularis*)?
A) Mebendazole (Vermox)
B) Permethrin (Elimite)
C) Metronidazole (Flagyl)
D) Oral vancomycin (Vancocin)
E) Tetracycline (Achromycin)

Answer and Discussion

The answer is A. Pinworms is a common pediatric infection caused by the parasite *Enterobius vermicularis*. The parasite is a small (1 cm) white worm that lives in the bowel (usually the cecum) and often migrates out of the anus at night to deposit eggs on the perianal skin, giving rise to severe and intense pruritus. Children aged 5 to 10 years are predominantly affected. Young children may not be able to sleep, and rectal and vulvar inflammation may be evident. In many cases, the entire family may be affected through a fecal–oral route. Diagnosis can be made by visualizing the worms or applying cellophane tape to the anal area in the morning before bathing and observing for ova with microscopy (cellophane tape test). Treatment involves the administration of mebendazole (Vermox) in one dose, followed by a repeat dose 2 weeks later. Albendazole or pyrantel pamoate may be substituted for mebendazole. In most cases, the entire household should be treated. Other treatment recommendations include laundering of all bedclothes and underwear.

Additional Reading: Pinworms. *Nelson Textbook of Pediatrics,* 19th ed. Philadelphia, PA: Elsevier/Saunders; 2011.

Category: Nonspecific system

> Treatment of pinworms (*Enterobius vermicularis*) involves the administration of mebendazole (Vermox) in one dose, followed by a repeat dose 2 weeks later.

80. Which of the following drugs is concentrated in breast milk and should be avoided by women who are breast-feeding?
A) Heparin
B) Alcohol
C) Digoxin
D) Penicillin
E) Amitriptyline

Answer and Discussion

The answer is B. Medications that are classified as weak bases are usually concentrated in breast milk. Contraindicated drugs include anticancer drugs, therapeutic doses of radiopharmaceuticals, ergot and its derivatives (e.g., methysergide), lithium, chloramphenicol, atropine, thiouracil, iodides, and mercurials. These drugs should not be used in nursing mothers, or nursing should be stopped if any of these drugs is essential. Other drugs to be avoided in the absence of studies on their excretion in breast milk are those with long half-lives, those that are potent toxins to the bone marrow, and those given in high doses long term. However, drugs that are so poorly absorbed orally that they are given (to the mother) parenterally pose no threat to the infant, who would receive the drug orally but not absorb it.

Nicotine and alcohol are concentrated in breast milk and should be avoided by mothers who are breast-feeding. Other drugs, including heparin, acetaminophen, insulin, diuretics, digoxin, β-blockers, penicillins, cephalosporins, most over-the-counter cold remedies, amitriptyline, codeine, and ibuprofen, do not show up in significant amounts in breast milk. Some oral contraceptives can depress lactation (particularly large-dose, estradiol-containing birth control pills), but in most cases are considered safe.

Additional Reading: Strategies of breastfeeding success. *Am Fam Physician.* 2008;78(2):225–232.

Category: Patient/population-based care

81. A 3-year-old who attends day school is seen in the middle of June. The parent reports that the child has had profuse watery diarrhea. Laboratory tests of the stool sample show leukocytes, red blood cells (RBCs), and small comma-shaped bacteria that have a corkscrew motion. The most likely diagnosis is
A) *Salmonella* infection
B) *Shigella* infection
C) *Rotavirus* infection
D) *Campylobacter* infection
E) *Escherichia coli* infection

Answer and Discussion

The answer is D. *Campylobacter* is an intestinal infection that can lead to profuse watery diarrhea. It is considered one of the most common causes of bacterial gastroenteritis. In many cases, it affects young infants, particularly those in day care centers; it is more common in the summer months. Associated foods include contaminated milk or water, poultry, and beef. Chickens are the classic source of *Campylobacter;* however, essentially all food sources can harbor the bacteria. In addition, pets can carry *Campylobacter*. Symptoms include loose, watery stools or bloody and mucus-containing stools. Fever, vomiting, malaise, and myalgia are common. Abdominal pain is usually periumbilical and cramping in nature. Children severely affected may show signs of dehydration. Laboratory tests of stool samples show leukocytes, RBCs, and small comma-shaped bacteria that have a characteristic corkscrew motion. In most cases, antibiotics are unnecessary; however, antibiotics such as the quinolones (not used in children), erythromycin, doxycycline, and gentamicin are recommended for patients with the dysenteric form of the disease, high fever or severe course and for immuosuppressed, underlying diseases or carrier state. Sepsis is treated with parenteral aminoglycoside, meropenem or imipenem. After treatment, repeat stool cultures should be performed to ensure eradication. Fecal shedding of the organisms can last up to 2 to 3 weeks in untreated patients. Severe cases or those immunosuppressed should be treated.

Additional Reading: *Campylobacter. Nelson Textbook of Pediatrics,* 19th ed. Philadelphia, PA: Elsevier/Saunders; 2011.

Category: Gastrointestinal system

82. In the United States, deficiencies of which of the following are common in adolescents?
A) Iron
B) Vitamin B_{12}
C) Folate
D) Thiamine
E) Calcium

Answer and Discussion

The answer is E. In the United States, only a minority of adolescents receive the recommended daily allowance of calcium. As a result, there is the possibility of a future epidemic of osteopenia or even osteoporosis in normal individuals who have calcium deficiency.

Additional Reading: Rickets and hypervitaminosis D: calcium deficiency. *Nelson Textbook of Pediatrics*, 19th ed. Philadelphia, PA: Elsevier/Saunders; 2011.

Category: Patient/population-based care

83. A 6-month-old infant is brought in for a well-child visit. The growth chart shows the child's growth has slowed when compared with the growth curve expected for his age despite adequate caloric intake. The most appropriate action is
A) To increase feeding amounts
B) To reassure the family that this is a common finding and that no further workup is necessary
C) To order laboratory tests, including a CBC, electrolyte levels, serum glucose levels, and urinalysis
D) To consult social services
E) To start nutritional supplement

Answer and Discussion
The answer is C. Failure to thrive in childhood is a state of undernutrition due to inadequate caloric intake, inadequate caloric absorption, or excessive caloric expenditure. In the United States, it is seen in 5% to 10% of children in primary care settings. A combination of anthropometric criteria more accurately identify children at risk of failure to thrive (FTT). Weight for length is a better indicator of acute undernutrition and identifies children who need prompt nutritional treatment. Weight less that 70% of the 50th percentile on the weight-for-length curve is indicator of severe malnutrition.

Most cases involved not only behavioral or psychosocial issues but also biologic and environmental processes. It is a very important part to obtain an accurate account of the child's eating habits and caloric intake. Routine laboratory testing is not generally recommended. Reasons for hospitalization include failure of outpatient management, suspicion of abuse or neglect, or severe psychosocial impairment of caregiver. Multidisciplinary treatment approach, including home nursing visits and nutritional support, has been shown to improve weight gain, parent–child relationship, and cognitive development.

Additional Reading: Failure to thrive: an update. *Am Fam Physician.* 2011;83(7):829–834.

Category: Endocrine system

84. Variation in a young patient's electrocardiogram pattern is noted with respiration. The rhythm remains sinus rhythm. The most appropriate action is
A) Reassurance to patient and family
B) Holter monitoring
C) Cardiology consultation
D) Administration of β-blockers
E) Synchronized cardioversion

Answer and Discussion
The answer is A. Sinus arrhythmia is usually noted in young, healthy patients and represents no concern for underlying pathology. The variation in heart rate is affected by normal respirations and is associated with the alternating increases and decreases in vagal and sympathetic tone. Patients report no symptoms, and no treatment is required.

Additional Reading: Disturbances of rate and rhythm of the heart. *Nelson Textbook of Pediatrics*, 19th ed. Philadelphia, PA: Elsevier/Saunders; 2011.

Category: Cardiovascular system

85. A 3-year-old boy is diagnosed with constitutional growth delay. The workup is unremarkable. The most appropriate management is
A) Vitamin E supplementation
B) Administration of prednisone
C) Monitoring of thyroid function tests every 3 months
D) Reassurance to parents
E) Nutritional consult

Answer and Discussion
The answer is D. Constitutional growth delay is one variant of normal growth. Length and weight measurements of affected children are normal at birth, and growth is normal for the first 4 to 12 months of life. Growth then decelerates to near or below the third percentile for height and weight. By 2 to 3 years of age, growth resumes at a normal rate of 5 cm/year or more. The majority of these children is male and have a bone age that is appropriate for height age but are delayed relative to their chronologic age. Some of these children experience delayed puberty but eventually complete normal development without complications. Reassurance to the parent is the most appropriate management for children who are at Tanner stage 2 or 3, do not have underlying chronic disease, and have skeletal age-appropriate height as they grow older. The parents can be reassured that the child will go through a growth spurt in the near future, and no further testing is warranted. Although the child may end up being shorter than his or her peers, the child usually follows growth patterns of the parents. Only in extremely severe cases, medications such as anabolic and androgenic steroids are considered.

Additional Reading: Hypopituitarism. *Nelson Textbook of Pediatrics*, 19th ed. Philadelphia, PA: Elsevier/Saunders; 2011.

Category: Endocrinology

86. A 3-year-old child presents with high fever, prostration, and purpuric rash. Appropriate management should be
A) Administration of oral antibiotics with next-day follow-up
B) Hospitalization, intravenous antibiotics, and close observation
C) To obtain throat culture and treat if positive for strep
D) Symptomatic measures for likely viral infection
E) To check Lyme's disease titers

Answer and Discussion
The answer is B. Meningococcemia is a severe infection that is caused by *Neisseria meningitidis*. The mode of transmission is through infected respiratory secretions. The onset is usually abrupt, and the course can be fulminant despite treatment. Symptoms include fever, chills, fatigue, and prostration. A distinctive petechial or purpuric rash develops. Fulminant disease can result in disseminated intravascular coagulopathy and septic shock. Children younger than 5 years are the most commonly affected. In many cases, meningitis results and can be fatal (5% of patients). Diagnosis can be made with an antigen detection test of the blood, cerebrospinal fluid, and urine. Cultures can also be used but typically require longer amounts of time. Treatment involves the use of high-dose intravenous penicillin G, ampicillin, central nervous system–penetrating cephalosporins, and chloramphenicol in an intensive care unit setting. Exposed household, day school, or school contacts should receive chemoprophylaxis with rifampin. Ceftriaxone and ciprofloxacin are also prophylactic substitutes for adults. Meningococcal vaccination should be given to individuals at risk (e.g., asplenic individuals, travelers in high-risk areas, college students living in dorms, military recruits, and patients with complement deficiencies). Newer recommendations may include universal administration.

Additional Reading: Bacterial meningitis. *Nelson Textbook of Pediatrics*, 19th ed. Philadelphia, PA: Elsevier/Saunders; 2011.

Category: Nonspecific system

87. Which statement regarding metatarsus adductus is true?
A) Metatarsus adductus is the rarest of foot disorders to affect children.
B) Intoeing rarely occurs as a result of metatarsus adductus.
C) Boys are more commonly affected.
D) Surgery is rarely needed.
E) Stretching exercises are rarely effective.

Answer and Discussion

The answer is D. Metatarsus adductus is the most common congenital foot deformity seen in children. Girls are more commonly affected, and the left side is more commonly affected. The most likely cause is positioning while in utero. Examination reveals adduction of the forefoot with a convex lateral border. The ankle has normal motion. The foot should be assessed for flexibility by holding the heel in neutral position and abducting the forefoot to at least a neutral position. If this cannot be done, then the deformity is rigid (i.e., metatarsus varus). The majority of cases of metatarsus adductus noted at birth resolve without treatment by 1 year of age. Flexible metatarsus adductus is managed by stretching exercises during the first 8 months of life. Parents are instructed to hold the infant's hindfoot in one hand, the forefoot in the other, and stretch the midfoot, opening the "C"-shaped curve and slightly overcorrecting it. Flexible deformities that persist beyond 8 months, and rigid deformities, may need a cast application. Improved results occur if treatment is started before 8 months of age. Casts should be changed biweekly with correction usually achieved after three or four casts. Residual adductus causes no long-term disability. Surgery is not typically recommended because of the risk of complications.

Additional Reading: The foot and toes. *Nelson Textbook of Pediatrics*, 19th ed. Philadelphia, PA: Elsevier/Saunders; 2011.

Category: Musculoskeletal system

88. Which of the following immunizations may result in a false-negative purified protein derivative (PPD) tuberculosis test?
A) Tetanus
B) Hepatitis B
C) Pneumococcal
D) Influenza
E) MMR

Answer and Discussion

The answer is E. Some persons (e.g., anergic patients, those with recent viral infections or those recently treated with live virus vaccines) may not react to the tuberculin skin test even though they are truly infected with *Mycobacterium tuberculosis*. Of those discussed, only the MMR is a live virus.

Additional Reading: Tuberculosis: tuberculin skin testing. *Nelson Textbook of Pediatrics*, 19th ed. Philadelphia, PA: Elsevier/Saunders; 2011.

Category: Patient/population-based care

89. Which of the following is the treatment of choice for pertussis?
A) Penicillin G
B) Amphotericin B
C) Erythromycin
D) Ciprofloxacin
E) Metronidazole

Answer and Discussion

The answer is C. Pertussis is a highly contagious (gram-negative rod) bacterial disease caused by *Bordetella pertussis*. The disease is characterized by a short paroxysmal cough that ends with an inspiratory whoop. The incubation period is usually 7 to 21 days. Transmission occurs through a respiratory route. The disease is divided into three stages:

1. The *catarrhal stage* is characterized by sneezing, lacrimation, decreased appetite, fatigue, coryza, and a cough that usually becomes diurnal and lasts 10 to 14 days.
2. The *paroxysmal stage* is characterized by the whooping cough; vomiting as a result of the persistent cough may occur; this stage may last up to 4 weeks.
3. The *convalescent stage* involves a slow improvement of the cough and constitutional symptoms.

The entire episode may last up to 3 months. Diagnosis is made with a nasopharyngeal swab. Treatment involves the use of erythromycin. Household or other close contacts should also be treated with oral erythromycin. Most patients may return to their regular activity 5 days after the administration of erythromycin. In adults and infants younger than 6 months, the classic whoop may not occur, but the diagnosis should be considered with a cough lasting more than 2 weeks. Parapertussis, caused by *Bordetella parapertussis,* is a similar illness and is clinically indistinguishable from pertussis, except it usually has a milder course and fewer complications.

Additional Reading: Pertussis. *Nelson Textbook of Pediatrics*, 19th ed. Philadelphia, PA: Elsevier/Saunders; 2011.

Category: Respiratory system

> Parapertussis, caused by *Bordetella parapertussis*, is a similar illness and is clinically indistinguishable from pertussis, except it usually has a milder course and fewer complications.

90. A 4-year-old presents with impetigo associated with the knee. No other areas are involved. The most appropriate treatment is
A) Topical mupirocin
B) Topical bacitracin
C) Topical neomycin
D) Topical polymyxin B
E) Oral cefalexin

Answer and Discussion

The answer is A. Impetigo is a contagious superficial skin infection most commonly seen in children, with a peak incidence between the ages of 2 and 6 years. The condition is the most common skin infection affecting children. Causative agents include group A beta-hemolytic streptococci (GABHS) and *Staphylococcus aureus*. Complications such as cellulitis, lymphangitis, and septicemia are rare and result from spread of the infection. The infection is transmitted via direct contact with the lesion. Antibiotic administration is the mainstay of therapy. If the area of affected skin is limited, mupirocin is an effective topical therapy and has been shown to be more effective than the other topical antibiotics (i.e., neomycin, bacitracin, polymyxin B, and gentamicin). There is insufficient evidence to determine whether oral antibiotics are better than topical agents in patients with more extensive disease, although there are obvious practical reasons to choose oral agents if large amounts of skin are involved. Antibiotic categories to consider include penicillins, cephalosporins, and macrolides. Oral antibiotics have significantly more side effects, especially GI effects, than topical agents.

Additional Reading: Impetigo. *Nelson Textbook of Pediatrics*, 19th ed. Philadelphia, PA: Elsevier/Saunders; 2011.

Category: Integumentary

91. Which of the following is the most appropriate management of an asymptomatic umbilical hernia in a newborn?
A) Immediate surgical correction
B) Reassurance to parents that most hernias resolve in 6 to 8 weeks
C) Surgical correction if the hernia does not resolve before school age
D) Application of an elastic support to the midabdomen
E) None of the above

Answer and Discussion

The answer is C. Umbilical hernias are more commonly seen in premature, female, and African American infants. The condition results from imperfect closure or weakness of the umbilical ring. If noted before 6 months of age, most resolve spontaneously before 1 year of age. Although rare, incarceration of the bowel is the most dangerous condition associated with abdominal hernias. If the hernia does not close before school age, incarcerates the bowel, or becomes symptomatic, surgical correction should be considered. Reduction of the hernia with strapping devices is not useful.

Additional Reading: The umbilicus. *Nelson Textbook of Pediatrics*, 19th ed. Philadelphia, PA: Elsevier/Saunders; 2011.

Category: Integumentary

92. Early breast-feeding is associated with
A) Improved growth in the first 2 months
B) Lower risk of aspiration
C) Less temperature instability
D) Fewer apneic spells
E) Higher rates of postpartum depression

Answer and Discussion

The answer is C. Mothers of newborn infants should initiate breast-feeding as soon as possible after giving birth. When mothers initiate breast-feeding within one-half hour of birth, the baby's suckling reflex is strongest, and the baby is more alert, which facilitates feeding. Early breast-feeding has been shown to be associated with fewer nighttime feeding problems and better mother–infant bonding. Additionally, infants who are breast-fed earlier have been shown to have higher core temperatures and less temperature instability.

Additional Reading: Strategies of breastfeeding success. *Am Fam Physician*. 2008;78(2):225–232.

Category: Patient/population-based care

93. A 5-year-old boy is brought in for a well-child visit. The child's parents are noted to be relatively short, and they have concerns because their child is shorter than most of the other children in his class. The child's skeletal maturation is consistent with his chronologic age. The most likely diagnosis is
A) Parental neglect
B) Hypothyroidism
C) Genetic short stature
D) Acromegaly
E) Dwarfism

Answer and Discussion

The answer is C. Genetic short stature is a delay in growth and development that patterns the parents' growth and development. Typically, if the child has tall parents, the child will eventually be tall; if the parents are short, the child will eventually be short. Also, if the parents developed late in adolescence, then the child will mirror this development. Constitutional growth delay can be differentiated from genetic short stature by the level of skeletal maturation, which is consistent with chronologic age in the latter condition. There is no treatment necessary; however, the family may need reassurance that the child is normal and that no further treatment or evaluation is necessary.

Additional Reading: Assessment of growth. *Nelson Textbook of Pediatrics*, 19th ed. Philadelphia, PA: Elsevier/Saunders; 2011.

Category: Endocrine system

94. A 40-year-old woman who received killed measles vaccination in 1965 presents with high fever, headaches, abdominal pain, and a rash that began on her arms and spread to her trunk and face. Which of the following factors makes you suspicious that this is not typical measles?
A) Development of cough
B) Development of high fever
C) Presence of abdominal pain
D) Distribution of rash
E) Development of headaches

Answer and Discussion

The answer is D. A typical measles syndrome occurs in individuals who were immunized with the original killed virus vaccine, which was administered from 1963 to 1967. Some cases have been linked to the newer, live attenuated vaccine that was improperly stored. The disease is thought to result from a hypersensitive response in persons who have partial immunity. Symptoms are similar to regular measles and include high fever, headache, abdominal pain, cough, and a rash that begins on the extremities (unlike regular measles in which the rash tends to form on the face first) 1 to 2 days after the onset of the initial symptoms. The rash may become purpuric or hemorrhagic. Koplik's spots are rarely seen in atypical measles.

Additional Reading: Measles. *Nelson Textbook of Pediatrics*, 19th ed. Philadelphia, PA: Elsevier/Saunders. 2011.

Category: Patient/population-based care

95. Which of the following is the most common malignancy diagnosed in childhood?
A) Wilm's tumor
B) Retinoblastoma
C) Melanoma
D) Acute lymphoblastic leukemia (ALL)
E) Osteosarcoma

Answer and Discussion

The answer is D. Leukemia is the most common malignancy diagnosed in childhood. ALL is the most common type of leukemia in children. ALL typically occurs in children between 1 and 10 years of age, although it can occur at any age. This leukemia is more common in male children and in Caucasians. Diagnosing ALL can be challenging. Frequently, the diagnosis is delayed because early symptoms are nonspecific and may resemble viral infections. Most children affected present with generalized malaise, loss of appetite, and a low-grade fever. Additional symptoms include pallor, petechiae or ecchymoses, bone pain, and significant weight loss. The physical examination may not be revealing, but significant lymphadenopathy or hepatosplenomegaly should raise suspicion for leukemia. Hepatosplenomegaly is always an abnormal finding. A practical approach to the child with suspicious findings is to obtain a CBC with a WBC differential and a reticulocyte count. The presence of blast cells on the peripheral smear is diagnostic of leukemia. However, many patients with leukemia only have blast cells in their bone marrow. The finding of anemia, especially if accompanied by reticulocytopenia or a high mean corpuscular volume, thrombocytopenia, leukopenia, or leukocytosis is likely associated with leukemia and deserves further evaluation. Illnesses that may mimic leukemia include infectious mononucleosis caused by Epstein–Barr virus or, less frequently, cytomegalovirus infection, collagen vascular disease, and aplastic anemia.

Additional Reading: Signs and symptoms of childhood cancer: a guide for early recognition. *Am Fam Physician*. 2013;88(3): 185–192.

Category: Patient/population-based care

96. Which of the following foods has/have been associated with the development of botulism in children younger than 1 year?
A) Corn syrup
B) Peanuts
C) Honey
D) Cereal
E) Animal crackers

Answer and Discussion

The answer is C. Botulism is caused by a toxin produced by the anaerobe *Clostridium botulinum*. Symptoms usually occur within 24 hours after ingestion of contaminated food (usually canned food). These symptoms include dry mouth, diplopia, dysarthria, dysphagia, decreased visual acuity, nausea, vomiting, abdominal cramps, and diarrhea. Neurologic disorders include weakness and eventual paralysis, which can lead to respiratory failure and death. Sensory function remains intact. Diagnosis is made by discovery of the botulinum toxin in the affected food or stool of affected patients. Treatment involves supportive therapy, including mechanical ventilation and the administration of a trivalent antitoxin. Mortality rates approach 25%. Prevention involves the use of pressure cookers, which provide temperatures higher than 100°C (212°F), for at least 10 minutes when canning vegetables; boiling food for at least 10 minutes before eating destroys any toxins present. Infant botulism is caused by the ingestion of botulinum spores, which produce the toxin in vivo. Unlike food-borne botulism, infant botulism is not caused by ingestion of a preformed toxin. Constipation is initially present in 90% of cases of infant botulism and is followed by neuromuscular paralysis beginning with the cranial nerves and proceeding to peripheral and respiratory musculature. Cranial nerve deficits typically include ptosis, extraocular muscle palsies, weak cry, poor suck, decreased gag reflex, pooling of oral secretions, and an expressionless face. Severity varies from mild lethargy and slowed feeding to severe hypotonia and respiratory insufficiency. Most infants affected are between the ages of 2 and 3 months. Finding *C. botulinum* toxin or organisms in the feces establishes the diagnosis. Honey has been shown to contain botulinum spores and thus should be avoided in children younger than 1 year. Administration of the antitoxin may be considered (not in infants). Additionally, antibiotics may be useful to treat secondary infections. Aminoglycosides should be avoided because they may potentiate the effects of the toxin. A clinical trial is being performed to determine the usefulness of human botulism immune globulin (derived from the plasma of persons immunized with *C. botulinum* toxoid) in the treatment of infant botulism.

Additional Reading: Botulism. *Nelson Textbook of Pediatrics*, 19th ed. Philadelphia, PA: Elsevier/Saunders; 2011.

Category: Nonspecific system

97. Which of the following is true regarding management of head lice?
A) Children should be kept out of school until no visible evidence of nits is noted.
B) Household members should only be treated if live lice or eggs are noted within 1 cm of the scalp.
C) Head lice programs have had a significant impact on lowering the incidence of head lice.
D) Cleaning of bedding has little impact on lice eradication.
E) The health of those exposed is more important than the confidentiality of the child affected.

Answer and Discussion

The answer is B. Practice guidelines published by the AAP state that if a case of head lice is identified, all household members should be checked, and only those with live lice or eggs within 1 cm of the scalp should be treated. It is recommended to treat family members who share a bed with the person who is infected and to adequately clean hair care items and bed linens belonging to that person. A child with active head lice has likely had the infestation for a month or more by the time it is discovered and poses little risk to others. The child does not have a resulting hygiene or health problem and should stay in class but be discouraged from close, direct head contact with others. The child's parents should be notified immediately, and confidentiality should be maintained so the child is not embarrassed. A child should be allowed to return to school after proper treatment and should not miss school because of head lice. Head lice screening programs have not had a significant effect on the incidence of head lice in the school setting over time and are not cost-effective.

Additional Reading: Pediculosis and scabies: a treatment update. *Am Fam Physician*. 2012;86(6):535–541.

Category: Patient/population-based care

98. Which of the following statements about osteoid osteoma is true?
A) It is a malignant tumor of long bones.
B) It is more common in girls.
C) It usually presents as a pathologic fracture.
D) Radiographs show radiolucent areas surrounded by sclerosis.
E) Treatment involves systemic chemotherapy.

Answer and Discussion

The answer is D. Osteoid osteoma is a benign tumor that usually involves the long bones of pediatric and adolescent patients. They are found more commonly in boys. Most cases present with pain, not fracture. Radiographs show a characteristic radiolucent area surrounded by sclerosis, which is usually associated with the ends of the tibia or femur. Technetium bone scans are helpful in determining the area involved. Treatment for severe refractory cases involves surgical resection, which is curative. Anti-inflammatory drugs are often helpful for mild cases and can relieve the pain.

Additional Reading: Benign tumors and tumor-like processes of bone. *Nelson Textbook of Pediatrics*, 19th ed. Philadelphia, PA: Elsevier/Saunders; 2011.

Category: Musculoskeletal system

99. Which of the following is *not* a suitable treatment for molluscum contagiosum (MC)?
A) Curettage
B) Cryotherapy
C) Trichloroacetic acid
D) Imiquimod (Aldara)
E) 5-fluorouracil

Answer and Discussion

The answer is E. MC is a benign superficial eruption resulting from viral infections of the skin. MC eruptions are usually self-limited and without sequelae, although they can be more extensive especially in immunocompromised persons. In patients with HIV, MC infection frequently is not self-limited and can be much more extensive and even disfiguring. MC may serve as a cutaneous marker of severe immunodeficiency and sometimes is the first indication of HIV infection. Lesions usually spontaneously disappear but treatment by local destruction or immunologic modulation can shorten the disease course. Spontaneous disappearance of MC lesions with no residual scarring is common. This may occur after a period of inflammation and minor tenderness. Autoinoculation is associated with scratching of the lesions and transmission to others can occur. Lesion destruction may be mechanical (curettage, laser, or cryotherapy with liquid nitrogen or nitrous oxide cryogun), chemical (trichloroacetic acid, tretinoin), or immunologic (imiquimod). Advantages to imiquimod therapy include minimal side effects and convenience of application.

Additional Reading: Cutaneous viral infections. *Nelson Textbook of Pediatrics*, 19th ed. Philadelphia, PA: Elsevier/Saunders; 2011.

Category: Integumentary

> MC lesion destruction may be mechanical (curettage, laser, or cryotherapy with liquid nitrogen or nitrous oxide cryogun), chemical (trichloroacetic acid, tretinoin), or immunologic (imiquimod).

100. Which of the following statements about lead poisoning in children is true?
A) Symptoms include vomiting, irritability, weight loss, and abdominal pain.
B) Repeated ingestion of small amounts of lead is less dangerous than a single large ingestion.
C) All paints used in the home should be <25% lead.
D) It is treated with deferoxime.
E) Neurologic deficits are not routinely associated with lead poisoning.

Answer and Discussion

The answer is A. Lead poisoning is a particular concern for young children. Also known as *plumbism,* the condition is characterized by generalized weakness, vomiting, irritability, weight loss, changes in personality, ataxia, headache, and abdominal pain. Radiographic particles are often seen on abdominal films, and there is usually a visible lead line on the gums and involving bones at the metaphyseal zone. Further complications include delayed development with diminished IQ, decreased hearing, peripheral neuropathy, seizures, and coma in severe cases. The syndrome usually affects children younger than 5 years who have ingested lead. Some common sources of lead include leaded paint chips, solder, glazed pottery, and fumes from burning batteries. Repeated ingestion of small amounts of lead (>0.5 mg of lead absorbed per day) is more dangerous than one single large dose. All paints used in the home should be <1% lead. Drinking water is another important source of lead exposure if there are lead pipes or lead fixtures or fittings. Universal screening by blood lead testing of all children at ages 12 months and 24 months was the standard. Given the national decline in the prevalence, recommendations have been revised to target high-risk populations. Departments of heath are responsible for determining the local prevalence of lead poisoning; if this information is absent, the practitioner should continue to test all children ages 12 months and 24 months. Risk factors include living in a house built before 1950, living in a house built before 1978 with ongoing renovations, sibling or playmate with lead poisoning, lead-based industry in the child's neighborhood, recent immigrant, pica, developmental delay, and all Medicaid-eligible children. Venous sampling is preferred to capillary.

Screening value at or above 2 µg/dL is exposure and requires diagnostic testing to determine appropriate intervention. If the BLL is elevated, further testing is required depending on the value. BLL of 45 µg/dL or higher requires prompt chelation therapy.

Four drugs are available: dimercaptosuccinic acid, penicillamine, edatate calcium disodium, and dimercaprol. The choice of agent is guided by the severity of lead poisoning, effectiveness of the drug, and ease of administration. Close monitoring should be instituted to watch for renal failure and the development of seizures. Children should not be allowed to return to lead-contaminated environments until they are deemed safe by environmental agents.

Additional Reading: Lead poisoning. *Nelson Textbook of Pediatrics*, 19th ed. Philadelphia, PA: Elsevier/Saunders; 2011.

Category: Patient/population-based care

101. The first solid food (iron-fortified cereal) should typically be administered to an infant at
A) 2 to 4 months
B) 4 to 6 months
C) 6 to 8 months
D) 8 to 12 months
E) Only after 1 year

Answer and Discussion

The answer is B. Iron-fortified cereals should be the first solid food introduced to young infants at 4 to 6 months of age. These can be continued until approximately 18 months of age. When to start solid foods depends on the infant's needs and readiness, but infants do not need solids before 6 months of age. Neurologic development has progressed sufficiently for tongue and mouth movement to handle solids at approximately 4 months in full-term infants. Solid feedings given earlier than 4 months of age are extremely difficult to manage because the infant's extrusion reflex causes the tongue to push solid food out of the mouth. Other foods, including fruit and vegetable baby food, may be started soon after the introduction of cereal. Typically one new food is added per week. Baby food meats can be added at 6 to 7 months; table food can be added at 8 to 12 months. Foods easily aspirated such as chunks of meat, popcorn, or nuts should be avoided. Whole milk can replace formula or breast milk at 12 months of age. And reduced-fat milk is usually given at 2 years of age. To prevent food sensitivities, peanuts, eggs, and cow's milk should be avoided until the child is 1 year old. Honey should be avoided in children <1 year of age because of the risk of infant botulism.

Additional Reading: Feeding during the first year of life. *Nelson Textbook of Pediatrics,* 19th ed. Philadelphia, PA: Elsevier/Saunders; 2011.

Category: Gastroenterology system

102. A 4-year-old girl complains of vaginal itching, especially at night when she is going to bed. The most likely diagnosis is
A) Ascariasis
B) Cutaneous larva migrans
C) Pinworms
D) Pubic lice
E) MC

Answer and Discussion

The answer is C. *Enterobius* (pinworms) is the most common parasite affecting children in the United States. Its prevalence approaches 100% in institutionalized children. Infestation usually results from hand-to-mouth transfer of ova from the perianal area to fomites (clothing, bedding, furniture, rugs, toys), from which the ova are picked up by the new host, transmitted to the mouth, and swallowed. Although less common, airborne ova may be inhaled and then swallowed. The pinworms reach maturity in the lower GI tract within 2 to 6 weeks. The female worm migrates to the perianal region (usually at night) to deposit ova. Movements of the female worm cause pruritus. The ova can survive on fomites as long as 3 weeks under normal conditions. Most persons who harbor pinworms have no symptoms or signs. Some will, however, experience the perianal itching and develop perianal excoriations from persistent scratching. Vaginitis in young girls may be due to irritation from pinworms. Pinworm infestation can be diagnosed by finding the female worm, which is about 10-mm long (males average 3 mm), in the perianal region 1 or 2 hours after the child goes to bed at night or by microscopic identification of the ova. The ova are obtained in the early morning before the child arises by patting the perianal skinfolds with a strip of transparent adhesive tape. This procedure should be repeated on five successive mornings if necessary to rule out pinworm infestation. A single dose of mebendazole (regardless of age) is effective in eradicating pinworms (but not ova) in about 90% of cases. Pyrantel pamoate is also used and repeated after 2 weeks. Because multiple infestations within the household are the rule, treatment of the entire family is recommended. Extensive handwashing and housekeeping have little effect on the control or treatment of pinworm infestation.

Additional Reading: Enterobiasis. *Nelson Textbook of Pediatrics*, 19th ed. Philadelphia, PA: Elsevier/Saunders; 2011.

Category: Nonspecific system

103. Retinopathy of prematurity (ROP) is associated with
A) Gestational diabetes
B) Excessive oxygen administration
C) Maternal hypothyroidism
D) Maternal rubella infection
E) Development of congenital cataracts

Answer and Discussion

The answer is B. Retinopathy of prematurity, or *retrolental fibroplasia*, is thought to be related to exposure of retinal vessels of premature infants to excessive oxygen concentrations; the condition rarely occurs otherwise. Other risk factors include respiratory distress, apnea, bradycardia, heart disease, infection, hypoxia, hypercarbia, acidosis, anemia, and the need for transfusion. Most affected infants weigh <1,500 g, and the mechanism of injury is believed to be excessive oxygen exposure leading to the development of free radicals and neovascularization and eventual retinal detachment. Occasionally, if the neovascularization is mild, the abnormal vessels may spontaneously regress, preserving vision but usually leaving the infant with significant myopia. Prevention is aimed at carefully monitoring oxygen supplementation in minimal amounts to preserve brain tissue and, ultimately, preventing premature birth. However, oxygen alone is neither sufficient nor necessary to produce retinopathy of prematurity and no safe level of oxygen has been determined. Treatment involves the use of cryotherapy and laser photocoagulation, which may be beneficial in select cases. All infants who weigh <1,500 g should be evaluated by an ophthalmologist before discharge from the hospital and at least once at 6 months after birth.

Additional Reading: Disorders of the retina and vitreous. *Nelson Textbook of Pediatrics*, 19th ed. Philadelphia, PA: Elsevier/Saunders; 2011.

Category: Special sensory

104. The definition of delayed sexual maturation in boys includes
A) No testicular development by age 10 years
B) More than 5 years between the initial and completed growth of genitalia
C) Lack of axillary hair growth by 13 years of age
D) Lack of pubic hair growth 1 year after the growth spurt
E) No pubertal-related voice changes before age 15 years

Answer and Discussion

The answer is B. Delayed sexual maturation is defined as follows:

- *In boys:* No testicular development by age 14 years, no pubic hair by age 15 years, and more than 5 years between the initial and completed growth of the genitalia
- *In girls:* No breast development by age 13 years, no pubic hair before age 14 years, and no menstruation within 5 years of the development of breast buds, or if menstruation does not occur by age 16

One of the major causes is *constitutional delay,* which is defined as an inherited delayed maturation affecting the child and which is also often noted in the parents. In these cases, the prepubertal growth is normal, but the skeletal growth and adolescent growth spurt is delayed. Those affected develop sexually late but are considered completely normal. The condition is more common in boys and can be treated with the use of testosterone supplementation. Girls with severe pubertal delay should be investigated for primary amenorrhea.

Additional Reading: Hypopituitarism. *Nelson Textbook of Pediatrics*, 19th ed. Philadelphia, PA: Elsevier/Saunders; 2011.

Category: Patient/population-based care

105. Which of the following is a negative predictor for streptococcal pharyngitis?
A) Fever >38.3°C (100.9°F)
B) Exposure to a known *Streptococcus* pharyngitis contact
C) Pharyngeal or tonsillar exudates
D) Recent cough

Answer and Discussion

The answer is D. According to the Walsh Prediction Scale, the following are given equal weightage in the diagnosis of strep pharyngitis:

- Fever >38.3°C (100.9°F)
- Exposure to a known *Streptococcus* pharyngitis contact
- Pharyngeal or tonsillar exudates, enlarged or tender nodes

Recent cough actually was a negative predictor for strep pharyngitis. In patients with a low probability of streptococcal pharyngitis (score of −1), only follow-up is needed. Those in the intermediate group (score of 0 or 1) could be tested further, treated, or followed, depending on physician preference. Patients with a high probability of disease (score of 2 or 3) should be treated empirically with an antibiotic.

Additional Reading: Clinical practice. Streptococcal pharyngitis. *N Engl J Med.* 2011;364(7):648.

Category: Respiratory system

106. Which of the following statements about posterior urethral valves is true?
A) They affect only male children.
B) They cannot be detected by prenatal ultrasound.
C) Most cases are resolved spontaneously.
D) They are secondary to abnormal valves found in the posterior calices of the kidney, giving rise to urinary diverticula.
E) They are not detected by a voiding cystourethrogram.

Answer and Discussion

The answer is A. Children with UTIs do not always present with symptoms such as urinary frequency, dysuria, or flank pain. Infants may present with fever and irritability or other subtle symptoms such as lethargy. Older children may also have nonspecific symptoms such as abdominal pain or unexplained fever. A urinalysis should be obtained in a child with unexplained fever or symptoms that suggest a UTI.

Posterior urethral valves are commonly the cause of UTIs in young boys only. These valves are secondary to abnormal folds in the prostatic urethra that enlarge with voiding and cause obstruction of the urethral lumen. Symptoms include decreased urinary stream, overflow incontinence, and UTIs with dysuria. Affected boys can be identified prenatally with maternal ultrasound, which shows bilateral hydronephrosis; a distended bladder; and, if obstruction is severe, oligohydramnios. UTIs noted in boys suspected of posterior urinary valves should undergo further evaluation, including voiding cystourethrogram, or perineal ultrasound, as soon as the diagnosis is suspected; this will help reduce the risk of kidney damage. Treatment involves surgical resection of the valves.

Additional Reading: Posterior urethral valves. *Nelson Textbook of Pediatrics,* 19th ed. Philadelphia, PA: Elsevier/Saunders; 2011.

Category: Nephrologic system

107. Of the following, the most appropriate treatment for cradle cap is
A) Topical ketoconazole
B) Aloe vera shampoo
C) Topical moisturizers
D) Vitamin E
E) Topical hydrocortisone

Answer and Discussion

The answer is E. Newborns frequently develop seborrheic dermatitis, with a thick, yellow, crusted scalp lesion (cradle cap); fissuring and yellow scaling behind the ears; red facial papules; and an irritated diaper rash. In infants, a baby shampoo is used daily and 1% hydrocortisone cream is applied twice daily. Additionally, the dermatitis usually responds to frequent zinc or tar shampoos.

Additional Reading: Eczematous disorders: seborrheic dermatitis. *Nelson Textbook of Pediatrics,* 19th ed. Philadelphia, PA: Elsevier/Saunders; 2011.

Category: Integumentary system

108. A 4-year-old boy swallows a small button battery. The child undergoes a chest radiograph and abdominal series. The battery is located in the lower esophagus, above the lower esophageal ring. The most appropriate management is
A) Observation
B) Endoscopy to remove the battery
C) Barium-swallow study
D) Ipecac administration
E) None of the above

Answer and Discussion

The answer is B. Children younger than 4 years are at particular risk for the ingestion of foreign bodies such as button batteries used in wristwatches and cameras. If a child ingests a battery, a radiograph of the child's chest and abdomen is indicated to locate the battery's position. If the battery is located distal to the lower esophageal ring, no further therapy is needed; however, if the battery is larger than 1.5 cm, a follow-up radiograph should be performed 48 hours later to make sure the battery has passed through the pylorus. If the battery is lodged in the esophagus, endoscopy should be performed to remove the foreign body. A battery lodged in the esophagus can lead to perforation if left for more than 4 hours.

Additional Reading: Ingestions: foreign bodies in the esophagus. *Nelson Textbook of Pediatrics,* 19th ed. Philadelphia, PA: Elsevier/Saunders; 2011.

Category: Gastroenterology system

109. A 12-year-old boy presents with pain over the tibial tubercle. His mother reports a recent growth spurt. The most likely diagnosis is
A) Legg–Calvé–Perthes disease
B) Shin splints
C) Osgood–Schlatter disease
D) Osteosarcoma
E) Stress fracture

Answer and Discussion

The answer is C. Osgood–Schlatter disease is caused by inflammation of the tibial tubercle that usually occurs at the time of a child's growth spurt. It is aggravated by strenuous physical activity such as climbing or running. Boys are more affected than girls, the condition is usually unilateral, and most patients are between 10 and 15 years of age. Symptoms include pain, swelling, and tenderness over the tibial tubercle. The cause is repeated traction of the inferior patellar tendon on the developing epiphyseal insertion. Radiographs of the knee, although unnecessary for the diagnosis, usually show bone fragments at the site of the tibial tubercle. Treatment includes rest (especially from deep-knee bends), ice therapy, and anti-inflammatory drugs. In severe cases, more aggressive therapy, including casting, cortisone injections, and surgery, to remove loose bodies may be necessary but is infrequent.

Additional Reading: The knee: Osgood–Schlatter disease. *Nelson Textbook of Pediatrics,* 19th ed. Philadelphia, PA: Elsevier/Saunders; 2011.

Category: Musculoskeletal system

110. A 4-year-old boy is brought to your office by his mother. The child has evidence of a stomatitis and a vesicular rash that affects his hands and feet. The most likely cause is
A) Coxsackievirus
B) Adenovirus
C) Syphilis
D) Varicella
E) Measles

Answer and Discussion

The answer is A. The coxsackievirus is responsible for several infections that usually affect the pediatric population. There are two types of the virus:

- Coxsackievirus A
  - A16 is responsible for hand, foot, and mouth disease, which is characterized by stomatitis and a vesicular rash that affects

the hands and feet. It is usually mild, affects young children, and may occur in epidemics.

- A2, A4, A5, A6, A7, and A10 are responsible for herpangina, which is a more severe febrile illness that sometimes leads to febrile seizures. Other symptoms include a severe sore throat; vesiculoulcerative lesions that affect the tonsils, soft palate, and posterior pharynx; headaches; myalgias; and vomiting.

- Coxsackievirus B

  - B1, B2, B3, B4, and B5 are responsible for pleurodynia with pain associated with the area of diaphragmatic attachment. Other symptoms include fever, headache, sore throat, malaise, and vomiting. Orchitis and pleurisy may also occur.

Coxsackievirus B infection is rare in persons older than 60 years and is more common in children and young adults. The infection is transmitted by hand-to-mouth contact and may become widespread in certain populations. This virus has been called "the great pretender" because of the variety of clinical syndromes it can produce. Many infections that are caused by the virus are subclinical. More serious conditions caused by coxsackievirus B include myocarditis, orchitis, myalgia, and pleurodynia. Pleurodynia may be severe and can occur in epidemics referred to as *Bornholm disease,* named after the original description of an early epidemic on the Danish island of Bornholm. Patients with pleurodynia are usually children or young adults who present with severe pleuritic pain, tachypnea, and systemic upset. The condition is usually self-limiting, but there can be serious, though rare, long-term sequelae. In most cases, the treatment of coxsackievirus is symptomatic, and most infections are self-limited. Antibiotics are usually unnecessary unless concomitant bacterial infection is suspected.

Additional Reading: Nonpolio enteroviruses: hand-foot-and-mouth disease. *Nelson Textbook of Pediatrics,* 19th ed. Philadelphia, PA: Elsevier/Saunders; 2011.

Category: Nonspecific system

> **In most cases, the treatment of coxsackievirus is symptomatic, and most infections are self-limited.**

111. The most common cause of metabolic pancreatitis in children is
A) Type I diabetes mellitus
B) Primary hyperparathyroidism
C) Primary hyperthyroidism
D) Diabetes insipidus
E) Cushing's syndrome

Answer and Discussion

The answer is B. Hypercalcemia and hyperlipidemia are two recognized causes of pancreatitis, both in children and in adults. The hypercalcemia may be masked by the transient calcium-lowering effect of acute pancreatitis. Primary hyperparathyroidism related to adenoma or hyperplasia (sometimes secondary to multiple endocrine neoplasia, type IIa) is the most common cause of the hypercalcemia.

Additional Reading: Pancreatitis. *Nelson Textbook of Pediatrics,* 19th ed. Philadelphia, PA: Elsevier/Saunders; 2011.

Category: Patient/population-based care

112. A 3-month-old boy is brought to your office by his parents. The child has an erythematous perineal rash that spares the skin folds of the groin area. The most likely diagnosis is
A) Diaper dermatitis
B) Yeast dermatitis
C) Heat rash
D) Varicella
E) Childhood eczema

Answer and Discussion

The answer is A. Diaper dermatitis, also known as *primary irritant dermatitis,* results from chronic exposure to urine and feces and its subsequent skin irritation. It is a shiny, erythematous rash that spares the skin folds in the groin area and usually affects infants after 3 months of age. In severe cases, the skin may ulcerate. Treatment involves adequate drying of the area with exposure to air. Frequent diaper changes may also speed recovery, as well as application of petroleum jelly and zinc oxide to the affected areas. If the condition lasts more than a few days, the diagnosis of candidiasis must be considered. Rubber or plastic pants inhibit moisture evaporation and should be avoided.

Additional Reading: Diaper dermatitis. *Nelson Textbook of Pediatrics,* 19th ed. Philadelphia, PA: Elsevier/Saunders; 2011.

Category: Integumentary system

113. The anterior fontanel usually closes at
A) 3 months
B) 6 months
C) 12 months
D) 2 years
E) 5 years

Answer and Discussion

The answer is C. The diagnosis of an abnormal fontanel requires the physician to appreciate the wide variation of normal. At birth, an infant has six fontanels. The anterior fontanel is the largest and most important for clinical evaluation. The average size of the anterior fontanel is 2.1 cm, and the median time of closure is around 1 year of age. The most common causes of a large anterior fontanel or delayed fontanel closure are achondroplasia, hypothyroidism, Down's syndrome, increased intracranial pressure, and rickets. A bulging anterior fontanel can be a result of increased intracranial pressure or intracranial and extracranial tumors, and a sunken fontanel usually is a sign of dehydration. A physical examination helps the physician determine which imaging modality, such as plain films, ultrasonography, CT scan, or magnetic resonance imaging, to use for diagnosis.

Additional Reading: Neurologic evaluation: head. *Nelson Textbook of Pediatrics,* 19th ed. Philadelphia, PA: Elsevier/Saunders; 2011.

Category: Neurologic

114. An adequate level of fluoride supplementation in drinking water is equal to
A) 1,000 parts per million (ppm)
B) 500 ppm
C) 100 ppm
D) 10 ppm
E) 1 ppm

Answer and Discussion

The answer is E. Fluoride helps reduce the formation of dental caries. It is most effectively administered in drinking water. The need for supplementation depends on the amount of fluoride in the drinking water. Adequate levels are usually 1 ppm. Water with levels <0.6 ppm may require supplementation. Fluoride toothpaste is not a suitable alternative supplement. Supplementation should be initiated for infants given ready-to-feed formulas that do not contain fluoride and for infants who are breast-fed after 6 months of age. Excessive fluoride supplementation can cause fluorosis. The following recommendations are given by the AAP:

Supplemental Fluoride Dosage Schedule

Fluoride in Home Water (ppm)

Age	<0.3	0.3–0.6	>0.6
Birth–6 mo	0[a]	0	0
6 mo–3 yr	0.25	0	0
3–6 yr	0.50	0.25	0
6–16 yr	1.0	0.50	0

[a]Milligrams of fluoride per day

> **Additional Reading:** Micronutrient mineral deficiencies. *Nelson Textbook of Pediatrics*, 19th ed. Philadelphia, PA: Elsevier/Saunders; 2011.

> **Category:** Nonspecific system

115. The most appropriate treatment for school avoidance is
A) To return the child to school and then determine reasons for school avoidance
B) To allow the child to remain at home until reasons for avoidance are determined
C) To prescribe methylphenidate
D) To begin inpatient psychotherapy
E) To change teachers or schools

Answer and Discussion

The answer is A. School avoidance/refusal is a problem encountered in many family physicians' offices. Children may manifest numerous complaints to their parents and teachers to avoid attending school. The beginning of the school year appears to increase significantly the incidence of headache. The first step in the treatment of a child refusing to go to school is to get him or her back into the classroom and, once that is accomplished, identify reasons why the child is avoiding school. Some common problems include difficulty with peer relationships, family discord at home, and poor school performance that may be caused by attention-deficit disorder, dyslexia, and visual or hearing difficulties. Working closely with the child's family and teachers can be beneficial.

> **Additional Reading:** School refusal in children and adolescents. *Am Fam Physician*. 2003;68(8):1555–1561.

> **Category:** Psychogenic system

116. The normal heart rate for newborns is
A) 60 to 100 beats/minute
B) 100 to 120 beats/minute
C) 120 to 160 beats/minute
D) 140 to 160 beats/minute

Answer and Discussion

The answer is C. The normal heart rate in newborns is 120 to 160 beats/minute.

> **Additional Reading:** Cardiovascular compromise in the newborn infant. *Nelson Textbook of Pediatrics*, 19th ed. Philadelphia, PA: Elsevier/Saunders; 2011.

> **Category:** Cardiovascular system

117. Which of the following is a description of Prader–Willi syndrome?
A) Tall, large arm span, increased risk of aortic rupture
B) Obese, hypotonic, mental retardation, hypogonadism
C) Short, obese, frontal bossing, precocious puberty
D) Normal size, mental retardation, precocious puberty

Answer and Discussion

The answer is B. Prader–Willi syndrome is characterized by decreased fetal activity, obesity, hypotonia, mental retardation, and hypogonadotropic hypogonadism. The syndrome is caused by a defect on the proximal long arm of the paternal chromosome 15 or by a defect on the maternal chromosome 15. Associated features include failure to thrive due to hypotonia and feeding difficulties, which generally improve after 6 to 12 months of age. From about 12 to 18 months and beyond, uncontrollable appetite causes worsening weight gain as well as psychological problems, as insatiable hunger with significant obesity becomes the most noticeable feature. Rapid weight gain continues but with ultimate short stature in adulthood. Behavioral features include emotional lability, poor gross motor skills, cognitive impairment, and insatiable hunger. Facial abnormalities include a narrow bitemporal dimension, almond-shaped eyes, and a mouth with thin upper lips and downturned corners. Hypogonadotropic hypogonadism, cryptorchidism, and a hypoplastic penis and scrotum in male children or hypoplastic labia in female children are present. Skeletal abnormalities include scoliosis, kyphosis, and osteopenia. Limb abnormalities include small hands and feet.

> **Additional Reading:** Cytogenetics. *Nelson Textbook of Pediatrics*, 19th ed. Philadelphia, PA: Elsevier/Saunders; 2011.

> **Category:** Patient/population-based care

118. A 6-month-old is brought to your office in mid-January. The child's mother reports that the infant has had a low-grade fever, wheezing with coughing, and diminished appetite. The most likely diagnosis is
A) Bronchiolitis secondary to RSV
B) Pneumonia secondary to *S. pneumoniae*
C) Aspiration pneumonia
D) Asthma
E) Bronchitis secondary to *H. influenzae*

Answer and Discussion

The answer is A. Bronchiolitis is a common disease of the lower respiratory tract of infants and results from inflammatory obstruction of the small airways. The condition affects young children (younger than 2 years), and the peak incidence is in infants 6 months of age. Bronchiolitis is caused in most cases (>50%) by RSV. Other causes include parainfluenza virus and adenoviruses and *Mycoplasma*. It most commonly occurs in the winter months. Signs and symptoms include coughing, wheezing, fever, nasal flaring, tachypnea, delayed expiration, and chest wall retractions. The WBC count and differential are usually normal. Nasal swabs can be used for RSV cultures, and rapid antigen assays may be performed to aid in diagnosis. Chest radiographs are usually normal; however, hyperinflation and increased interstitial markings in the perihilar area may be noted. Treatment is accomplished with bronchodilators, humidified oxygen via a croup tent, and intravenous fluids. In severe cases, ribavirin aerosol, an antiviral agent, can be administered. Bronchiolitis is more likely to develop in infants who are exposed to cigarette smoke. RSV immune globulin given just before and during RSV season is effective in preventing severe RSV disease in at-risk infants with chronic lung disease.

Additional Reading: Wheezing, bronchiolitis and bronchitis. *Nelson Textbook of Pediatrics*, 19th ed. Philadelphia, PA: Elsevier/Saunders; 2011.

Category: Respiratory system

119. Most children affected with rotavirus are
A) Younger than 6 months
B) Between 6 months and 2 years of age
C) Older than 2 years
D) Between 2 and 4 years of age
E) Between 5 and 7 years of age

Answer and Discussion

The answer is B. Rotavirus is a viral intestinal infection commonly seen in children, predominantly during the winter months. Epidemics are common in day care centers. Most of the children affected are between 6 months and 2 years of age, but any child can be affected. Symptoms include profuse, watery diarrhea with the absence of blood, mild fevers, mild abdominal cramping, and vomiting (which may precede the onset of diarrhea). Some children may have associated respiratory complaints. The diagnosis is usually made by the clinical presentation but can be confirmed with viral antigen detection kits. Stool tests for WBCs are negative, supporting the diagnosis of a viral infection. Treatment involves oral rehydration for mild cases and intravenous fluid replacement for moderate to severe dehydration. Lactose-containing foods should be avoided if they appear to exacerbate the symptoms. Breast-feeding should be continued during rehydration. The bananas, rice, cereal, applesauce, and toast diet has not been shown to be superior to a regular diet. Most cases resolve in 5 to 7 days. The rotavirus vaccine approved in 1998 was suspended from use in July 1999 because of an association of intussusception. In 2006 and 2008, newer vaccines were released. Since the one (Rotarix) has been found to have parts of an extraneous virus and the Food and Drug Administration has recommended suspension of its use. The other (RotaTeq) is still recommended.

Additional Reading: Caliciviruses and astroviruses. *Nelson Textbook of Pediatrics,* 19th ed. Philadelphia, PA: Elsevier/Saunders; 2011.

Category: Gastroenterology system

> Stool tests for WBCs are negative with rotavirus, supporting the diagnosis of a viral infection.

120. Which of the following congenital heart defects (CHD) is considered a cyanotic lesion?
A) Ventricular septal defect
B) Atrial septal defect
C) Patent ductus arteriosis
D) Coarctation of the aorta
E) Tetralogy of Fallot

Answer and Discussion

The answer is E. CHDs are classified into two broad categories: acyanotic and cyanotic lesions. The most common acyanotic lesions are ventricular septal defect, atrial septal defect, atrioventricular canal, pulmonary stenosis, patent ductus arteriosus, aortic stenosis, and coarctation of the aorta. Congestive heart failure is the primary risk in infants with acyanotic lesions.

- *Ventricular septal defect:* Ventricular septal defect is the most common CHD. It may occur in any location on the septal wall. The significance of a ventricular septal defect is related to the size of the defect and ranges from insignificant to severe. Spontaneous closure within the first 6 months of life occurs in 30% to 40% of defects and is more likely to occur in smaller defects than in larger defects. Congestive heart failure, which may begin to develop at 6 to 8 weeks of age, is managed with diuretics and digoxin (Lanoxin). Indications for surgical closure include impaired growth that is not responsive to medical management and development of pulmonary hypertension. Postoperative complications include conduction defects, such as transient right bundle branch block.
- *Atrial septal defect:* Atrial septal defects may occur as sinus venosus, secundum, or primum type. The overall rate of spontaneous closure of the secundum type of atrial septal defect is approximately 85% in the first 4 years of life. Primum and sinus venosus types with defects >8 mm rarely close spontaneously, and surgical intervention is usually necessary. Most children with an atrial septal defect remain asymptomatic, but in those who develop congestive heart failure, medical management with diuretics and digoxin can be beneficial. Indications for surgical closure are persistence of the defect beyond 4 years of age, refractory congestive heart failure, and the presence of other associated defects, such as ventricular septal defect or valvular anomalies. Cardiac dysrhythmias and mitral valve prolapse may be late sequelae of treated or untreated atrial septal defect in children or adults. Pulmonary hypertension may develop in adults with an untreated atrial septal defect. Atrial flutter or fibrillation may also occur in adults with a history of atrial septal defect, regardless of the treatment.
- *Atrioventricular canal:* Atrioventricular canal is characterized by a combination of a primum type of atrial septal defect, a common atrioventricular valve, and an inlet type of ventricular septal defect. Most of the hemodynamic problems associated with this abnormality are caused by the ventricular septal defect, although mitral regurgitation or left-ventricle-to-right-atrium regurgitation, or both, may lead to pulmonary overload. The treatment of congestive heart failure in association with atrioventricular canal, the indications for surgical repair, and the postoperative complications are similar to those described for ventricular septal defect. Surgery should be performed before the onset of pulmonary vascular occlusive disease. Palliative pulmonary artery banding may be performed in infants who have refractory congestive heart failure and are too small for definitive repair.
- *Pulmonary stenosis:* Pulmonary stenosis may be valvular, subvalvular, or supravalvular. The clinical manifestations of pulmonary stenosis may vary from an asymptomatic lesion to frank congestive heart failure. Newborns may respond to prostaglandin E_1 infusion. Balloon valvuloplasty, performed during cardiac catheterization, is the preferred method of treatment for the valvular type of pulmonary stenosis. If this treatment is not successful, surgery is necessary.
- *Patent ductus arteriosus:* Patent ductus arteriosus is a common problem in premature infants. Closure may be spontaneous; if medical closure is required, indomethacin is effective. In term infants, spontaneous closure is unlikely, and indomethacin is not effective. Congestive heart failure and recurrent pneumonia are

likely complications if the flow through the ductus is substantial. Surgical ligation remains the preferred method of closure and should be performed as soon as possible. Cardiopulmonary bypass is not necessary. Nonsurgical techniques for correction of patent ductus arteriosus, such as catheter placement of an embolic device in term infants and indomethacin therapy in premature infants, are gaining popularity. Patent ductus arteriosus is the only CHD that may be considered surgically "cured," with no long-term sequelae.

- *Aortic stenosis:* Aortic stenosis may be valvular, subvalvular, or supravalvular. It may be asymptomatic or may cause symptoms of congestive heart failure. The pressure gradient across the stenosis increases with the child's growth, as the cardiac output increases. Surgical correction is the preferred treatment. Timing of the surgery is dependent on the child's cardiopulmonary status, the type of procedure planned (valvulotomy vs. valve replacement), and the size of the valve if a graft is needed. Lifelong anticoagulation therapy is required if a prosthetic valve replacement is performed.

- *Coarctation of the aorta:* Narrowing of the aorta may occur anywhere along its length, but the vast majority of cases occur just below the origin of the left subclavian artery. The classic clinical sign of coarctation of the aorta is a higher blood pressure in the arms than in the legs and pulses that are bounding in the arms but decreased in the legs. Surgical repair is usually performed between the ages of 2 and 4 years. Urgent surgical repair is performed in cases of circulatory shock, cardiomegaly, severe hypertension, or severe congestive heart failure.

- The most common cyanotic lesions are tetralogy of Fallot and transposition of the great arteries. In infants with cyanotic lesions, hypoxia is more of a problem than congestive heart failure.

- *Tetralogy of Fallot:* Tetralogy of Fallot is the most common CHD seen after infancy, with surgical repair usually undertaken when the child reaches 3 years of age. It consists of a large ventricular septal defect, right outflow tract obstruction, right ventricular hypertrophy, and overriding of the aorta. The classic clinical presentation is characterized by hyperpnea, irritability, cyanosis, and decreased murmur intensity. Squatting decreases systemic venous return by trapping blood in the legs, breaking the overload–hypoxia cycle. If this maneuver is ineffective, pharmacologic treatment may be necessary. Medical management of tetralogy of Fallot includes education on ways to treat the symptoms, prevention of anemia, and prophylaxis for subacute bacterial endocarditis. Surgical palliation consists of placement of a shunt from the subclavian artery to the ipsilateral pulmonary artery. Several different types of shunt procedures are currently performed. Total repair includes placement of a ventricular septal defect patch and right ventricular outflow tract widening. Total repair is performed before the child is 4 years of age.

- *Transposition of the great arteries:* Complete transposition of the great arteries occurs in a small percentage of children with CHD. The aorta and pulmonary arteries are transposed so that the two circulations are separate and parallel rather than in sequence. Infants with transposition of the great arteries are cyanotic at birth and often have congestive heart failure. Associated defects such as an atrial septal defect or patent ductus arteriosus, which permit the mixing of blood from the two sides of the vascular tree, are necessary for the infant's survival. Transposition of the great vessels requires that the ductus should be kept open by prostaglandin infusion until surgery can be performed. Metabolic abnormalities and severe hypoxia should be corrected

before surgical repair is undertaken. The definitive surgical procedure of choice is the arterial switch operation in which the aorta and the pulmonary artery are divided and reattached to their proper positions, resulting in a physiologic repair. It should be performed as soon as possible. Associated defects, such as ventricular septal defect, pulmonary stenosis, and patent ductus arteriosus, may necessitate a staged repair. Late complications of surgical repair include pulmonary or aortic stenosis, coronary artery obstruction, ventricular dysfunction, arrhythmias, and mitral regurgitation.

Suspicion of a congenital heart defect should be raised by the presence of feeding difficulties in association with tachypnea, sweating and subcostal recession, or severe growth impairment. More frequent follow-up is required if congestive heart failure is present.

Additional Reading: Cyanotic congenital heart disease; acyanotic congenital heart disease. *Nelson Textbook of Pediatrics,* 19th ed. Philadelphia, PA: Elsevier/Saunders; 2011.

Category: Cardiovascular system

121. Which of the following is true regarding hepatitis B vaccination in healthy infants?
A) The first immunization should be given by 2 months of age, second immunization 1 to 2 months later, and third immunization between 6 and 18 months.
B) Injections should be given in the buttock to increase immunogenicity.
C) Only infants at risk should receive hepatitis B vaccination.
D) Two doses will provide optimal results.
E) None of the above.

Answer and Discussion
The answer is A. Hepatitis B immunizations currently available in the United States are recombinant vaccines (Recombivax-HB, Engerix-B). Three intramuscular doses are required to induce optimal protective antibody responses. The vaccine should be administered in the anterolateral thigh muscle in infants and in the deltoid muscle in children, adolescents, and adults; injection in the buttocks or via the intradermal route may lead to diminished immunogenicity with lower seroconversion rates and serologic titers. Universal vaccination of infants is recommended. A three-dose schedule is required and should be initiated during the newborn period or by 2 months of age, a second dose given 1 to 2 months later, and a third dose given by 6 to 18 months of age. Most school districts now require hepatitis B immunization before admission to kindergarten or first grade. Susceptibility testing before vaccination is not routinely indicated, and postvaccination testing for immunity is not necessary after routine immunization.

Additional Reading: Viral hepatitis. *Nelson Textbook of Pediatrics,* 19th ed. Philadelphia, PA: Elsevier/Saunders; 2011.

Category: Gastroenterology system

122. A child is found to have higher blood pressures in the arms than in the legs and pulses are bounding in the arms but decreased in the legs. The most likely condition is
A) Ventricular septal defect
B) Tetralogy of Fallot
C) Transposition of the great arteries
D) Coarctation of the aorta
E) Aortic stenosis

Answer and Discussion

The answer is D. Coarctation of the aorta involves narrowing of the aorta that may occur anywhere along its length, but the vast majority of cases occur just below the origin of the left subclavian artery. The classic clinical sign of coarctation of the aorta is a higher blood pressure in the arms than in the legs and pulses that are bounding in the arms but decreased in the legs. Surgical repair is usually performed between the ages of 2 and 4 years. Emergent surgical repair is performed in cases of circulatory shock, cardiomegaly, severe hypertension, or severe congestive heart failure.

> **Additional Reading:** Systemic hypertension. *Nelson Textbook of Pediatrics,* 19th ed. Philadelphia, PA: Elsevier/Saunders; 2011.

Category: Cardiovascular system

123. A 4-year-old girl is brought to the emergency room. The mother reports that the child recently recovered from a viral URI, but over the past few days she has developed nosebleeds and bleeding from the gums. She also has noticed bruising of the extremities. The most likely diagnosis is
A) Meningococcemia
B) Idiopathic thrombocytopenic purpura (ITP)
C) Hemophilia A
D) Ingestion of warfarin
E) Vitamin K deficiency

Answer and Discussion

The answer is B. ITP is a disorder that usually affects children between 2 and 6 years of age. Boys and girls are equally affected. The condition usually follows a febrile, viral illness (particularly varicella, Epstein–Barr, and cytomegalovirus) during the winter months. Petechiae, purpura, and bleeding from mucous membranes develop within 3 weeks after the infection. Laboratory results often show thrombocytopenia (platelet counts <20,000 mm^3), and bone marrow studies show an increase in megakaryocytes. Prothrombin time and partial thromboplastin time are normal, but bleeding times are increased. No treatment is necessary in mild cases. In more severe cases with platelet counts below 20,000 mm^3 or with active bleeding, corticosteroids, 7-globulin, or other immunosuppressant agents that transiently elevate the platelet count can be used, but they do not alter the course of the illness. In severe cases, splenectomy or plasmapheresis may be necessary to achieve remission. Intracranial hemorrhage is the primary cause of death in severe cases. Most cases are mild, and patients recover completely without complications.

There is a chronic form of ITP that usually affects patients between 20 and 50 years of age; women tend to be affected more than men. Treatment for this form is similar to acute ITP, and psychosocial issues involving the chronic state are similar to those of hemophilia.

> **Additional Reading:** Platelet and blood vessel disorders. *Nelson Textbook of Pediatrics,* 19th ed. Philadelphia, PA: Elsevier/Saunders; 2011.

Category: Hematologic system

124. Which of the following CHDs can be surgically cured with no permanent sequelae?
A) Coarctation of the aorta
B) Tetralogy of Fallot
C) Patent ductus arteriosis
D) Ventricular septal defect
E) Transposition of the great vessels

Answer and Discussion

The answer is C. Patent ductus arteriosus is the only congenital heart defect that may be considered surgically "cured," with no long-term sequelae.

> **Additional Reading:** Cyanotic congenital heart disease; acyanotic congenital heart disease. *Nelson Textbook of Pediatrics,* 19th ed. Philadelphia, PA: Elsevier/Saunders; 2011.

Category: Cardiovascular system

125. A 2-year-old is seen in your office. The parent reports that the child shows in-toeing when walking. On examination, the child exhibits femoral anteversion. The most appropriate treatment is
A) Reassurance to the parent that the condition usually corrects itself as the child grows older
B) Referral to an orthopaedist
C) Referral to a physical therapist
D) Bracing to correct internal rotation of the femurs
E) Fitting for corrective shoes

Answer and Discussion

The answer is A. Femoral anteversion is a common orthopaedic finding in young children. The condition results when femoral anteversion leads to excessive internal rotation of the femur. As a result, the child may exhibit "kissing knees," toeing in, and the appearance of lack of coordination of the lower extremities. Maximal femoral anteversion occurs between 1 and 3 years of age. This abnormality usually corrects itself as the child becomes older. Significant abnormalities found after 8 years of age should be referred to an orthopaedist. Activities that may help correct the condition include ballet, bicycling, and skating because of the rotation exercises involved. In most cases, bracing is not beneficial. Severe cases may require osteotomy for rotational correction.

> **Additional Reading:** Torsional and angular deformities. *Nelson Textbook of Pediatrics,* 19th ed. Philadelphia, PA: Elsevier/Saunders; 2011.

Category: Cardiovascular system

126. A 2-year-old is brought into your office. The parent reports a purulent, malodorous, bloody discharge from the child's left nostril. The most likely diagnosis is
A) Foreign body in the nose
B) Acute sinusitis
C) Wegener's granulomatosis
D) Cerebrospinal fluid leak
E) Chronic tonsillitis

Answer and Discussion

The answer is A. Young children often lodge foreign bodies in their noses. Symptoms include unilateral purulent, malodorous, and often bloody nasal discharge. Other symptoms include nasal congestion and abnormal nasal sounds. Some children with clear nasal discharge or mild sinus congestion may harbor a foreign body. Foreign bodies should be removed anteriorly. An attempt at lavage should not be made because of the risk of pushing the foreign body further into the nasal cavity. Radiographs of the nasal area and sinuses may help localize the foreign body. There are several methods to remove nasal foreign bodies, including the use of an alligator forceps, ear curettes, and a Fogarty catheter (which is slipped behind the foreign body, inflated, and removed pulling the foreign body along with it); if the foreign body does not appear to have sharp edges, the practitioner can simply have the child blow the nose, forcing the foreign body out. If removal is unsuccessful, ear, nose, and throat referral and perhaps general anesthesia is in order. Inspection of the unaffected side and the ears should also be performed to ensure they are unaffected.

Additional Reading: Foreign bodies of the airway. *Nelson Textbook of Pediatrics,* 19th ed. Philadelphia, PA: Elsevier/Saunders; 2011.

Category: Cardiovascular system

127. Varicella-zoster immunoglobulin (VZIG) is recommended for which of the following groups?
A) All newborns
B) Newborns of mothers with onset of varicella 5 days before delivery
C) Hospitalized premature infants older than 28 weeks' gestation, regardless of the mother's history of chickenpox
D) Pregnant women just before delivery who have no history of varicella and were exposed at the time of conception
E) Newborns >4,500 g regardless of exposure history or mother's exposure history

Answer and Discussion
The answer is B. VZIG is indicated for the prevention of varicella and zoster infections in the following groups:

- Full-term infant born to mother who has chickenpox <1 week before delivery
- Every premature infant born to a mother with active chickenpox (even if present longer than 1 week)
- Newborns whose mothers had onset of varicella 5 days before delivery or within 2 days after delivery who are exposed to varicella
- Hospitalized premature infants (gestation of 28 weeks or more) whose mothers have no history of chickenpox
- Hospitalized premature infants (gestation of <28 weeks or <1,000 g) regardless of maternal history

VZIG is given by intramuscular injection. One vial (125 U) is given for each 10 kg of body weight, with a maximum dose of 625 U (five vials). For maximal effectiveness, VZIG should be given within 48 hours and preferably not more than 96 hours after exposure. Side effects are usually related to local discomfort at the injection site.

Current recommendations include routine vaccination of all infants with a single dose of live varicella virus vaccine (Varivax) at 12 to 18 months of age. Those older than 13 years with negative varicella titers require two doses given 4 to 8 weeks apart. The live virus is contraindicated in immunocompromised children. Varicella may occur in up to 6% of patients despite immunization; however, the illness is usually mild.

Additional Reading: Vaccines and preventable diseases: varicella (Chickenpox) Vaccination 2012. From: http://www.cdc.gov/vaccines/ on 10/03/2013.

Category: Patient/population-based care

128. The most common cause of lead exposure is
A) Playing with toys made with lead
B) Exposure to water from lead pipes
C) Breathing lead particles from the atmosphere
D) Ingesting food contaminated with lead
E) Ingesting contaminated paint chips or house dust

Answer and Discussion
The answer is E. More than 4% of children in the United States have lead poisoning. In the United States, an estimated 310,000 children younger than 5 years have elevated BLLs. Rates of lead poisoning are even higher in large cities and among people with low incomes. The most common cause of lead poisoning today is old paint with increased lead content. Lead has not been used in house paint since 1978. However, many older houses and apartment buildings (especially those built before 1960) have lead-based paint on their walls. Children can get lead poisoning by chewing on pieces of peeling paint or by swallowing house dust or soil that contains tiny chips of the leaded paint from these buildings (pica). Lead can also be in air, water, and food. Lead levels in the air have gone down greatly since lead was taken out of gasoline in the 1970s. Lead is still found in some old water pipes, although using lead solder to mend or put together water pipes is no longer allowed in the United States. Lead can also be found in food or juice stored in foreign-made cans or improperly fired ceramic containers.

Additional Reading: Lead poisoning in children. *Am Fam Physician.* 2010;81(6):751–757.

Category: Patient/population-based care

129. Which of the following statements about night terrors is true?
A) They affect adults more than children.
B) They are often remembered in vivid detail.
C) They occur during stages 3 and 4 of non–rapid eye movement (NREM) sleep.
D) They occur during rapid eye movement (REM) sleep.
E) They are unaffected by benzodiazepines.

Answer and Discussion
The answer is C. Night terrors occur more frequently in children than in adults. Boys between 5 and 7 years are more commonly affected. Symptoms include sudden onset, fearful, screaming episodes that disrupt stages 3 and 4 NREM sleep cycle. They may accompany sleepwalking. They differ from nightmares in that nightmares occur during REM sleep and are frequently remembered in vivid detail, whereas night terrors are not remembered. A short course of diazepam (which suppresses stages 3 and 4 of sleep) or imipramine (Tofranil) is often helpful in patients with severe night terrors but is not helpful for patients who suffer from nightmares. An underlying emotional disorder should be investigated in children with persistent or prolonged night terrors.

Additional Reading: Sleep medicine. *Nelson Textbook of Pediatrics,* 19th ed. Philadelphia, PA: Elsevier/Saunders; 2011.

Category: Psychogenic

> Symptoms of night terrors include sudden onset, fearful, screaming episodes that occur during stages 3 and 4 NREM sleep cycle. Night terrors are not remembered.

130. Which of the following statements is true regarding short stature in children?
A) Those with short stature and delayed bone age are considered to have constitutional short stature.
B) Those with genetic short stature rarely reach the height of their parents.
C) Those with constitutional short stature should undergo a comprehensive evaluation looking for secondary causes.
D) Chromosome studies should be performed on children suspected of genetic short stature.
E) Children with constitutional growth delay rarely reach normal adult height.

Answer and Discussion

The answer is A. Assessment of a child's growth rate is necessary when evaluating short stature. Most children in or below the fifth percentile for height have normal growth rates. In the absence of other clinical findings, no further assessment is needed; however, the child should be followed to ensure that the growth rate remains normal. Among children with short stature but normal growth rates, two specific groups can be identified on the basis of bone age: (1) those with genetic short stature and (2) those with constitutional short stature. Children with short stature who have normal growth rates and normal bone age are considered to have genetic short stature. Their eventual adult stature will likely be similar to that of their parents. On the other hand, children with short stature and delayed bone age are considered to have constitutional short stature. Following a period of decreased growth rate in infancy, the growth rate in these children will return to normal for the remainder of their childhood. While these children may be considered short at some points during their childhood, they can be expected to eventually acquire normal adult height. In both groups, no further medical assessment or treatment is necessary. Children with short stature and decreased growth rates warrant a comprehensive evaluation for an underlying pathologic condition. The assessment should include a CBC, a urinalysis, a chemistry profile, and thyroid studies. Children should undergo a sweat chloride test if they have a history of recurrent pulmonary or GI symptoms. Chromosome studies should be obtained if there are physical signs of Turner's syndrome. Growth hormone studies should not consist of a single random determination. Growth hormone stimulation methods are necessary. Consultation is warranted if the initial evaluation fails to reveal an etiology for the decreased stature.

Additional Reading: The skeletal dyplasias. *Nelson Textbook of Pediatrics,* 19th ed. Philadelphia, PA: Elsevier/Saunders; 2011.

Category: Endocrine system

131. Measles (rubeola) is associated with which of the following conditions?
A) Small erythematous ulcerations on the tongue
B) Joint pain, rash, infertility
C) Unexplained brain deterioration with seizure formation, behavioral and intellectual deterioration, motor abnormalities, and possible death years after a measles attack
D) Petechial rash that develops on the trunk and spreads to involve the face and extremities
E) Disseminated intravascular coagulopathy

Answer and Discussion

The answer is C. Measles is a highly contagious disease that was common in children before the advent of immunization. Symptoms include the three Cs (cough, coryza, conjunctivitis), high fever, maculopapular rash, and pathognomonic Koplik's spots (small white spots that resemble flecks of sand surrounded by areas of erythema) on the buccal mucosa, usually opposite the first and second upper molar. The cause is a paramyxovirus that is spread by respiratory secretions. The disease is communicable 2 to 4 days before the onset of the characteristic rash, which usually develops on the face and spreads to involve the entire body approximately 2 weeks from the time of exposure. In 3 to 5 days, the patient usually improves and the fever and rash subside. Measles is usually self-limited and has a low mortality rate unless significant complications develop. Complications include pneumonia, bacterial superinfection, acute thrombocytopenic purpura, encephalitis, and subacute sclerosing panencephalitis (unexplained brain deterioration with seizure formation, motor abnormalities, and possible death years after the measles attack). Treatment for measles is directed toward the relief of symptoms and appropriate medication for any secondary infections. The use of immunoglobulin may also be indicated. Children should be immunized with the live attenuated MMR vaccination at 12 to 15 months and again at age 4 to 6 years. Measles vaccine is not recommended for pregnant women, immunocompromised patients, or HIV patients.

Additional Reading: Measles. *Nelson Textbook of Pediatrics,* 19th ed. Philadelphia, PA: Elsevier/Saunders; 2011.

Category: Patient/population-based care

132. Diagnosis of mental retardation is
A) Easily identified by clinicians
B) Typically made by chromosomal analysis
C) Dependent on a complete history, physical examination, and developmental assessment of the child
D) Easily associated with an underlying etiology

Answer and Discussion

The answer is C. Mental retardation in young children is often missed by clinicians. The condition is present in 2% to 3% of the population, either as an isolated finding or as part of a syndrome or broader disorder. Causes of mental retardation are numerous and include genetic and environmental factors. In at least 30% to 50% of cases, physicians are unable to determine etiology despite thorough evaluation. Diagnosis is highly dependent on a comprehensive personal and family medical history, a complete physical examination, and a careful developmental assessment of the child. These will guide appropriate evaluations and referrals to provide genetic counseling, resources for the family, and early intervention programs for the child. The family physician is encouraged to continue regular follow-up visits with the child to facilitate a smooth transition to adolescence and young adulthood.

Additional Reading: Language development and communcation disoders. *Nelson Textbook of Pediatrics,* 19th ed. Philadelphia, PA: Elsevier/Saunders; 2011.

Category: Neurologic

133. Which of the following conditions is associated with congenital cataracts?
A) Maternal rubella infection
B) Maternal varicella infection
C) Congenital hypothyroidism
D) Acromegaly
E) Fetal hydrops

Answer and Discussion

The answer is A. A cataract is a proteinaceous opacity of the lens. Causes of congenital cataracts include ocular trauma, maternal rubella, diabetes mellitus, galactosemia, Marfan's syndrome, and Down's syndrome. Monocular cataracts should be corrected as soon as possible (within the first 3 months of birth) so that vision can develop properly. Delayed intervention can lead to development of abnormal vision. Treatment of the amblyopia may be the most demanding and difficult step in the visual rehabilitation of infants and children with cataracts.

Additional Reading: Rubella. *Nelson Textbook of Pediatrics,* 19th ed. Philadelphia, PA: Elsevier/Saunders; 2011.

Category: Special sensory

134. A child with Down's syndrome is born, and you explain to the family

A) Heart defects are very rare in Down's syndrome children.
B) Some women are fertile; however, there is a 50% chance their children will have Down's syndrome.
C) Fertility is not affected in men.
D) IQ scores are rarely affected in Down's syndrome children.
E) The most common site for heart defects is associated with the atrial septum.

Answer and Discussion

The answer is B. Newborns affected with Down's syndrome are often placid, rarely cry, and demonstrate muscular hypotonia. Excess skin around the neck is common and can be detected by fetal ultrasound as edema of the neck. Physical and mental development are impaired; the mean IQ is about 50. Microcephaly, a flattened occiput, and short stature are characteristic. The outer sides of the eyes are slanted upward, and epicanthal folds at the inner corner of the eye usually are present. Brushfield's spots (gray to white spots resembling grains of salt around the periphery of the iris) usually are visible and disappear during the first 12 months of life. The bridge of the nose is flattened; the mouth is often kept open because of a large protruding tongue that is furrowed and lacks the central fissure; and the ears are small and rounded. Hands are short and broad and often have a single palmar crease (simian crease); the fingers are short, with clinodactyly (incurving) of the fifth finger, which often has only two phalanges. The feet may have a wide gap between the first and second toes, and a plantar furrow often extends backward on the foot. Hands and feet show characteristic dermal prints (dermatoglyphics). Congenital heart disease, most commonly affecting the ventricular septum or the atrioventricular canal, occurs in about 40% of affected newborns. There is an increased incidence of almost all other congenital anomalies, particularly duodenal atresia. Many people with Down's syndrome develop thyroid problems, which may be difficult to detect unless blood tests are done. Additionally, they are prone to developing hearing problems and problems with vision. Regular screening may be appropriate. At autopsy, all adult Down's syndrome brains show the microscopic findings of Alzheimer's disease, and many persons also develop the associated clinical signs. Some affected women are fertile, and they have a 50% chance that their fetus will also have Down's syndrome; however, many of these affected fetuses abort spontaneously. All men with Down's syndrome are infertile.

Additional Reading: Cytogenetics. *Nelson Textbook of Pediatrics,* 19th ed. Philadelphia, PA: Elsevier/Saunders; 2011.

Category: Nonspecific system

135. Which of the following findings is most commonly associated with fetal alcohol syndrome?

A) Low birth weight
B) Seizures
C) Palmar erythema
D) Peripheral neuropathy
E) Cirrhosis

Answer and Discussion

The answer is A. Fetal alcohol syndrome is a constellation of symptoms in a newborn and is a result of maternal alcohol consumption. Physical findings include low birth weight, short palpebral fissures, midface hypoplasia, abnormal palmar creases, and cardiac abnormalities. Varying degrees of mental retardation may be present. Severe symptoms are usually the result of heavy ethanol consumption (i.e.,

5 or more drinks daily); however, milder effects may be associated with consumption of smaller amounts. Because a safe level of alcohol consumption during pregnancy has not been established, pregnant women should be counseled to avoid all alcohol use during pregnancy.

Additional Reading: Metabolic disturbances. *Nelson Textbook of Pediatrics,* 19th ed. Philadelphia, PA: Elsevier/Saunders; 2011.

Category: Patient/population-based care

136. Klinefelter's syndrome is associated with

A) Short stature and hirsutism
B) Tall stature with disproportionately long arms and legs
C) Delayed onset of puberty
D) Low urinary excretion of FSH
E) Universal cognitive defects

Answer and Discussion

The answer is B. Klinefelter's syndrome occurs in about 1 of 800 live male births. The extra X chromosome comes from the mother in 60% of cases. Affected persons tend to be tall, with disproportionately long arms and legs. They often have small, firm testes, and about one-third develop gynecomastia. Puberty usually occurs at the normal age, but facial hair growth is often light. There is a predisposition for learning difficulties, and many have significant deficits. However, clinical variation is varied, and many 47, XXY men are normal in appearance and intellect and are found in the course of an infertility workup (probably all 47, XXY men are sterile) or in chromosomal surveys of normal populations. Boys from the latter group have been followed developmentally. Testicular development varies from nonfunctional tubules to some production of spermatozoa, and urinary excretion of follicle-stimulating hormone is frequently increased. Some affected have 3, 4, and even 5 X chromosomes along with the Y. The more X chromosomes, the greater the severity of mental retardation.

Additional Reading: Cytogenetics. *Nelson Textbook of Pediatrics,* 19th ed. Philadelphia, PA: Elsevier/Saunders; 2011.

Category: Nonspecific system

137. A 5-year-old child has a chronic relapsing and pruritic superficial inflammation of the skin that affects the antecubital and popliteal fossas. The most likely diagnosis is

A) *Rhus* dermatitis
B) Atopic dermatitis
C) Hereditary angioedema
D) Cushing's disease
E) Lyme's disease

Answer and Discussion

The answer is B. Atopic dermatitis is a condition characterized by chronic relapsing, superficial inflammation of the skin. The skin disorder is associated with severe pruritus and eczematous changes with erythematous papules or plaques that may show excoriations or lichenification. Many patients may show three different stages. The first stage is an infantile stage that begins at 2 to 3 months of age and lasts until 18 months of age. The eczematous rash affects the cheeks and scalp, may form oval-shaped patches on the trunk, and may eventually affect the extensor surfaces. The inflammation resolves in most cases. However, in 33% of patients, the rash progresses into stage 2, which is usually referred to as *childhood eczema*. The rash during this stage usually affects the flexor surfaces of the antecubital and popliteal fossas. Other areas of involvement include the neck, wrists, and, occasionally, the hands and feet. The third stage is adolescent eczema, which usually occurs around the age of 12 years. Only 33% of children with childhood eczema progress to adolescent eczema, which usually only involves the hands. Atopic dermatitis is less common after 30 years of age. The condition appears to be associated with asthma, hay fever, elevated IgE levels, and urticaria. There also appears to be a genetic predisposition to develop atopic dermatitis. Triggering factors include certain foods (e.g., cheese, wheat, nuts, legumes, egg whites) and inhaled irritants (e.g., pollens, perfumes, toxic fumes). Treatment involves the use of antihistamines, corticosteroid creams, emollients (Eucerin or Aquaphor), wet-to-dry dressing changes with Burow's solution, and antibiotics for secondary bacterial infections. Bathing should be kept to a minimum. A short course of oral steroids may be helpful for severe cases. The avoidance of triggering factors is also important. Extremes of temperature and humidity should be avoided.

Additional Reading: Atopic dermatitis, an Overview. *Am Fam Physician*. 2012;86(1):35–42.

Category: Integumentary system

138. A child is born with excessive dorsal lymphedema of the hands and feet and with lymphedema or loose folds of skin over the posterior aspect of the neck. There is a low hairline on the back of the neck, ptosis, a broad chest with widely spaced nipples, multiple pigmented nevi, short fourth metacarpals and metatarsals, prominent finger pads, hypoplasia of the nails, and coarctation of the aorta. Based on the findings, the most likely diagnosis is
A) Klinefelter's syndrome
B) Turner's syndrome
C) Down's syndrome
D) Marfan's syndrome
E) Prader–Willi syndrome

Answer and Discussion

The answer is B. Affected newborns with Turner's syndrome may present with excessive dorsal lymphedema of the hands and feet and with lymphedema or loose folds of skin over the posterior aspect of the neck. However, many female children with Turner's syndrome are very mildly affected. Typically, short stature, webbing of the neck, low hairline on the back of the neck, ptosis, a broad chest with widely spaced nipples, multiple pigmented nevi, short fourth metacarpals and metatarsals, prominent finger pads, hypoplasia of the nails, coarctation of the aorta, bicuspid aortic valve, and increased carrying angle at the elbow occur. Renal anomalies and hemangiomas are common. Occasionally, telangiectasia occurs in the GI tract, with resultant intestinal bleeding. Mental retardation is rare, but many have some diminution of certain perceptual ability and thus score poorly on performance tests and in mathematics, even though they score average or above in verbal IQ tests. Gonadal dysgenesis with failure to go through puberty, develop breast tissue, or begin menses occurs in the majority of affected persons. Replacement with female hormones will bring on puberty. The ovaries are replaced by bilateral streaks of fibrous stroma and are usually devoid of developing ova. However, 5% to 10% of affected girls do go through menarche spontaneously, and very rarely, affected women have been fertile and have had children.

Additional Reading: Cytogenetics. *Nelson Textbook of Pediatrics,* 19th ed. Philadelphia, PA: Elsevier/Saunders; 2011.

Category: Nonspecific system

139. Which of the following conditions is associated with atopic dermatitis?
A) Asthma
B) Vasomotor rhinitis
C) Elevated IgA levels
D) Melanoma
E) Retinitis pigmentosa

Answer and Discussion

The answer is A. Atopic dermatitis is a chronic inflammatory condition of the skin that occurs in persons of all ages but is more common in children. The condition is characterized by intense pruritus and a course associated with exacerbations and remissions. Atopic dermatitis has been reported to affect as many as 10% of children. In the United States, the symptoms of atopic dermatitis typically resolve by adolescence in 50% of affected children, but the condition can persist into adulthood. Poor prognostic features include a family history of the condition, early disseminated infantile disease, female gender, and coexisting allergic rhinitis and asthma. The diagnosis of atopic dermatitis is based on the findings of the history and physical examination. Exposure to possible exacerbating factors, such as aeroallergens, irritating chemicals, foods, and emotional stress, can cause exacerbations. There are no specific laboratory findings or histologic features that define atopic dermatitis, although elevated IgE levels are found in a majority of affected patients. In infants and young children with atopic dermatitis, pruritus commonly is present on the scalp, face (cheeks and chin), and extensor surfaces of the extremities. More than 50% of patients with atopic dermatitis have or develop asthma or allergic rhinitis. The majority of patients have a positive family history of atopy. Even if atopic dermatitis resolves with age, the predisposition for asthma and rhinitis persists.

Additional Reading: Atopic dermatitis, an overview. *Am Fam Physician*. 2012;86(1):35–42.

Category: Integumentary system

140. Which of the following would concern a physician about a child's development?
A) Rolls over at 4 months
B) First words at 15 months
C) Walks at 12 months
D) Ties shoes at 5 years
E) Copies a circle at 3 years

Answer and Discussion

The answer is B. Some important developmental milestones for children include the following:

- *4 to 5 months:* Rolls over to supine position
- *6 months:* Sits without support
- *9 months:* Says "mama" and "dada" indiscriminately
- *9 months:* Creeps and crawls, pulls to stand, waves bye-bye
- *10 months:* Says "mama" and "dada" discriminately
- *12 months:* Walks alone
- *15 months:* Creeps upstairs, builds two-block towers, walks independently
- *18 months:* Points to four body parts
- *24 months:* Jumps, kicks ball, removes coat, verbalizes wants
- *3 years:* Copies circle; gives full name, age, and gender; throws ball overhand
- *4 years:* Hops on one foot, dresses with little assistance, shoes on the correct feet
- *5 years:* Ties shoes, prints first name, plays competitive games

Impairments in hearing can relate to delayed development. Therefore, the first step in the evaluation of a child with language delay is hearing assessment.

Additional Reading: Important growth and developmental milestones. *Nelson Textbook of Pediatrics*, 19th ed. Philadelphia, PA: Elsevier/Saunders; 2011.

Category: Nonspecific system

141. Which of the following statements about measles immunizations is true?
A) Allergies to eggs or neomycin are not contraindications to the measles vaccine.
B) Those who received killed virus immunization between 1963 and 1967 should receive a live attenuated booster vaccination.
C) Infants receiving vaccination before 15 months of age do not need booster vaccinations.
D) The present immunization is a genetically derived recombinant vaccine.
E) Those born before 1956 should receive a measles booster vaccination.

Answer and Discussion

The answer is B. Measles immunization is accomplished with a live attenuated virus given at 12 to 15 months of age in the MMR vaccine and then as a booster with the preschool physical at 4 to 6 years of age. Those vaccinated with the killed virus (available in the United States from 1963 to 1967) should be given the live attenuated vaccine, because ineffectiveness is associated with the killed virus given during that period. Those born before 1956 are, in most cases, immune as a result of natural infection and therefore require no additional vaccination. Also, infants vaccinated before 12 months of age should receive two additional boosters. Prior anaphylactic reactions to eggs or neomycin are relative contraindications to the administration of the measles vaccine. A pediatric allergist or immunologist should be consulted before administration.

Additional Reading: Vaccination options for preventing measles, mumps, rubella, and varicella; 2012. From: http://www.cdc.gov/vaccines/

Category: Patient/population-based care

142. Premature infants are at increased risk for kernicterus. Which of the following statements is true regarding bilirubin in these children?
A) Decreased bowel motility increases the amount of excreted bilirubin in the stools.
B) Early feedings increase bowel motility and promote bilirubin excretion.
C) Feeding has little impact on the level of bilirubin excretion.
D) Enterohepatic circulation does not occur until the infant reaches 40 weeks.
E) Delayed clamping of the umbilical cord allows for better excretion of bilirubin.

Answer and Discussion

The answer is B. Premature infants develop hyperbilirubinemia more often than do full-term infants, and kernicterus may occur at serum bilirubin levels as low as 10 mg/dL (170 µmol/L) in underweight premature infants who are ill. The higher bilirubin levels in premature infants may be partially due to inadequately developed hepatic excretion mechanisms, including deficiencies in bilirubin's uptake from the serum, its hepatic conjugation to bilirubin diglucuronide, and its excretion into the biliary tree. Decreased bowel motility enables more bilirubin diglucuronide to be deconjugated within the intestinal lumen by enterohepatic circulation of bilirubin. On the other hand, early feedings increase bowel motility and reduce bilirubin reabsorption and can thereby significantly decrease the incidence and severity of physiologic jaundice. Uncommonly, delayed clamping of the umbilical cord can also increase the risk of significant hyperbilirubinemia by allowing the transfusion of a large RBC mass; RBC breakdown and bilirubin production are thus increased.

Additional Reading: Digestive system disorders: kernicterus. *Nelson Textbook of Pediatrics*, 19th ed. Philadelphia, PA: Elsevier/Saunders; 2011.

Category: Hematologic system

143. Which of the following statements about insulin-dependent diabetes mellitus type I is true?
A) It usually develops in patients older than 30 years.
B) The disease is associated with insensitivity of the body's tissues to insulin.
C) Ninety percent of those affected present in nonketotic hyperosmolar coma.
D) There is a lack of insulin production as a result of destruction to the β cells in the islets of Langerhans.
E) Diabetic ketoacidosis is not associated with insulin-dependent diabetes mellitus type I.

Answer and Discussion

The answer is D. Insulin-dependent diabetes is the result of an insulin deficiency and appears to be a chronic autoimmune destruction of the β cells of Langerhans' islets. There is an increased risk among family members, and it is more common in individuals younger than 30 years. The most common symptoms are polyphagia, polyuria, polydipsia, increased thirst, weight loss despite increased appetite, fatigue, and blurred vision. One-third of patients have diabetic ketoacidosis at the time of presentation. Signs include severe dehydration, labored respirations (Kussmaul's respirations), altered mental status, abdominal pain, enuresis, and fruity breath. Laboratory results show hyperglycemia and glycosuria. Treatment involves the administration of exogenous insulin. Many patients (approximately 66%) experience a period of total or partial remission ("honeymoon period") within a few weeks or months after initiation of medication. The goals of treatment are replacing insulin, instituting diet and exercise regimens, and monitoring glucose levels.

Additional Reading: Diabetes mellitus. *Nelson Textbook of Pediatrics*, 19th ed. Philadelphia, PA: Elsevier/Saunders; 2011.

Category: Endocrine system

144. Which of the following is not associated with the development of acne?
A) Excessive sebum production
B) Diets high in fat
C) Hyperkeratinization with development of microcomedo
D) Accumulation of lipids and cellular debris
E) Bacterial colonization

Answer and Discussion

The answer is B. Acne is a disease associated with the pilosebaceous units in the skin. It is thought to be caused by four important factors:

1. Excessive sebum production secondary to sebaceous gland hyperplasia.
2. Subsequent hyperkeratinization of the hair follicle prevents normal shedding of the follicular keratinocytes, which then obstruct the follicle and form an inapparent microcomedo.

3. Lipids and cellular debris soon accumulate within the blocked follicle.
4. This microenvironment encourages colonization of *Propionibacterium acnes,* which provokes an immune response through the production of numerous inflammatory mediators. Inflammation is further enhanced by follicular rupture and subsequent leakage of lipids, bacteria, and fatty acids into the dermis.

Additional Reading: Diagnosis and treatment of acne. *Am Fam Physician.* 2012;86(8):734–740.

Category: Integumentary

145. A 4-year-old boy is brought to the emergency room by his parents. They report that the child swallowed a penny. On examination, the child has no abdominal tenderness. Radiographs of the abdomen localize the coin in the duodenum. The appropriate management includes
A)` Laxative administration
B) Esophagogastroduodenoscopy with removal of the coin
C) Ipecac administration
D) Charcoal administration
E) Observation

Answer and Discussion

The answer is E. It is not uncommon for infants and small children who swallow coins to present to the family physician's office or emergency room. Most children are completely asymptomatic. A radiograph of the chest, neck, and abdominal area should help locate the radiopaque coin. If it is found below the diaphragm, the child only needs to be observed until the coin is passed. If the coin is lodged in the esophagus or if the child exhibits symptoms related to the ingested coin, an esophagogastroduodenoscopy may be necessary to remove the foreign body. In most cases, sharp objects should be retrieved by endoscopy (if possible) if they have not entered the small intestine. Follow-up radiographs of the abdomen can help locate and mark the progress of coins in the intestines. Handheld metal detectors have also been used to locate the position of the coin. The use of ipecac, charcoal, or laxatives is not indicated.

Additional Reading: Foreign bodies in the GI tract. *The Merck Manual of Diagnosis and Therapy.* 19th ed. Merck Research Laboratories; 2011.

Category: Gastroenterology system

146. Which of the following statements is true regarding breast-feeding and nipple confusion?
A) The World Health Organization recommends avoiding the use of pacifiers or bottle-feeding to establish successful breast-feeding.
B) There is compelling evidence that pacifier use and bottle-feeding are detrimental to successful breast-feeding.
C) Early pacifier use is associated with increased breast-feeding at 1 month.
D) Supplementation with a cup or bottle increases the duration of breast-feeding.
E) Cup feeding was associated with a shorter duration of breast-feeding in comparison with bottle-feeding in mothers who had cesarean sections.

Answer and Discussion

The answer is A. The UNICEF/World Health Organization Baby Friendly Hospital Initiative recommends avoiding the use of pacifiers or bottle-feeding to ensure successful breast-feeding; however, the evidence supporting this recommendation is limited. Cup feeding has been advocated as a safe alternative to bottle-feeding in breast-fed infants who require supplemental feedings to prevent "nipple confusion" or future problems with breast-feeding. Researchers conclude that early pacifier introduction is associated with fewer mothers exclusively breast-feeding at 1 month and decreased overall breast-feeding duration when compared with later pacifier introduction. Supplementation by cup or bottle led to a decrease in overall breast-feeding duration compared with infants receiving no supplementation. In mothers who had cesarean delivery, cup feeding was significantly associated with higher rates of exclusive breast-feeding and overall duration of breast-feeding compared with bottle-feeding.

Additional Reading: Risks and benefits of pacifiers. *Am Fam Physician.* 2009;79(8):681–685.

Category: Nonspecific system

147. Which of the following statements about scoliosis is true?
A) The most common form is congenital.
B) The patient has a normal Adam's test.
C) Patients with abnormalities >5 degrees should be referred to an orthopaedist.
D) Most curvature is to the right in the thoracic spine, causing the right shoulder to be higher than the left.
E) Syringomyelia is not associated with scoliosis.

Answer and Discussion

The answer is D. *Scoliosis* is defined as the presence of a lateral spinal curvature of 11 degrees or more. Its prevalence during adolescence is estimated to be between 2% and 3%. Curvatures >100 degrees can contribute to restrictive pulmonary disease; however, deviations of this magnitude are extremely rare. Scoliosis is classified as idiopathic (80% of cases), congenital (5%), neuromuscular (10%), or miscellaneous (5%). Severe scoliosis is more common in female patients. Idiopathic scoliosis is an inherited autosomal-dominant condition that occurs with variable penetrance. Most patients are asymptomatic; however, they may report backaches. The child should be examined with his or her back facing the examiner. The patient is asked to flex forward, and the scapula height is observed (known as the Adam's test). If scoliosis is present, asymmetry in scapular height is noted. In most cases, the right shoulder is higher than the left because of a convex curve of the spine to the right in the thoracic area and to the left in the lumbar area. Hip height and symmetry may also be affected. Radiographs should only be considered when a patient has a curve that might require treatment or could progress to a stage requiring treatment (usually 40 to 100 degrees). Radiographs should include posteroanterior and lateral views of the spine with the patient standing. Magnetic resonance imaging should be obtained in patients with an onset of scoliosis before 8 years of age, rapid curve progression of more than 1 degree/month, an unusual curve pattern such as left thoracic curve, neurologic deficit, or pain. Treatment depends on the degree of curvature. The primary goal of treating adolescent idiopathic scoliosis is preventing progression of the curve magnitude. Curves <10 to 15 degrees require no active treatment and can be monitored, unless the patient's bones are very immature and progression is likely. Moderate curves between 25 and 45 degrees in patients lacking skeletal maturity used to be treated with bracing, but this treatment has never been proven to prevent curve progression. Poor compliance with wearing a brace obviates any potential usefulness of the therapy. Much controversy surrounds brace indications, and trends since the mid-1980s have moved toward no bracing or bracing only the more significant curves (20 to 50 degrees). In more severe cases, braces (e.g., Milwaukee brace) or surgery may be indicated. Painful scoliosis may indicate underlying neurologic problems, such as syringomyelia or spinal cord lesion, and is less likely to be idiopathic.

Additional Reading: Screening for idiopathic scoliosis in adolescents. *J Bone Joint Surg Am.* 2008;90(1):195–198.

Category: Musculoskeletal system

> When evaluating for scoliosis, the patient is asked to flex forward and the scapula height is observed (known as the Adam's test). If scoliosis is present, asymmetry in scapular height is noted.

148. Which of the following organisms is most commonly associated with dental caries in children?

A) *Staphylococcus aureus*
B) *Bacteroides fragilis*
C) *Pasteurella multicida*
D) *Eikenella corrodens*
E) *Streptococcus mutans*

Answer and Discussion

The answer is E. The mutans streptococci (i.e., *Streptococcus mutans* and *Streptococcus sobrinus)* have been reported as the principal bacteria responsible for the initiation of dental caries in humans.

Additional Reading: Dental caries. *Nelson Textbook of Pediatrics,* 19th ed. Philadelphia, PA: Elsevier/Saunders; 2011.

Category: Special sensory

149. Which of the following is recommended in pediatric adolescent screening?

A) Lipid profiles for all teenagers before age 18 years
B) Blood chemistries to include electrolytes and CBC determination
C) Routine screening for STDs in sexually active teens
D) Tuberculosis screening for all teens
E) Urinalysis for all girls above the age of 18 years

Answer and Discussion

The answer is C. Guidelines for adolescent preventive services (GAPS) consists of 24 recommendations that encompass health care delivery, health guidance, screening, and immunizations. The objective of GAPS is to improve health care delivery to adolescents using primary and secondary interventions to prevent and reduce adolescent morbidity and mortality. Following are the 24 recommendations made:

1. From ages 11 to 21 years, all adolescents should have an annual routine health visit.
2. Preventive service should be age and developmentally appropriate and should be sensitive to individual and sociocultural differences.
3. Physicians should establish office policies regarding confidential care for adolescents.
4. Parents or other adult caregivers of adolescents should receive health guidance at least once during early adolescence, once during middle adolescence, and, preferably, once during late adolescence.

5. All adolescents should receive general health guidance annually.
6. All adolescents should receive guidance annually to promote the reduction of injuries.
7. All adolescents should receive guidance annually about dietary habits.
8. All adolescents should receive guidance annually about the benefits of exercise and should be encouraged to engage in safe exercise on a regular basis.
9. All adolescents should receive guidance annually regarding responsible sexual behaviors, including abstinence. Latex condoms to prevent STDs (including HIV infection) and appropriate methods of birth control should be made available with instructions on ways to use them effectively.
10. All adolescents should receive guidance annually to promote avoidance of tobacco, alcohol and other abusable substances, and anabolic steroids.
11. All adolescents should be screened annually for hypertension according to the protocol developed by the National Heart, Lung, and Blood Institute's Task Force on Blood Pressure Control in Children.
12. Selected adolescents should be screened to determine their risk of developing hyperlipidemia and adult coronary heart disease, following the protocol developed by the Expert Panel on Blood Cholesterol Levels in Children and Adolescents.
13. All adolescents should be screened annually for eating disorders and obesity.
14. All adolescents should be asked annually about their use of tobacco products, including cigarettes and smokeless tobacco.
15. All adolescents should be asked annually about their use of alcohol and other abusable substances and about their use of over-the-counter or prescription drugs, including anabolic steroids, for nonmedical purposes.
16. All adolescents should be asked annually about involvement in sexual behaviors that may result in unintended pregnancy and STDs, including HIV infection.
17. Sexually active adolescents should be screened for STDs.
18. Adolescents at risk for HIV infection should be offered confidential HIV screening. (Newer guidelines recommend longer screening intervals.)
19. Female adolescents who are sexually active and women 18 years or older should be screened annually for cervical cancer by use of a Papanicolaou test.
20. All adolescents should be asked annually about behaviors or emotions that indicate recurrent or severe depression or risk of suicide.
21. All adolescents should be asked annually about a history of emotional, physical, or sexual abuse.
22. All adolescents should be asked annually about learning or school problems.
23. Adolescents should receive a tuberculin skin test if they have HIV, have been exposed to active tuberculosis, have lived in a homeless shelter, have been incarcerated, have lived in or come from an area with a high prevalence of tuberculosis, or currently work in a health care setting.
24. All adolescents should receive prophylactic immunizations according to the guidelines established by the federally convened Advisory Committee on Immunization Practices.

Additional Reading: Adolescent health screening and counseling. *Am Fam Physician.* 2012;86(12):1109–1116.

Category: Patient/population-based care

150. The most likely suspected cause for positional head deformities in children is
A) Supine positioning
B) Premature birth
C) Genetic influences
D) Child abuse
E) Poorly developed sternocleidomastoid muscle

Answer and Discussion

The answer is A. In 1993, the American Society of Craniofacial Surgeons documented an increase in the incidence of posterior cranial deformities (occipital plagiocephaly) in infants who had no predisposing risk factors. The relationship of this increased incidence to the "Back to Sleep" campaign was proposed in 1996 and was supported by evidence of a rapid increase in positional head deformity without any significant change in the rate of synostotic plagiocephaly.

> **Additional Reading:** Congenital anomalies of the central nervous system. *Nelson Textbook of Pediatrics,* 19th ed. Philadelphia, PA: Elsevier/Saunders; 2011.

> Category: Neurologic

151. Which of the following statements about Duchenne's muscular dystrophy is true?
A) Girls are affected more commonly than boys.
B) Early symptoms include mental retardation.
C) Distal muscles are affected before proximal muscles, and pseudohypertrophy of muscles can occur.
D) Creatinine kinase levels are low or undetectable.
E) Cardiomyopathy may result.

Answer and Discussion

The answer is E. Duchenne's muscular dystrophy is a genetically linked disorder (usually X-linked recessive) that usually affects boys between 2 and 5 years of age. The condition is caused by a mutation at the Xp21 locus, which results in the absence of dystrophin, a protein found inside the muscle cell membrane. It affects 1 in 3,600 live male births. Becker's muscular dystrophy is the same fundamental disease with a genetic defect at the same locus but a milder clinical disease.

Many affected individuals have no family history of the disorder. Early manifestations include rapid fatigue on ambulation or running, clumsiness, waddling gait, and a distinctive pattern of climbing up on the legs from a sitting to standing position known as *Gowers' maneuver.* The proximal muscles are usually affected before the distal muscles; pseudohypertrophy of the gastrocnemius (seen in 90% of patients), triceps, and vastus lateralis may occur. Cardiomyopathy and mental retardation may occur in advanced cases, although intellectual impairment occurs in all patients. Diagnosis is usually accomplished by muscle biopsy, which shows degeneration of muscle fibers and proliferation in connective tissue. Electromyelography studies often distinguish between neuropathic and myopathic processes. Laboratory tests show a significantly elevated creatinine kinase level. Dystrophin analysis of muscle samples is also very helpful in the diagnosis; dystrophin is extremely low (<3%) or undetectable in patients with Duchenne's dystrophy. Mutation analysis of DNA isolated from peripheral blood leukocytes identifies deletions or duplications in the dystrophin gene in approximately 65% of patients and point mutations in approximately 25% of patients. Treatment involves physical therapy and braces. The prognosis is usually poor, with most patients dying of pneumonia before the age of 20 years.

> **Additional Reading:** Muscular dystrophies. *Nelson Textbook of Pediatrics,* 19th ed. Philadelphia, PA: Elsevier/Saunders; 2011.

> Category: Musculoskeletal system

152. Pseudostrabismus is best diagnosed using a
A) Snellen's eye chart
B) Funduscopic examination
C) Cover/uncover test
D) Corneal light reflex test
E) Slit-lamp examination

Answer and Discussion

The answer is D. Visual acuity improves as children become older. All children older than 8 years should be able to achieve 20/20 visual acuity using eyeglass correction. Younger children should be referred to an ophthalmologist if there is a difference between the right and left eyes of two or more lines on a Snellen's chart visual evaluation. Strabismus is the most common cause of amblyopia (decreased visual acuity). All infants should have consistent, synchronized eye movement by 5 to 6 months of age. Strabismus most often results from an altered reflex arc in the central nervous system. It can also result from cranial nerve palsies, neuromuscular disorders, or structural abnormalities. Amblyopia is not necessarily related to the degree of strabismus. Small deviations can result in significant vision loss. Strabismus is categorized as medial deviation (esotropia), lateral deviation (exotropia), or vertical deviation (hypertropia). Vertical deviation is the least common type. Deviations that are always manifested are called *tropias,* whereas those that are only elicited by provocative testing are called *phorias.* Intermittent strabismus occurs when there is inconsistent alignment. Usually, the angle between the normal eye and the strabismic eye stays constant through all directions of eye movement and is not influenced by the eye used for fixation. This is termed *concomitant strabismus.* When the eye divergence worsens in some gaze directions, the strabismus is nonconcomitant. This is characteristic of restrictive or paralytic etiologies. In the majority of cases, strabismus develops between 18 months and 6 years of age. Pseudostrabismus is an apparent esotropia that occurs when a child has a wide nasal bridge and prominent epicanthal folds. The corneal light reflex is symmetric with pseudostrabismus. No treatment is needed. Amblyopia is treated by forcing the use of the suppressed eye with a patch over the preferred eye. A schedule whereby the patch is removed for 1 to 2 waking hours each day reduces the risk of a deprivation amblyopia in the good eye. Once the visual goal is achieved, part-time patching is needed to prevent relapse and is often continued for many months to years. The shorter the time that amblyopia is present and the later the age at which it began, the better the prognosis.

> **Additional Reading:** Disorders of eye movement and alignment. *Nelson Textbook of Pediatrics,* 19th ed. Philadelphia, PA: Elsevier/Saunders; 2011.

> Category: Special sensory

153. Which of the following statements is true regarding sexual abuse in children?
A) Less than 10% of girls at age 18 years have been sexually abused.
B) Sexual acting out is a normal child activity and represents little concern.
C) Secondary enuresis can be a symptom of sexual abuse.
D) Physicians should make a careful decision if there is enough evidence to report parents suspected of sexual abuse.
E) A person who reports sexual abuse may be held liable if no abuse is found.

Answer and Discussion

The answer is C. It is estimated that by the age of 18 years, 12% to 25% of girls and 8% to 10% of boys become victims of sexual abuse. With this high prevalence, it is likely that primary care physicians will encounter child victims of abuse in their practice. Suspicion of sexual abuse should be raised when children exhibit behavioral changes or have anogenital or other medical problems. Behavioral changes include sexual acting out, aggression, problems in school, regression (e.g., return to thumb sucking, use of a security blanket), sleep disturbances, depression, and eating disturbances. Sexual acting-out behavior is the most specific indicator of possible sexual abuse. Medical problems include anogenital trauma, bleeding, irritation or discharge, dysuria, frequent UTIs, encopresis, enuresis (especially after continence has been achieved), pregnancy, diagnosis of an STD, and oral trauma. Children may present with somatic complaints such as recurrent abdominal pain or frequent headaches resulting from the psychological stress. Physicians are mandated to report suspected cases of child sexual abuse to the local child protective services agency. When sexual abuse is suspected or when a child discloses a sexual abuse event, a report should be made. In most states, the person who reports the suspected abuse case will not be held liable if the report is made in "good faith."

> **Additional Reading:** Child abuse: approach and management. *Am Fam Physician.* 2007;75(2):221–228.
>
> Category: Patient/population-based care

154. Which of the following statements regarding colic is true?
A) Infants affected with colic are usually <10% on height and weight growth curves.
B) Symptoms are usually more severe at night.
C) The onset of colic occurs at birth.
D) Symptoms of colic last for approximately 1 year.
E) Colic has lasting negative effects on maternal mental health.

Answer and Discussion

The answer is B. Infant colic is characterized by excessive and inconsolable crying, hypertonicity, and wakefulness, mainly in the evening. An estimated 5% to 28% of infants have colic during the first few months of life. The widely cited "rule of threes" defines a colicky infant as one who is healthy and well-fed but cries for a total of at least 3 hours/day, more than 3 days in any 1 week. Onset is usually between the second and sixth weeks of life, and remission of symptoms generally occurs by 3 months of age. Although colic is thought to be a self-limited condition, it can be overwhelming to parents over a substantial number of weeks. One concern, moreover, is the potential lasting impact of colic on maternal mental health. Studies have shown that colic usually is a self-limited condition that does not result in long-lasting negative effects on maternal mental health.

> **Additional Reading:** Sequelae of infant colic. Evidence of transient infant distress and absence of lasting effects on maternal mental health. *Arch Pediatr Adolesc Med.* 2002;156:1183–1188.
>
> Category: Patient/population-based care

155. Which of the following statements regarding colic in infants is true?
A) Newborns are usually noted to be colicky before discharge from the hospital.
B) Inadequate parenting is a common cause of colic.
C) Treatment consists of swaddling the infant firmly in a blanket.
D) Infants rarely respond to being held, rocked, or being patted.
E) Colic rarely occurs at predictable times of day.

Answer and Discussion

The answer is C. The term *infant colic* is referred to as a symptom constellation that consists of paroxysms of crying, apparent abdominal pain, and irritability. Colic can begin shortly after a baby comes home from the hospital but more often begins some weeks later and may persist until age 3 or 4 months. Typically, the colicky infant eats and gains weight well. He or she may seem excessively hungry and often sucks vigorously on almost anything available. However, bouts of crying may represent significant stress to the family and parents. Colic often occurs at a predictable time of day or night, but a few infants cry almost incessantly. Excessive crying causes aerophagia, which results in flatulence and abdominal distention. The diagnosis of colic is a diagnosis of exclusion. Identifiable conditions must be ruled out by physical examination, blood count, urinalysis, or other studies as needed. In most cases no testing is necessary. Parents should be reassured that the baby's irritability is not due to poor parenting. The infant may respond to being held, rocked, or patted gently. An infant with a strong sucking urge who fusses soon after a feeding may need to suck more. A pacifier also may quiet the infant. A very active, restless infant may respond to being swaddled firmly with a small blanket. A milk-substitute formula may be tried briefly to ascertain whether milk intolerance exists. Parents should be assured that the colicky infant is healthy, that this behavior will cease in a few weeks, and that too much crying is not harmful.

> **Additional Reading:** Evaluation and management of colic. In: Basow DS, ed. *UpToDate.* Waltham, MA: UpToDate; 2013.
>
> Category: Gastroenterology system

156. An 8-year-old with a 5-year history of cystic fibrosis comes in to your office with increasing respiratory symptoms consisted with infection. Which of the following organisms is most likely involved?
A) *Streptococcus pneumoniae*
B) *Haemophilus influenzae*
C) *Mycoplasma pneumoniae*
D) *Pseudomonas aeruginosa*
E) *Moraxella catarrhalis*

Answer and Discussion

The answer is D. Early in the course of cystic fibrosis, *Staphylococcus aureus* is the pathogen most often isolated from the respiratory tract, but as the disease progresses, *Pseudomonas aeruginosa* is most frequently isolated. A mucoid variant of *Pseudomonas* is uniquely associated with cystic fibrosis.

> **Additional Reading:** Cystic fibrosis. *The Merck Manual of Diagnosis and Therapy*, 19th ed. Merck Research Laboratories; 2011.
>
> Category: Respiratory system

> Early in the course of cystic fibrosis, *Staphylococcus aureus* is the pathogen most often isolated from the respiratory tract, but as the disease progresses, *Pseudomonas aeruginosa* is most frequently isolated.

157. Which of the following conditions may represent a contraindication for immunization?
A) Increase in body temperature to 38.5°C (101°F) after previous immunization
B) Allergy to neomycin
C) Recent mild URI in an otherwise healthy child
D) Current antibiotic use
E) Family history of seizure disorder

Answer and Discussion

The answer is B. The following conditions are in most cases contra-indications to immunization practices:

- Previous severe reaction to the vaccine (anaphylaxis or persistent temperature >40.5°C [105°F])
- Allergy to eggs for influenza, yellow fever, and MMR vaccines
- Allergy to neomycin for MMR vaccine
- Immunocompromised patients or contacts for live attenuated vaccines such as MMR and varicella
- Chronic steroid therapy at moderate or high doses

Some health care providers inappropriately consider certain circumstances to be contraindications to immunization. For example,

- Reaction to a previous DTaP dose that involved only soreness, redness, or swelling at the site of the injection or a temperature <105°F (40.5°C)
- Mild acute illness with low-grade fever in an otherwise healthy child
- Current antibiotic use
- Prematurity (however, hepatitis B immunization in most cases should be delayed)
- History of nonspecific allergies
- Allergies to duck meat or feathers
- Family history of convulsion in persons considered for pertussis or measles vaccination

Additional Reading: Vaccines and immunizations. From: http://www.cdc.gov/vaccines/

Category: Patient/population-based care

---

158. A 15-year-old presents with a painful area of her lower right leg. She is a volleyball player for her high school team. The pain is described as a dull, aching pain that has been present for the last several months. Recently, it has become worse and is especially present at night. The most likely diagnosis is

A) Osteosarcoma
B) Shin splints
C) "Growing pains"
D) Osgood–Schlatter's disease
E) Stress fracture

Answer and Discussion

The answer is A. Patients with osteosarcoma typically present with dull, aching pain of several months' duration that may suddenly become more severe. The increase in pain severity may correlate with tumor penetration of cortical bone and irritation of the periosteum, or with pathologic fracture. Night pain is common and may awaken the patient from sleep. Chronic indolent night pain should not be dismissed as "growing pains," especially when it is unilateral. Patients frequently have a history of a minor injury, sprain, or muscle pull incurred while participating in a sport. The physical examination may reveal localized tenderness, restricted range of motion of the adjacent joint, and a limp or muscle atrophy and may confirm the presence of a mass, swelling, or deformity. Children frequently have referred pain; therefore, it is essential to perform a comprehensive examination of the joint above and below the area of complaint, as well as spinal and reflex examinations.

Additional Reading: Neoplasms of bone. *Nelson Textbook of Pediatrics,* 19th ed. Philadelphia, PA: Elsevier/Saunders; 2011.

Category: Musculoskeletal system

---

159. A 2-year-old girl is brought in by her mother. The child has evidence of high fever for the past 9 days, conjunctivitis (without exudate), erythematous pharynx, and swollen lips that have fissured and cracked. The child is also noted to have a generalized erythematous, maculopapular rash associated with the hands and feet and early desquamation of the superficial layer of skin. The most likely diagnosis is

A) Lyme's disease
B) Scarlet fever
C) Kawasaki's disease
D) Henoch–Schonlein purpura
E) Herpangina

Answer and Discussion

The answer is C. Kawasaki's disease, or mucocutaneous lymph node syndrome, is a disease of young children and is associated with an idiopathic vasculitis of the small- and medium-size blood vessels. The condition is characterized by prolonged high fever (>39°C [102°F]) that is often not relieved with antipyretics and the following:

- Conjunctival injection without exudate
- Erythematous mouth and pharynx, with the development of strawberry tongue and red swollen lips, which may progress to fissuring and cracking by day 6 of disease
- Generalized maculopapular rash
- Induration of the hands and feet with erythema associated with the feet and hands, with desquamation during the second and third week of disease
- Unilateral cervical lymphadenopathy

For the diagnosis to be made, patients must have a fever for 5 days or more plus at least four of the aforementioned criteria. The rash appears within 3 days of the onset of fever and can vary in character. Frequently, the rash is scarlatiniform on the trunk and erythematous on the palms and soles with subsequent distal desquamation. Mucous membrane involvement is common and includes hyperemic bulbar conjunctiva; injected oropharynx; dry, cracked lips; and a strawberry tongue. Other symptoms include sterile pyuria, arthritis or arthralgias, aseptic meningitis, carditis with congestive heart failure, hydrops of the gallbladder, pericardial effusion, and arrhythmias. The physical examination may reveal nonsuppurative cervical lymphadenopathy (>1.5 cm in diameter). Coronary artery abnormalities develop in 20% to 25% of patients with Kawasaki's disease. Cardiovascular complications are the major cause of short-term and long-term morbidity and mortality. Laboratory findings include leukocytosis with a bandemia, anemia, thrombocytosis, and an elevated erythrocyte sedimentation rate. Most affected individuals are younger than 5 years, with peak occurrence between 1 and 2 years of age. The condition is rare in children younger than 6 months and older than 12 years. Treatment involves supportive care and the use of aspirin and intravenous γ-globulin. Steroid use is contraindicated and may increase the risk for coronary aneurysms. Antibiotics are unnecessary. Close follow-up with electrocardiography, chest radiographs, and echocardiography is necessary. Some patients may require coronary angiography to rule out aneurysm formation.

Additional Reading: Kawasaki disease. *Nelson Textbook of Pediatrics,* 19th ed. Philadelphia, PA: Elsevier/Saunders; 2011.

Category: Nonspecific system

---

160. An appropriate first step in the management of gastroesophageal reflux for an infant is

A) H₂-receptor antagonist
B) Prokinetic agent
C) Proton pump inhibitor
D) Thickening feedings with dry rice cereal added to formula

Answer and Discussion

The answer is D. A common condition in infants is gastroesophageal reflux (GER), which causes parental anxiety resulting in numerous visits to the physician. The term GER implies a physiologic process in a healthy infant with no underlying systemic abnormalities. GER is a common condition involving regurgitation, or "spitting up," which is the passive return of gastric contents retrograde into the esophagus. The prevalence of GER peaks between 1 and 4 months of age and usually resolves by 6 to 12 months of age. There is no gender predilection or definite peak age of onset beyond infancy. A more severe form is gastroesophageal reflux disease (GERD). GERD is a pathologic process in infants manifested by poor weight gain, signs of esophagitis, persistent respiratory symptoms, and changes in neurobehavior. After the first year of life, GERD is more resistant to complete resolution. Risk factors for GERD include a history of esophageal atresia with repair; neurologic impairment and delay, hiatal hernia, bronchopulmonary dysplasia, asthma, and chronic cough. GERD is also associated with pulmonary aspiration, chronic bronchitis, and bronchiectasis. Conservative treatment for mild symptoms of GERD involves thickened feedings and positional changes in infants, and dietary modification in children. Healthy infants who regurgitate without signs of GERD may be managed by thickening feedings with dry rice cereal added to formula. Thickened feeding reduces regurgitation and fussiness, and increases daily caloric intake. Smaller, more frequent feedings are recommended in older infants and children. The medications used for GERD include H_2-receptor antagonists, prokinetic agents, and proton pump inhibitors for patients with persistent esophagitis. Lansoprazole is also available in a liquid alkaline form for use in the childhood population.

Additional Reading: Gastroesophageal reflux disease. *Nelson Textbook of Pediatrics,* 19th ed. Philadelphia, PA: Elsevier/Saunders; 2011.

Category: Gastroenterology system

161. The primary bacteria associated with the development of dental caries is
A) *Streptococcus mutans*
B) *Staphylococcus aureus*
C) *Streptococcus pneumoniae*
D) *Enterobacter species*
E) *Streptococcus viridans*

Answer and Discussion

The answer is A. Dental caries occur when the tooth's surface is susceptible to injury, bacteria are present, and there is a food source from which the bacteria can live and reproduce. The primary bacteria is *S. mutans,* which can manufacture lactic acid, damaging the tooth's protective covering. Excessive and repeated consumption of dietary carbohydrates places the patient at risk for the development of dental caries. Symptoms may include sensitivity to hot and cold fluids or foods, persistent pain, or visible caries formation. Diagnosis is usually made by probing the dental pits with a sharp dental instrument and detecting softened enamel. Radiographs may also show radiolucent areas. Treatment involves removal of the damaged enamel and replacement with restorative material. Prophylaxis involves proper brushing and flossing technique two times per day, combined with the use of fluoride and regular dental checkups to remove plaque buildup.

Additional Reading: Dental caries. *Nelson Textbook of Pediatrics,* 19th ed. Philadelphia, PA: Elsevier/Saunders; 2011.

Category: Special sensory

162. A 1-week-old is diagnosed with breast milk jaundice. You should instruct the mother to
A) Maintain breast pumping and switch the child to formula feeding and monitor bilirubin levels
B) Stop breast-feeding and start phototherapy
C) Continue breast-feeding and start phototherapy
D) Schedule an exchange transfusion
E) Avoid any future breast-feeding and switch to formula feeding

Answer and Discussion

The answer is A. Breast milk jaundice usually peaks in the 6th to 14th days of life. This late-onset jaundice may develop in up to one-third of healthy breast-fed infants. Total serum bilirubin levels vary from 12 to 20 mg/dL (340 µmol/L) and are not considered pathologic. The underlying cause of breast milk jaundice is not entirely known. Substances in maternal milk, such as β-glucuronidases, and nonesterified fatty acids may inhibit normal bilirubin metabolism. The bilirubin level usually decreases continually after the infant is 2 weeks old, but it may remain persistently elevated for 1 to 3 months. If the diagnosis of breast milk jaundice is in doubt or the total serum bilirubin level becomes markedly elevated, breast-feeding may be temporarily interrupted, although the mother should continue to express breast milk to maintain production. With formula substitution, the total serum bilirubin level should decline rapidly over 48 hours (at a rate of 3 mg/dL [51 µmol/L]/day), confirming the diagnosis. Breast-feeding may then be resumed.

Additional Reading: Jaundice associated with breastfeeding. *Nelson Textbook of Pediatrics,* 19th ed. Philadelphia, PA: Elsevier/ Saunders; 2011.

Category: Gastroenterology system

163. A 15-year-old female dancer presents with pain, swelling, and a "give away" sensation in her knee. The patient reports that going up- and downstairs aggravates the pain. Physical examination shows an increased Q angle. The most likely diagnosis is
A) Anterior cruciate ligament rupture
B) Osgood–Schlatter disease
C) Patellofemoral syndrome
D) Tibial plateau fracture
E) Iliotibial band syndrome

Answer and Discussion

The answer is C. Patellofemoral syndrome is a common overuse injury associated with the anterior knee. It commonly affects young women. In most cases, the syndrome is associated with poor conditioning and the initiation of a new activity, particularly running, but also other activities including dancing, gymnastics, and figure skating. Symptoms include pain, swelling, and a "give away" sensation associated with the knee. Ascending or descending hills or stairs and repeated squatting or weight bearing on a semiflexed knee tend to aggravate symptoms. The contributing factor is weakness of the quadriceps muscles and particularly the vastus medialis. The condition is also associated with an increased Q angle (the angle formed from a line down the femur and a line formed by the patellar tendon) and a high-riding patella (patella alta). Radiographs (sunrise view) of the knees may show patellofemoral malalignment but are not necessary for the diagnosis. Treatment involves rest, ice, nonsteroidal anti-inflammatory agents, and quadriceps-strengthening exercises. Knee braces have shown no significant benefit in terms of symptom relief.

Additional Reading: Management of patellofemoral pain syndrome. *Am Fam Physician.* 2007;75(2):194–202.

Category: Musculoskeletal system

164. Of the following, the drug of choice for a pertussis infection is
A) Penicillin
B) Tetracycline
C) Ciprofloxacin
D) Chloramphenicol
E) Erythromycin

Answer and Discussion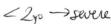

The answer is E. Pertussis is a potentially serious illness in children younger than 2 years. Mortality is about 1% to 2% in children younger than 1 year of age (highest in the first month of life). Most deaths are caused by bronchopneumonia and cerebral complications. Pertussis is troublesome but rarely serious in older children and adults, except in the elderly. Patients should be quarantined, particularly from susceptible infants, for at least 1 month from disease onset or until symptoms have subsided. Hospitalization is recommended for seriously ill infants to assess progression of disease and prevent and treat complications. Antibiotics given in the catarrhal stage may ameliorate the disease. After paroxysms are established, antibiotics usually have no discernible effect but are recommended to limit spread. The drug of choice is a macrolide antibiotic (e.g., erythromycin or azithromycin). Antibiotics should also be used for any bacterial complications such as bronchopneumonia and otitis media.

Additional Reading: Pertussis: a disease affecting all ages. *Am Fam Physician.* 2006;74(3):420–426.

Category: Respiratory system

165. Which of the following statements about isotretinoin is true?
A) It is recommended in the treatment of mild to moderate acne.
B) It has potential detrimental effects on the kidney.
C) It has beneficial effects on cholesterol levels.
D) Documentation of a negative pregnancy test is mandatory before its use in women.
E) A common side effect is tinnitus.

Answer and Discussion

The answer is D. Isotretinoin is used for moderate to severe nodulocystic acne unresponsive to conventional therapy. Therapy usually lasts 16 to 20 weeks followed by an 8-week drug vacation before the administration of the next course. It is absolutely contraindicated in pregnancy, and 2 to 3 contraceptive methods should be instituted before its administration. In addition, female patients should have a documented negative pregnancy test before isotretinoin administration. Side effects include xerosis, cheilitis, epistaxis, myalgias, and arthralgias. The effects of the drug may also alter the liver function test, blood counts, blood glucose, uric acid, and cholesterol and triglyceride levels, all of which may require frequent monitoring. There has been an association with pseudotumor cerebri development in patients who use isotretinoin. The administration is required to be monitored by certified provider.

Additional Reading: Drugs for acne, rosacea and psoriasis. *Treat Guidel Med Lett.* 2013;11(125):1–8.

Category: Integumentary

 The effects of isotretinoin may also alter the liver function test, blood counts, blood glucose, uric acid, and cholesterol and triglyceride levels, all of which may require frequent monitoring.

166. Which of the following is an acceptable criterion for discharging a premature infant from the neonatal unit?
A) Body temperature is maintained in an open crib.
B) The child is maintaining its birth weight.
C) The child is gaining weight of 5 g/day.
D) The child can tolerate tube feeds.
E) The child can react to external stimuli.

Answer and Discussion

The answer is A. Because of the increased survival rate and because many neonatal intensive care units now allow early discharge, family physicians are increasingly likely to provide care to small, premature infants after discharge from the hospital. Most neonatal units have no minimum weight requirement for discharge (although most are at least 1,800 to 2,100 g). Medical guidelines for discharge are as follows:

- Body temperature is maintained while the infant is in an open crib, usually at 34 weeks of gestational age or at 2,000 g (4 lb, 6 oz) of weight.
- The infant feeds by mouth well enough to have a weight gain of 10 to 30 g/day.
- The infant is not receiving medications that require hospital management.
- No recent major changes in medications or oxygen administration have occurred.
- No recent episodes of apnea or bradycardia have occurred.

During the first 2 years of life, growth is plotted using age corrected for prematurity. Growth charts for the "average" premature infant have been designed for this purpose. After the infant reaches 2 years of age, a standard growth chart for chronologic age may be used. The infant's development during the first 2 years should be plotted from the infant's estimated due date rather than the infant's birth date. The Denver Prescreening Developmental Questionnaire, the Denver Developmental Screening Test, and the Gesell Screening Inventory are all accepted tests. Using a standardized developmental test is more important than the choice of test. The timing of immunizations in the physician's office should be based on the infant's chronologic age (not the gestational age). The only exception is hepatitis B vaccination. The AAP Committee on Infectious Diseases has issued a statement indicating that it may be advisable to delay administration of hepatitis B vaccine until the infant weighs 2,000 g (4 lbs, 6 oz). The full dose of all immunizations should be given. As with term infants, premature infants should be given the acellular pertussis vaccine. Influenza vaccine should be given to infants older than 6 months with chronic medical problems, especially lung disease. With all premature infants, consideration should also be given to administering influenza vaccine before the influenza season to parents and other frequent visitors in the home. Administration of the pneumococcal vaccine at 2 years of age may be beneficial in infants with chronic problems such as lung disease; more recently, the heptavalent vaccine (Prevnar) has been given.

Additional Reading: Outpatient care of the premature infant. *Am Fam Physician.* 2007;76(8):1159–1164.

Category: Patient/population-based care

167. Which of the following statements about enuresis in children is true?
A) Primary enuresis is defined as the onset of bed-wetting after a 6-month period of dryness.
B) Bed-wetting usually occurs in stage 1 of NREM sleep.
C) Most outgrow the condition before 12 years of age.
D) There is no approved treatment for enuresis.
E) Diagnosis should consist of cystoscopy to rule out structural causes.

Answer and Discussion

The answer is C. Nocturnal enuresis beyond 5 years of age in girls and 6 years of age in boys is a relatively common problem. Primary enuresis is defined as a patient who has never had an extended period of dryness since birth. Secondary enuresis is the onset of bed-wetting after 6 months of dryness. The condition is more common in young boys and firstborn children, and there is usually a positive family history. Bed-wetting usually occurs during the first REM sleep cycle, when sleep is relatively light. It may also occur in other stages, except for stage 1. The family and patient should be reassured that this is a common problem and is not associated with any underlying disorder. Diagnostic tests are usually limited to urinalysis to rule out infection. The bladder is usually a normal structural size but is functionally small. The physician should keep in mind that primary nocturnal enuresis is a diagnosis of exclusion, and all other causes of bed-wetting must be ruled out. Causes of secondary enuresis include neurogenic bladder and associated spinal cord abnormalities, UTIs, and the presence of posterior urethral valves in boys or an ectopic ureter in girls. Posterior urethral valves cause significant voiding symptoms such as straining to void and diminished urinary stream. An ectopic ureter causes constant wetting. Treatment consists of observation. In older children, imipramine, oxybutynin (Ditropan), or nasal desmopressin (DDAVP) can be used. Other forms of treatment for older children include bell-and-pad conditioning. Most patients outgrow the condition before 12 years of age. Daytime enuresis may indicate underlying pathology or voiding dysfunction and requires further evaluation.

Additional Reading: Voiding dysfunction. *Nelson Textbook of Pediatrics*, 19th ed. Philadelphia, PA: Elsevier/Saunders; 2011.

Category: Nephrologic system

168. The majority of cases of occult bacteremia are caused by
A) *Streptococcus pneumoniae*
B) *Neisseria meningitidis*
C) *Staphylococcus aureus*
D) *Haemophilus influenzae* type B (Hib)
E) *Salmonella*

Answer and Discussion

The answer is A. Occult bacteremia is caused by *Streptococcus pneumoniae* in 65% to 75% of cases, and the remainder by other bacteria, including *Neisseria meningitidis*, *Salmonella* spp., and *Staphylococcus aureus*. The incidence of bacteremia due to *Haemophilus influenzae* type B (Hib) has decreased substantially where Hib conjugate vaccine is part of routine childhood immunization. Occult bacteremia is detected in about 4% to 17% of febrile infants between 1 and 24 months of age. The majority of cases occur in infants between 6 and 24 months of age. Children who look well enough to be managed as outpatients but who are later found to be bacteremic are usually younger than 24 months of age. Incidence does not vary with sex or race.

Additional Reading: Bacteremia and septic shock. *Nelson Textbook of Pediatrics*, 19th ed. Philadelphia, PA: Elsevier/Saunders; 2011.

Category: Nonspecific system

169. Substances that are contraindicated during breast-feeding include all of the following *except*
A) Alcohol
B) Tetracycline
C) Penicillin
D) Ciprofloxacin
E) Bromocriptine

Answer and Discussion

The answer is C. Certain medications are contraindicated during breast-feeding, including quinolone antibiotics, tetracycline, chloramphenicol, bromocriptine, cyclosporine, cyclophosphamide, doxorubicin, methotrexate, lithium, and ergotamine. Other drugs that have relative contraindications include metronidazole, sulfonamides, salicylates, phenobarbital, other psychotropic medication, and antihistamines. Caffeine in large amounts should also be avoided. In addition, recreational drugs (e.g., alcohol, cocaine, marijuana) should be avoided.

Additional Reading: Strategies for breastfeeding success. *Am Fam Physician*. 2008;78(2):225–232.

Category: Nonspecific system

170. Which of the following is not usually associated with autism?
A) Normal IQs
B) Echolalia
C) Repetitive movements
D) Self-injury behaviors
E) Seizures

Answer and Discussion

The answer is A. The impairments noted in autistic persons are varied and result in good skills in some areas and poor skills in others. Echolalia, the involuntary repetition of a word or a sentence just spoken by another person, is a common feature of language impairment that, when present, may cause language skills to appear better than they really are. There may also be deficiencies in symbolic thinking, stereotypic behaviors (e.g., repetitive nonproductive movements of hands and fingers, rocking, meaningless vocalizations), self-stimulation, self-injury behaviors, and seizures. Mental retardation is not a diagnostic criterion, but it is frequently present in the moderate to severe range.

Additional Reading: Primary care for children with autism. *Am Fam Physician*. 2010;81(4):453–460.

Category: Nonspecific system

171. Which of the following statements about otitis media is true?
A) The most common organisms causing otitis media in newborns are *Streptococcus pneumoniae*, *Haemophilus influenzae*, and *Moraxella catarrhalis*.
B) Ten percent of otitis media cases with *H. influenzae* as the causative organism are resistant to amoxicillin.
C) Close to 100% of otitis media cases with *M. catarrhalis* as the causative organism are resistant to amoxicillin.
D) The treatment of otitis media should include the use of antibiotics and an antihistamine/decongestant preparation.
E) Analgesic medication is rarely needed in the treatment of otitis media.

Answer and Discussion

The answer is C. Otitis media is one of the most frequent reasons parents bring their children to the physician. The condition occurs more frequently in the winter months and affects bottle-fed infants (especially those put to bed with bottles) more frequently than other infants; it also affects boys more often than girls, as well as premature infants or those enrolled in day care more often than other infants. Infants with cleft palate or Down's syndrome are also at increased risk. The most common etiologic agents for otitis media are as follows:

- *Streptococcus pneumoniae*
- *Moraxella (Branhamella) catarrhalis*
- Nontypeable *H. influenzae*

Newborns are more likely to be affected with *E. coli* and *S. aureus*. Children older than 5 years are less frequently affected by *Klebsiella pneumoniae*, and *Bacteroides* rarely cause otitis media. Viruses, including RSV, rhinovirus, and adenovirus, can also cause otitis media and are often complicated with secondary bacterial organisms.

The major factor that contributes to otitis media is eustachian tube dysfunction and anatomic immaturity, which allows fluid and bacteria to reflux into the middle ear. Symptoms of otitis media include pain, fever, and occasionally purulent drainage if the tympanic membrane has ruptured. Younger children may be fussy, irritable, and show decreased appetite or sleep disturbances. Pulling at the ears may also be a sign of otitis media. Physical examination usually shows a bulging erythematous tympanic membrane with a loss of tympanic landmarks and lack of mobility with pneumatoscopy. Treatment involves the use of analgesics and first-line antibiotics, including amoxicillin, trimethoprim–sulfamethoxazole, and erythromycin. Amoxicillin remains the antibiotic of first choice, although a higher dosage (80 mg/kg/day) may be indicated to ensure eradication of resistant *S. pneumoniae*. Oral cefuroxime or amoxicillin–clavulanate and intramuscular ceftriaxone are suggested second-line choices for treatment failure.

Thirty percent to 60% of *S. pneumoniae* and close to 100% of *M. catarrhalis* strains are β-lactamase producers and are resistant to amoxicillin. Resistance may vary according to locality. If β-lactamase–producing infections are suspected, amoxicillin–clavulanate, erythromycin, trimethoprim–sulfamethoxazole, or cephalosporins are recommended. The use of antihistamines and decongestants has little or no benefit in the treatment of otitis media.

Additional Reading: The diagnosis and management of acute otitis. *Pediatrics.* 2013;131(3):e964–e999.

Category: Special sensory

172. According to the AAP, at what age should a child begin formal swimming lessons?
A) After 1 year of age
B) After 2 years of age
C) After 3 years of age
D) After 4 years of age
E) After 5 years of age

Answer and Discussion

The answer is D. Children who are near water are at higher risk of drowning. The AAP has updated its policy about swimming programs for infants and toddlers. While some aquatic programs may include water safety instructions for parents and children, these programs are clearly not designed to teach children how to swim. In fact, swimming skills are not the same as water safety skills, and parents should be clear about what is developmentally possible in different age groups. Rudimentary swimming movements (e.g., the dog paddle) are possible in a 1-year-old child, but traditional swimming strokes do not occur until a child is about 5 years of age. Children who have not yet reached their fourth birthday will not have the neuromuscular capability to adequately learn swimming skills. Taking swimming lessons at an earlier age does not mean that the child will master water skills earlier or be more proficient than children who take such lessons later. Training programs have been shown to improve water survival skills, but safety training has not been shown to decrease the risk of drowning. In fact, programs that emphasize making the child stop fearing water may, in fact, encourage children to enter the water without supervision. Therefore, the AAP recommends that children do not begin formal swimming lessons until after they are 4 years of age. Parents should not be encouraged to believe that a child's participation in an aquatic program will decrease the risk of drowning, and they should remain within arm's reach or able to touch the swimmer at all times (also known as *touch supervision*).

Additional Reading: American academy of pediatrics committee on sports medicine and fitness and committee on injury and poison prevention. Prevention of drowning. *Pediatrics.* 2010;126(1):e253–e262.

Category: Patient/population-based care

173. The most common cause of septic joint in an immigrant 3-year-old boy with no prior immunizations is
A) *Neisseria gonorrhea*
B) *Pasteurella multocida*
C) *Mycoplasma pneumoniae*
D) *Streptococcus pneumoniae*
E) *Haemophilus influenzae*

Answer and Discussion

The answer is E. Bacterial infections are usually responsible for septic joints. In children (between 2 and 5 years of age), the most common pathogen associated with osteomyelitis is *Staphylococcus aureus*; other causes include *Staphylococcus*, *Streptococcus*, and gram-negative bacteria. In sexually active teenagers and young adults, *Neisseria gonorrhea* is a common cause. Additionally, *Staphylococcus*, group A *Streptococcus*, and *Streptococcus pneumoniae* are causes. Other agents include viruses, mycobacteria, or fungi. *H. influenzae* type B was most common before universal vaccination and may affect unimmunized immigrants. *Salmonella* and *S. aureus* are the two most common causes of osteomyelitis in children with sickle cell anemia. Patients with rheumatoid arthritis are at particular risk for septic joints. In adults, the most common joint affected is the knee, whereas, in children, the hip and knee are the most commonly affected. Typically, the child with a septic joint will have pain with any range of motion of the joint, whereas patients with trauma or toxic synovitis will allow some range of motion of the joint. Laboratory tests show an elevated WBC count and elevated sedimentation rate. Culture and Gram's stain of the joint fluid should be performed. Blood cultures are positive in 30% to 40%. Treatment involves surgical débridement as soon as possible if a bacterial source is suspected.

Additional Reading: Septic arthritis. *Nelson Textbook of Pediatrics,* 19th ed. Philadelphia, PA: Elsevier/Saunders; 2011.

Category: Musculoskeletal system

> In sexually active teenagers and young adults, *Neiserria gonorrhea* is a common cause of septic joints.

174. Which of the following sounds is associated with a positive Ortolani's sign when assessing for developmental dysplasia of the hip (DDH)?
A) "Snap"
B) "Click"
C) "Clunk"
D) "Pop"
E) "Grinding"

Answer and Discussion

The answer is C. The AAP has issued a clinical practice guideline about early detection of DDH. It is important to remember that no physical examination finding is pathognomonic for DDH. The neonate should have a normal range of motion of abduction to 75 degrees and adduction to 30 degrees. A physical assessment should include evaluation for asymmetry as well as assessing Ortolani's and Barlow's signs. The Ortolani's maneuver is performed with the infant supine and the hip flexed to 90 degrees. The leg is held in neutral rotation with the physician's index and middle finger along the greater trochanter and the thumb along the inner thigh. The hip is abducted as the leg is lifted anteriorly. A "clunk" (not a high-pitched click) indicates a positive Ortolani's sign and occurs as the dislocated femoral head is reduced into the acetabulum. A positive Barlow's sign occurs when there is a palpable "clunk" (or movement) of the femoral head being dislocated. Again, the infant has the hip flexed to 90 degrees; the leg is adducted while posterior pressure on the knee is applied to detect an unstable hip dislocation. High-pitched clicks are common with extension and flexion and are insignificant. With the infant prone, the physician should check for limb length discrepancy or asymmetric gluteal or thigh folds. In an older infant (about 3 months of age), limited abduction of the hip is a reliable sign of DDH. Again, asymmetry should be sought. Physical examination screening for DDH should occur at 2 to 4 days and at each well-child visit (1, 2, 4, 6, 9, and 12 months) until the child is 1 year old or is reliably able to walk.

Additional Reading: Screening for developmental dysplasia of the hip: a systematic literature review for the US Preventive Services Task Force. *Pediatrics.* 2006; 117:3.

Category: Musculoskeletal system

175. Erythema infectiosum (fifth disease) is caused by
A) Parvovirus
B) Adenovirus
C) Rhinovirus
D) Paramyxovirus
E) Herpes virus

Answer and Discussion

The answer is A. Parvovirus B19 is the causative agent responsible for erythema infectiosum, or fifth disease. The incubation period is 6 to 14 days. Outbreaks frequently occur at day schools, elementary schools, or junior high schools, and they frequently occur in the spring. Symptoms include a distinctive facial rash that has a "slapped-cheek" appearance, fever, arthralgias, and fatigue. Within 2 days, the facial rash gives rise to a generalized lacelike macular rash that involves the trunk. It has become increasingly clear over the past several years that parvovirus B19 causes arthritis and arthralgias in adults and children. Although parvovirus infections in adults are most commonly asymptomatic, an estimated 50% to 60% of women with symptomatic disease manifest arthropathy. Men appear to be affected much less frequently. Blood cell counts during the illness show leukopenia, lymphopenia, and thrombocytopenia with decreased reticulocytes. Because parvovirus B19 infects erythroid progenitor cells in the bone marrow and causes temporary cessation of RBC production, patients who have underlying hematologic abnormalities (and thus depend on a high rate of erythropoiesis) are prone to cessation of RBC production if they become infected. This can result in a transient aplastic crisis, which may occur in persons with chronic hemolytic anemia and conditions of bone marrow stress. Thus, patients with sickle cell anemia, thalassemia, acute hemorrhage, and iron-deficiency anemia are at risk. The diagnosis of erythema infectiosum is made clinically, and laboratory studies are not needed under normal circumstances. Serologic tests are usually relied on for the diagnosis of parvovirus B19 infection in patients with transient aplastic crisis or arthropathy; a positive parvovirus B19–specific IgM antibody or a significant rise in parvovirus B19–specific IgG titer is indicative of an acute or recent infection. Exposure during pregnancy can lead to fetal hydrops, spontaneous abortion, and fetal death. Supportive care during an attack of fifth disease is usually adequate, and the illness is self-limited. The risk of respiratory transmission is decreased significantly when the rash starts to fade. Children with erythema infectiosum are not infectious and can attend school and day care.

Additional Reading: Parvovirus B19. *Nelson Textbook of Pediatrics,* 19th ed. Philadelphia, PA: Elsevier/Saunders; 2011.

Category: Nonspecific system

176. Simultaneous administration of what other vaccine can diminish the effectiveness of the varicella vaccine?
A) MMR vaccine
B) Hepatitis B vaccine
C) *Haemophilus influenzae* vaccine
D) Pneumococcal vaccine
E) Influenza vaccine

Answer and Discussion

The answer is A. Varicella is a highly contagious illness manifested by fever and a 3-to-5-day rash. Experts recommend live attenuated varicella-zoster vaccine for healthy susceptible children (12 months and older), adolescents, and adults because of its high efficacy rate. Widespread use of the varicella vaccine has substantially decreased the rates of chickenpox and vaccine-related complications. Vaccinated persons develop milder symptoms with fewer skin lesions, which are more likely to be macular than vesicular. Residual scarring also is less common. However, atypical cases are making the diagnosis of varicella more difficult. Recent varicella exposure is the most useful clinical diagnostic hint because demonstration of viral antigen in skin scrapings or vesicular fluid is rarely available to the physician. It also is important to exclude similarly presenting conditions and to note that breakthrough varicella infection can be communicated to susceptible persons. Vaccination may be less effective in children younger than 15 months. However, because children 12 to 15 months of age are at risk and may not return at a later age for vaccination, the present recommendation remains to vaccinate at 12 months of age. Studies have found that children given a varicella vaccine within 30 days or less of receiving an MMR vaccine are at an increased risk of developing breakthrough varicella infection. Therefore, guidelines suggest separating the MMR and varicella-zoster vaccines by 28 days if not given simultaneously.

Additional Reading: Varicella-Zoster virus infections. *Nelson Textbook of Pediatrics,* 19th ed. Philadelphia, PA: Elsevier/Saunders; 2011.

Category: Patient/population-based care

177. Transposition of the great vessels is associated with which of the following?
A) An aorta that arises from the left atrium
B) Cyanosis at birth with an intact ventricular septum
C) A pulmonary vein that empties into the right ventricle
D) A pulmonary artery that arises from the right ventricle
E) A superior vena cava that empties directly into the pulmonary circulation

Answer and Discussion

The answer is B. Transposition of the great vessels is a cause of cyanotic heart disease. Male term infants are more commonly affected than their female counterparts, as are infants of diabetic mothers. The condition is associated with an aorta that arises from the right ventricle and a pulmonary artery that arises from the left ventricle. There are basically two types:

- Transposition with an intact septum
- Transposition with a ventricular septal defect

Because the systemic blood must mix with the pulmonary circulation, an intact ventricular septum leads to immediate cyanosis and death if not treated. In many cases, the ductus arteriosus remains open for several days, and cyanosis does not develop until it has fully closed. In most cases, congestive heart failure develops and can lead to death. Retardation of growth and development is common. Many (but not all) children will have an associated systolic murmur, and some show significant cyanosis at the time of birth. Chest radiographs may be normal but can show mild cardiomegaly with an egg-shaped heart with a narrow superior mediastinum and increased pulmonary vascular markings ("egg on a string"). Cardiac catheterization is used for the diagnosis, and surgery is performed to return the normal anatomic circulation or to place an intra-atrial shunt to redirect blood flow to the appropriate circulation.

> **Additional Reading:** Cyanotic congenital heart disease. *Nelson Textbook of Pediatrics,* 19th ed. Philadelphia, PA: Elsevier/Saunders; 2011.

> Category: Cardiovascular system

178. The most common organism isolated in periorbital cellulitis in vaccinated children in the absence of trauma is

A) *H. influenzae* type B
B) *Streptococcus pneumoniae*
C) *Moraxella catarrhalis*
D) *Staphylococcus aureus*
E) *Pseudomonas aeruginosa*

Answer and Discussion

The answer is B. Periorbital and orbital cellulitis may be caused by trauma (e.g., a wound, an insect bite), an associated infection (e.g., sinusitis), or seeding from bacteremia. Before widespread immunization, *Haemophilus influenzae* type B was the most common cause secondary to bacteremia (about 80% of cases) and remains so in non-immunized populations. *Streptococcus pneumoniae* accounted for most of the remaining 20% of cases. *S. pneumoniae* is the most likely agent in *Haemophilus influenzae* type B-vaccinated patients when sinusitis is present. The most common pathogens associated with external foci (trauma) are *Staphylococcus aureus* and *Streptococcus pyogenes,* but these are seldom isolated from the blood. In general, a bacterial pathogen is isolated from the blood in <33% of patients with periorbital cellulitis.

> **Additional Reading:** Differential diagnosis of the swollen red eyelid. *Am Fam Physician.* 2007;76(12):1815–1824.

> Category: Special sensory

179. A 4-year-old boy is noted to have impaired language development, compulsive repetitive behavior, impaired intelligence, and a preoccupation with inanimate objects. The most likely diagnosis is

A) Conductive hearing loss
B) Attention-deficit disorder
C) Autism
D) Manic–depressive disorder
E) Dyslexia

Answer and Discussion

The answer is C. *Autism* is a condition that is associated with abnormal social relationships, impaired language development and understanding, compulsive repetitive behavior with a resistance to change, and impaired intelligence; most affected individuals are in the mentally retarded range. The condition affects boys more frequently than girls and, in most cases, manifests itself before 1 year of age. Symptoms include a lack of attachment; preoccupation with inanimate objects; avoidance of eye contact; resistance to change; outbursts of temper; repetitive, often self-destructive acts; delayed speech development or total muteness; and seizures in severely impaired children. Neurologic examination fails to show focal findings. CT scans of the head may show enlargement of the ventricles, and EEG studies are usually unremarkable. Most children are brought to their doctors because of poor speech development. Treatment involves psychotherapy; however, results have been limited with regard to improving the child's deficiencies and behavior. Most children require special schooling. Mainstream treatment consists of early, intensive education for parents, focusing on behavior and communication disorders. A highly structured environment with intensive individual instruction should be encouraged. Laboratory, metabolic, or genetic tests and diagnostic imaging provide little useful information, although an EEG is indicated in children in whom epilepsy is suspected. No specific pharmacologic therapies are available, but many patients do not require medication. When needed, medication is generally used for a particular manifestation or constellation of symptoms. Families may benefit from ongoing counseling and support and specific instructions for dealing with tantrums and destructive behavior. Parents should be cautioned about costly and often questionable dietary, medical, and other unconventional therapies.

> **Additional Reading:** Primary care for children with autism. *Am Fam Physician.* 2010;81(4):453–460.

> Category: Patient/population-based care

180. An 18-year-old woman presents with swelling, warmth, and spreading redness at the upper part of her ear, where she recently underwent an ear piercing. Appropriate antibiotic coverage includes

A) Cephalexin
B) Ciprofloxacin
C) Azithromycin
D) Penicillin
E) Tetracycline

Answer and Discussion

The answer is B. The popularity of body piercing at sites other than the earlobe has grown since the mid-1990s. The tongue, lips, nose, eyebrows, nipples, navel, and genitals are areas frequently used for piercing. Complications include local and systemic infections, poor cosmetic results, and foreign body rejection. Swelling and damage to the dentition are common problems after tongue piercing. Minor infections, allergic contact dermatitis, keloid formation, and traumatic tearing may occur after piercing of the earlobe. "High" ear piercing through the ear cartilage is associated with more serious infections and disfigurement. Fluoroquinolone antibiotics are advised for treatment of auricular perichondritis because of their antipseudomonal activity. Navel, nipple, and genital piercings often have prolonged healing times.

> **Additional Reading:** Complications of body piercing. *Am Fam Physician.* 2005;72:2029–2034, 2035–2036.

> Category: Special sensory

181. Which of the following is not a contraindication for diphtheria–pertussis–tetanus (DPT) immunization?
A) Fever of 105°F (40.4°C) or higher within 48 hours after previous DPT dose
B) Current mild viral infection
C) Continuous crying for more than 3 hours after previous DPT dose
D) Convulsions within 3 days of a previous DPT dose
E) Progressive neurologic disorder that is not diagnosed

Answer and Discussion

The answer is B. Several conditions are a contraindication to the DTaP immunization:

- Fever of 105°F (40.4°C) or higher within 48 hours after previous dose
- Previous anaphylaxis to the vaccine
- Moderate to severe current illness; febrile illness
- Encephalopathy within 7 days after a previous DTaP dose
- Progressive neurologic disorder that is not diagnosed
- Continuous crying for more than 3 hours within 48 hours after a previous DTaP dose
- Convulsions occurring within 3 days after a previous DTaP dose

> **Additional Reading:** Contraindications and precautions to commonly used vaccines. National Center for Immunization and Respiratory Diseases. From: http://www.cdc.gov/vaccines/

Category: Patient/population-based care

182. Which of the following medications has been shown to shorten hospital stays in children with croup?
A) Epinephrine
B) Dexamethasone
C) Albuterol
D) Antiviral medication
E) Ipratropium bromide

Answer and Discussion

6mo–6yo

The answer is B. Viral croup is the most common form of airway obstruction in children 6 months to 6 years of age. For children with mild croup, symptomatic care and mist therapy may be all that are necessary. Epinephrine has been used in the past to treat more severe cases of croup, but recent meta-analyses have found that glucocorticoid use is associated with shorter hospital stays, improvement in croup scores, and less use of epinephrine. Studies have shown that treatment with oral dexamethasone is as effective as intramuscular dexamethasone or nebulized budesonide. While more studies are needed to establish guidelines, oral dexamethasone can be used to treat mild to moderate croup with close follow-up and instructions for further care, if needed.

> **Additional Reading:** Croup: an overview. *Am Fam Physician.* 2011;83(9):1067–1073.

Category: Respiratory system

> Glucocorticoid use in children with croup is associated with shorter hospital stays, improvement in croup scores, and less use of epinephrine.

183. A 3-month-old girl is brought into your office. The parent reports that she has been having excessive nonpurulent tearing from the left eye for the past 4 weeks. The most likely diagnosis is
A) Congenital cataracts
B) *Chlamydia trachomatis* infection
C) Dacryostenosis
D) Glaucoma
E) Viral conjunctivitis

Answer and Discussion

2–12 wks old

The answer is C. Congenital stenosis of the nasolacrimal duct is associated with excessive tearing of usually one eye. The condition is rather common and usually affects children between 2 and 12 weeks of age. In most cases, the condition resolves by 6 months of age. Parents should be instructed to massage the duct two to three times daily. If no relief occurs by 12 months of age, the duct may need to be probed with the aid of anesthesia. Topical antibiotics should be administered if purulent discharge or conjunctivitis develops.

> **Additional Reading:** Anatomy, imaging, and pathology of the lacrimal apparatus. *Nelson Textbook of Pediatrics,* 19th ed. Philadelphia, PA: Elsevier/Saunders; 2011.

Category: Special sensory

184. Which of the following (otherwise healthy) age groups is considered a priority group when administering influenza vaccine?
A) Birth to 6 months
B) 6 months to 23 months
C) 2 years to 5 years
D) Children below 7
E) Children in elementary school

Answer and Discussion

The answer is B. Given the uncertainties in doses and distribution, the American Academy of Family Physicians and the CDC recommend that the following priority groups receive trivalent inactivated influenza vaccine (TIV):

- Persons aged ≥65 years with comorbid conditions
- Residents of long-term care facilities
- Persons aged 2 to 64 years with comorbid conditions
- Persons aged ≥65 years without cormorbid conditions
- Children aged 6 to 23 months
- Pregnant women
- Health care personnel who provide direct patient care
- Household contacts and out-of-home caregivers of children aged ≤6 months

> **Additional Reading:** Key facts about seasonal flu vaccines. Centers for Disease Control and Prevention; 2013. From: http://www.cdc.gov/vaccines/

Category: Patient/population-based care

185. Which of the following statements about transient cortical blindness is true?
A) It usually lasts 3 to 5 days.
B) It can be associated with head trauma.
C) It is associated with cerebral edema seen on CT scans.
D) It is associated with permanent slowing seen on EEG.
E) It is commonly associated with other neurologic findings.

Answer and Discussion

The answer is B. Transient cortical blindness is blindness without other focal neurologic signs that resolves in 24 hours; it is usually caused by mild head trauma. Head CT scans are unremarkable, and there is no evidence of skull fractures. EEG results initially show some slowing, which resolves spontaneously as the blindness dissipates.

Additional Reading: Retrochismal disorders. *Nelson Textbook of Pediatrics,* 19th ed. Philadelphia, PA: Elsevier/Saunders; 2011.

Category: Special sensory

186. Which of the following medications is *not* approved for the treatment of influenza A in a 15-year-old adolescent?
A) Amantadine
B) Rimantadine
C) Zanamivir
D) Oseltamivir

Answer and Discussion

The answer is B. Four influenza antiviral agents are available in the United States: amantadine, rimantadine, zanamivir, and oseltamivir. Amantadine and rimantadine are chemically related antiviral drugs known as adamantanes, with activity against influenza A viruses but not influenza B viruses. Amantadine was approved in 1966 for chemoprophylaxis of influenza type A virus infections among adults and children 1 year or older. Rimantadine was approved in 1993 for treatment and chemoprophylaxis of influenza A infection among adults and prophylaxis among children. Although rimantadine is approved only for chemoprophylaxis of influenza A infection among children, rimantadine treatment for influenza A among children can be beneficial. Zanamivir and oseltamivir are chemically related antiviral drugs known as neuraminidase inhibitors that have activity against both influenza A and B viruses. Both zanamivir and oseltamivir were approved in 1999 for treating uncomplicated influenza infections. Zanamivir is approved for treating persons 7 years or older, and oseltamivir is approved for treatment of persons 1 year or older. In 2000, oseltamivir was approved for chemoprophylaxis of influenza among persons 13 years or older.

Additional Reading: Key facts about seasonal flu vaccines. Centers for Disease Control and Prevention, 2013. From: http://www.cdc.gov/vaccines/

Category: Patient/population-based care

187. A painless, cystic structure in the scrotum that transilluminates but is not associated with the presence of sperm is most likely a
A) Spermatocele
B) Hydrocele
C) Varicocele
D) Epididymis
E) Testicular tumor (Leydig's cell)

Answer and Discussion

The answer is B. Hydrocele is a common condition in which a collection of fluid forms between the tunica vaginalis and the tunica albuginea surrounding the testicle. It is usually noted as a painless, enlarging, cystic structure that transilluminates. It is usually an idiopathic congenital finding but can be associated with injury, infection, and, rarely, tumor. Most cases require no further treatment unless the patient is symptomatic or a hernia occurs; surgical consultation is then recommended. Ultrasound examination is usually not necessary, unless there is a question about the diagnosis or the mass does not transilluminate; in these cases, other conditions such as testicular tumors should be ruled out. In some cases, a communicating hydrocele may start out small in the early morning and enlarge throughout the day, or it may enlarge with Valsalva-type maneuvers (e.g., coughing, crying, changing position). Most hydroceles seen in newborns resolve during the first year, and parents need only to be reassured about the condition.

Additional Reading: Disorders and anomalies of scrotal contents. *Nelson Textbook of Pediatrics,* 19th ed. Philadelphia, PA: Elsevier/Saunders; 2011.

Category: Reproductive system

188. Which of the following statements regarding inhalant abuse is true?
A) Approximately 5% of children in middle school and high school have experimented with inhaled substances.
B) No associated fetal abnormalities have been associated with inhalant abuse during pregnancy.
C) Drug testing can help aid in the diagnosis of inhalant abuse.
D) Inhalant abuse can become addictive.
E) Reversal of inhalant effects can be achieved with the administration of naloxone (Narcan).

Answer and Discussion

The answer is D. Inhalant abuse is a prevalent and common form of substance abuse in teenagers. Study results consistently show that nearly 20% of children in middle school and high school have experimented with inhaled substances. The method of delivery is inhalation of a solvent from its container, a soaked rag, or a bag. Solvents include almost any household cleaning agent or propellant, paint thinner, glue, or lighter fluid. Inhalant abuse typically can cause a euphoric feeling and can become addictive. Acute effects include sudden sniffing death syndrome, asphyxia, and serious injuries (e.g., falls, burns, frostbite). Chronic inhalant abuse can damage cardiac, renal, hepatic, and neurologic systems. Inhalant abuse during pregnancy can cause fetal abnormalities. Diagnosis of inhalant abuse is difficult and relies almost entirely on a thorough history and a high index of suspicion. No specific laboratory tests confirm solvent inhalation. Treatment is generally supportive because there are no reversal agents for inhalant intoxication. Education of young persons and their parents is essential to decrease experimentation with inhalants.

Additional Reading: Inhalant abuse in children and adolecents. In: Basow DS, ed. *UpToDate.* Waltham, MA: UpToDate; 2013.

Category: Nonspecific system

189. Tick paralysis is associated with all of the following *except*
A) The bite of the *Dermacentor* or *Amblyomma* species of ticks
B) Muscle weakness, anorexia, lack of coordination, ascending flaccid paralysis
C) A bacteria harbored by the tick that serves as its vector
D) A neurotoxin produced by the tick's salivary gland
E) Rapid recovery once the tick is removed

Answer and Discussion

The answer is C. Ticks are capable of carrying many diseases. The *Dermacentor* and *Amblyomma* species of ticks found in North America have been linked to a condition called *tick paralysis.* Children, especially those with long hair that can hide ticks, are usually those affected. Manifestations include muscle weakness, anorexia, lack of coordination, lethargy, nystagmus, and an ascending flaccid paralysis. Sensory examinations and lumbar punctures are normal. In severe cases, respiratory and bulbar paralysis can occur. The paralysis is thought to be caused by inoculation of a neurotoxin that is found in the tick's salivary gland; it is not thought to represent a disease carried by the tick. Therefore, antibiotics are not indicated for affected patients; removal of the tick usually starts the recovery. Treatment of tick paralysis is symptomatic. In severe cases, mechanical ventilation may be necessary if respiratory paralysis occurs. Mortality rates can be as high as 10% for those with severe cases that go untreated. Removal of the tick usually results in improvement within a few hours and total recovery in a few days.

Additional Reading: Spotted fever and transitional group rickettsioses. *Nelson Textbook of Pediatrics,* 19th ed. Philadelphia, PA: Elsevier/Saunders; 2011.

Category: Neurologic

190. Which of the following is true regarding *Neisseria meningitidis*?
A) Serogroup B that accounts for the highest incidence of disease in young infants is prevented with administration of the vaccine.
B) Young adults affected with *Neisseria meningitidis* typically have better outcomes than other age groups.
C) Eleven- to 18-year-old adolescents should be vaccinated against *Neisseria meningitidis.*
D) Antibiotic prophylaxis is only recommended for household contacts.
E) Even high-risk adults should not receive *Neisseria meningitidis* vaccination because of potential side effects.

Answer and Discussion

The answer is C. *Neisseria meningitidis* has an average annual incidence of one case per 100,000 in the United States. The disease can cause rapid death or result in severe neurologic and vascular damage despite antibiotic therapy. Antibiotic chemoprophylaxis with rifampin, ciprofloxacin, or ceftriaxone is recommended for household and other close contacts. The majority of cases of meningococcal disease are sporadic, but outbreaks can occur, and vaccination of the affected population is often required. Serogroup B accounts for the highest incidence of disease in young infants but is not included in any vaccine licensed in the United States. Adolescents and young adults 15 to 24 years of age have a higher incidence of disease and a higher fatality rate than other populations. Because 70% to 80% of these infections in the United States are caused by meningococcal serogroups C, Y, and W-135, which are contained in the tetravalent meningococcal vaccines, they can be prevented. The U.S. Food and Drug Administration recently approved a meningococcal conjugate vaccine containing serogroups A, C, Y, and W-135. The Advisory Committee on Immunization Practices recommends that this vaccine be given to 11- and 18-year-old adolescents, to adolescents entering high school, and to college freshmen living in dormitories. The vaccine may also be given to persons 11 to 55 years of age who belong to certain high-risk groups.

Additional Reading: ACIP issues revised recommendations on meningococcal conjugate vaccine. *Am Fam Physician.* 2007; 76(9):1402.

Category: Patient/population-based care

191. Syringomyelia may expand during adolescent years. Typically, the first neurologic deficit is with
A) Coordination
B) Motor function
C) Pain and temperature sensation
D) Lower extremity reflexes
E) Mentation

Answer and Discussion

The answer is C. A syringomyelia is a fluid accumulation that involves the spinal canal and is usually associated with the cervical area; however, it may extend to involve the entire spinal cord. The lesion may expand during adolescent years and can give rise to symptoms including loss of sensation involving the distal extremities, upper shoulders, and back; spasticity; asymmetric or absent reflexes; and weakness with muscle wasting. Pain and temperature sensation are usually lost first. A rapidly progressing scoliosis may be the initial manifestation of syringomyelia. The congenital abnormality is associated with an Arnold–Chiari malformation, with cerebellar tissue extending into the spinal canal. Diagnosis involves the use of CT scans, magnetic resonance imaging (the test of choice), and myelography. Treatment involves surgery to remove the pocket of fluid.

Additional Reading: Spinal cord disorders. *Nelson Textbook of Pediatrics,* 19th ed. Philadelphia, PA: Elsevier/Saunders; 2011.

Category: Neurologic

192. Which of the following conditions is associated with meconium ileus?
A) Pyloric stenosis
B) Malrotation
C) Cystic fibrosis
D) Duodenal atresia
E) Hirshsprung's disease

Answer and Discussion

The answer is C. Meconium ileus is almost always an early sign of cystic fibrosis. The thick meconium in meconium ileus is easily differentiated from the rubbery meconium plug of meconium plug syndrome. In meconium ileus, the meconium adheres to the bowel mucosa and causes obstruction at the level of the terminal ileum. Distal to the obstruction, the colon is narrow in diameter and contains dry meconium pellets. The relatively empty colon of small caliber is termed a *microcolon.* Loops of distended small bowel can sometimes be palpated through the abdominal wall.

Additional Reading: Digestive tract disorders: meconium ileus in cystic fibrosis. *Nelson Textbook of Pediatrics,* 19th ed. Philadelphia, PA: Elsevier/Saunders; 2011.

Category: Gastroenterology system

> Meconium ileus is almost always an early sign of cystic fibrosis.

193. Which of the following statements about immunoglobulin A (IgA) deficiency is true?
A) It is the most common immunodeficiency.
B) It is associated with influenza vaccination administration.
C) Symptoms include night blindness, skin necrosis, and joint pain.
D) Treatment involves (scheduled) monthly antibiotic administration.
E) Most individuals affected die before age 20 years.

Answer and Discussion

The answer is A. IgA deficiency is the most common immunodeficiency and results in a lack of IgA in secretions. It is the mildest form of immunodeficiency and affects 1 in 600 individuals. The condition has been associated with phenytoin administration, congenital intrauterine infections, and abnormalities of chromosome 18. Most affected individuals are asymptomatic. However, some affected individuals may have decreased immune status resulting in frequent respiratory infections, allergies, recurrent diarrhea, and various autoimmune disorders (e.g., lupus erythematosus, rheumatoid arthritis). In most cases, treatment is unnecessary. However, patients with recurrent respiratory infections may use antibiotics frequently. In some cases, the patient may experience spontaneous remission. Some patients may have antibody development to IgA, which can lead to anaphylactic reactions during blood transfusion.

Additional Reading: Primary defects of antibody production. *Nelson Textbook of Pediatrics,* 19th ed. Philadelphia, PA: Elsevier/Saunders; 2011.

Category: Nonspecific system

194. When do symptoms of pyloric stenosis usually become noticeable?
A) After the first few feedings
B) Within the first week
C) At 4 to 6 weeks after birth
D) At 3 to 4 months of age
E) Pyloric stenosis does not typically cause symptoms

Answer and Discussion

The answer is C. Pyloric stenosis may cause almost complete gastric outlet obstruction. Hypertrophy is rare at birth but develops over the initial 4 to 6 weeks of life, when signs of upper intestinal obstruction usually first appear. Male children are affected more than female children (4:1). Forceful projectile vomiting of feedings (without bile) usually begins late in the first month of life. Delayed diagnosis may lead to repeated vomiting, dehydration, failure to gain weight, and hypochloremic metabolic alkalosis (from losses of hydrochloric acid). Diagnosis is suspected by palpation of a discrete, 2- to 3-cm, firm, movable pyloric "olive-like mass" deep in the right side of the epigastrum and confirmed by identification of the hypertrophied pyloric muscle by abdominal ultrasonography. If the diagnosis is uncertain, a barium swallow will show delayed gastric emptying and the typical "string sign" of a markedly narrowed, elongated pyloric lumen. The treatment of choice is a longitudinal pyloromyotomy, which leaves the mucosa intact and separates the incised muscle fibers. Postoperatively, the infant usually tolerates feedings within a few days.

Additional Reading: Pyloric stenosis and other congenital anomalies of the stomach. *Nelson Textbook of Pediatrics,* 19th ed. Philadelphia, PA: Elsevier/Saunders; 2011.

Category: Gastroenterology system

195. The most important recommendation a family physician can make regarding reducing the risk of death while riding a bicycle is
A) Always wear shoes while riding
B) Look both ways before crossing an intersection
C) Use proper hand signals
D) Make sure the bike is properly fitted
E) Wear a helmet while riding

Answer and Discussion

The answer is E. The peak incidence of bicycle-related injuries and fatalities is in the 9- to 15-year age group with a male-to-female ratio of 3:1. Important risk factors for bicycle-related injuries include not wearing a helmet, crashes involving motor vehicles, and an unsafe riding environment. In adolescents and young adults, alcohol and substance abuse can be associated with bicycle injury. Most injuries

occur in boys and are associated with riding at high speed; most serious injuries and fatalities result from collisions with motor vehicles. Although superficial soft tissue injuries and musculoskeletal trauma are the most common injuries, head injuries are responsible for most fatalities and long-term disabilities. Overuse injuries may contribute to a variety of musculoskeletal complaints, compression neuropathies, perineal complaints, and genital complaints. Physicians treating such patients should consider medical factors and suggest adjusting various components of the bicycle, such as the seat height and handlebars. Encouraging bicycle riders to wear helmets is key to preventing injuries; protective clothing and equipment and general safety advice also may offer some protection.

Additional Reading: Maximizing children's health: screening, anticipatory guidance, counselling. *Nelson Textbook of Pediatrics,* 19th ed. Philadelphia, PA: Elsevier/Saunders; 2011.

Category: Patient/population-based care

196. Which of the following is true regarding lice infestations?
A) They are obligate human parasites.
B) They frequently jump onto new hosts.
C) Person-to-person contact is not necessary for transmission.
D) Head and pubic lice may cause systemic disease.
E) The incidence of head lice is decreasing.

Answer and Discussion

The answer is A. The three lice species that infest humans are *Pediculus humanus capitis* (the head louse), *Phthirus pubis* (the crab or pubic louse), and *Pediculus humanus corpus* (the body louse). All three species are obligate human parasites. Contrary to popular belief, these insects do not hop, jump, or fly. Instead, they are transmitted by person-to-person contact. Despite the introduction of new treatments, the frequency of lice infestation may be increasing. One explanation may be the development of resistance to current treatments. Fortunately, head and pubic lice do not transmit systemic disease. Hence, treatment is directed at relieving symptoms and preventing reinfestation and transmission.

Additional Reading: Pediculosis and scabies: a treatment update. *Am Fam Physician.* 2012;86(6):535–541.

Category: Integumentary

197. Which of the following is the antibiotic of choice for treating infected dog bites?
A) Amoxicillin
B) Cephalexin
C) Azithromycin
D) Penicillin
E) Amoxicillin–clavulanate

Answer and Discussion

The answer is E. Almost one-half of all dog bites involve an animal owned by the victim's family or neighbors. A large percentage of dog bite victims are children. Although some breeds of dogs have been identified as being more aggressive than other breeds, any dog may attack when threatened. All dog bites carry a risk of infection, but immediate copious irrigation can significantly decrease that risk. Only 15% to 20% of dog bite wounds become infected. Crush injuries, puncture wounds, and hand wounds are more likely to become infected than scratches or tears. Most infected dog bite wounds yield polymicrobial organisms. *P. multocida* and *S. aureus* are the most common aerobic organisms. Amoxicillin–clavulanate potassium is the antibiotic of choice for an infected dog bite. For patients who are allergic to penicillin, doxycycline is an acceptable alternative, except for children younger than 8 years and pregnant women. Erythromycin can also be used, but the risk of treatment failure is greater because of antimicrobial resistance. Assessment for the risk of tetanus and rabies virus infection should be made. The dog bite injury should be documented with photographs and diagrams when appropriate. Patients who have been bitten by a dog should be instructed to elevate and immobilize the involved area. Most bite wounds should be reexamined in 24 to 48 hours, especially bites to the hands. Family physicians should educate parents and children on ways to prevent dog bites.

Additional Reading: Animal and human bites. *Nelson Textbook of Pediatrics*, 19th ed. Philadelphia, PA: Elsevier/Saunders; 2011.

Category: Nonspecific system

198. A 7-year-old with a history of mild asthma presents to your office complaining of wheezing and shortness of breath that have developed over the last 24 hours. She has not used any medication. Which of the following medications would be initially indicated?

A) Albuterol
B) Salmeterol
C) Cromolyn sodium
D) Inhaled corticosteroids
E) Theophylline

Answer and Discussion

The answer is A. The prevalence of asthma in children has increased 160% since 1980, and the disease currently affects nearly 5 million children in the United States. Asthma triggers include allergens from dust mites or mold spores, animal dander, cockroaches, pollen, indoor and outdoor pollutants, irritants (e.g., tobacco smoke, smoke from wood-burning stoves or fireplaces, perfumes, cleaning agents), pharmacologic triggers (e.g., aspirin or other NSAIDs, β-blockers, sulfites), physical triggers (e.g., exercise, hyperventilation, cold air), and physiologic factors (e.g., stress, gastroesophageal reflux, respiratory infection [viral, bacterial], rhinitis). The National Asthma Education and Prevention Program provides guidelines for improved asthma care. The four components of asthma management include regular assessment and monitoring, control of factors that contribute to or aggravate symptoms, pharmacologic therapy, and education of children and their caregivers. The guidelines recommend a stepwise approach to pharmacologic treatment, starting with aggressive therapy to achieve control and followed by a "step down" to the minimal therapy that maintains control. Quick relief of symptoms can be achieved preferentially by the use of short-acting β2-agonists. Medications for long-term control should be considered for use in children with persistent symptoms. Inhaled corticosteroids are the most potent long-term anti-inflammatory medications. Other options include long-acting β2-agonists (usually reserved for patients when other treatments have failed), cromolyn sodium and nedocromil, antileukotriene agents, and theophylline. All have advantages and disadvantages in individual situations. Poor compliance is a major problem in pediatric asthma management, and several factors play a role in this. These include the route of administration (oral therapy is preferred to inhaled medication), frequency of dosing (once- or twice-daily regimens are preferred), medication effects (a slow onset of action and long duration on discontinuance have poor adherence rates), and the risk or concern of side effects. The goals of pharmacologic therapy are to minimize daytime and nocturnal symptoms, the number of asthma episodes, and the use of short-acting β2-agonists to improve peak exploratory flow to 80% or more of personal best and to allow the child to maintain normal activities without producing adverse medication side effects.

Additional Reading: Current guidelines for the management of asthma in young children. *Allergy Asthma Immunol Res.* 2010; 2(1):1–13.

Category: Respiratory system

QUESTIONS

Each of the following questions or incomplete statements below is followed by suggested answers or completions. Select the ONE BEST ANSWER in each case.

1. Which of the following is considered first-line therapy for primary dysmenorrhea?

A) Nonsteroidal anti-inflammatory drugs (NSAIDs)
B) Selective serotonin reuptake inhibitors (SSRIs)
C) Antiestrogens
D) Acupuncture
E) Tricyclic antidepressants

Answer and Discussion

The answer is A. Primary dysmenorrhea is associated with cramping pain in the lower abdomen occurring just before and/or during menstruation, in the absence of other conditions such as endometriosis. The initial presentation of primary dysmenorrhea typically occurs in adolescence. The condition is associated with increased production of endometrial prostaglandin, resulting in increased uterine tone and stronger, more frequent uterine contractions. A diagnostic evaluation is unnecessary in women with typical symptoms and in the absence of risk factors for secondary causes. Nonsteroidal anti-inflammatory drugs are the most effective treatment, with the addition of oral contraceptive pills (OCPs) when necessary. About 10% of affected women do not respond to these measures. In these cases, it is important to consider secondary causes of dysmenorrhea in affected women. Acupuncture is also used as an alternative treatment.

> **Additional Reading:** Dysmenorrhea. *Am Fam Physician.* 2012; 85(4):386–387.

Category: Reproductive system

2. A 21-year-old woman who is 12 weeks pregnant with her first child presents to your office. A urinalysis shows evidence of bacteriuria. She is completely asymptomatic. Appropriate management at this time includes which one of the following?

A) No treatment at this time; repeat urinalysis at her next visit.
B) Reassure the patient that antibiotic administration is not necessary unless she should develops symptoms.
C) No antibiotic treatment; ask the patient to drink more fluids and cranberry juice daily.
D) Discontinue urinalysis at OB visits because of the high rate of false positives.
E) Treat the patient with a 7-day course of amoxicillin.

Answer and Discussion

The answer is E. Asymptomatic bacteriuria, defined as more than 100,000 colonies of a single bacterial species per milliliter of urine, cultured from midstream sample, is present in 2% to 7% of pregnant women. The most commonly associated bacteria is *Escherichia coli.* Pregnancy does not increase the incidence of asymptomatic bacteriuria; however, pyelonephritis develops in a significant number of pregnant women with untreated asymptomatic bacteriuria. Asymptomatic bacteriuria in women is associated with a higher preterm delivery rate than women without bacteriuria. Treatment of group B *Streptococcus* (GBS) bacteriuria has also been shown to decrease the rate of preterm delivery. Additionally, GBS bacteriuria has been associated with heavy GBS genitourinary colonization. The Centers for Disease Control and Prevention (CDC) recommends that pregnant women with GBS bacteriuria be treated at the time of diagnosis and during labor. Intrapartum antibiotic prophylaxis is used to prevent early GBS infection in newborns. In most cases, women who do not have asymptomatic bacteriuria at the initial prenatal visit will not develop bacteriuria later in the pregnancy. Accordingly, routine screening for asymptomatic bacteriuria should be performed at the initial prenatal visit. Treatment options include a 3- to 7-day course of (1) oral amoxicillin, (2) nitrofurantoin (Macrobid), or (3) cephalexin (Keflex). After therapy is completed, a urine culture should be repeated to ensure eradication of infection. This repeat culture also identifies patients with persistent or recurrent bacteriuria. For patients who have persistent or recurrent bacteriuria, consideration should be given to administering suppressive doses of antibiotics.

> **Additional Reading:** Urinary tract infections and asymptomatic bacteriuria in pregnancy. In: Basow DS, ed. *UpToDate.* Waltham, MA: UpToDate; 2013.

Category: Nephrologic system

Asymptomatic bacteriuria in women is associated with a higher preterm delivery rate than women without bacteriuria.

3. *Preterm labor* is defined as regular contractions with cervical change before
A) 40 weeks' gestation
B) 39 weeks' gestation
C) 38 weeks' gestation
D) 37 weeks' gestation
E) 36 weeks' gestation

Answer and Discussion

The answer is D. According to the American College of Obstetricians and Gynecologists (ACOG), *preterm labor* is defined as regular contractions associated with cervical change before 37 weeks' gestation.

Additional Reading: American College of Obstetricians and Gynecologists. Assessment of risk factors for preterm birth. *ACOG Practice Bulletin* no. 31. From: http://www.acog.org/Resources_And_Publications/Committee_Opinions_List

Category: Reproductive system

4. Which of the following bacterial infections is *not* generally associated with preterm labor?
A) *Ureaplasma urealyticum*
B) *Mycoplasma hominis*
C) *Gardnerella vaginalis*
D) *Bacteroides* species
E) All are associated with preterm labor.

Answer and Discussion

The answer is E. Several bacterial infections have been associated with preterm labor, including *Ureaplasma urealyticum, Mycoplasma hominis, Gardnerella vaginalis,* and *Peptostreptococcus* and *Bacteroides* species. These organisms are usually of low virulence, and it is unclear whether they are etiologic or associated with an acute inflammatory response of another etiology.

Additional Reading: American College of Obstetricians and Gynecologists. Assessment of risk factors for preterm birth. *ACOG Practice Bulletin* no. 31. From: http://www.acog.org/Resources_And_Publications/Committee_Opinions_List

Category: Reproductive system

5. Which of the following tests has been shown to be a good predictor of preterm birth in women presenting with symptomatic preterm uterine contractions, and thus help guide the pharmacologic management of preterm labor patients?
A) Screening for genitourinary infections
B) Measurement of salivary estriol
C) Cervical length measurement
D) Fetal fibronectin screening
E) Both C and D

Answer and Discussion

The answer is E. A positive fetal fibronectin testing combined with a shortened cervical length in women presenting with symptoms of preterm labor can be a useful predictor of preterm birth. These screening tests have been shown to have a high sensitivity and high positive predictive value, as well as a high negative predictive value so they are useful in guiding decisions regarding steroid and tocolytic administration in women who have positive results and allow avoidance of these therapies in women with negative results.

Additional Reading: Improving the screening accuracy for preterm labor: is the combination of fetal fibronectin and cervical length in symptomatic patients a useful predictor of preterm birth? A systematic review. *Am J Obstet Gynecol.* 2013;208(3):233; and Preterm labor. *Am Family Physician.* 2010;81(4):477–484.

Category: Reproductive system

6. Which of the following sports is contraindicated in pregnancy?
A) Walking
B) Stationary bicycle
C) Low-impact aerobics
D) Snow skiing
E) Swimming

Answer and Discussion

The answer is D. Concerns have been raised about the safety of some forms of exercise during pregnancy. Because of the body changes associated with pregnancy as well as the hemodynamic response to exercise, some precautions should be observed. Pregnant women should avoid exercise that involves the risk of abdominal trauma, falls, or excessive joint stress, as in contact sports, gymnastics, horseback riding, and skiing. In the absence of any obstetric or medical complications, ACOG recommends at least 30 minutes of exercise most or all days of the week during pregnancy. Studies have shown that exercise may contribute to prevention of gestational diabetes in obese women and that exercise can help women with gestational diabetes achieve euglycemia when diet alone is insufficient.

Additional Reading: Exercise during pregnancy. *ACOG Committee Opinion* no. 267. From: http://www.acog.org/Resources_And_Publications/Committee_Opinions_List

Category: Reproductive system

7. During pregnancy, it is important to counsel pregnant patients to add an additional _____ calories to their dietary intake for normal activity.
A) 150
B) 300
C) 500
D) 1,000
E) 1,500

Answer and Discussion

The answer is B. An increase of 300 calories per day is required in pregnancy. Caloric demands with exercise are even higher, although no studies have focused on exact requirements. If a mother is exercising while pregnant, she may need to further increase her caloric intake to assure adequate maternal weight gain. Competitive athletes and women with a history of prior growth-restricted infants should be followed especially closely for adequate fetal growth.

Additional Reading: Prenatal care: nutrition. *Williams Obstetrics,* 23rd ed. New York, NY: McGraw-Hill; 2010.

Category: Reproductive system

8. Which of the following is *not* a contraindication to aerobic exercise during pregnancy?

A) Pregnancy-induced hypertension (PIH)
B) Incompetent cervix
C) Preterm labor during a prior pregnancy
D) Placenta previa
E) Twin gestation

Answer and Discussion

The answer is **C**. Although supportive data are limited, there appears to be no reason why women who are in good health should not be permitted to engage in exercise while pregnant. However, women with medical or obstetric complications should be encouraged to avoid vigorous physical activity. Contraindications to exercise during pregnancy include hemodynamically significant cardiac disease, restrictive lung disease, gestational hypertension, pre-eclampsia, preterm rupture of membranes, preterm labor during the current pregnancy, incompetent cervix or cerclage placement, multiple gestation at risk of preterm labor, persistent second- or third-trimester bleeding, and placenta previa at >26 weeks gestational age.

> **Additional Reading:** Prenatal care: common concerns. *Williams Obstetrics,* 23rd ed. New York, NY: McGraw-Hill; 2010.
>
> **Category:** Reproductive system

9. Maternal temperature elevations above _____ can be detrimental to the fetus in the first trimester of pregnancy.

A) 37°C (98.6°F)
B) 37.8°C (100.0°F)
C) 38.3°C (101.0°F)
D) 38.9°C (102.0°F)
E) Maternal temperature has no detrimental effects on the fetus.

Answer and Discussion

The answer is **D**. Some data suggest a teratogenic potential when maternal temperatures rise above 38.9°C (102°F), especially in the first trimester.

> **Additional Reading:** Tergenic causes of malformations. *Ann Clin Lab Sci.* 2010;40(2):99–114.
>
> **Category:** Reproductive system

10. Which of the following over-the-counter medications is generally avoided during pregnancy?

A) Acetaminophen
B) Chlorpheniramine
C) Pseudoephedrine
D) Dextromethorphan
E) Aspirin

Answer and Discussion

The answer is **E**. High-dose aspirin has been theoretically associated with increased perinatal mortality, neonatal hemorrhage, decreased birth weight, prolonged gestation and labor, and possible birth defects and in general should be avoided in pregnancy. Low-dose aspirin in combination with heparin has been used successfully in the treatment of antiphospholipid syndrome in pregnancy. The other medications on the list are considered safe in pregnancy, though patients are encouraged to avoid all nonessential medication use in the first trimester and use the lowest possible doses of necessary medications for the limited periods of time for relief of symptoms throughout the remainder of pregnancy.

> **Additional Reading:** Over-the-counter medications in pregnancy. *Am Fam Physician.* 2003;67(12):2517–2524.
>
> **Category:** Reproductive system

> High-dose aspirin has been associated theoretically with increased perinatal mortality, neonatal hemorrhage, decreased birth weight, prolonged gestation and labor, and possible birth defects and in general should be avoided in pregnancy.

11. During labor, the fetal heart tracing shows repeated late decelerations. You suspect

A) Uteroplacental insufficiency
B) Abnormal presentation
C) Head engagement
D) Rapid descent of the fetus
E) Normal progression of labor

Answer and Discussion

The answer is **A**. Repetitive late decelerations of the fetal heart rate (FHR) may signal uteroplacental insufficiency.

> **Additional Reading:** Electronic fetal monitoring. *Williams Obstetrics,* 23rd ed. New York, NY: McGraw-Hill; 2010.
>
> **Category:** Reproductive system

12. Repetitive variable decelerations noted on fetal heart tracings suggest

A) Umbilical cord compression
B) Placenta previa
C) Uterine rupture
D) Polyhydramnios
E) Normal progression of labor

Answer and Discussion

The answer is **A**. Repetitive variable decelerations suggest umbilical cord compression, especially in the presence of oligohydramnios or amniotomy.

> **Additional Reading:** Electronic fetal monitoring. *Williams Obstetrics,* 23rd ed. New York, NY: McGraw-Hill; 2010.
>
> **Category:** Reproductive system

13. A 26-year-old primiparous woman pushed effectively during a 2-hour second stage with subsequent delivery of the infant's head followed by a "turtle sign" with inability to deliver the infant's shoulders with the normal amount of downward traction and maternal expulsive efforts. You diagnose shoulder dystocia and ask the mother to stop pushing and alert staff to this emergency. The next appropriate step is

A) Place the mother in the left lateral position
B) Perform McRoberts' maneuver
C) Apply fundal pressure
D) Use a rotational maneuver, either the Rubin II or Wood's corkscrew
E) Perform a cesarean section

Answer and Discussion

The answer is **B**. The recommended sequence for reducing shoulder dystocia begins with calling for help and asking the mother to stop her pushing efforts. The first step is the McRoberts' maneuver, in which assistants hyperflex the mother's hips against her abdomen, thereby rotating the symphysis pubis anteriorly and decreasing the forces needed to deliver the fetal shoulders. A retrospective study found this maneuver to be the safest and most successful technique for relieving shoulder dystocia. An assistant can add gentle posterolateral suprapubic pressure while the physician continues moderate posterior traction on the fetal head. Fundal pressure should be avoided, because it tends to increase the impaction. Rotational maneuvers may be tried next, beginning with the Rubin II maneuver which is done by inserting the fingers of one hand vaginally behind the posterior aspect of the anterior shoulder of the fetus and rotating the shoulder toward the fetal chest. This will adduct the fetal shoulder girdle, reducing its diameter. If the Rubin II maneuver is unsuccessful, the Woods corkscrew maneuver may be attempted. Two fingers are placed on the anterior aspect of the fetal posterior shoulder, applying gentle upward pressure around the circumference of the arc in the same direction as with the Rubin II maneuver. The Rubin II and Woods corkscrew maneuvers may be combined to increase forces by using two fingers behind the fetal anterior shoulder and two fingers in front of the fetal posterior shoulder.

> **Additional Reading:** Shoulder dystocia. *Williams Obstetrics,* 23rd ed. New York, NY: McGraw-Hill; 2010; and Shoulder dystocia. *Am Fam Physician.* 2004;69(7):1707–1714.

> **Category:** Reproductive system

14. The drug of choice for controlling eclamptic seizures is
A) Hydralazine
B) Phenobarbital
C) Phenytoin
D) Diazepam
E) Magnesium sulfate

Answer and Discussion

The answer is E. In the United States, magnesium sulfate is considered the drug of choice for controlling eclamptic seizures. Fewer intubations are required in the neonates of eclamptic women who are treated with magnesium sulfate. In addition, fewer newborns require placement in neonatal intensive care units. In the treatment of eclampsia and preeclampsia, magnesium sulfate is often given according to established protocols. If serum magnesium levels exceed 10 mEq/L (5 mmol/L), respiratory depression can occur. This problem may be counteracted by the rapid intravenous infusion of 10% calcium gluconate. Magnesium sulfate should be used with caution in patients with impaired renal or cardiac status. It should not be used in patients with myasthenia gravis.

> **Additional Reading:** Eclampsia. *Williams Obstetrics,* 23rd ed. New York, NY: McGraw-Hill; 2010.

> **Category:** Reproductive system

15. The current diagnosis of preeclampsia consists of which of the following?
A) Elevated blood pressure and proteinuria
B) Elevated blood pressure, proteinuria, and edema
C) Elevated blood pressure, proteinuria, edema, and seizures
D) Elevated blood pressure, proteinuria, edema, seizure, and headaches

Answer and Discussion

The answer is A. The classic preeclamptic triad include elevated blood pressure, proteinuria, and edema. More recently, edema has been removed as part of the criteria. Seizures are the distinguishing component of eclampsia.

> **Additional Reading:** Pregnancy hypertension. *Williams Obstetrics,* 23rd ed. New York, NY: McGraw-Hill; 2010.

> **Category:** Reproductive system

16. The most common cause of postpartum bleeding is
A) Retained placenta
B) Vaginal laceration
C) Uterine atony
D) Coagulopathy
E) HELLP syndrome

Answer and Discussion

The answer is C. Hemorrhage after placental delivery should prompt vigorous fundal massage while the patient is rapidly given oxytocin in their intravenous fluid. If the fundus does not become firm, uterine atony is the presumed (and most common) diagnosis. While fundal massage continues, the patient may be given methylergonovine (Methergine) intramuscularly, with the dose repeated at 2- to 4-hour intervals if necessary. Methylergonovine may cause cramping, headache, and dizziness. The use of this drug is contraindicated in patients with hypertension. Carboprost (Hemabate), 15-methyl prostaglandin F_{2a}, may be administered intramuscularly or intramyometrially every 15 to 90 minutes, up to a maximum dosage. As many as 68% of patients respond to a single carboprost injection, with 86% responding by the second dose. Another prostaglandin that is increasingly used in the treatment of postpartum hemorrhage is misoprostol which is most commonly administered rectally in a 800-to-1,000-mcg dose, though it can also be administered buccally or vaginally.

> **Additional Reading:** Obstetrical hemorrhage. *Williams Obstetrics,* 23rd ed. New York, NY: McGraw-Hill; 2010; and Prevention and management of postpartum hemorrhage. *Am Fam Physician.* 2007;75(6):875–882.

> **Category:** Reproductive system

17. An 18-year-old woman pregnant with her first child is in the second stage of labor. She complains of abdominal pain between uterine contractions. You suspect
A) Posterior presentation
B) Breech presentation
C) Abruption placenta
D) Vasa previa
E) Uterine atony

Answer and Discussion

The answer is C. The patient in labor who develops abdominal pain between uterine contractions or a tender uterus must be presumed to have abruptio placentae. Ultrasound examination has a high false-negative rate in diagnosing abruption and as a result this complication is diagnosed clinically. In one prospective study, 78% of patients with abruptio placentae presented with vaginal bleeding, 66% with uterine or back pain, 60% with fetal distress, and only 17% with uterine contractions or hypertonus. The management of abruptio placentae is primarily supportive and entails both aggressive hydration and monitoring of maternal and fetal well-being. Coagulation studies should be performed, and fibrinogen and D-dimers or fibrin-degradation products should be measured to screen for disseminated intravascular coagulation (DIC). Packed red blood cells should be typed and held. If the fetus appears viable but compromised, urgent cesarean delivery should be considered.

Additional Reading: Placental abruption. *Williams Obstetrics,* 23rd ed. New York, NY: McGraw-Hill; 2010.

Category: Reproductive system

18. A 25-year-old presents to your office complaining of abnormal vaginal bleeding. Your first consideration in the differential diagnosis is
A) Infection
B) Trauma
C) Foreign body
D) Pregnancy
E) Coagulopathy

Answer and Discussion

The answer is D. Pregnancy is the first consideration in women of childbearing age who present with abnormal uterine bleeding.

Additional Reading: Evaluation and management of abnormal uterine bleeding in premenopausal women. *Am Fam Physician.* 2012;85(1):35–43.

Category: Reproductive system

19. All patients undergoing cesarean section should
A) Always receive a preoperative antibiotic within 1 hour of start of surgery
B) Not receive antibiotics because of the risk of resistant infections
C) Receive antibiotics only if the surgery is prolonged (>1.5 hours)
D) Not receive antibiotics if they are considered low risk
E) Receive antibiotics only if infection is suspected

Answer and Discussion

The answer is A. According to ACOG, all patients undergoing cesarean delivery should receive prophylaxis with narrow-spectrum antibiotics such as a first-generation cephalosporin within the hour prior to surgical skin incision. Infection is the most common complication of cesarean delivery and can occur in 10% to 40% of women who have a cesarean compared with 1% to 3% of women who deliver vaginally. Although antibiotics have been given to women having cesareans to reduce their risk of postoperative infections, they have generally been given after the baby was born and the umbilical cord was clamped. This was based on concern that the antibiotics that made it into the baby's bloodstream from the mother would interfere with newborn lab tests or could lead to antibiotic-resistant infections. Newer studies have shown that prophylactic antibiotics given before initiation of cesarean section significantly reduces maternal infection and does not cause harm to newborns.

Additional Reading: Antimicrobial prophylaxis for cesarean delivery: timing of administration. *ACOG Committee Opinion* no. 465. From: http://www.acog.org/Resources_And_Publications/Committee_Opinions_List

Category: Reproductive system

20. In discussing the risk of placing an epidural during labor, you explain to your patient that
A) The ACOG recommends that epidural anesthesia in nulliparous women is not recommended until cervical dilation has reached 4 to 5 cm regardless of maternal request.
B) Early epidural anesthesia increases the risk of cesarean section.
C) Epidural anesthesia may increase the rate of vacuum extraction.
D) Epidural anesthesia has no effect on the length of the second stage of labor.
E) Epidural anesthesia is of little help with pain management in early labor.

Answer and Discussion

The answer is C. Epidural analgesia during labor is an effective pain reliever for labor that has become much more commonly used. Despite wide acceptance of this use, the timing of epidural placement remains controversial, with conflicting reports on the risk for subsequent cesarean deliveries and the length of the latent phase of labor. There are data from several studies suggesting that epidural anesthesia does lengthen the duration of the second stage of labor and may increase the rate of instrumented vaginal deliveries. Previously, ACOG recommended using other forms of analgesia in nulliparous women until they reach dilatation of 4 to 5 cm. However, some institutions did not follow these guidelines for all women in labor, so ACOG released a follow-up report recommending that maternal request is a sufficient indication for epidural analgesia during labor and that it should not be denied on the basis of cervical dilatation.

Additional Reading: Hawkins JL. Epidural anesthesia for labor and delivery. *NEJM.* 2010;362:1503–1510.

Category: Reproductive system

> Maternal request is a sufficient indication for epidural analgesia during labor. It should not be denied on the basis of cervical dilatation.

21. When using a vacuum extractor, the procedure should be abandoned after
A) 3 disengagements "pop-offs" of vacuum head
B) 20 minutes
C) 3 consecutive pulls to not produce any progress
D) 3 consecutive pulls to not produce infant's delivery
E) Any of the above

Answer and Discussion

The answer is E. Use of vacuum should be halted when there are three disengagements of the vacuum (or "pop-offs"), more than 20 minutes have elapsed, or three consecutive pulls result in no progress or delivery.

Additional Reading: Vacuum-assisted vaginal delivery. *Am Fam Physician.* 2008;78(8):953–960.

Category: Reproductive system

22. Proper placement of the vacuum extractor is
A) Placed as far anteriorly as possible
B) Over the sagittal suture extending to the posterior fontanel
C) Covering the posterior fontanel
D) Over the sagittal suture and 3 cm in front of the posterior fontanel
E) Anywhere on the exposed cranium

Answer and Discussion

The answer is D. When the vacuum extractor is placed on the fetal scalp, the center of the cup should be over the sagittal suture and about 3 cm (1.2 in.) in front of the posterior fontanel. As a general guide, the cup is generally placed as far posteriorly as possible. This cup placement maintains flexion of the fetal head and avoids traction over the anterior fontanel. In positioning the cup, the physician should be careful to avoid trapping maternal soft tissue (e.g., labia) between the cup and the fetal head.

Additional Reading: Vacuum extraction. *Williams Obstetrics,* 23rd ed. New York, NY: McGraw-Hill; 2010.

Category: Reproductive system

23. Pregnant patients with established human immunodeficiency virus (HIV) infection
A) Should avoid all antiviral medications because of their teratogenic potential
B) Should receive only zidovudine at the time of delivery
C) Do not need to switch off efavirenz if taking it when pregnancy is diagnosed
D) Should avoid zidovudine because of its limited effectiveness
E) Should receive only zidovudine if their CD4+ counts are unacceptably low

Answer and Discussion
The answer is C. Several important changes were made in the July 2012 update of the U.S. Department of Health and Human Services' Recommendations for Use of Antiretroviral Drugs in Pregnant HIV-1-Infected Women for Maternal Health and Interventions to Reduce Perinatal HIV Transmission in the United States (see summary and link below), particularly pertaining to zidovudine and efavirenz.

Zidovudine (AZT) no longer must be a part of a pregnant patient's antiretroviral therapy regimen (ART), nor is it necessary to administer intravenous AZT during delivery if she is on effective ART with an HIV RNA <400 copies/mL near delivery (BII). Because the risk of neural tube defects is restricted to the first 5 to 6 weeks of gestation when pregnancy is rarely diagnosed, and unnecessary antiretroviral drug changes during pregnancy may be associated with loss of viral control and increased risk of perinatal transmission, efavirenz (pregnancy category D) can be continued in pregnant women receiving an efavirenz-based regimen who present for antenatal care in the first trimester, provided the regimen produces virologic suppression (CIII). There are several ART medications recognized to be generally safe in pregnancy, and all pregnant women should be offered ART (AI). The decision whether to start the regimen in the first trimester or delay until 12 weeks' gestation will depend on CD4-cell count, HIV RNA levels, and maternal conditions such as nausea and vomiting (AIII). Earlier initiation of a combination antiretroviral regimen may be more effective in reducing transmission, but benefits must be weighed against potential fetal effects of first-trimester drug exposure.

> **Additional Reading:** Recommendations for use of antiretroviral drugs in pregnant HIV-1-infected women for maternal health and interventions to reduce perinatal HIV transmission in the United States. From: http://www.aidsinfo.nih.gov/guidelines/html/3/perinatal-guidelines/0

Category: Reproductive system

24. When repairing perineal lacerations, it has been shown that
A) Skin sutures may increase the incidence of perineal pain.
B) Skin sutures are required for adequate skin approximation.
C) Interrupted transcutaneous sutures are superior to running subcuticular sutures.
D) Sutures should begin at the anterior point of the skin laceration.
E) Repair with skin sutures leads to better outcomes.

Answer and Discussion
The answer is A. When the perineal muscles are repaired anatomically, the overlying skin is usually well approximated, and skin sutures are generally not required. Skin sutures have been shown to increase the incidence of perineal pain at 3 months after delivery. If the skin requires suturing, running subcuticular sutures have been shown to be superior to interrupted transcutaneous sutures.

Synthetic rapidly absorbable sutures are preferable to catgut, standard absorbable sutures, and these sutures should start at the posterior apex of the skin laceration and should be placed approximately 3 mm from the edge of the skin.

> **Additional Reading:** Absorbable suture materials for primary repair of episiotomy and second degree tears. *Cochrane Database Syst Rev.* 2010;6:CD000006.

Category: Reproductive system

25. Laser conization and LEEP procedures have been associated with
A) Premature rupture of membranes (PROM)
B) Increased peripartum mortality
C) Increased cesarean rates
D) Higher rates of endometritis during pregnancy
E) No adverse effects during pregnancy

Answer and Discussion
The answer is A. While there is an increased risk of PROM and preterm labor following laser conization or LEEP, there is not an associated increase in overall preterm deliveries. Although PROM leads to preterm deliveries, these were higher in the untreated group after adjustments compared with the treated group. The authors attribute this incongruity to the higher rate of iatrogenic preterm deliveries in the untreated group. The authors of the study suggest careful adherence to CIN (Cervical Intraepithelial Neoplasia) management guidelines, avoidance of unnecessary excisions, and appropriate counseling of previously treated women when they become pregnant.

> **Additional Reading:** Treatment for cervical intraepithelial neoplasia and risk of preterm delivery. *JAMA.* 2004;291:2100–2106.

Category: Reproductive system

26. A 39-year-old mother presents to your office for preconception counseling. She has one child affected with neural tube defect. Appropriate counseling concerning folic acid supplementation should include _____ daily.
A) 100 mcg
B) 400 mcg
C) 1 mg
D) 4 mg
E) None needed on the basis of her current age

Answer and Discussion
The answer is D. Taking folic acid supplementation before conception reduces the incidence of neural tube defects, including spina bifida and anencephaly. The average woman receives about 100 mcg of folic acid per day, mostly from fortified breads and grains. Supplementation should begin at least 1 month before conception and continue through the first 3 months of pregnancy; women should take a daily vitamin supplement containing at least 400 mcg of folic acid. Higher dosages are indicated for special-risk groups. A dosage of 1 mg per day is recommended for women with diabetes mellitus or epilepsy. Mothers who have given birth to children with neural tube defects should take 4 mg of folic acid per day for subsequent pregnancies.

> **Additional Reading:** Folic acid for the prevention of neural tube defects. *Am Fam Physician.* 2010;82(12):1533–1534.

Category: Neurologic

27. A 36-year-old woman has a history of a prior deep venous thrombosis (DVT). She is pregnant for the first time. In view of her prior history of DVT, you should recommend
A) Warfarin (Coumadin)
B) Heparin
C) Aspirin
D) Clopidogrel (Plavix)
E) No prophylaxis is necessary

Answer and Discussion

The answer is B. Women who have a personal or family history of venous thromboembolism should be offered testing for coagulopathy before pregnancy. Women with a prior history of DVT have a 7% to 12% risk of recurrence during pregnancy. Heparin (in regular or low-molecular-weight form) is indicated for prophylaxis and should be started as early in pregnancy as possible. Women receiving warfarin as maintenance therapy for DVT should be switched to heparin before conception because warfarin is teratogenic.

Additional Reading: ACOG Practice Bulletin no. 123. Thromboembolism in pregnancy. *Obstet Gynecol.* 2011;118(3):718–729.

Category: Cardiovascular system

28. When advising mothers concerning antiseizure medications during pregnancy, which of the following statements is true?
A) Multiple medications are preferred to maintain lower levels of medication.
B) Antiseizure medications should be discontinued at the time pregnancy is determined.
C) Seizure activity in mothers has no impact on fetal outcomes.
D) Most antiseizure medications are considered safe (category B).
E) Single agents are preferred to multiple medications.

Answer and Discussion

The answer is E. Children of mothers with epilepsy have a 4% to 8% risk of congenital anomalies, which may be caused by anticonvulsant medication or may be related to an increased genetic risk. These children also have an increased risk of developing epilepsy. Preconception counseling should include optimizing seizure control, prescribing folic acid supplements of 1 to 4 mg per day, and offering referral to a genetic counselor. Tonic-clonic seizures in pregnancy can lead to hypoxia in the fetus, and pregnant women with any type of seizure are also at risk for trauma (e.g., falls), which can also adversely impact the fetus. The therapeutic goal for women with seizure disorders who are pregnant is to prevent seizures while minimizing teratogenic damage to the fetus. When possible, use of multiple anticonvulsants (polytherapy) should be discouraged. It is advisable to aim to use the best single agent for the seizure type at the lowest protective level. A committee assembled by the American Academy of Neurology reassessed the evidence related to the care of women with epilepsy during pregnancy, including antiepileptic drug (AED) teratogenicity. Some of the conclusions published by this committee related to specific medication concerns are as follows:

1. It is probable that intrauterine first-trimester valproate (VPA) exposure has higher risk of major congenital malformations (MCMs) compared with carbamazepine, and possibly compared with phenytoin and lamotrigine.
2. AED polytherapy probably contributes to the development of major congenital malformations and reduced cognitive outcomes compared with monotherapy. Intrauterine exposure to VPA monotherapy probably reduces cognitive outcomes.

3. If possible, avoidance of VPA and AED polytherapy during the first trimester of pregnancy should be considered to decrease the risk of major congenital malformations. If possible, avoidance of VPA and AED polytherapy throughout pregnancy should be considered to prevent reduced cognitive outcomes.
4. If the patient has been seizure-free for 2 years or longer, drug discontinuation with a long taper period (3 months) may be successful.

Additional Reading: Management issues for women with epilepsy-focus on pregnancy (an evidence-based review): II. Teratogenesis and perinatal outcomes: report of the Quality Standards Subcommittee and Therapeutics and Technology Subcommittee of the American Academy of Neurology and the American Epilepsy Society. *Epilepsia.* 2009;50(5):1237–1246.

Category: Neurologic

29. Which of the following statements is true regarding smoking during pregnancy?
A) Smoking increases the risk of attention-deficit disorder in the child.
B) Nicotine patches are a safe alternative during pregnancy.
C) Bupropion (Zyban) should be avoided during pregnancy.
D) Regardless of when she stops smoking, infants born to mothers with a smoking history are more at risk for neonatal complications.
E) When compared with total abstinence, reducing the number of cigarettes smoked has no effect on fetal outcomes.

Answer and Discussion

The answer is A. Smoking increases the risk of miscarriage, low birth weight, perinatal mortality, and attention-deficit disorder in the child. If the mother smokes less than 1 pack of cigarettes per day, the risk of a low-birth-weight infant increases by 50%; with more than 1 pack per day, the risk increases by 130%. If the mother quits smoking by 16 weeks of pregnancy, the risk to the fetus is similar to that of a nonsmoker. Behavioral techniques, support groups, and family assistance may be beneficial. Nicotine patches or gum may be helpful before conception, but most authorities recommend avoiding them during pregnancy. Bupropion may be used during pregnancy after a discussion of risks and benefits. If the patient cannot stop smoking, the physician should help her establish a goal to decrease her number of cigarettes to fewer than 7 to 10 per day because many of the adverse effects are dose related.

Additional Reading: Smoking cessation in pregnancy (2013). *ACOG committee opinion paper* no. 471, 2013. From: http://www.acog.org/Resources_And_Publications/Committee_Opinions_List

Category: Patient/population-based care

30. The use of benzodiazepines during pregnancy has been associated with
A) Polydactily
B) Cleft lip
C) Spina bifida
D) Growth retardation
E) Developmental delay

Answer and Discussion

The answer is B. Maternal use of benzodiazepines during pregnancy has been associated with anomalies such as cleft lip and palate, as well as a withdrawal syndrome in the newborn.

Additional Reading: ACOG guidelines on psychiatric medication use during pregnancy and lactation. *Am Fam Physician.* 2008;78(6):772–778.

Category: Reproductive system

> 🌀 Maternal use of benzodiazepines during pregnancy has been associated with anomalies such as cleft lip and palate, as well as a withdrawal syndrome in the newborn.

31. Which of the following is *not* associated with maternal obesity during pregnancy?
A) Hydrocephalus
B) Maternal hypertension
C) Preeclampsia
D) Maternal diabetes
E) Macrosomic infant

Answer and Discussion
The answer is A. Obesity and being underweight increase pregnancy risks. Obesity increases the risks of maternal hypertension, preeclampsia, diabetes, and delivering a macrosomic infant. Women who are obese should diet before conception and then alter their consumption to a maintenance diet of 1,800 calories per day while trying to conceive.

Additional Reading: Obesity in Pregnancy. *ACOG Committee Opinion* no. 549, 2013. From: http://www.acog.org/Resources_And_Publications/Committee_Opinions_List

Category: Endocrine system

32. A 26-year-old primigravida presents to your office. She is pregnant with a twin gestation and is in her third trimester. She complains of pruritic, vesicular skin lesions that have developed on her abdomen. Her face, palms, and soles are spared. You suspect
A) Varicella
B) Scabies
C) Pruritic urticarial papules and plaques of pregnancy (PUPPP)
D) Herpes zoster
E) Hyperbilirubinemia

Answer and Discussion
The answer is C. Pruritic urticarial papules and plaques of pregnancy, also known as *polymorphic eruption of pregnancy,* is the most common dermatologic complaint of pregnancy, occurring in up to 1 in 160 pregnancies, with an increased incidence in multiple gestations. It usually occurs in primigravidas in the third trimester and recurrence in subsequent pregnancies is unusual. The rash may first appear postpartum. Pruritic urticarial papules and plaques of pregnancy typically have a marked pruritic component, the onset of which coincides with the skin lesions. The rash typically begins over the abdomen, commonly involving the striae gravidarum, and may spread to the breasts, upper thighs, and arms. The face, palms, soles, and mucosal surfaces are usually spared. The lesions typically consist of polymorphous, erythematous, nonfollicular papules, plaques, and sometimes vesicles. The lesions can be painful. The rash usually resolves near term or in the early postpartum period. Topical moisturizers and moderately potent steroids in combination with oral antihistamines can provide symptomatic relief.

Additional Reading: The skin disorders of pregnancy: a family physician's guide. *J Fam Pract.* 2010;59(2):89–96.

Category: Integumentary

33. What is the correct response to a Category III FHR tracing?
A) Expectant management
B) Attempt fetal scalp stimulation and if increase in FHR is not observed, continue to watch the patient closely and reattempt scalp stimulation in 30 minutes
C) Begin in utero resuscitation and proceed to cesarean section within 30 minutes if FHR tracing does not improve
D) Proceed to cesarean section immediately
E) Increase pitocin to vaginal delivery more rapidly

Answer and Discussion
The answer is C. Because of high interobserver variability in the interpretation of FHR tracings, the ACOG, the Society for Maternal-Fetal Medicine (SMFM), and the United States National Institute of Child Health and Human Development (NICHD) convened a workshop in 2008 to standardize definitions and interpretation for electronic fetal monitoring (EFM), propose management guidelines, and develop research questions. Major outputs from this workshop were a clear standard for FHR interpretation and a three-tier system (Categories I, II, and III) for the categorization of intrapartum electronic fetal monitoring.

A category III tracing is defined by either of the following criteria:

1. Absent baseline FHR variability and (any of the following):
   a. Recurrent late decelerations
   b. Recurrent variable decelerations
   c. Bradycardia

OR

2. A sinusoidal pattern

Category III tracings are abnormal and associated with an increased risk of fetal hypoxic acidemia. Patients with category III tracings should be prepared for delivery while initiating resuscitative measures. If there is no improvement in the tracing after resuscitative measures (such as IV fluid bolus, oxygen administration, left-sided positioning, discontinuation of uterotonics, consideration of tocolytics, and request for anesthesia to administer alpha adrenergic agonist if patient has recently received an epidural) and scalp stimulation does not result in FHR acceleration, delivery should be accomplished expeditiously, ideally within 30 minutes of the beginning of the Category III tracing.

Additional Reading: American College of Obstetricians and Gynecologists. ACOG Practice Bulletin no. 106: Intrapartum fetal heart rate monitoring: nomenclature, interpretation, and general management principles. *Obstet Gynecol.* 2009;114:192.

Category: Reproductive system

34. A 26-year-old woman who is 30 weeks pregnant is involved in a motor vehicle accident. She has suspected neck trauma and is in need of transport. You suggest placing her
A) In the left lateral decubitus position
B) In the Trendelenberg position
C) Prone position on a backboard
D) Supine on a backboard with her right hip elevated
E) Supine on a backboard

Answer and Discussion
The answer is D. After 20 weeks of gestation, the enlarged uterus may compress the great vessels when a pregnant woman is in a supine position. This compression can cause a decrease of up to

30 mm Hg in maternal systolic blood pressure, a 30% decrease in stroke volume, and a consequent decrease in uterine blood flow. Manual deflection of the uterus laterally or placement of the patient in the lateral decubitus position avoids uterine compression. Because of suspected neck trauma in this patient, placing her supine on a backboard with her right hip elevated 4 to 6 in. with towels is the safest treatment.

Additional Reading: Blunt trauma in pregnancy. *Am Fam Physician.* 2004;70:1303–1310, 1313.

Category: Reproductive system

35. Which of the following statements about the evaluation of infertility is true?
A) The woman should be evaluated before the man with a postcoital test.
B) A hysterosalpingogram should be performed as the first step in an infertility workup.
C) The first step is evaluation of the male factor with a sperm analysis.
D) Hormone level determination is the first test that should be ordered for the woman before the workup for the man.
E) An endometrial biopsy on the woman is the first test to consider in the workup of infertility.

Answer and Discussion
The answer is C. Infertility affects as many as 10% to 15% of couples in the United States and appears to be increasing in incidence. The definition of infertility is the lack of conception after 1 year of unprotected intercourse. As many as 40% of infertility cases are the result of the male factor (i.e., inadequate sperm production, abnormal sperm motility, or abnormally formed sperm). Other factors involve the female factor and include previous pelvic infections with fallopian tube damage, anovulation, low progesterone levels, hypothyroidism, hyperprolactinemia, or the presence of antisperm antibodies. In the evaluation of infertility, the man is usually evaluated first with a sperm analysis, because the female evaluation may be more extensive. If the sperm is found to be adequate, the woman can be evaluated with a postcoital test, hormone level determination, endometrial sampling, and hysterosalpingogram, which determine patency of the fallopian tubes. Measurement of basal body temperature may show a 0.5°F to 1.0°F increase in temperature-supporting ovulation. Further evaluation may require endocrine testing or computed tomography (CT) scanning of the head to rule out pituitary tumors or testing to rule out polycystic ovary disease.

Additional Reading: Infertility. *Am Fam Physician.* 2007;75(6): 849–856.

Category: Reproductive system

36. Which of the following conditions is characterized by infarction of the pituitary gland during labor and delivery?
A) Asherman's syndrome
B) Stein–Leventhal syndrome
C) Sheehan's syndrome
D) Cushing's disease
E) Nelson's syndrome

Answer and Discussion
The answer is C. Sheehan's syndrome is a complication of childbirth that results from shock and excessive peripartum bleeding. During pregnancy the pituitary gland usually enlarges and is vulnerable to infarction if excessive bleeding compromises blood flow. Necrosis of the pituitary can occur with varying loss of pituitary function. Symptoms of Sheehan's syndrome include lack of postpartum milk production as a result of low prolactin levels, breast atrophy, loss of pubic or axillary hair, amenorrhea, depressed mental status, low blood pressure, loss of libido, and lack of sweating. Laboratory findings include evidence of hypothyroidism, adrenal insufficiency, and decreased gonadotropin hormone secretion. Treatment involves the replacement of inadequate hormones, including thyroxine, glucocorticoids, and sex hormones. Asherman's syndrome is the development of adhesions, also known as "uterine synechiae," within the endometrial cavity, most commonly as a result of instrumentation such as D + C postpartum or from intrauterine infection. Stein-Leventhal is an older term for polycystic ovary syndrome (PCOS) characterized by anovulation, oligo or amenorrhea, excess androgens, obesity, insulin resistance, and infertility. Cushing's disease is a condition that is caused by excess corticosteroids, especially cortisol, usually from adrenal or pituitary hyperfunction and is characterized by obesity, hypertension, muscular weakness, and easy bruising. Nelson's syndrome refers to a spectrum of symptoms and signs arising from an adrenocorticotropin (ACTH)-secreting pituitary macroadenoma after a therapeutic bilateral adrenalectomy.

Additional Reading: Sheehan syndrome. *Williams Obstetrics,* 23rd ed. New York, NY: McGraw-Hill; 2010.

Category: Endocrine system

37. Which of the following is NOT a risk factor for early-onset neonatal sepsis?
A) Preterm birth
B) Maternal Group B Strep colonization
C) Macrosomia
D) Prolonged rupture of membranes >18 hours
E) Low socioeconomic status

Answer and Discussion
The answer is C. The major risk factors for early-onset neonatal sepsis are preterm birth, maternal colonization with GBS rupture of membranes >18 hours, and maternal signs or symptoms of intra-amniotic infection. Other variables include ethnicity (i.e., black women are at higher risk of being colonized with GBS), low socioeconomic status, male sex, and low Apgar scores. Preterm birth/low birth weight is the risk factor most closely associated with early-onset sepsis. Infant birth weight is inversely related to risk of early-onset sepsis, so large-for-gestational age infants would be less likely to get early-onset sepsis. In the United States, the most common pathogens responsible for early-onset neonatal sepsis are GBS and *Escherichia coli.* A combination of ampicillin and an aminoglycoside (usually gentamicin) is generally used as initial therapy, and this combination of antimicrobial agents also has synergistic activity against GBS and *Listeria monocytogenes.* Third-generation cephalosporins (e.g., cefotaxime) represent a reasonable alternative to an aminoglycoside. However, several studies have reported rapid development of resistance when cefotaxime has been used routinely for the treatment of early-onset neonatal sepsis, and extensive/prolonged use of third-generation cephalosporins is a risk factor for invasive candidiasis. Because of its excellent cerebrospinal fluid (CSF) penetration, empirical or therapeutic use of cefotaxime should be restricted for use in infants with meningitis attributable to gram-negative organisms. Ceftriaxone is contraindicated in neonates because it is highly protein bound and may displace bilirubin, leading to a risk of kernicterus.

Additional Reading: Management of neonates with suspected or proven early-onset bacterial sepsis. *Pediatrics.* 2012;129(5):1006–1015.

Category: Reproductive system

38. Which of the following statements is true regarding seat belt use in pregnancy?
A) The use of correctly positioned seat belts can increase the risk of fetal injury.
B) The lap belt should be placed under the gravid uterus and over the thighs with the shoulder harness placed between the breast and over the uterus.
C) The air bag should be disabled.
D) Seat belt-restrained women who are in motor vehicle crashes have the same fetal mortality rate as women who are not in motor vehicle crashes.
E) The shoulder harness should not be used during pregnancy.

Answer and Discussion

The answer is D. Proper seat belt use is the most significant preventive measure in decreasing maternal and fetal injury and mortality after motor vehicle crashes. Seat belt-restrained women who are in motor vehicle crashes have the identical fetal mortality rate as women who are not in motor vehicle crashes, but, unrestrained women who are in crashes are more than twice as likely to lose their fetuses. Prenatal care should include three-point seat belt instruction. The lap belt should be placed under the gravid abdomen, snugly over the thighs, with the shoulder harness off to the side of the uterus, between the breasts and over the midline of the clavicle. Seat belts placed directly over the uterus can cause fetal injury. Airbags should not be disabled during pregnancy.

Additional Reading: Blunt trauma in pregnancy. *Am Fam Physician.* 2004;70:1303–1310, 1313.

Category: Patient/population-based care

39. A patient presenting for care in the first-trimester of pregnancy requests information on what types of noninvasive testing are available to detect Down's syndrome in her fetus at an early stage in her pregnancy. You inform her that
A) A combination of an ultrasound done in the first trimester measuring a specific anatomical area of her fetus and maternal blood testing on the same day will help identify if she is at increased risk for Down's syndrome.
B) Only an amniocentesis done in the early second trimester can give her the information that she is looking for.
C) She should wait until the second trimester to have a maternal quadruple screen and an ultrasound to look at fetal anatomy.
D) Only patients who wish to terminate their pregnancies for abnormal fetuses should pursue genetic testing.
E) There are now too many prenatal tests available for this indication and that she will need to meet with a genetic counselor to help decide what testing she would like to have.

Answer and Discussion

The answer is A. American College of Obstetrics and Gynecology recommends that all pregnant women are offered aneuploidy screening before 20 weeks. Currently available screening includes the ultrasound measurement of fetal nuchal translucency in the late first trimester which, when enlarged, is associated with a variety of trisomies, most notable trisomy-21, as well as fetal congenital anomalies such as cardiac defects. Combining the nuchal translucency with 1st trimester biochemical markers allows identification of a population of pregnant women at high risk for aneuploidy early in their pregnancies, and these women should receive genetic counseling and be offered first-trimester chorionic villus sampling (CVS) or second-trimester amniocentesis. If no increased risk is identified with first-trimester screening, this information can be combined later in pregnancy with second-trimester maternal serum screening to increase the sensitivity of testing for aneuploidy and decrease the false positive rate of either of these forms of testing done separately. If either a fetal anatomical survey done by second-trimester U/S (Ultra Sound) sug-gests a major congenital anomaly and/or if a high risk for aneuploidy is detected on combined first- and second-trimester aneuploidy screening, the patient should receive genetic counseling and offered diagnostic fetal chromosomal testing via amniocentesis. A relatively new option for women is to be offered noninvasive prenatal testing (NIPT) as an alternative to amniocentesis. NIPT allows the isolation of cell-free fetal DNA from the plasma of pregnant women as another detection tool for fetal aneuploidy. Counseling regarding the limitations of NIPT should include a discussion that the screening test provides information regarding only trisomy 21 and trisomy 18 and, in some laboratories, trisomy 13. It does not replace the precision obtained with diagnostic tests, such as chorionic villus sampling or amniocentesis, and currently does not offer other genetic information.

Additional Reading: Screening for fetal chromosomal abnormalities. *ACOG Practice Bulletin* no. 77, 2007; and Noninvasive prenatal testing for fetal aneuploidy. *ACOG Practice Bulletin* no. 545, and 2012. From: http://www.acog.org/Resources_And_Publications/Committee_Opinions_List

Category: Reproductive system

40. Pregnant women should avoid contact with cat litter because of the risk for developing
A) Cryptococcus
B) Cytomegalovirus
C) Toxoplasmosis
D) Coccidioidomycosis
E) Erythema infectiosum

Answer and Discussion

The answer is C. Toxoplasmosis is a granulomatous disease caused by the protozoan *Toxoplasmosis gondii*, which affects the central nervous system (CNS). The disease is extremely common, and affected patients are usually asymptomatic. Symptoms, when present, mimic mononucleosis and include malaise, fever, myalgias, rashes, and cervical and axillary lymphadenopathy. Laboratory and physical findings include mild anemia, leukopenia, lymphocytosis, elevated liver function tests, and hypotension. A more severe form may occur in patients with acquired immunodeficiency syndrome (AIDS) or other patients who are immunocompromised; complications include hepatitis, pneumonitis, meningoencephalitis, and myocarditis. Chronic toxoplasmosis can lead to retinochoroiditis, persistent diarrhea, muscular weakness, and headache. Congenital toxoplasmosis can lead to spontaneous abortion or stillbirths. A multitude of congenital defects may occur, including blindness and severe mental retardation. Diagnosis is usually made by serologic tests with fluorescent antibody techniques. CT examination of the brain may show enhancing lesions, and biopsies can be taken to look for the organisms microscopically. Treatment is reserved for more severe cases and consists of the combined use of pyrimethamine, sulfadiazine, and folinic acid (leucovorin). Immunocompromised patients require maintenance treatment for life. Because the protozoan is found in cat feces, pregnant women should avoid handling cat litter.

Misoprosol → IV pitocin

Additional Reading: Pet-related infections. *Am Fam Physician.* 2007;76(9):1314–1322.

Category: Nonspecific system

41. What percentage of babies born to HIV-positive mothers is HIV positive?
A) 0% to 1%
B) 20% to 30%
C) 50% to 75%
D) 90% to 100%
E) 100%

Answer and Discussion

The answer is B. Prenatal screening for HIV should be offered to all pregnant women. Approximately 25% of newborns born to HIV-positive mothers will be infected with HIV, and another approximately 10% to 15% will become infected if breast-fed. Hence, breast-feeding is discouraged if there is access to clean water and formula. In the United States, Cesarean section is recommended if the maternal viral load exceeds 1,000 copies/mL, but this is controversial and some centers do this at any detectable viral load close to delivery. After delivery, the infant should be screened repeatedly using HIV DNA or RNA polymerase chain reaction (PCR) assays. Maternal HIV antibody crosses the placenta and will be detectable in all HIV-exposed infants up to age 18 months; therefore, standard antibody tests should not be used for HIV diagnosis in newborns until that time. HIV RNA or DNA PCR should be performed within the first 14 to 21 days of life, at 1 to 2 months, and at 4 to 6 months of age. Some experts also perform a virologic test at birth, especially in women who have not had good virologic control during pregnancy or if adequate follow-up of the infant may not be assured. A positive HIV virologic test should be confirmed as soon as possible with a second HIV virologic test on a different specimen. Two positive HIV tests constitute a diagnosis of HIV infection. All HIV-exposed infants should receive 6 weeks of zidovudine, and some centers add either a single or repeated doses of nevirapine if the mother was not fully virally suppressed before delivery.

Additional Reading: U.S. Department of Health and Human Services' Recommendations for Use of Antiretroviral Drugs in Pregnant HIV-1-Infected Women for Maternal Health and Interventions to Reduce Perinatal HIV Transmission in the United States. From: http://www.aidsinfo.nih.gov/guidelines/html/3/perinatal-guidelines/0

Category: Reproductive system

42. The most appropriate management for intrauterine fetal demise in the 3rd trimester includes
A) Observation for up to 4 weeks until the mother goes into labor
B) Immediate cesarean section
C) Administration of intravenous oxytocin (Pitocin) after serial misoprostol 25 to 50 mcg every 4 hours until cervix ripened
D) High-dose misoprostol (200 to 400 mcg every 4 hours)
E) Heparin plus antibiotic prophylaxis and observation for up to 4 weeks

Answer and Discussion

The answer is C. The risk of disseminated intravascular coagulation is increased if a dead fetus has been retained in utero for more than 4 weeks. Therefore, it is practical to provide expectant management for patients with in utero fetal demise for up to 1 to 3 weeks. However, because many mothers experience significant psychological stress from carrying a dead fetus, patients who have

experienced a fetal demise should be offered hospital admission and induction of labor. Induction is most effective if vaginal prostaglandins such as misoprosol are given first to provide cervical ripening followed by intravenous pitocin. Doses of misoprostol for cervical ripening in the third trimester of pregnancy are typically 25 to 50 mcg through vagina every 4 hours, while higher doses (200 to 400 mcg every 4 hours) can be used to achieve uterine evacuation for second-trimester intrauterine fetal demise.

Additional Reading: Diagnosis and management of stillbirth. In: Basow DS, ed. *UpToDate.* Waltham, MA: UpToDate; 2013.

Category: Reproductive system

43. A standard dose of Rh immune globulin (300 μg) prevents sensitization from fetomaternal hemorrhage of up to
A) 30 mL of whole blood
B) 60 mL of whole blood
C) 100 mL of whole blood
D) 500 mL of whole blood
E) Any amount of whole blood

Answer and Discussion

The answer is A. Rh immune globulin (RhIg) must be administered to an Rh-negative mother immediately after abortion or delivery (live or stillborn) unless the infant is Rh_o (D) and D^u negative, the mother's serum already contains anti-Rh_o (D), or the mother refuses. The standard dose of intramuscular RhIg (300 μg) prevents sensitization from fetomaternal hemorrhage of up to 30 mL whole blood. It is necessary to identify women with fetomaternal hemorrhage to calculate the doses needed to prevent sensitization via a screening rosette test, which, if positive, is followed by a quantitative test (e.g., Kleihauer–Betke).

Additional Reading: Evidence-based prenatal care: Part II. Third-trimester care and prevention of infectious diseases. *Am Fam Physician.* 2005;71:1555–1562.

Category: Hematologic system

44. Which of the following statements regarding varicella during pregnancy is true?
A) If a pregnant woman has no history of varicella and tests negative for antibodies, she should be immunized as soon as possible.
B) Varicella vaccination should be avoided in breast-feeding women.
C) Susceptible pregnant women who are exposed to varicella are candidates for varicella zoster immune globulin.
D) Pregnancy should be delayed 6 months after varicella vaccination.
E) A single dose of varicella vaccine is safe during pregnancy and can be administered to help protect the fetus.

Answer and Discussion

The answer is C. If varicella testing is performed in the preconception period, women can be offered two doses of varicella vaccine at least 1 month apart. Pregnancy should be delayed 1 month after vaccination. Varicella vaccine is contraindicated in pregnant women. Women found to be nonimmune during pregnancy should be counseled to avoid exposure to chickenpox and to report exposure immediately. Susceptible pregnant women who are exposed to varicella are candidates for varicella zoster immune globulin. Nonimmune women should be offered postpartum varicella vaccination. The vaccine is considered safe in breast-feeding women.

Additional Reading: Evidence-based prenatal care: Part II. Third-trimester care and prevention of infectious diseases. *Am Fam Physician.* 2005;71:1555–1562.

Category: Patient/population-based care

45. Rho(D) immune globulin (RhoGAM) is indicated when
A) The mother has type AB blood
B) The father is Rh negative
C) The mother is Rh positive
D) None of the above

Answer and Discussion

The answer is D. If the antibody test is negative, Rh-negative mothers should be given an immune globulin preparation at 28 weeks' gestation to prevent erythroblastosis fetalis. If the father is also Rh negative, the administration is unnecessary; however, extramarital pregnancies should be considered. A dose of RhoGAM should also be given at the time of delivery, depending on the blood type of the infant. If the infant is Rh negative, the mother's dose can be determined by the Kleihauer–Betke (FetalDex) test, which measures the amount of fetal erythrocytes in the maternal blood. If the newborn is Rh negative, there is no need for immune globulin administration. The immune globulin should also be given to Rh-negative women after elective or spontaneous abortion, placental abruption, ectopic pregnancy, or amniocentesis. Typically, the standard dose is 300 μg, which protects up to 10 mL of Rh-positive fetal red cells.

Additional Reading: Evidence-based prenatal care: Part II. Third-trimester care and prevention of infectious diseases. *Am Fam Physician.* 2005;71:1555–1562.

Category: Hematologic system

46. When there is first-trimester bleeding, fetal viability can be definitely determined by which of the following tests?
A) Qualitative β-human chorionic gonadotropin (hCG) determination
B) Serial quantitative β-hCG measurements
C) Transvaginal ultrasonography
D) Serum progesterone levels
E) Both B and C

Answer and Discussion

The answer is C. Approximately 25% of pregnant women experience vaginal spotting or heavier bleeding during the first trimester of pregnancy, and 25% to 50% of these pregnant women experience spontaneous abortion. Genetic anomalies are the most common cause of spontaneous abortion in the first trimester. Qualitative hCG determination only gives a diagnosis of the positive presence of hCG, usually at a level of >25 mIU/mL, but does not give any information regarding the viability or location of an actual pregnancy. When first-trimester bleeding is present, potential viability of the pregnancy can be determined with a quantitative β-hCG determination, which is repeated 3 to 5 days later. The β-hCG level should double every 48 hours when a normal pregnancy is present, but does not definitively diagnose an intrauterine viable pregnancy until confirmed by ultrasound. A fetus should be seen with vaginal ultrasound by the 33rd to 35th day after the last menstrual period, or when the β-hCG level has reached 1,500 to 2,000 mIU/mL. If the β-hCG level exceeds 1,500 to 2,000 mIU/mL and no intrauterine pregnancy is found with

vaginal ultrasound, an ectopic pregnancy should be suspected, especially if an adnexal mass is palpated on physical examination or the expecting mother experiences lower abdominal pain. Progesterone levels of <5 ng/dL usually indicate a nonviable pregnancy but progesterone measurements are not generally used for diagnosis of viability.

Additional Reading: First trimester bleeding. *Am Fam Physician.* 2009;79(11):985–992.

Category: Reproductive system

47. A 27-year-old woman presents for her annual examination. Her body mass index (BMI) is 31 and she has hirsutism and reports difficulty with conception. She does not have monthly menses, and typically has a period only every 5 to 6 months. Based on her likely diagnosis, which of the following malignancies is she most at increased risk for?
A) Ovarian carcinoma
B) Colon cancer
C) Pancreatic cancer
D) Endometrial carcinoma
E) Breast cancer

Answer and Discussion

The answer is D. PCOS is the most common endocrine abnormality in women of reproductive age. The syndrome is associated with chronic anovulation, oligomenorrhea, and infertility. Macrovascular diseases such as type 2 diabetes mellitus, hypertension, and atherosclerotic heart disease are more likely in women with PCOS. In addition, chronic anovulation predisposes women to endometrial hyperplasia and carcinoma. Symptoms that prompt women to seek attention include irregular menses, hirsutism, or infertility. The earliest manifestations of PCOS are noted around the time of puberty. Adolescent girls affected with PCOS often have early puberty and show hyperandrogenism and insulin resistance. In the early reproductive period, chronic anovulation results in difficulty with fertility. If pregnancy is achieved, it frequently terminates in spontaneous first-trimester loss or is associated with gestational diabetes. More than 50% of those affected are obese. Abnormal androgen production declines as menopause approaches (as it does in women without PCOS), and menstrual patterns may normalize. However, perimenopausal and postmenopausal women with a history of PCOS have increased rates of type 2 diabetes, hypertension, and coronary artery disease compared with control patients. PCOS appears to follow a familial distribution. Luteinizing hormone (LH) and follicle-stimulating hormone (FSH) levels are often elevated in PCOS, with the LH:FSH ratio greater than 3:1. Individualized therapy should incorporate steroid hormones, antiandrogens, and insulin-sensitizing agents such as metformin. Metformin increases ovulation rates in some women with PCOS and also may reduce fasting insulin concentrations, lower blood pressure, and reduce low-density lipoprotein cholesterol. Weight loss by way of reduced carbohydrate intake and exercise is the most important intervention; this step alone can restore menstrual regularity and fertility and provide long-term prevention against diabetes and heart disease.

Additional Reading: Clinical manifestations of polycystic ovary syndrome in adults. In: Basow DS, ed. *UpToDate.* Waltham, MA: UpToDate; 2013.

Category: Endocrine system

48. A 29-year-old woman is now in her 14th week of pregnancy and developed an initial outbreak of genital herpes. You explain to her
A) Genital herpes (herpes simplex virus [HSV]) is a sexually transmitted disease (STD) that can be treated in such a way as to prevent future recurrences.
B) The risk for transmission to the neonate is high among women who newly acquire genital herpes near term and low among women who acquire genital HSV during the first half of pregnancy.
C) Termination of the pregnancy should be considered.
D) Cesarean section will be needed for her delivery, irrespective of whether she has recurrent herpetic lesions at that time or not.
E) Antiviral medications such as acyclovir (Zovirax) cannot be used in pregnancy if she develops recurrent attacks.

Answer and Discussion
The answer is B. HSV is a sexually transmitted infection (STI) that is not curable and has a varying rate of recurrence in all individuals. In pregnancy, the highest risk for neonatal transmission (30% to 50%) is among infants of women with their first outbreak of genital HSV close to the time of delivery. The risk of neonatal transmission is low (<1%) for pregnant women who have recurrences near term; however, because recurrent genital HSV is much more common than initial HSV infection in pregnancy, the proportion of neonatal HSV infections acquired from mothers with recurrent herpes is still significant. Prevention of neonatal HSV infection is best accomplished by preventing the acquisition of new genital HSV infection during late pregnancy, decreasing the recurrence rate of HSV infections near term for pregnant women with a history of prior genital HSV infection, and avoiding exposure of the infant to herpetic lesions during delivery. Suppressive antiviral treatment late in pregnancy reduces the frequency of cesarean sections among women who have recurrent genital herpes by diminishing the frequency of recurrences at term. Women with recurrent HSV infection should be counseled about the use of antiviral therapy such as acyclover close to term to decrease the rate of cesarean delivery. They should also be informed about the role of cesarean delivery in decreasing vertical transmission, which is typically only offered in the presence of active HSV genital lesions at the time of labor. For women with active lesions after delivery, care should be taken to avoid postpartum transmission to the infant through direct contact.

> **Additional Reading:** Diseases characterized by genital, anal or perianal ulcers. *CDC Sexually Transmitted Disease Treatment Guidelines*; 2010.

Category: Reproductive system

49. Which of the following is not a risk factor for group B β-streptococcal infection in the neonate?
A) Twin gestation
B) Less than 37 weeks' gestation
C) Prolonged rupture of membranes
D) Maternal fever
E) Maternal Group B-streptococcal anogenital colonization

Answer and Discussion
The answer is A. GBS infection is responsible for a significant amount of neonatal morbidity and mortality. Up to 30% of women are colonized by GBS. Risk factors for neonatal infection include less than 37 weeks' gestation, prolonged rupture of membranes (>18 hours), and maternal fever. Multiple organizations recommend that all women be offered GBS screening by vaginorectal culture at 35 to 37 weeks' gestation and that colonized women be treated with appropriate intravenous antibiotics at the time of labor or rupture of membranes. GBS bacteriuria indicates heavy maternal colonization. Women with GBS bacteriuria in their current pregnancy or a previous infant with GBS infection should be offered intrapartum antibiotics routinely and therefore do not require vaginorectal culture.

> **Additional Reading:** Prevention of perinatal group B streptococcal disease: updated CDC guideline. *Am Fam Physician.* 2012;86(1):59–65.

Category: Reproductive system

50. Patients who have difficulty with infertility may have antisperm antibodies. Which one of the following medications may help lower antisperm antibodies?
A) Medroxyprogesterone (Depo-Provera)
B) OCPs
C) Gonadotropin-releasing hormone (GnRH) agonist
D) Corticosteroids
E) None of the above

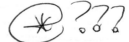

Answer and Discussion
The answer is D. Immunologic infertility can occur in women as a result of the development of local and circulating antisperm antibodies. In men, there may also be circulating antibodies that prevent conception. Men with previous vasectomies have an increased risk of antisperm antibodies. Immunologic tests are now available for the detection of these antibodies. In some cases, spontaneous remission of antibodies has occurred. In cases in which they persist, steroids may be useful in lowering the levels of antibodies, thus allowing pregnancy.

> **Additional Reading:** Evaluation of male infertility. In: Basow DS, ed. *UpToDate.* Waltham, MA: UpToDate; 2013.

Category: Reproductive system

51. A 26-year-old woman presents to your office with questions regarding an intrauterine device (IUD) for birth control. Which of the following statements is true?
A) IUD use is decreasing in the United States.
B) Failure rates can be as high as 10%.
C) IUDs currently available in the United States pose little risk for pelvic inflammatory disease (PID) in appropriate candidates.
D) Placement of an IUD may affect future fertility.
E) Both copper and levonorgestrel-containing IUDs produce similar bleeding patterns in users.

Answer and Discussion
The answer is C. An IUD is a contraceptive method that involves placing a foreign body through the cervical os and into the uterus. Interest in the IUD started in the 1960s and its use in this country increased over the next decade. A 1974 study, however, linked the Dalkon Shield to maternal death and found it to have a disproportionately higher rate of infection than any other IUD. The cause of infection was the multifilament string (or tail), which was a modification of the monofilament tails used by other IUDs. This multifilament tail provided a pathway for bacteria, enabling them to bypass the immunologic barrier provided by the endocervix. This design flaw caused a fivefold increase in PID and an increase in septic abortion. After the Dalkon Shield was removed from the market, the use of IUDs declined in the United States. Currently, there are two IUDs on the market in the United State, both of which have an improved

design and research has shown them to be a safe and efficacious form of birth control. The availability of these types of IUDs and their improved safety record has led to increased use of IUDs in the United States over the past 10 to 20 years. The "ParaGard" copper T308A is a type of IUD that is marketed for use for 10 years. A common side effect of the copper IUD is menorrhagia, which necessitates its removal in some women. The "Mirena" levonorgestrel-secreting IUD is effective for at least 5 years, and some sources suggest that it may effectively prevent pregnancy for up to 7 years. The levonorgestrel exerts a direct effect on the uterus, which diminishes menstrual bleeding. Combined failure rates of both types of IUDs are <1% to 1.9% over 10 years, which is comparable to female sterilization. Contraindications for the use of IUDs include current cervical or uterine infections and pregnancy. Multiple studies conclude that the IUD poses little or no increased risk of PID or infertility when used by appropriately selected patients. Multiple studies have shown no increased risk for cervical or uterine malignancies in IUD users.

> Additional Reading: Long-acting reversible contraception: implants and intrauterine devices. *ACOG Practice Bulletin* no. 1, 2011. From: http://www.acog.org/Resources_And_Publications/Committee_Opinions_List

Category: Reproductive system

52. An 18-year-old woman has noted diffuse darkened areas of skin on her face following the initiation of oral contraceptives. The most likely diagnosis is
A) Melasma
B) Lupus pernio
C) Malignant melanoma
D) Sebaceous hyperplasia
E) Acne

Answer and Discussion

The answer is A. Melasma occurs in some women taking oral contraceptives. The condition is characterized by areas of darkened pigmentation that may affect the face. The condition is also seen in pregnancy. The condition is more common in African Americans and Latinas. Sun exposure can worsen the condition. Usually, the areas fade when pregnancy is complete or oral contraceptives are discontinued. Lupus pernio is a chronic, raised, indurated lesion of the skin, often purplish in color and associated with underlying sarcoidosis. Melanoma lesions are typically dark black and are not associated with oral contraceptive use. Sebaceous hyperplasia is a disorder of the sebaceous glands in which they become enlarged, sometimes in response to the hormones of pregnancy, producing yellow shiny bumps on the face, but do not alter the pigmentation of the skin. Oral contraceptives can both predispose patients to acne or improve it; however, acne lesions do typically appear as dark areas, except in cases of postacne scar formation.

> Additional Reading: Common skin conditions during pregnancy. *Am Fam Physician.* 2007;75(2):211–218.

Category: Integumentary

53. Which of the following is the drug of choice for use in Group B streptococcal colonized pregnant women in labor for the prevention of group B streptococcal infection in the neonate?
A) Intramuscular ceftriaxone
B) Oral ciprofloxacin
C) Intravenous penicillin G
D) Intravenous vancomycin
E) Oral amoxicillin

Answer and Discussion

The answer is C. Intravenous penicillin G is the preferred antibiotic for the prevention of group B β-streptococcal infection in newborns, with ampicillin as an alternative. Penicillin G should be administered at least 4 hours before delivery for maximum effectiveness. Cefazolin is recommended in women allergic to penicillin who are at low risk of anaphylaxis. Clindamycin and erythromycin are options for women at high risk for anaphylaxis if testing shows that their GBS isolates are sensitive to these agents. Vancomycin should be used in women allergic to penicillin and whose cultures indicate resistance to clindamycin and erythromycin or when susceptibility is unknown.

> Additional Reading: Prevention of perinatal group B streptococcal disease. Revised guidelines from CDC 2010. *MMWR Recomm Rep.* 2010;59(RR-10):1–32.

Category: Reproductive system

54. The diagnostic test of choice for the detection of ectopic pregnancy is
A) A single quantitative β-hCG level
B) CT of pelvis
C) Magnetic resonance imaging (MRI) of the pelvis
D) Transvaginal pelvic ultrasonography
E) Laparoscopy

Answer and Discussion

The answer is D. Ectopic pregnancy occurs in 1.5% to 2% of pregnancies and is potentially life threatening. Although there has been decreased mortality associated with this condition due to early detection and treatment before rupture, ectopic pregnancy still accounts for 0.5 deaths per 1,000 pregnancies, which represents 6% of all maternal deaths. Risk factors for ectopic pregnancy include prior PID, tubal surgery, and previous ectopic pregnancy. If a pregnancy occurs in the presence of an IUD, there is a higher risk that it will be ectopic. When diagnosed early, ectopic pregnancy may be treated medically rather than surgically. Therefore, ectopic pregnancy should be considered and quickly ruled out in all women of reproductive age who present with abdominal pain or vaginal bleeding. Transvaginal ultrasonography used in conjunction with quantitative hCG levels is the best method for diagnosis of ectopic pregnancy.

> Additional Reading: Ectopic pregnancy *NEJM.* 2009;361: 379–387.

Category: Reproductive system

55. Which of the following statements about molar pregnancy is true?
A) Malignant transformation is monitored by serial α-fetoprotein levels.
B) Further pregnancies should be discouraged after a molar pregnancy.
C) It is usually associated with hyperemesis gravidarum.
D) Risk for recurrent molar pregnancy is not increased in women who have had previous molar pregnancies.
E) The majority of molar pregnancies result in malignant transformation.

Answer and Discussion

The answer is C. A molar pregnancy (hydatidiform mole) occurs when the placenta undergoes trophoblastic transformation and results in a neoplasm of the placenta. The abnormal placenta is usually swollen, edematous, and vesicular, resembling a cluster of grapes. The condition usually affects women younger than 20 and older than 40 years of age, and those with a prior history of hydatidiform mole are at increased risk. Hydatidiform moles are usually associated with hyperemesis gravidarum and preeclampsia that occurs before the third trimester. Other associated conditions include vaginal bleeding; signs and symptoms of hyperthyroidism; trophoblastic embolization that may cause cough, tachypnea, and cyanosis; enlarged uterus associated with gestation; and theca lutein cysts resulting in ovarian enlargement. In 80% of patients, the molar pregnancy resolves after dilation and curettage without complications; however, in 20%, there is a malignant transformation of the tissue. Therefore, serum hCG determination (which is usually significantly elevated at time of diagnosis) should be monitored every 2 weeks after evacuation of the uterus until the value drops to nonpregnant values and then every 1 to 2 months for 1 year. Repeated pelvic examinations should be performed on a monthly basis after a molar pregnancy for the first year. In addition, a chest x-ray should be performed at the time of evacuation and 4 to 8 weeks after evacuation to check for metastasis. The lungs are the most common sites for metastasis. Patients should avoid pregnancy for at least 1 year after the development of a molar pregnancy. Those who have had prior molar pregnancies have an increased risk for recurrent molar pregnancies, and those who have recurrent molar pregnancies are at an increased risk for malignant transformation. Malignant transformation is usually treated with methotrexate.

> **Additional Reading:** Gestational trophoblastic neoplasia. *Williams Obstetrics,* 23rd ed. New York, NY: McGraw-Hill; 2010.

Category: Reproductive system

> Hydatidiform moles are usually associated with hyperemesis gravidarum and preeclampsia that occur before the third trimester.

56. A 44-year-old woman presents with irregular vaginal bleeding. Appropriate initial management includes
A) Endometrial biopsy
B) Trial of oral contraceptives
C) Medroxyprogesterone injection
D) Surgical referral

Answer and Discussion

The answer is A. Women who are reproductively mature, are older than 40, and experience irregular vaginal bleeding should be evaluated with endometrial biopsy to rule out endometrial hyperplasia or carcinoma. In addition, other tests to rule out thyroid dysfunction and bleeding disorders should be considered. Adolescents with abnormal vaginal bleeding can be regulated with oral contraceptive medications once pregnancy and infection have been ruled out. Vaginal bleeding before the age of 9 and after the age of 52 in the absence of hormone replacement is a cause for concern and requires investigation.

> **Additional Reading:** Evaluation and management of abnormal uterine bleeding in premenopausal women. *Am Fam Physician.* 2012;85(1):35–43.

Category: Reproductive system

57. In the management of a pregnant patient, medications are classified based on their risk to the fetus. Category C medications
A) Should never be given during pregnancy
B) Are considered safe during pregnancy
C) Should only be given in life-threatening situations
D) Have unknown risk for the fetus
E) Are associated with teratogenicity in animals

Answer and Discussion

The answer is D. The following medication classifications are used to determine the risk of their use during pregnancy:

- *Category A:* Controlled studies in women fail to demonstrate risk to the fetus in the first trimester; considered safe with no harmful effects on the fetus.
- *Category B:* Animal studies do not indicate a risk; however, there are no human studies. Considered relatively safe during pregnancy.
- *Category C:* Unknown fetal risk with no human studies to support or disprove safety.
- *Category D:* Some risk has been proved for the fetus; these drugs should be used only in life-threatening situations.
- *Category X:* Proven harm to the fetus; should not be used in pregnancy.

> **Additional Reading:** Briggs GG, Freeman RK, Yaffe SJ. *Drugs in Pregnancy and Lactation: A Reference Guide to Fetal and Neonatal Risk.* Philadelphia, PA: Lippincott Williams & Wilkins; 2011.

Category: Reproductive system

58. Which of the following medications has been shown to be comparable to laparoscopic salpingostomy in the treatment of small ectopic pregnancy that has not ruptured?
A) Bromocriptine
B) Methotrexate
C) Thalidomide
D) Misoprostol
E) Oxytocin

Answer and Discussion

The answer is B. In recent years, intramuscular methotrexate has been advocated as an alternative to salpingostomy for management of ectopic pregnancy. In addition, there is also interest in using serum hCG or progesterone levels to monitor resolution of ectopic pregnancy after intervention. On the basis of study results, a single dose of intramuscular methotrexate is comparable to laparoscopic salpingostomy for the treatment of a small, unruptured ectopic pregnancy. The fact that serum progesterone levels resolved faster than serum hCG levels suggests that serum progesterone may be a better marker for monitoring resolution of ectopic pregnancy. Guidelines have been developed to choose appropriate candidates for medical treatment of ectopic versus surgical. The good candidate for methotrexate must be hemodynamically stable, with no evidence of pending or current rupture of the ectopic, preferably with hCG level < 5000 K, ectopic mass size <3 to 4 cm, and able to comply with follow-up. Patients with abnormal renal or hepatic function at baseline or certain gastric or hematologic disorders are not generally candidates for this therapy.

> **Additional Reading:** Medical management of ectopic pregnancy. *ACOG Practice Bulletin* no. 94, 2008. From: http://www.acog.org/Resources_And_Publications/Committee_Opinions_List

Category: Reproductive system

59. Which of the following medications can be safely used for cervical ripening for term pregnancies?
A) Terbutaline
B) Methotrexate
C) Thalidomide
D) Misoprostol
E) Bromocriptine

Answer and Discussion

The answer is D. Misoprostol (Cytotec) is a synthetic prostaglandin E1 analog that has been U.S. Food and Drug Administration (FDA) approved and marketed for gastric protection, not for use in labor patients. However, this drug has been extensively investigated for use in cervical ripening and labor induction. Low-dose (25 mcg) intravaginal misoprostol appears to be safe and effective for cervical ripening in term pregnancy for patients without a history of cesarean section. Compared with other cervical ripening methods, misoprostol has an increased rate of vaginal delivery within 24 hours without significant differences in cesarean section rates or fetal outcomes. A 50-mcg dose of intravaginal misoprostol causes increased rates of uterine hyperstimulation and may be associated with an increased cesarean section rate. Because of a potential increased risk of uterine rupture, use of misoprostol for labor induction in women with a previous cesarean section is relatively contraindicated.

> **Additional Reading:** Vaginal misoprostol for cervical ripening in term pregnancy. *Am Fam Physician.* 2006;73(3):511–512.

> **Category:** Reproductive system

60. Which of the following statements about uterine adenomyosis is true?
A) The condition is associated with the invasion of myometrial tissue into the peritoneal cavity.
B) The condition commonly causes intense pelvic pain, dysuria, and dyspareunia.
C) Those affected with uterine adenomyosis have an increased risk of endometrial cancer.
D) The condition is considered benign and usually causes no associated symptoms.
E) The condition results from uterine atony after delivery.

Answer and Discussion

The answer is D. Uterine adenomyosis is defined as the invasion of endometrial tissue into the myometrium. This common disorder is benign and usually causes no symptoms. Those who do have symptoms complain of menorrhagia, irregular vaginal bleeding, pelvic pain, and bladder or rectal discomfort. Pelvic examination may reveal an enlarged uterus that feels softer in consistency; there may be associated fibroid tumors. Hysterectomy may be indicated for those beyond their childbearing years if symptoms are severe. Oral contraceptives and GnRH agonists are not very effective in treatment. Uterine adenomyosis is more likely to cause secondary dysmenorrhea than fibroids, endometrial polyps, cervical papillomas, or polycystic ovary disease.

> **Additional Reading:** Adenomyosis. In: Domino F, ed. *The 5-Minute Clinical Consult.* Philadelphia, PA: Lippincott Williams and Wilkins; 2014.

> **Category:** Reproductive system

61. A 17-year-old girl is seen in the emergency room. She reports high fever, nausea, vomiting, myalgias, and lethargy. On examination, she is found to have hypotension and a generalized erythematous rash and desquamation of the hands and feet. Laboratory tests show an increased white blood cell count, increased blood urea nitrogen, and increased serum creatinine with decreased urine output. The most likely diagnosis is
A) Gonorrhea
B) Lyme disease
C) Toxic shock syndrome
D) Tertiary syphilis
E) PID

Answer and Discussion

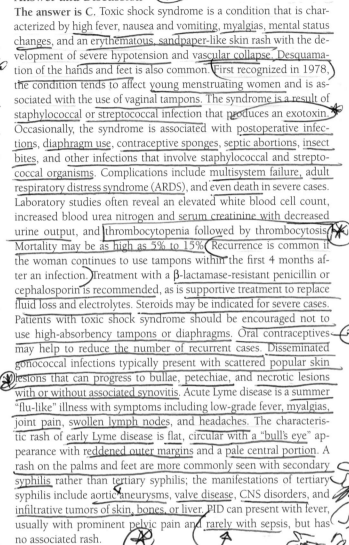

The answer is C. Toxic shock syndrome is a condition that is characterized by high fever, nausea and vomiting, myalgias, mental status changes, and an erythematous, sandpaper-like skin rash with the development of severe hypotension and vascular collapse. Desquamation of the hands and feet is also common. First recognized in 1978, the condition tends to affect young menstruating women and is associated with the use of vaginal tampons. The syndrome is a result of staphylococcal or streptococcal infection that produces an exotoxin. Occasionally, the syndrome is associated with postoperative infections, diaphragm use, contraceptive sponges, septic abortions, insect bites, and other infections that involve staphylococcal and streptococcal organisms. Complications include multisystem failure, adult respiratory distress syndrome (ARDS), and even death in severe cases. Laboratory studies often reveal an elevated white blood cell count, increased blood urea nitrogen and serum creatinine with decreased urine output, and thrombocytopenia followed by thrombocytosis. Mortality may be as high as 5% to 15%. Recurrence is common if the woman continues to use tampons within the first 4 months after an infection. Treatment with a β-lactamase-resistant penicillin or cephalosporin is recommended, as is supportive treatment to replace fluid loss and electrolytes. Steroids may be indicated for severe cases. Patients with toxic shock syndrome should be encouraged not to use high-absorbency tampons or diaphragms. Oral contraceptives may help to reduce the number of recurrent cases. Disseminated gonococcal infections typically present with scattered popular skin lesions that can progress to bullae, petechiae, and necrotic lesions with or without associated synovitis. Acute Lyme disease is a summer "flu-like" illness with symptoms including low-grade fever, myalgias, joint pain, swollen lymph nodes, and headaches. The characteristic rash of early Lyme disease is flat, circular with a "bull's eye" appearance with reddened outer margins and a pale central portion. A rash on the palms and feet are more commonly seen with secondary syphilis rather than tertiary syphilis; the manifestations of tertiary syphilis include aortic aneurysms, valve disease, CNS disorders, and infiltrative tumors of skin, bones, or liver. PID can present with fever, usually with prominent pelvic pain and rarely with sepsis, but has no associated rash.

> **Additional Reading:** Staphylococcal toxic shock syndrome. In: Domino F, ed. *The 5-Minute Clinical Consult.* Philadelphia, PA: Lippincott Williams and Wilkins; 2014.

> **Category:** Reproductive system

62. A 35-year-old woman presents to your office complaining of a copious white vaginal discharge. Microscopic examination shows evidence of pseudohyphae. The most appropriate treatment is
A) Penicillin G
B) Doxycycline
C) Terconazole (Terazol) vaginal cream
D) Metronidazole (Flagyl)
E) Topical acyclovir

Answer and Discussion

The answer is C. Yeast vaginitis (monilial vaginitis) is caused by *Candida albicans.* Predisposing factors include the recent use of wide-spectrum antibiotics, the use of oral contraceptives, pregnancy, menstruation, diabetes mellitus, constrictive undergarments, the use of immunosuppressive drugs (e.g., steroids), or immunodeficient states (e.g., AIDS). As part of their vaginal flora, 20% of women harbor *C. albicans* and are asymptomatic. Symptoms include intense vulvar irritation, pruritus, and vaginal discomfort. Erythema that affects the

Yeast: acidic pH

vulvar area, vaginal lining, and cervix is usually present. A copious, white, cottage cheese-like vaginal discharge also generally occurs. Diagnosis is made by microscopic examination of vaginal secretions following the application of potassium hydroxide to a glass slide. Characteristic budding yeast-like cells are noted with projections of pseudohyphae. Vaginal pH is less than 4.5. Treatment consists of local antifungal vaginal cream (miconazole [Monistat], terconazole, and others) applied nightly for 3 to 7 days; the newer oral antifungals usually produce satisfactory results. Incorrect diagnosis of yeast vaginitis and administration of antibiotics such as penicillin, doxycycline, and metronidazole can allow further overgrowth of yeast in the vagina and increase symptoms. Acylovir, given either topically or orally, is a usual treatment for symptomatic genital herpes simplex infections.

Additional Reading: Vaginitis: diagnosis and treatment. *Am Fam Physician*. 2011;83(7):807–815.

Category: Reproductive system

63. Which of the following is not true of oxytocin administration?
A) The drug must be given through a controlled infusion device.
B) Oxytocin must be administered as a continuous infusion or in "pulsed" doses.
C) The medication can have a diuretic effect with high doses.
D) Hyperstimulation can result from oxytocin administration.

Answer and Discussion

The answer is C. Oxytocin is mixed for use by placing 10 U in 1 L of isotonic intravenous solution to achieve a concentration of 10 mU/mL. Because severe hypotension can occur, especially during rapid intravenous administration, and because the drug is infused into the main intravenous line, a controlled infusion device must be used to determine its rate. It can be administered as a continuous infusion or in "pulsed" doses. Oxytocin's effect is noted within 3 to 5 minutes, and a steady state is achieved within 15 to 30 minutes. Studies show a wide range of effective dosages and change intervals, and no regimen has been shown to be clearly superior. Oxytocin has many advantages. The medication is potent and easy to titrate, has a short half-life (1 to 5 minutes), and is generally well tolerated. Dose-related adverse effects can occur. Because oxytocin is close to vasopressin in structure, it has an antidiuretic effect when given in high dosages (40 mU/min); thus, water intoxication is a possibility in prolonged inductions. Uterine hyperstimulation and uterine rupture can also occur. When the resting uterine tone remains >20 mm Hg, uteroplacental insufficiency and fetal hypoxia can result. This outcome emphasizes the importance of continuous fetal monitoring while administering oxytocin.

Additional Reading: Oxytocin augmentation during labor with epidural analgesia. *Am Fam Physician*. 2013;87(11):760–761.

Category: Reproductive system

64. Which of the following medications has been used with success in gestational diabetes?
A) Glipizide (Glucotrol)
B) Glyburide (Micronase, Diabeta)
C) Glimepiride (Amaryl)
D) Rosiglitazone (Avandia)
E) Repaglinide (Prandin)

Answer and Discussion

The answer is B. Gestational diabetes mellitus (GDM) is carbohydrate intolerance that occurs during pregnancy. Those affected are at risk of developing diabetes and related conditions later in life and face

a range of complications during pregnancy, including hypertension, preeclampsia, and cesarean delivery. Macrosomia is more common in infants exposed to GDM, as are the risks of operative delivery, shoulder dystocia, birth trauma, and obesity during childhood. Although the U.S. Preventive Services Task Force (USPSTF) concluded both in 2003 and 2008 that there was insufficient evidence to recommend universal screening for GDM, >90% of obstetric physicians report screening all patients. Screening based on risk factors such as obesity, family or personal history of diabetes, or previous adverse pregnancy outcome misses approximately one-half of mothers with GDM. The most commonly used test is the 50-g 1-hour glucose challenge. The accepted optimal limits vary, but at the recommended level of 130 mg/dL (7.2 mmol/L), the screening test has an estimated sensitivity of 79% and a specificity of 87%. The diagnostic test specific to pregnancy and with the most supporting data is the 100-g 3-hour oral glucose tolerance test, which is commonly given to women who have had an abnormal 1-hour glucose challenge test. Women with GDM are often treated initially with diets designed to achieve normal glycemic levels and avoid ketoacidosis. However, an acceptable diet has not been determined, and calorie restriction may increase the chance of ketosis. Several trials have demonstrated reduced fetal macrosomia if the mother is treated with insulin. Although insulin treatment is common in GDM, only 9% to 40% of treated mothers benefit. Treatment aims to achieve glucose levels of 120 mg/dL 2 hours postprandially and <90 mg/dL when fasting. Oral hypoglycemic agents, with the exception of glyburide, are contraindicated in pregnancy. In one study, glyburide provided outcomes comparable to those achieved with insulin in patients with GDM who had failed to achieve adequate glycemic control with diet alone. Clinical experience and the evidence published thus far also support the safety and efficacy of metformin use in pregnancy with respect to the immediate pregnancy outcomes. However, the long-term impact—positive or negative—of metformin use is still largely an unknown quantity, so this is not yet an agent routinely used in women with GDM who fail diet and need pharmacologic therapy. When glycemic control is satisfactory and no complications occur, mothers with GDM routinely do not require early or operative delivery. Nevertheless, the high incidence of macrosomia and other complications often results in cesarean or other operative delivery.

Additional Reading: Diagnosis and management of gestational diabetes mellitus. *Am Fam Physician*. 2009;80(1):57–62; and Metformin therapy during pregnancy: good for the goose and good for the gosling too? *Diabetes Care*. 2011;34(10):2329–2330.

Category: Endocrine system

Macrosomia is more common in infants exposed to GDM, as are the risks of operative delivery, shoulder dystocia, birth trauma, and obesity during childhood.

65. The diagnosis of endometriosis is generally made by
A) Detection of increased estrogen levels
B) Endometrial biopsy
C) Pelvic ultrasound
D) Laparoscopy
E) CT of the pelvis

Answer and Discussion

The answer is D. Endometriosis is the presence of endometrial tissue outside the uterus. Locations include the ovaries, fallopian tubes, uterosacral ligaments, peritoneal cul-de-sac, and uterovesical peritoneum.

Rare locations include the nasal mucosa and lungs. Theories for the development of endometriosis are abundant and include the migration of endometrial tissue through the fallopian tubes and into the peritoneal cavity or transformation of existing epithelium into endometrial-type tissue. Symptoms include dysmenorrhea, dyspareunia, infertility, dysuria, irregular vaginal bleeding, and pelvic pain. As many as 33% of affected individuals have no symptoms. Risk factors include nulliparity and a positive family history. Most patients have normal examination results; however, some have a tender retroverted uterus or adnexal masses that are tender with palpation. Diagnosis is usually accomplished with laparoscopy. Treatment involves the use of analgesics, progesterone, and oral contraceptives to regulate cycles for mild disease. More advanced disease can be treated with danazol (Danocrine), an anabolic steroid that has androgen activity. Side effects of danazol therapy include weight gain, fluid retention, fatigue, acne, chloasma, irregular vaginal bleeding, cholestatic jaundice with prolonged use, and hepatic dysfunction in patients who receive high doses. GnRH agonists are also used for treatment. Severe cases may require surgery.

Additional Reading: Evaluation and treatment of endometriosis. *Am Fam Physician.* 2013;87(2):107–113.

Category: Reproductive system

66. Symptoms that present the greatest concern in pregnant women include
A) Chronic vomiting
B) Nausea
C) Heartburn
D) Abnormal cravings
E) Mild edema

Answer and Discussion

The answer is A. Symptoms noted in early pregnancy that present concern to the physician include vaginal bleeding or fluid vaginal discharge, severe headaches, visual disturbances, chronic vomiting, fever or chills, dysuria, swelling of the face or hands, and pelvic pain. Abnormal cravings, nausea, mild lower extremity edema, and heartburn are common complaints of pregnancy.

Additional Reading: Hyperemesis gravidarum. *Williams Obstetrics,* 23rd ed. New York, NY: McGraw-Hill; 2010.

Category: Reproductive system

67. Which of the following statements about primary dysmenorrhea is true?
A) The condition usually worsens with the use of oral contraceptives.
B) It is thought to be associated with excessive prostaglandin activity.
C) The onset of symptoms typically begins after 30 years of age.
D) Endometriosis is a common cause.
E) The condition is related to adenomyosis.

Answer and Discussion

The answer is B. Primary dysmenorrhea is defined as menstrual-related pain that occurs during menstruation with the absence of pelvic pathology. The onset is usually before 20 years of age, and it affects women during the first day or two after the onset of menstruation. The cause is thought to be secondary to excessive prostaglandin activity, which leads to uterine contractions and ischemia, giving rise to pelvic discomfort. Other symptoms include headache, nausea, and occasionally vomiting, constipation, diarrhea, and urinary frequency. Premenstrual symptoms, including water retention, irritability, nervousness, and depression, may also persist during the early period of menstruation. Treatment

usually involves reassurance, nonsteroidal anti-inflammatory agents, and heating pads to the lower abdomen. A trial of oral contraceptives may be beneficial. In women who do not desire hormonal contraception, there is some evidence of benefit with the use of the Japanese herbal remedy toki-shakuyaku-san; thiamine, vitamin E, and fish oil supplements; a low-fat vegetarian diet; and acupressure.

In secondary dysmenorrhea, patients report the same symptoms as those of primary dysmenorrhea, except that there is evidence of pelvic pathology (i.e., endometriosis, fibroids, chronic PID, IUD use, cervical stenosis, or adenomyosis). The age of onset is usually older than 20 years, and the course can be progressive. The treatment is correction of the underlying cause.

Additional Reading: Dysmenorrhea. *Am Fam Physician.* 2005;71:285–292.

Category: Reproductive system

68. A 33-year-old woman who delivered last week presents to your office with questions about her gestational diabetes that developed during the first trimester. You explain
A) Her risk of developing type 2 diabetes in the future is no different from anyone else.
B) She should be screened for diabetes with either fasting blood glucose measurements or a 2-hour glucose tolerance test 6 weeks postpartum and yearly thereafter.
C) No further monitoring is necessary unless she develops symptoms of diabetes.
D) She should be tested for diabetes 6 months after delivery via fasting blood glucose measurements on two occasions or a 2-hour oral 75-g glucose tolerance test.

Answer and Discussion

The answer is B. Women with gestational diabetes are at sevenfold higher risk for developing type 2 diabetes in the future and should be tested for diabetes 6 weeks after delivery via fasting blood glucose measurements on two occasions or a 2-hour oral 75-g glucose tolerance test. Normal values for a 2-hour glucose tolerance test are less than 140 mg/dL. Values between 140 and 200 mg/dL (11.1 mmol/L) represent impaired glucose tolerance, and greater than 200 mg/dL are diagnostic of diabetes. Screening for diabetes should be repeated annually thereafter, especially in patients who had elevated fasting blood glucose levels during pregnancy.

Additional Reading: Gestational diabetes after delivery: short-term management and long-term risks. *Diabetes Care.* 2007;30(suppl 2):S225–S235.

Category: Endocrine system

69. Which of the following medications is contraindicated for the management of hypertension in pregnancy?
A) Methyldopa
B) Hydralazine
C) Labetalol
D) Nifedipine XL
E) Losartan

Answer and Discussion

The answer is E. Most hypertensive women of childbearing age have stage I or II hypertension (systolic blood pressure of 140 to 179 mm Hg or diastolic blood pressure of 90 to 109 mm Hg) without target organ damage. Therefore, the risk for acute cardiovascular consequences during pregnancy is very low. Improved maternal or neonatal outcomes with antihypertensive therapy have not been documented in this group. Accordingly, the Working Group advises that antihypertensive medication might be safely withheld in such patients, provided that blood pressure remains less than 150 to 160 mm Hg systolic and 100 to 110 diastolic while the patient is off medications. Continuing previous antihypertensive medication is another option, although angiotensin-converting enzyme (ACE) inhibitors and angiotensin-receptor blockers should not be used during pregnancy. Because methyldopa (Aldomet) has the longest track record of safety in pregnancy, it is preferred by many clinicians. Hydralazine, nifedipene, and labetalol are also used.

> **Additional Reading:** Update on the use of antihypertensive drugs in pregnancy. *Hypertension.* 2008;51:960–969.

Category: Cardiovascular system

70. Which of the following is most commonly associated with nongonococcal urethritis?
A) Herpes simplex
B) Ureaplasma
C) Chlamydia
D) Trichomonas
E) Syphilis

Answer and Discussion

The answer is C. Nongonococcal urethritis is diagnosed when exam or microscopy findings indicate inflammation without the presence of the gram-negative intracellular diplococci (GNID) that cause gonorrhea. This is commonly caused by chlamydia infections (approximately 15% to 40% of cases). Chlamydia is currently the most common STD in the United States. Other causes include *Trichomonas vaginalis*, HSV, *Mycoplasma genitalium*, and *Adenovirus*. Symptoms include clear vaginal or penile discharge, dysuria, pruritus, and occasionally meatal erythema. Women are often completely asymptomatic. Symptoms, when they are present, include vaginal discharge, dysuria, frequency, pelvic pain, and dyspareunia. The incubation period is between 7 and 28 days. Diagnosis of chlamydia infections has historically been difficult because it is an obligate intracellular parasite; however, advances in testing technology have made nucleic acid hybridization tests as well as nucleic acid amplification tests (NAATs) widely available. NAATs are currently the preferred method for diagnosing chlamydia infection due to their higher sensitivity, ability to be used for to detect chlamydia in urine samples, and ease of testing concurrently for chlamydia and gonorrhea from the same sample. Rapid and accurate diagnosis is essential due to need for partner notification and referral to treatment. Chlamydia can result in PID and infertility in women, and complications for men include epididymitis and Reiter's syndrome. Chlamydia is adequately treated either with single-dose azithromycin 1 g or doxycycline 100 mg bid × 7 days. Single-dose azithromycin, especially with witnessed dosing in medical clinics, is associated with a high treatment success rates.

> **Additional Reading:** Diseases characterized by urethritis and cervicitis. *CDC Sexually Transmitted Disease Treatment Guidelines*; 2011.

Category: Reproductive system

71. Dysfunctional uterine bleeding is most common
A) During pregnancy
B) After sexual intercourse
C) At the time of menopause
D) With the development of PID
E) In premenarchal girls

Answer and Discussion

The answer is C. Dysfunctional uterine bleeding is defined as abnormal uterine bleeding in the absence of inflammation, pregnancy, or tumors. The condition is most commonly associated with anovulation. It usually occurs just after menarche or around the time of menopause. Treatment depends on the age of the patient, the desire for fertility and contraception, and the duration and severity of bleeding. If the patient is young and healthy and the bleeding is not profuse, she can be treated medically with high-dose oral estrogens every 6 hours, which usually stops the bleeding within the first 24 hours. After the cessation of bleeding, the patient should continue with daily estrogen for the rest of the month, followed by the administration of progesterone during the final 10 days of the month. After the addition of the progesterone, withdrawal bleeding should occur within a few days, and the patient can then begin OCPs to regulate her menstrual cycles. If bleeding continues, further evaluation with an endometrial biopsy or dilation and curettage may be necessary. Older women in the perimenopausal state may initially need endometrial biopsy and possible dilation and curettage to rule out endometrial hyperplasia or endometrial cancer.

> **Additional Reading:** Evaluation and management of abnormal uterine bleeding in premenopausal women. *Am Fam Physician.* 2012;85(1):35–43.

Category: Reproductive system

72. Which of the following statements about exercise-induced amenorrhea is true?
A) The condition is rarely reversible with weight gain.
B) It usually affects women who weigh >115 lb or those who have gained >10% to 15% in muscle mass.
C) Osteoporosis can be associated.
D) It is usually associated with prolactinomas.
E) Hormone therapy is contraindicated in those affected.

Answer and Discussion

The answer is C. Exercise-induced amenorrhea is a condition that is noted in competitive female athletes. The cause appears to be associated with the athlete's weight and weight loss. Menstrual irregularities or amenorrhea are most likely to develop in women who weigh <115 lb or those who have lost >10 lb (10% to 15% of normal weight) while training. The basis of amenorrhea is unknown but may be associated with hypothalamic dysfunction. In most cases, weight gain reverses the condition; however, many women are unwilling to gain the additional weight. The female athlete triad is defined as the combination of disordered eating, amenorrhea, and osteoporosis. This disorder often goes unrecognized. The consequences of lost bone mineral density (BMD) can be devastating for the female athlete. Premature osteoporotic fractures can occur, and lost BMD may never be regained. Athletes with prolonged oligomenorrhea or amenorrhea lasting for at least 6 months should undergo bone density evaluation with a dual-energy x-ray absorptiometry (DEXA) scan. DEXA screening should also be performed on female athletes who have normal menstrual cycles but have experienced two or more stress fractures. Early recognition of the female athlete triad can be accomplished by the family physician through risk factor assessment and screening questions. Instituting an appropriate diet and moderating the frequency of exercise may result in the natural return of menses. Hormone therapy should be considered early to prevent the loss of bone density.

Additional Reading: Health-related concerns of the female athlete: a lifespan approach. *Am Fam Physician.* 2009;79(6):489–495.

Category: Nonspecific system

73. Painless and profuse vaginal bleeding in the third trimester is most likely
A) Placenta acreda
B) Placenta previa
C) Vaso previa
D) Bloody show
E) Cervical ripening

Answer and Discussion

The answer is B. Painless hemorrhage is the hallmark sign of placenta previa. Although spotting may occur during the first and second trimesters of pregnancy, the first episode of hemorrhage usually begins at some point after the 28th week and is characteristically described as being sudden, painless, and profuse. With the onset, clothing or bedding is saturated by an impressive amount of bright red, clotted blood, but the blood loss usually is not extensive, seldom produces shock, and is almost never fatal. In about 10% of cases, there is some initial pain because of coexisting placental abruption, and spontaneous labor may be expected over the next few days in 25% of patients. In rare cases, bleeding is less dramatic or does not begin until after spontaneous rupture of the membranes or the onset of labor. Occasionally, nulliparous patients can reach term without bleeding, possibly because the placenta has been protected by an intact cervix.

Additional Reading: Placenta previa. *Williams Obstetrics,* 23rd ed. New York, NY: McGraw-Hill; 2010.

Category: Reproductive system

74. The normal amount of blood loss for a vaginal delivery is
A) 250 mL
B) 500 mL
C) 1,000 mL
D) 1,500 mL
E) 2,000 mL

Answer and Discussion

The answer is B. The normal pregnant patient typically loses 500 mL of blood at the time of vaginal delivery and 1,000 mL during a cesarean delivery. Appreciably more blood can be lost without clinical evidence of a volume deficit as a result of the 40% expansion in blood volume that occurs by the 30th week of pregnancy.

Additional Reading: Postpartum hemorrhage. *Williams Obstetrics,* 23rd ed. New York, NY: McGraw-Hill; 2010.

Category: Reproductive system

75. Which of the following statements about epidural anesthesia is true?
A) It provides anesthesia only for lumbar and sacral nerve roots.
B) It should only be used for multigravida women.
C) It can be used in hemophiliacs.
D) It can be associated with hypotension.
E) Placement of the catheter should be at the L2–L3 level.

Answer and Discussion

The answer is D. Epidural anesthesia is used as a regional block during childbirth. The procedure is performed by inserting a needle in the L3–L4 interspace and threading a catheter into the epidural space. The catheter is then aspirated to check for the presence of cerebrospinal fluid. If this occurs, the catheter must be repositioned. A test dose is then administered to reconfirm position. When position is confirmed, a full dose of anesthetic is administered through the catheter. Analgesia is usually established with fentanyl plus a small dose of bupivacaine. Fentanyl works better for the visceral pain that is associated with labor, whereas bupivacaine is more effective for somatic pain. The dose may need to be repeated to maintain anesthesia during delivery. In most cases, a full dose provides anesthesia of nerve roots T10–S5. Risks that are involved with epidural anesthesia include drug reaction, hypotension, and rare neurologic complications. If the dura is penetrated, a spinal headache eventually develops in many patients. Contraindications to epidural anesthesia include adverse effects to anesthesia, bleeding tendency, infection of the lumbar area, or underlying neurologic defects. Some studies have reported that epidural anesthesia may prolong labor, leading to an increased cesarean delivery rate.

Additional Reading: Hawkins JL. Epidural anesthesia for labor and delivery. *NEJM.* 2010;362:1503–1510.

Category: Reproductive system

76. Which of the following statements regarding anencephaly is true?
A) Intracerebral shunts can be used effectively in preventing CNS complications.
B) The condition should be suspected with elevations in α-fetoprotein levels.
C) Children who are affected may need additional tutoring during school.
D) Nicotinic acid may help prevent anencephaly when given antepartum.
E) Urinary tract infections are common in those affected.

Answer and Discussion

The answer is B. The condition of anencephaly occurs when the cerebral hemispheres are absent. In some cases, there may be some cystic neural remnants. In many instances, the spinal cord and brainstem are affected. Diagnosis is suspected with elevated α-fetoprotein levels obtained at 16 to 18 weeks' gestation and confirmed with ultrasound examination. Unfortunately, the condition is incompatible with life, and these infants are usually stillborn or die within a few hours or days after birth. The use of prenatal vitamins that contain at least 0.4 mg folic acid can help prevent neural tube defects such as anencephaly.

Additional Reading: Acrania/Anencephaly. *Williams Obstetrics,* 23rd ed. New York, NY: McGraw-Hill; 2010.

Category: Reproductive system

77. Which of the following medications is *not* used in the treatment of preterm labor?
A) Ritodrine
B) Magnesium sulfate
C) Terbutaline
D) Propanolol
E) Nifedipene

Answer and Discussion

The answer is D. *Tocolysis* is the process of stopping preterm labor contractions with medication. Medications that are used for tocolysis include β-sympathomimetics, magnesium sulfate, prostaglandin synthetase inhibitors (indomethacin), and calcium-channel blockers *(handwritten top margin: inl preg.: varied (↓/↑) AFP levels)*

(nifedipine). Of these, ritodrine (Yutopar), a β-sympathomimetic, although still used, is not used as frequently for labor tocolysis, and terbutaline is now often utilized because of its ease of administration. Tocolysis is usually not successful if the cervix has dilated to >4 cm and should be reserved for pregnancies between viability and 34 weeks' gestation. Contraindications to tocolysis include fetal distress, fetal anomalies, significant risk to the mother, abruptio placentae, or placenta previa with heavy bleeding.

Additional Reading: Preterm labor. *Am Fam Physician.* 2010; 81(4):477–484.

Category: Reproductive system

78. Which of the following is *not* considered as part of the Amsel criteria for diagnosing bacterial vaginosis (BV)?
A) Milky, homogeneous, adherent discharge
B) Vaginal pH greater than 4.5
C) Positive whiff test
D) Presence of clue cells on light microscopy
E) Vaginal itching

Answer and Discussion
The answer is E. The Amsel criteria are considered to be the standard diagnostic approach to BV and continue to be used for the diagnosis. The criteria include the following: milky, homogeneous, adherent discharge; vaginal pH ≥4.5; positive whiff test (the discharge typically has a fishy smell); and presence of clue cells in the vaginal fluid on light microscopy. If three of the four criteria are met, there is a 90% likelihood of BV.

Additional Reading: Vaginitis: diagnosis and treatment. *Am Fam Physician.* 2011;83(7):807–815.

Category: Reproductive system

79. Which of the following screening tests has been shown to reduce breast cancer-related mortality in average-risk women?
A) Mammogram
B) Mammogram with clinical breast exam
C) Breast self-examination
D) MRI
E) Screening for BRCA mutation

Answer and Discussion
The answer is A. Breast cancer is the most common nonskin cancer and the second leading cause of cancer death in North American women. Mammography is the only screening test shown to reduce breast cancer–related mortality. There is general agreement that screening should be offered at least biennially to women 50 to 74 years of age. For women 40 to 49 years of age, the risks and benefits of screening should be discussed, and the decision to perform screening should take into consideration the individual patient risk, values, and comfort level of the patient and physician. Information is lacking about the effectiveness of screening in women 75 years and older. The decision to screen women in this age group should be individualized, keeping the patient's life expectancy, functional status, and goals of care in mind. For women with an estimated lifetime breast cancer risk of more than 20% or who have a BRCA mutation, screening should begin at 25 years of age or at the age that is 5 to 10 years younger than the earliest age that breast cancer was diagnosed in the family. Screening with MRI may be considered in high-risk women, but its impact on breast cancer

mortality is uncertain. Clinical breast examination plus mammography seems to be no more effective than mammography alone at reducing breast cancer mortality. Teaching breast self-examination does not improve mortality and is not recommended; however, women should be aware of any changes in their breasts and report them promptly.

Additional Reading: Breast cancer screening update. *Am Fam Physician.* 2013;87(4):274–278.

Category: Integumentary

80. Which of the following statements about neural tube defects is true?
A) Laboratory testing is not useful in the diagnosis of neural tube defects.
B) Elevated α-fetoprotein levels should be further evaluated by obstetric ultrasound.
C) Nicotinic acid has been shown to help prevent neural tube defects.
D) α-Fetoprotein testing should be done at 24 to 28 weeks' gestation.
E) Elevated α-fetoprotein levels are not associated with normal pregnancies.

(handwritten: αFP (AFP))

Answer and Discussion
The answer is B. Neural tube defects (e.g., spina bifida, meningomyelocele, anencephaly) can be screened for by performing a serum α-fetoprotein blood test, which is done at 16 to 18 weeks' gestation. Evaluation is based on maternal weight and length of gestation. The accuracy of the test approaches 95%. Causes for elevations of maternal α-fetoprotein include inaccurate gestation dates, multiple gestations, abdominal wall defects in the fetus, congenital nephrotic syndrome, fetal demise, and neural tube defects. In addition, normal pregnancies may be associated with elevations in α-fetoprotein levels. Low levels of α-fetoprotein are associated with inaccurate gestation dates, chromosome trisomy such as Down's syndrome, molar pregnancy, and fetal demise. In addition, normal pregnancies may exhibit low α-fetoprotein levels. In most cases, an obstetric ultrasound should be performed if the α-fetoprotein level is abnormal. Recent studies have shown that the administration of folic acid before pregnancy may help to prevent neural tube defects. The current recommendations are that women who plan to conceive should consume at least 0.4 mg folate/day (which is usually contained in a prenatal vitamin). Preconception counseling should include a discussion of folic acid supplementation.

Additional Reading: Folic acid for the prevention of neural tube defects: recommendation statement. *Am Fam Physician.* 2010;82(12):1526–1527.

Category: Neurologic

81. A 28-year-old woman with a recent new sexual partner presents with pelvic pain, fever, vaginal discharge, and nausea with vomiting. Examination shows a significant cervical motion tenderness. The most likely diagnosis is
A) Ectopic pregnancy
B) Pyelonephritis
C) PID
D) BV
E) Yeast vaginitis

Answer and Discussion

The answer is C. PID is a condition that includes infection of the fallopian tubes, cervix, endometrium, or ovaries. It is usually seen in women younger than 30 years of age who are sexually active. The use of condoms lowers the risk of PID. The use of IUDs and multiple sex partners increases the risk.

Causative agents include chlamydia, gonorrhea, and multiple organisms found in normal vaginal flora. Many cases involve polymicrobial infections. Acute symptoms include pelvic pain, fever, vaginal discharge, dyspareunia, nausea, and vomiting, though some cases of PID present with more mild or subtle symptoms. Physical examination reveals adnexal, uterine, and cervical motion tenderness (positive Chandelier sign). Laboratory findings include elevations of white blood counts, elevated erythrocyte sedimentation rate, and elevated C-reactive protein. Increased white blood cells on microscopy of cervical secretions as well as positive testing for chlamydia and/or gonorrhea in the lower genital tract is often present, though negative gonorrhea or chlamydia testing does not rule out PID. The differential diagnosis includes appendicitis, ectopic pregnancy, urinary tract infection, and peritonitis from other causes. Complications of PID include chronic PID, infertility, and ectopic pregnancy. Parenteral treatment for a patient who is unable to tolerate oral medications consists of cefotetan or cefoxitin plus doxycycline. Outpatient therapy with oral antibiotics can be used in the majority of patients with PID and includes a single dose of ceftriaxone 250 mg IM and oral doxycycline 100 mg bid for 14 days with or without metronidazole 500 mg bid for 14 days. Follow-up care must be available within 72 hours to evaluate the response to treatment.

Additional Reading: Pelvic inflammatory disease. CDC Sexually Transmitted Disease Treatment Guidelines; 2010.

Category: Reproductive system

82. A 27-year-old asymptomatic pregnant woman at 8 weeks gestational age is found to have hyperthyroidism. Which of the following medications is the drug of choice for treatment in the first trimester?
A) Propylthiouracil (PTU)
B) Radioactive iodine
C) Methimazole
D) Propranolol
E) Levothyroxine

Answer and Discussion

The answer is A. Hyperthyroidism during pregnancy is usually associated with Graves' disease. Other causes include toxic nodular goiter, choriocarcinoma, hydatidiform mole, ovarian teratoma, and iatrogenic thyrotoxicosis. Symptoms may include weight loss, tachycardia, exophthalmos, pretibial myxedema, generalized weakness, and tremor. Laboratory findings include an elevated triiodothyronine, thyroxine, and low-sensitive thyroid-stimulating hormone (TSH). Treatment depends on the situation. Antithyroid medications readily cross the placenta and inhibit fetal thyroid function. PTU and methimazole cross the placenta but are used in the treatment of hyperthyroidism during pregnancy. Due to reports of possible teratogenic effects of methimazole, PTU is the drug of choice in the first trimester. Some experts are now recommended a change to methimazole from PTU at the beginning of the second trimester, due to an association of PTU with liver failure. Beta blockers can be used to control tremor and tachycardia but should be limited to 2-to-6-week duration if possible to minimize impact on fetal growth. Radioactive iodine ablation of the thyroid is contraindicated during pregnancy. Close monitoring of thyroid hormones is required when administering antithyroid medications during pregnancy. Side effects of the medications include rash, urticaria, arthralgias, and agranulocytosis, which may predispose to maternal infection. Surgery is reserved for severe refractive cases. Untreated hyperthyroidism during pregnancy can lead to premature delivery, neonatal thyrotoxicosis, and spontaneous abortion.

Additional Reading: Hyperthyroidism during pregnancy: treatment. In: Basow DS, ed. *UpToDate*. Waltham, MA: UpToDate; 2013.

Category: Endocrine system

83. Which of the following is a characteristic of atrophic vaginitis?
A) Vaginal pH of 5 to 7
B) Milky discharge
C) Increased vaginal rugae
D) Endometrial cells noted on wet-mount microscopic examination
E) Increased glycogen levels

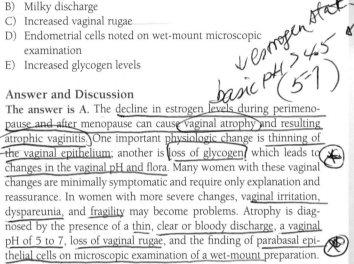

↓ estrogen state
↓ acidic pH > 4.5
basic PH (5-7)

Answer and Discussion

The answer is A. The decline in estrogen levels during perimenopause and after menopause can cause vaginal atrophy and resulting atrophic vaginitis. One important physiologic change is thinning of the vaginal epithelium; another is loss of glycogen, which leads to changes in the vaginal pH and flora. Many women with these vaginal changes are minimally symptomatic and require only explanation and reassurance. In women with more severe changes, vaginal irritation, dyspareunia, and fragility may become problems. Atrophy is diagnosed by the presence of a thin, clear or bloody discharge, a vaginal pH of 5 to 7, loss of vaginal rugae, and the finding of parabasal epithelial cells on microscopic examination of a wet-mount preparation.

Additional Reading: Clinical manifestations and diagnosis of vaginal atrophy. In: Basow DS, ed. *UpToDate*. Waltham, MA: UpToDate; 2013.

Category: Reproductive system

84. A 45-year-old woman is noted to have four yeast infections in 1 year. Appropriate management of this patient should be
A) Continued observation and treatment only if symptomatic
B) Further evaluation for hypothyroidism
C) Blood test to look for the presence of diabetes and HIV infection
D) Prophylactic therapy with weekly metronidazole
E) Examination for endometrial structural abnormalities

Answer and Discussion

The answer is C. Recurrent vulvovaginal candidiasis is defined as four or more yeast infections in 1 year. The possibility of uncontrolled diabetes mellitus or immunodeficiency should be considered in women with recurrent vulvovaginal candidiasis. When it has been determined that no reversible causes are present (e.g., antibiotic therapy, uncontrolled diabetes, OCP use) and initial therapy has been completed, maintenance therapy may be appropriate. Selected long-term regimens include the use of clotrimazole and fluconazole. The role of boric acid and lactobacillus therapy remains in question.

Additional Reading: Treatment of recurrent vulvovaginal candidiasis. *Am Fam Physician.* 2011;83(12):1482–1484.

Category: Reproductive system

> The possibility of uncontrolled diabetes mellitus or immunodeficiency should be considered in women with recurrent vulvovaginal candidiasis.

85. Which of the following statements about dysfunctional uterine bleeding is true?
A) The condition is most common during the middle of a woman's reproductive years.
B) It typically occurs during pregnancy.
C) Most cases are seen with anovulatory cycles.
D) Gynecologic malignancies are related to dysfunctional uterine bleeding.
E) Inflammation is a commonly associated condition.

Answer and Discussion
The answer is C. Dysfunctional uterine bleeding is defined as abnormal uterine bleeding in the absence of inflammation, pregnancy, or tumors. It is the most common form of abnormal uterine bleeding and is seen most commonly at the extremes of the reproductive cycle (menarche and menopause). Most cases are seen with anovulatory cycles. Causes include exogenous estrogen use, PCOS, hyperthyroidism, and hypothyroidism.

Additional Reading: Terminology and evaluation of abnormal uterine bleeding in premenopausal women. In: Basow DS, ed. *UpToDate.* Waltham, MA: UpToDate; 2013.

Category: Reproductive system

86. An 18-year-old woman presents to your office complaining of pelvic pain, dysuria, and a purulent yellowish-green vaginal discharge. A Gram's stain of cervical secretions shows gram-negative diplococci. The most appropriate medication is
A) Ceftriaxone + azithromycin
B) Penicillin G + azithromycin
C) Cefuroxime + tetracycline
D) Cefoxitin + doxycycline
E) Metronidazole + doxycycline

Answer and Discussion
The answer is A. Gonorrhea is caused by a gram-negative diplococcus, *Neisseria gonorrhoeae*. Symptoms include purulent, yellowish-green vaginal, rectal, or penile discharge; urethritis; and genital irritation and discomfort. Other symptoms include scrotal pain, abdominal or pelvic pain, and pharyngeal discomfort. Some patients, especially women, are completely asymptomatic. Disseminated gonococcal infection can give rise to polyarthralgias, tenosynovitis, and a hemorrhagic papular or pustular skin rash that affects the genitalia, hands, feet, and other areas of the body. The disease is spread by sexual contact. Incubation is 2 to 14 days for men and 7 to 21 days for women. Diagnosis is accomplished with Gram's stains that show leukocytes with intracellular gram-negative diplococci and more accurately with cultures made on Thayer–Martin chocolate agar media. Urogenital *N. gonorrhoeae* infections can also be diagnosed nonculture (e.g., the NAAT) techniques that can simultaneously test for chlamydia infection. For patients with uncomplicated genital, rectal, and pharyngeal gonorrhea, CDC now recommends combination therapy with ceftriaxone 250 mg as a single intramuscular dose, plus either azithromycin 1 g orally in a single dose *or* doxycycline 100 mg orally twice daily for 7 days. There are times, however, when it may be necessary to use an alternative antibiotic regimen that does not

include ceftriaxone. In instances where ceftriaxone is not available, CDC recommends cefixime 400 mg orally, plus either azithromycin 1 g orally *or* doxycycline 100 mg orally twice daily for 7 days. For patients with a severe allergy to cephalosporins, CDC recommends a single 2-g dose of azithromycin orally. In both of these circumstances, CDC recommends a test of cure for these patients 1 week after treatment and partners should also be located and treated.

Other STDs (e.g., syphilis, HIV, hepatitis) may also coexist and need appropriate diagnosis and treatment, though chlamydia infection will be adequately covered by these suggested regimens.

Additional Reading: Update to *CDC's Sexually Transmitted Diseases Treatment Guidelines*, 2010: oral cephalosporins no longer a recommended treatment for gonococcal infections. *MMWR.* 2012;61(31):590–594.

Category: Reproductive system

87. The maximum acceptable cumulative dose of ionizing radiation during pregnancy is
A) 100 rads
B) 50 rads
C) 10 rads
D) 5 rads
E) 1 rad

Answer and Discussion
The answer is D. The accepted cumulative dose of ionizing radiation during pregnancy is 5 rads, and no single diagnostic study exceeds this maximum. In utero exposure to ionizing radiation can be teratogenic, carcinogenic, or mutagenic. The effects are directly related to the level of exposure and stage of fetal development. The fetus is most susceptible to radiation during organogenesis (2 to 7 weeks after conception) and in the early fetal period (8 to 15 weeks after conception). Nonurgent radiologic testing should be avoided during this time. Noncancer health effects have not been detected at any stage of gestation after exposure to ionizing radiation of less than 5 rad. The risk of childhood cancer (e.g., leukemia) is increased regardless of the dose. Pregnant women should be counseled that radiation exposure from a single diagnostic imaging procedure does not increase the risk of fetal anomalies or pregnancy loss. Spontaneous abortion, growth restriction, and mental retardation may occur at higher exposure levels. Appropriate counseling of patients before radiologic studies are performed is critical. Physicians should carefully weigh the risks and benefits of any radiographic study and include the mother in the decision-making process whenever possible. In utero exposure to nonionizing radiation is not associated with significant risks; therefore, ultrasonography is safe to perform during pregnancy.

Additional Reading: Health effects of prenatal radiation exposure. *Am Fam Physician.* 2010;82(5):488–493.

Category: Reproductive system

88. You perform a Pap smear on a premenopausal 48-year-old woman and the results reveal the presence of benign appearing endometrial cells. She reports normal monthly menses with no menorrhagia, intermenstrual vaginal bleeding, or any other associated symptoms. Appropriate management consists of
A) Endometrial biopsy
B) Ultrasound examination of the uterus
C) Dilation and curettage
D) Colposcopy
E) No further evaluation

Answer and Discussion

The answer is E. The presence of endometrial cells on a Pap smear are reported for all women above age 40. If a woman is still menstruating, the presence of benign endometrial cells are rarely associated with any significant underlying pathology, and such women do not need additional evaluation. Current evidence supports further evaluation in a postmenopausal woman above age 40 with benign endometrial cells on a Pap test. This evaluation may occur with transvaginal ultrasound, office endometrial biopsy, or both. Hormone-replacement therapy (HRT) may increase the rate of benign endometrial shedding, but postmenopausal women on hormone-replacement therapy still require evaluation for this finding. The presence of atypical endometrial cells on a Pap require additional evaluation, regardless of age or menopausal status of the woman.

Additional Reading: Endometrial cells in cervical cytology: review of cytological features and clinical assessment. American Society for Colposcopy and Cervical Pathology. *J Low Genit Tract Dis.* 2006;10(2):111–122.

Category: Reproductive system

89. A 56-year-old woman presents for her well-woman exam. She has been seen yearly for the last 10 years with normal cytology on her routine annual Pap smears and is otherwise healthy. She has not had any STDs and is in a monogamous relationship with her husband of 30 years. She has never had testing for the presence of high-risk human papillomavirus (HPV) infection. She inquires about her Pap smear. An appropriate response is

A) A yearly Pap smear is necessary in her age group because of the risk of cervical cancer.
B) Pap smears are no longer required for women in her age group.
C) An appropriate interval for repeat Pap smear screening with HPV testing alone is 5 years.
D) An appropriate interval for Pap smear screening with cytology alone is 3 years.
E) She would need a repeat Pap smear only if she had another sexual partner.

Answer and Discussion

The answer is D. In March 2012 the American Cancer Society (ACS), the American Society for Colposcopy and Cervical Pathology (ASCCP), the American Society for Clinical Pathology (ASC), and the U.S. Preventive Services Task Force updated existing recommendations on cervical cancer screening. The recommendations are categorized by the age of the patient and are as follows: (1) Adolescents should not have any screening and cervical cancer prevention efforts should be focused on universal HPV vaccination; (2) Women ages 21 to 29 years should be screened every 3 years with Pap cytology alone. Routine co-testing for oncogenic (high-risk) HPV is not recommended; and (3) Women ages 30 to 65 years should have cytology screening every 3 years or cytology plus high-risk HPV testing every 5 years. Women above age 65 and those who have undergone removal of the cervix with hysterectomy and have no history of CIN II or greater or cervical cancer do not need Pap screening.

Additional Reading: New cervical cancer screening guidelines recommend less frequent assessment. *OBG Management.* 2012;24(4):1–5; and ACS, ASCCP, ASC screening guidelines for the prevention and early detection of cervical cancer. American Society for Colposcopy and Cervical Pathology. *J Low Genit Tract Dis.* 2012;16(3):1–29.

Category: Reproductive system

90. Live virus vaccines, such as measles, mumps, and rubella, should be administered to pregnant women
A) At the first prenatal visit following conception
B) At least 3 months before conception
C) During the second trimester
D) During the third trimester
E) At 18 to 20 weeks' gestation

Answer and Discussion

The answer is B. Immunizations with live attenuated vaccines, such as measles, mumps, rubella, varicella, and the oral vaccine for polio, are contraindicated in pregnancy and 3 months before conception. Immunizations with inactivated virus, such as influenza, *Pneumococcus*, tetanus, pertussis, rabies, and the injectable poliovirus, as well as the hepatitis B recombinant vaccine, are safe to administer.

Additional Reading: Guidelines for vaccinating pregnant women. From: http://www.cdc.gov/vaccines/pubs/preg-guide.htm

Category: Patient/population-based care

91. Women immunized for rubella should be counseled to avoid pregnancy for
A) 1 month
B) 3 months
C) 6 months
D) 1 year
E) Rubella immunization presents no dangers before or during pregnancy.

Answer and Discussion

The answer is B. Rubella ("German measles") is a highly contagious childhood disease that can affect pregnant mothers. As many as 15% of mothers do not have antibodies to the rubella virus. Symptoms include fever, cough, and conjunctivitis. Other symptoms include headaches, malaise, myalgias, arthralgias, and postauricular and suboccipital lymphadenopathy. An erythematous morbilliform rash usually develops on the face and spreads inferiorly. Generally, the symptoms of rubella are less severe than those of rubeola, and there is usually no prodrome seen with rubella (unlike with rubeola). Spontaneous abortion occurs two to four times more frequently in pregnancies that are complicated by rubella. Transmission to the fetus occurs by direct infection. If the woman is affected during the first trimester, the risk of birth defects is higher than if she is affected during the last two trimesters. Effects of the virus on the fetus (congenital rubella syndrome) include cataracts, glaucoma, blindness, cardiac abnormalities, deafness, mental retardation, cerebral palsy, growth retardation, hemolytic anemia, and cleft palate. In cases of maternal rubella, therapeutic abortion can be considered if infection occurs in the first two trimesters. All women should receive routine rubella testing during pregnancy. If negative, the patient should be vaccinated during the immediate postpartum period. Women who are immunized with the live attenuated virus should not become pregnant for 3 months following immunization. The use of immune globulin for pregnant women who are exposed to rubella is not recommended.

Additional Reading: Guidelines for vaccinating pregnant women. From: http://www.cdc.gov/vaccines/pubs/preg-guide.htm

Category: Patient/population-based care

92. An 18-year-old woman presents to your office complaining of irregular periods. On examination, she is found to be obese, has evidence of excessive facial hair, and reports that her mother had similar problems. Laboratory studies show normal estrogen levels, increased LH, low FSH, elevated testosterone level, and elevated urinary 17-ketosteroids. The most likely diagnosis is
A) Pregnancy
B) Cushing's disease
C) PCOS
D) Adrenal adenoma
E) Acromegaly

Answer and Discussion

The answer is C. PCOS (Stein–Leventhal syndrome) is an inherited condition characterized by cystic ovaries, hirsutism, amenorrhea, and obesity. It is the most common cause of anovulation and hirsutism. Some patients present with primary amenorrhea, some have abnormal irregular periods, and some have normal periods. Laboratory studies show normal or increased levels of estrogen, increased LH, normal or decreased FSH, normal or increased testosterone, and increased urinary 17-ketosteroids. Pelvic ultrasound can also aid in the diagnosis by demonstrating bilateral enlargement of the ovaries. Administration of progesterone usually results in withdrawal bleeding for patients with amenorrhea. Glucose intolerance with increased insulin levels may also be present. Therapy includes the use of oral contraceptives to suppress hirsutism and small doses of glucocorticoid (dexamethasone) at bedtime to suppress the adrenal gland. Bromocriptine has shown some benefit for the menstrual irregularities and hirsutism. Antiandrogens can be combined with OCPs for the treatment of hirsutism. If used alone, antiandrogens may produce irregular uterine bleeding. The most commonly used antiandrogens are spironolactone (Aldactone), flutamide (Eulexin), and cyproterone (Cyprostat). These agents should not be used in pregnant women. Spironolactone, in a dosage of 25 to 100 mg administered twice a day, is the most commonly used antiandrogen because of its safety, availability, and low cost. Flutamide is usually given in a dosage of 250 mg twice a day, and cyproterone is given in a dosage of 25 to 50 mg/day for 10 days each month.

GnRH analogs such as leuprolide (Lupron) should be reserved for use in women who do not respond to combination hormonal therapy or cannot tolerate OCPs. The GnRH analogs should be used cautiously, with particular attention given to long-term consequences (e.g., hot flushes, bone demineralization, atrophic vaginitis) that can occur secondary to hypoestrogenemia induced by these agents. Surgery (wedge resection of the ovary) has also been shown to restore ovulatory periods and fertility.

Cushing's disease is condition that is caused by excess corticosteroids, especially cortisol, usually from adrenal or pituitary hyperfunction and is characterized by obesity, hypertension, muscular weakness, and easy bruising. Many adrenal adenomas do not produce any symptoms of hormonal excess; however, when "active" or "functioning" they can lead to Cushing's disease or primary aldosteronism. Acromegaly is abnormal growth of the hands, feet, and face, caused by overproduction of growth hormone by the pituitary gland.

Additional Reading: Polycystic ovary syndrome. *Am Fam Physician.* 2009;80(6):579–580.

Category: Endocrine system

93. A 48-year-old otherwise healthy woman has undergone a hysterectomy secondary to abnormal vaginal bleeding. Pathology results confirm no evidence of malignancy. She asks you how often she should have a Pap smear. The appropriate response is
A) Yearly Pap smears for an additional 3 years are recommended.
B) Pap smears should be reinstituted if she develops atrophic vaginitis.
C) Pap smears should be repeated every 3 years.
D) Pap smears should be performed every 5 years.
E) No further Pap smears are necessary.

Answer and Discussion

The answer is E. Multiple studies have concluded that vaginal cuff smear testing is not necessary in women who have undergone hysterectomy for benign conditions.

Additional Reading: ACS, ASCCP, ASC screening guidelines for the prevention and early detection of cervical cancer. American Society for Colposcopy and Cervical Pathology. *J Low Genit Tract Dis.* 2012;16(3):1–29.

Category: Reproductive system

94. A Pap smear result in a 25-year-old woman shows atypical cells of undetermined significance (ACS-US). HPV typing is negative for high-risk HPV. Appropriate management at this time includes
A) Repeat Pap smear in 3 years
B) Repeat Pap smear at 6 months
C) Colposcopy
D) LEEP procedure
E) Repeat Pap smear in 1 year with high-risk HPV testing

Answer and Discussion

The answer is A. Women with ASC-US (Atypical Squamous Cells of Undetermined Significance) cytology and a negative high-risk HPV test should continue with routine screening as per age-specific guidelines. Data from published studies have shown that the risk of precancerous lesions following an HPV-negative, ASC-US cytology result is very low, and not qualitatively different from a negative co-test. Because of the very low cervical cancer risk observed in the HPV-negative, ASC-US cytology populations, continued routine screening is recommended for this group: 3-year interval for cytology only screening of women ages 21 to 65 or 5-year interval for co-testing (cytology plus high-risk HPV testing) of women ages 30 to 65.

Additional Reading: ACS, ASCCP, ASC screening guidelines for the prevention and early detection of cervical cancer. American Society for Colposcopy and Cervical Pathology. *J Low Genit Tract Dis.* 2012;16(3):1–29.

Category: Reproductive system

95. Which of the following ultrasound parameters is best used for estimating gestational age during the first trimester?
A) Crown–rump length
B) Biparietal diameter
C) Femur length
D) Head–foot length
E) Estimated weight

Answer and Discussion

The answer is A. An ultrasound can be used to measure crown–rump length, biparietal diameter, abdominal circumference, and femur length, all of which can be used to confirm dates. The crown–rump length is more accurate during the first trimester, whereas the biparietal diameter and femur length are used more during the second trimester. The ultrasound is best used in the first trimester for estimating age of the fetus. As pregnancy progresses, estimation of age is more difficult to assess using ultrasound examination.

Additional Reading: Initial prenatal assessment and first trimester prenatal care. In: Basow DS, ed. *UpToDate*. Waltham, MA: UpToDate; 2013.

Category: Reproductive system

96. The most common cause of galactorrhea is
A) Psychotropic medication
B) Hypothyroidism
C) Prolactinoma
D) Nipple stimulation
E) Sexual intercourse

Answer and Discussion

The answer is C. Galactorrhea is defined as the presence of lactation in the absence of pregnancy, so pregnancy testing should occur before any further workup. For nonpregnant patients, galactorrhea is most commonly caused by hyperprolactinemia, especially when associated with amenorrhea. The most common cause for hyperprolactinemia is a prolactinoma in the pituitary gland or other sellar or suprasellar lesions. Other causes include psychotropic medications, opioids, antihypertensive drugs (α-methyldopa), hypogonadism, nipple stimulation, bronchogenic carcinomas, herpes zoster, hypothyroidism, renal insufficiency, and trauma. After pathologic nipple discharge is ruled out, patients with galactorrhea should be evaluated by measurement of their prolactin level. The result can range from slightly elevated (>23 to 25 ng/mL) to a thousand times the upper limit of normal. In general, adenomas are more common when prolactin levels are >200 ng/mL and larger adenomas cause higher prolactin levels. Those with hyperprolactinemia should have their thyroid and renal function assessed.

Elevated prolactin levels should prompt CT or MRI scans of the sella turcica to exclude pituitary adenomas. Visual field defects may also be present if tumors impinge on the optic chiasm. Patients with prolactinomas are usually treated with dopamine agonists (bromocriptine or cabergoline); surgery or radiation therapy is rarely required. Medications causing hyperprolactinemia should be discontinued or replaced with a medication from a similar class with lower potential for causing hyperprolactinemia. Normoprolactinemic patients with idiopathic, nonbothersome galactorrhea can be reassured and do not need treatment; however, those with bothersome galactorrhea usually respond to a short course of a low-dose dopamine agonist.

Additional Reading: Evaluation and management of galactorrhea. *Am Fam Physician.* 2012;85(11):1073–1080.

Category: Endocrine system

97. The definition of *dyspareunia* is
A) Painful intercourse
B) Abnormal hip alignment
C) Disturbed pelvic sensation
D) Altered menstrual cycles
E) Difficult labor

Answer and Discussion

The answer is A. Dyspareunia is painful intercourse, and the causes can be organic or psychogenic. Organic causes include inflammatory diseases of the vulva or vagina; infections, including fungal, bacterial, and viral (herpes, condyloma); tight-fitting clothes; a contracted vaginal orifice (caused by scarring from previous episiotomy or trauma); atrophic vaginitis; lack of lubrication; foreign bodies; an intact or constricted hymen; or a reaction to chemicals that are involved in contraception, deodorant sprays, and douches. Other pelvic disorders, including pelvic infections, masses, or endometriosis, can lead to dyspareunia. Psychogenic causes may include fear, anxiety, disinterest, or previous abuse or rape. Treatment involves adequate lubrication, correction of organic causes, and psychotherapy and education for psychogenic causes.

Additional Reading: Dyspareunia. In: Domino F, ed. *The 5-Minute Clinical Consult.* Philadelphia, PA: Lippincott Williams and Wilkins; 2014.

Category: Reproductive system

98. A Pap smear result for a 23-year-old female patient comes back with atypical cells of undetermined significance and the report cannot exclude high-grade intraepithelial lesion. Atypical Squamous Cells, Cannot Rule Out High-Grade Squamous Intra-epithelial Lesion (ASC-H). Appropriate management at this time includes
A) Repeat Pap smear at 1 year
B) Repeat Pap smear at 6 months
C) Colposcopy
D) LEEP procedure
E) Cervical cryotherapy

Answer and Discussion

The answer is C. Although high-grade intraepithelial lesion is less common than ASC-US, the risk of underlying CIN II or III is higher and colposcopy is recommended. Women ages 21 to 24 years with no CIN II or III identified at the time of colposcopy should be observed with colposcopy and cytology every 6 months for up to 2 years, until 2 consecutive negative Pap tests are reported and no high-grade colposcopy abnormality is observed.

Additional Reading: 2012 updated consensus guidelines for the management of abnormal cervical cancer screening tests and cancer precursors. American Society for Colposcopy and Cervical Pathology. *J Low Genit Tract Dis.* 2013;17(5):S1–S27.

Category: Reproductive system

99. A 40-year-old woman's Pap smear result comes back as having atypical glandular cells (AGC). Appropriate management at this time includes
A) Repeat Pap smear at 1 year
B) Repeat Pap smear at 6 months
C) Colposcopy
D) Colposcopy with endocervical and endometrial sampling
E) HPV testing and colposcopy only if high-risk HPV identified

Answer and Discussion

The answer is D. For women with all subcategories of AGC except atypical endometrial cells, colposcopy with endocervical sampling is recommended regardless of HPV result. Accordingly, triage by reflex HPV testing is not recommended, and triage using repeat cervical cytology is unacceptable. Endometrial sampling is recommended in conjunction with colposcopy and endocervical sampling in women 35 years of age and older with all subcategories of AGC. Endometrial sampling is also recommended for women younger than 35 years with clinical indications suggesting they may be at risk for endometrial neoplasia. These include unexplained vaginal bleeding or conditions suggesting chronic anovulation. For women with atypical endometrial cells, initial evaluation limited to endometrial and endocervical sampling is preferred, with colposcopy acceptable either at the initial evaluation or deferred until the results of endometrial and endocervical sampling are known; if colposcopy is deferred and no endometrial pathology is identified, colposcopy is then recommended.

Additional Reading: 2012 updated consensus guidelines for the management of abnormal cervical cancer screening tests and cancer precursors. American Society for Colposcopy and Cervical Pathology. *J Low Genit Tract Dis.* 2013;17(5):S1–S27.

Category: Reproductive system

100. When testing fetal well-being, which of the following factors is *not* measured with a biophysical profile?
A) Fetal tone
B) Amniotic fluid
C) FHR
D) Fetal size
E) Body movements

Answer and Discussion

The answer is D. Biophysical profile testing is a more extensive method of testing fetal well-being than is nonstress testing. Indications include the following:

- Maternal hypertension
- Maternal diabetes
- Postterm pregnancies
- Multiple gestations
- Oligohydramnios
- Intrauterine growth retardation
- Placental abnormalities
- Decreased fetal movement
- Previous intrauterine fetal demise

The test involves the testing of five different aspects of fetal well-being with real-time ultrasound, including the following:

- Fetal breathing
- Body movements
- Fetal tone
- Amniotic fluid volume
- FHR monitoring (nonstress test)

Each aspect is given either a score of 0 for abnormal findings or 2 for normal findings. A score of 4 or less is a poor prognostic indicator, whereas a score of 8 or 10 is reassuring for fetal well-being. A score of 6 is suspicious for chronic asphyxia.

Additional Reading: The fetal biophysical profile. In: Basow DS, ed. *UpToDate.* Waltham, MA: UpToDate; 2013.

Category: Reproductive system

101. The most sensitive method to diagnose endometrial cancer is with
A) Papanicolaou (Pap) smear
B) Ultrasound
C) CT of the pelvis
D) Endometrial biopsy
E) Fractionated endometrial curettage

Answer and Discussion

The answer is E. Adenocarcinoma of the endometrium usually occurs in postmenopausal women between 50 and 60 years of age. It usually arises from the columnar cells of the endometrial lining.

Associated conditions that constitute risk factors include adenomatous hyperplasia; unopposed estrogen use; delayed menopause; infertility (nulliparity); Stein–Leventhal syndrome; previous breast, colon, or ovarian cancer; diabetes; chronic tamoxifen use; hypertension; and obesity. The hallmark symptom is unexplained irregular vaginal bleeding, particularly in postmenopausal women. The diagnosis can be made with Pap smears in 40% of patients; however, because of the relatively high rate of false-negative results, diagnosis is better made with endometrial biopsy, ultrasound, or the gold standard fractionated endometrial curettage. Treatment involves surgical excision with total abdominal hysterectomy and bilateral oophorectomy followed by lymph node sampling. Chemotherapy using cytotoxic drugs as well as progesterone and radiation is also used in the treatment of endometrial cancer. Prognosis depends on the stage and differentiation of the cancer. Well-differentiated, well-localized tumors have a 5-year survival rate of close to 95%, whereas poorly differentiated tumors with metastasis have less than a 20% 5-year survival rate.

Additional Reading: McGarry K. Endometrial cancer. *The 5-Minute Consult Clinical Companion to Women's Health.* Philadelphia, PA: Lippincott Williams and Wilkins; 2012.

Category: Reproductive system

102. Which of the following is recommended for postpartum breast engorgement?
A) Firm binding of breast with a comfortable wrap
B) Cabbage leaves
C) Bromocriptine
D) Initiation of oral contraceptives
E) Topical vitamin E

Answer and Discussion

The answer is A. The best way to prevent postpartum breast engorgement is to bind the breasts firmly with a comfortable wrap. Other suggestions include cold packs, analgesics, and the avoidance of direct warm water during showering. The use of bromocriptine (a dopamine agonist) to stop lactation is associated with rebound lactation after discontinuation of the medication, hypotension, hypertension, seizures, and stroke; it is no longer approved by the U.S. Food and Drug Administration for this use. Other medications, such as estrogen and testosterone combinations are not recommended because of their increased risk for thromboembolism and hair growth, respectively. In most cases, breast engorgement resolves within 72 hours.

Additional Reading: Treatments for suppression of lactation. *Cochrane Database Syst Rev.* 2012;9:CD005937.

Category: Integumentary

103. A 38-year-old woman has a Pap smear result of AGC-favor neoplasia. She undergoes colposcopy and no invasive disease is found. Appropriate management at this time includes
A) Repeat Pap smear at 1 year
B) Repeat Pap smear at 6 months
C) Repeat colposcopy at 6 months
D) LEEP procedure
E) Cold-knife conization procedure

Answer and Discussion

The answer is E. The category of AGC is divided into "not otherwise specified" (AGC-NOS) and "favor neoplasia" or adenocarcinoma in situ (AIS). For women with AGC "favor neoplasia" or endocervical AIS cytology, if invasive disease is not identified during the initial colposcopic workup, a diagnostic excisional procedure is recommended (AII). It is recommended that the type of diagnostic excisional procedure used in this setting provide an intact specimen with interpretable margins, such as a cold-knife cone procedure. Excision via a LEEP procedure may affect interpretation of specimen margins and so is not the preferred procedure. Endocervical sampling after excision is preferred.

> Additional Reading: 2012 updated consensus guidelines for the management of abnormal cervical cancer screening tests and cancer precursors. American Society for Colposcopy and Cervical Pathology. *J Low Genit Tract Dis.* 2013;17(5)S1–S27.

Category: Reproductive system

104. Which of the following medications is associated with an increased risk of endometrial carcinoma?
A) Bromocriptine (Parlodel)
B) Oral contraceptives
C) Progesterone
D) Alendronate (Fosamax)
E) Tamoxifen (Nolvadex)

Answer and Discussion
The answer is E. Risk factors for endometrial cancer include anovulatory cycles, obesity, nulliparity, age greater than 35 years, unopposed estrogen use, and tamoxifen therapy.

> Additional Reading: Ries LA, Eisner MP, Kosary CL, et al., eds. *SEER Cancer Statistics Review, 1975–2006.* Bethesda, MD: National Cancer Institute; 2009. From: http://seer.cancer.gov/studies/epidemiology/study14.html

Category: Reproductive system

> Risk factors for endometrial cancer include anovulatory cycles, obesity, nulliparity, age greater than 35 years, unopposed estrogen use, and tamoxifen therapy.

105. Which of the following is an absolute contraindication of tocolysis?
A) Chorioamnionitis
B) 4-cm cervical dilation
C) Biophysical profile score of 8
D) Oligohydramnios
E) Hyperthyroidism

Answer and Discussion
The answer is A. The arresting of labor has certain contraindications that must be ruled out before tocolytics are given. Absolute contraindications include the following:

- Severe abruptio placentae
- Infection (chorioamnionitis)
- Severe bleeding
- Severe pregnancy-induced hypertension
- Fetal anomalies that are incompatible with life
- Fetal death
- Severe growth retardation
- Fetal distress

Relative contraindications include the following:

- Hyperthyroidism
- Uncontrolled diabetes
- Maternal heart disease
- Hypertension
- Mild abruptio placentae
- Stable placenta previa
- Fetal distress
- Mild growth retardation
- Cervical dilation greater than 5 to 6 cm

Corticosteroids are recommended to help prevent respiratory distress syndrome (RDS) if there is PROM before 34 weeks' gestation. Delay of labor for >1 week after rupture of membranes is usually not recommended unless the fetus is very small (<1,250 g).

> Additional Reading: Preterm labor. *Am Fam Physician.* 2010; 81(4):477–484.

Category: Reproductive system

106. When testing fetal well-being, which of the following statements about the nonstress test is true?
A) Two or more fetal heart accelerations (at least 15 beats above baseline) that last for 15 seconds in a 20-minute period are reassuring.
B) Late decelerations are usually noted with fetal movements.
C) An abnormal nonstress test should be followed by a contraction stress test.
D) The presence of oligohydramnios is accurately predicted with the results of a nonstress test.
E) Nonstress tests should be routinely performed beginning at 38 weeks until delivery.

Answer and Discussion
The answer is A. Nonstress tests are used for antenatal well-being studies. Nonstress testing includes the use of a fetal heart monitor and contraction monitor. Testing is usually reserved for complicated pregnancies (e.g., intrauterine growth retardation, gestational diabetes, pregnancy-induced hypertension, multiple gestations, prior stillbirth) or postdate pregnancy. A reassuring nonstress test shows two or more FHR accelerations of at least 15 beats/second above the baseline that last for at least 15 seconds during a 20-minute period. If this criterion is not met, a biophysical profile should be performed. Late or variable decelerations are concerning findings. Oligohydramnios is a risk for cord compression but is not well predicted by nonstress testing. Simplistically, the nonstress test is primarily a test of fetal well-being, whereas the contraction stress test is a test of uteroplacental function.

> Additional Reading: Overview of fetal assessment. In: Basow DS, ed. *UpToDate.* Waltham, MA: UpToDate; 2013.

Category: Reproductive system

107. RhoGAM should be given to Rh-negative mothers at
A) First prenatal visit and at delivery
B) 12 and 36 weeks' gestation
C) 16 weeks' gestation and after delivery, depending on Rh status of the newborn
D) 28 weeks' gestation and after delivery, depending on Rh status of the newborn
E) 28 and 36 weeks' gestation

Answer and Discussion

The answer is D. The condition of erythroblastosis fetalis is the result of blood incompatibility between the mother and fetus. It results when an Rh-negative woman is impregnated by an Rh-positive man. Red blood cells (RBCs) cross the placenta into the mother's bloodstream and evoke the production of her antibodies to the child's RBCs. The antibodies can cross the placenta and result in severe anemia that may cause death to the fetus. To compensate, the fetal bone marrow releases immature RBCs and erythroblasts (thus, the name *erythroblastosis fetalis*). The condition rarely affects the first pregnancy, and the risk for sensitization increases with each pregnancy. As a result of the antibody destruction of RBCs, there is an increased production of bilirubin that can result in kernicterus, which is characterized by poor feeding, apnea, poor fetal tone, mental retardation, seizures, and death. In the United States, approximately 15% of marriages involve Rh-positive fathers and Rh-negative mothers, but the potential may be underestimated because of the number of children who are born out of wedlock with unknown fathers. Of this 15%, only 1 in 27 are affected with erythroblastosis fetalis. Prevention of the disease is accomplished by administering RhoGAM, an anti-Rh antibody, to the mother. RhoGAM attacks and destroys the fetal blood cells when they cross the placenta, before they can involve the production of antibodies. RhoGAM is administered at 28 weeks' gestation and then after delivery, if the infant is determined to be Rh positive. Mothers of Rh-negative infants do not need postpartum RhoGAM. It should also be given if abortion or ectopic pregnancy occurs or in any case in which there is fetal–maternal transfer of blood. All mothers should be screened for Rh status at their initial prenatal visit.

> **Additional Reading:** Evidence-based prenatal care: Part II. Third-trimester care and prevention of infectious diseases. *Am Fam Physician.* 2005;71:1555–1562.

Category: Hematologic system

108. A 17-year-old woman presents to your office complaining of dysfunctional uterine bleeding. Appropriate management consists of
A) Endometrial sampling
B) Ultrasound examination of the uterus
C) Endometrial sampling and ultrasound evaluation
D) Dilation and curettage
E) Use of oral contraceptives and observation

Answer and Discussion

The answer is E. Endometrial cancer is rare in 15- to 18-year-old women. Therefore, most adolescents with dysfunctional uterine bleeding can be treated safely with hormone therapy and observation, without diagnostic testing.

> **Additional Reading:** Evaluation and management of abnormal uterine bleeding in premenopausal women. *Am Fam Physician.* 2012;85(1):35–43.

Category: Reproductive system

109. Which of the following is used infrequently in the treatment of pubic lice (pediculosis) because of concerns regarding potential toxicity?
A) Malathion
B) Permethrin
C) Pyrethrins/piperonyl butoxide
D) Lindane
E) Ivermectin

Answer and Discussion

The answer is D. Pubic lice are readily transmitted sexually. There is some evidence that occasionally they may be transmitted through contaminated clothing or towels, although this is controversial. The presence of pubic lice should prompt an evaluation for other common STDs, such as chlamydial infection and gonorrhea. Treatment is the same as for head lice. Recommended treatments include permethrin 1% or pyrethrins 0.3%/piperonyl butoxide 4% as first-line agents, and alternative regimens of malathion 0.5% lotion or oral ivermectin at 250 mcg per kg, repeated in two weeks. Lindane is not recommended as first-line therapy because of potential toxicity. It should only be used as an alternative if the patient cannot tolerate other therapies or if other therapies have failed. The mainstay of treatment for body lice is laundering clothing and bedding in hot water and regular bathing. Sexual contacts also should be treated if infested.

> **Additional Reading:** Ectoparasitic infections. *CDC Sexually Transmitted Disease Treatment Guidelines*; 2010; and Pediculosis and scabies: a treatment update. *Am Fam Physician.* 2012;86(6):535–541.

Category: Integumentary

110. Fibroid tumors can be associated with which of the following conditions?
A) Amenorrhea
B) Renal lithiasis
C) Postpartum hemorrhage
D) Increased risk of ovarian carcinoma
E) Increased risk for endometrial hyperplasia

Answer and Discussion

The answer is C. Fibroid tumors are irregular enlargements of the uterus. They are the most common benign tumors of the female genital tract, with as many as 20% of 40-year-old women affected. The tumors are composed of smooth muscle and connective tissue. In most cases, the condition is asymptomatic; however, it can cause dysmenorrhea with heavy menstrual blood loss leading to anemia and irregular periods. Occasionally, the fibroids degenerate, giving rise to intense pelvic pain and the development of pelvic infections. In some cases, infertility can occur when a fibroma blocks the fallopian tube. Other complications include difficult pregnancies with dystocia and excessive postpartum hemorrhage and urinary frequency or difficulty in defecating when the tumors press on the bladder or colon. Diagnosis is usually made with ultrasound, CT scan, MRI, or hysteroscopy. Treatment involves GnRH analogs (leuprolide), which may decrease the size of the fibroid; however, regrowth often occurs after the medication is discontinued. For severe cases, surgery, including myomectomy or hysterectomy, may be indicated. Treatment with estrogen can produce growth of the tumors and worsening of symptoms.

> **Additional Reading:** Uterine myomas. In: Domino F, ed. *The 5-Minute Clinical Consult.* Philadelphia, PA: Lippincott Williams and Wilkins; 2014.

Category: Reproductive system

111. The most appropriate medication for the treatment of pyelonephritis in pregnancy is
A) Ampicillin + gentamicin
B) Trimethoprim-sulfamethoxazole
C) Tetracycline
D) Nitrofurantoin
E) Ciprofloxacin

Answer and Discussion

The answer is A. Pyelonephritis is one of the most common serious complications in pregnancy. It occurs in approximately 2% of pregnancies and more frequently in the third trimester. Symptoms include fever, chills, dysuria, flank pain, nausea, vomiting, and malaise. Pregnant women with acute pyelonephritis should be treated initially with a second- or third-generation cephalosporin, such as ceftriaxone 1 g every 12 hours, and then assessed to determine whether further treatment as an outpatient is appropriate. Ampicillin (2 g IV every 6 hours) and Gentamicin (1.5 mg/kg every 8 hours) is an acceptable alternative. Sulfonamides are contraindicated in the third trimester of pregnancy because of the risk of kernicterus in newborns. Quinolone antibiotics (e.g., ciprofloxacin) interfere with cartilage development and should be avoided. Tetracyclines are contraindicated because they can cause yellowish discoloration in the child's teeth. Nitrofurantoin is used frequently in pregnancy but can induce hemolysis in patients who are deficient in glucose-6-phosphate dehydrogenase (G6PD; affects approximately 2% of African Americans). Treatment of pyelonephritis is necessary because of the increased risk of premature labor. All pregnant patients with pyelonephritis should be hospitalized, and periodic fetal monitoring should be instituted. Follow-up cultures are indicated to ensure eradication.

Additional Reading: Diagnosis and treatment of acute pyelonephritis in women. *Am Fam Physician.* 2011;84(5):519–526; and Urinary tract infections and asymptomatic bacteriuria in pregnancy. In: Basow DS, ed. *UpToDate.* Waltham, MA: UpToDate; 2013.

Category: Nephrologic system

112. Which of the following tests is indicated at the time of the first prenatal visit in a healthy mother?
A) α-Fetoprotein testing
B) Quantitative β-hCG
C) Antibody test (indirect Coombs' test)
D) Glucose tolerance test
E) Free T4

Answer and Discussion

The answer is C. Prenatal testing is usually performed at the initial prenatal visit. Tests include Pap smear (if due based on age-appropriate screening intervals), complete blood count, urinalysis with culture, ABO blood type, Rh status, antibody test (indirect Coombs' test), rubella antibody titer, syphilis, HIV, and hepatitis B surface antigen testing. Other tests may include urine or cervical testing for chlamydia and gonorrhea, tuberculosis skin test, sickle cell prep, Hepatitis C antibody, varicella antibody, and TSH. α-fetoprotein testing is usually done with the maternal serum screening at 15 to 18 weeks' gestation, 1-hour glucose challenge test (glucola) at 24 to 28 weeks' gestation, and hematocrit and Rh antibody screening at 28 weeks' gestation. Patients at high risk for STDs may need repeated STD screening later in pregnancy. Vaginal rectal swab for Group B strep should be obtained from all pregnant women 35- to 37-week gestational age except those already known to have had Group B strep bacteriuria.

Additional Reading: Evidence-based prenatal care: Part I. General prenatal care and counseling issues. *Am Fam Physician.* 2005;71(7):1307–1316.

Category: Reproductive system

113. Which of the following would support the diagnosis of menopause in a woman taking no medications?
A) Vaginal pH >4.5
B) FSH level <10 mIU/mL
C) Endometrial cells noted on Pap smear
D) TSH >5.6
E) Progesterone >10 ng/dL

basic pH

Answer and Discussion

The answer is A. A vaginal pH >4.5 indicates menopause in women who are without vaginitis and are not receiving estrogen therapy. Studies have shown that vaginal pH is similar to FSH levels in establishing the diagnosis of low estrogen levels or menopause and that a vaginal pH of 4.5 or less can be used to monitor adequate response to estrogen-replacement therapy. BV can also cause a vaginal pH to be >4.5. FSH levels >40 mIU/mL typically indicate a menopausal state. Low progesterone levels <100 pg/mL are often seen in menopause though low progesterone levels can also be seen in women taking oral contraceptives.

Additional Reading: Roy S, Caillouette JC, Roy T. Vaginal pH is similar to follicle-stimulating hormone for menopause diagnosis. *Am J Obstet Gynecol.* 2004;190:1272–1277.

Category: Reproductive system

114. Which of the following is an absolute contraindication for the use of oral contraceptives in women above the age of 35?
A) Family history of stroke
B) Hypertension without vascular disease
C) Mild hyperlipidemia
D) Diabetes with neuropathy
E) Smoker (<10 cigarettes/day)

Answer and Discussion

The answer is D. Risks associated with combination OCPs may limit their use in women older than 35 years of age. Most concerns are based on early studies of oral contraceptive formulations with a high ethinyl estradiol content, rather than more recent studies of lower dose formulations. Although use of OCPs increases the risk of venous thromboembolism, the degree of risk appears to be the same in women taking formulations that contain 20 to 35 mcg of estrogen. The absolute risk of venous thromboembolism is very low (1 case per 10,000 OCP users per year). OCPs also contain progestins, including desogestrel and gestodene. These two progestins have been associated with an increased risk of venous thromboembolism. The risk of myocardial infarction may be increased in women using OCPs, especially if smoking (>10 cigarettes per day) or other cardiovascular risk factors are present. The association between OCP use and ischemic stroke is not clear, although increased risk has been demonstrated in OCP users who have migraines. There is no documentation of an increased risk of breast cancer in women who use OCPs. One study has found a slightly increased risk of gallstones, although the risk was lower in women older than 35 years of age than in younger women. The potential benefits of OCP use in women older than 35 years of age include effective birth control, reduced risk of ovarian and endometrial cancers, possible reduced risk of colon cancer, improvement of perimenopausal symptoms, improvement of acne, and increased BMD (although improved fracture rates have not yet been demonstrated). Before use of OCPs is initiated, a thorough medical history should be obtained and blood pressure should be measured. If a patient has risk factors for cardiovascular disease or a family history of dyslipidemia, a routine fasting lipid panel is recommended.

Mild lipid abnormalities do not contraindicate use of OCPs, but lipid levels should be monitored. Because OCPs can increase blood pressure, they should be prescribed with caution in patients with mild hypertension and patients who smoke. Absolute contraindications include the following:

- Pregnancy
- Postpartum less than 6 weeks and breast-feeding
- Age more than 35 years and heavy smoker (>15 cigarettes per day)
- Systolic blood pressure >160 mm Hg, diastolic blood pressure greater than 99 mm Hg
- Hypertension with vascular disease
- Diabetes with neuropathy, retinopathy, nephropathy, or vascular disease
- History of DVT or pulmonary embolism
- Major surgery with prolonged immobilization
- History of ischemic heart disease
- History of stroke
- Complicated valvular disease (with atrial fibrillation, pulmonary hypertension, bacterial endocarditis)
- Severe headaches with focal neurologic symptoms
- Current breast cancer
- Active viral hepatitis, severe cirrhosis, benign or malignant liver tumors

The best OCP in women above 35 is the one with the lowest effective estrogen dose. Side effects are most common during the first 3 months. The most frequent adverse effects are abnormal menstrual bleeding, nausea, weight gain, mood changes, breast tenderness, and headache. Follow-up should include annual blood pressure measurements, lipid profiles in patients with a baseline abnormality, and a review of symptoms that could signify an important adverse effect. Breakthrough bleeding is common and usually resolves spontaneously after a few months. The incidence of breakthrough bleeding appears to be higher with formulations containing lower estrogen doses.

Additional Reading: Prescribing oral contraceptives for women older than 35 years of age. *Ann Intern Med.* 2003;138:54–64.

Category: Reproductive system

> The potential benefits of OCP use in women older than 35 years of age include effective birth control, reduced risk of ovarian and endometrial cancers, possible reduced risk of colon cancer, improvement of perimenopausal symptoms, improvement of acne, and increased BMD (although improved fracture rates have not yet been demonstrated).

115. Which of the following is associated with preeclampsia?
A) Blood pressure elevations >140 systolic and >90 diastolic
B) Trace proteinuria
C) Mild edema
D) Seizures
E) Scotomata

Answer and Discussion
The answer is A. Preeclampsia is defined as follows:

- Hypertension (>90 mm Hg diastolic and >140 mm Hg systolic after 20 weeks on two separate occasions taken 6 hours apart)

- Proteinuria (>300 mg/24 hours or 1+ or greater on urine dipstick)
- Other laboratory abnormalities include increased creatinine and uric acid, thrombocytopenia, and elevated liver function test

Note: Edema has been removed from the criteria.

Risk factors include age younger than 20 or older than 40 years, primigravid state, previous preeclampsia, twin pregnancy, diabetes mellitus, hydatidiform mole, fetal hydrops, or chronic hypertension. *Eclampsia* is defined as the above criteria plus the development of seizures that cannot be attributed to other causes. Warning signs for the development of eclampsia may include severe headache, scotomas, blurred vision, and vomiting. HELLP syndrome (*h*emolysis, *e*levated *l*iver function tests, and *l*ow *p*latelets) may also occur.

Additional Reading: Preeclampsia, eclampsia, and hypertension. *Am Fam Physician.* 2009;79(10):895–896.

Category: Reproductive system

116. Gestational diabetic screening during pregnancy for women without risk factors for diabetes should take place
A) At the first prenatal visit
B) At 12 to 16 weeks' gestation
C) At 24 to 28 weeks' gestation
D) At 30 to 34 weeks' gestation
E) Randomly throughout pregnancy

Answer and Discussion
The answer is C. Diabetes during pregnancy is associated with a number of abnormalities that affect the fetus, including increased risk of spontaneous abortion, congenital anomalies (e.g., neural tube defects, cardiac defects, skeletal abnormalities, malformations of the intestinal and urinary tract), and fetal macrosomia. White's criteria are used to classify gestational diabetes:

- A1: gestational diabetes not requiring insulin
- A2: gestational diabetes requiring insulin
- B: onset in a patient older than 20 years of age or lasting less than 10 years
- C: onset at 10 to 20 years of age or duration of 10 to 20 years
- D: onset in patients younger than 10 years of age or duration of more than 20 years
- F: nephropathy
- R: proliferative retinopathy or vitreous hemorrhage
- H: atherosclerotic heart disease that is clinically evident
- T: renal transplant

Risk factors for gestational diabetes include maternal age older than 35 years, obesity, positive family history of diabetes, and prior history of gestational diabetes and/or macrosomia, and women with these risk factors should be screened early in pregnancy. All other pregnant women (and high-risk women with normal early screening) should be screened for diabetes between weeks 24 and 28 of gestation with the glucola (1-hour 50-g oral glucose) screening test. If values are >130 to 140 mg/dL, a 3-hour glucose tolerance test should be performed. Although most women experience a resolution of diabetes immediately postpartum, they are at increased risk of developing type II diabetes mellitus later in life, so should be screened for diabetes 6 weeks postpartum and annually thereafter.

Additional Reading: Diagnosis and management of gestational diabetes. *Am Fam Physician.* 2009; 80(1):57–62.

Category: Reproductive system

117. Which of the following test results is associated with pregnancy?
A) Increased white blood cell count
B) Decreased alkaline phosphatase
C) Increased hemoglobin
D) Decreased lactic dehydrogenase
E) Decreased fibrinogen level

Answer and Discussion

The answer is A. Many laboratory values are affected during pregnancy:

- Hemoglobin/hematocrit: decreased
- White blood cell count: increased
- Fibrinogen level: increased
- Erythrocyte sedimentation rate: increased
- Albumin level: decreased
- Fasting blood glucose: decreased
- Lactic dehydrogenase: increased
- Creatinine phosphokinase: increased
- Alkaline phosphatase: increased
- Calcium (total): decreased
- Cortisol: increased
- Prolactin: increased
- Thyroxine total: increased

Mild glycosuria and proteinuria are also common during pregnancy. Excessive amounts should prompt for further evaluation to rule out gestational diabetes and preeclampsia.

> **Additional Reading:** Maternal physiology. *Williams Obstetrics*, 23rd ed. New York, NY: McGraw-Hill; 2010.

> **Category:** Reproductive system

118. Studies have shown that the use of depot medroxyprogesterone acetate (DMPA) contraception is associated with
A) Reversible bone loss
B) Increased migraines
C) Increased endometrial cancer
D) Increased pregnancy risk
E) Increased teratogenicity in future pregnancies

Answer and Discussion

The answer is A. DMPA is associated with a decrease in BMD that is generally temporary and reversible. Data suggest that the loss in BMD is rapid within the first 2 years of use, but after approximately 2 years of use, loss of BMD slows dramatically. Although women have a decrease in BMD while using DMPA, studies have consistently demonstrated that BMD is regained back to baseline levels equivalent to that seen in non-DMPA users when DMPA is discontinued. There have been no randomized trials on DMPA use and fracture risk. The benefits of excellent protection against pregnancy that DMPA provides are felt to outweigh the risks of bone loss in most normal healthy women, women with conditions that place them at high risk for osteoporosis and fracture, such as chronic corticosteroid use, disorders of bone metabolism, a strong family history of or anorexia nervosa, may not be well suited for long-term DMPA use.

> **Additional Reading:** Hatcher RA, et al. Injectable contraceptives. *Contraceptive Technology,* 20th ed. New York, NY: Ardent Media; 2011.

> **Category:** Reproductive system

119. Which of the following findings would support the diagnosis of PCOS?
A) Irregular menstrual periods caused by anovulation or irregular ovulation
B) Lab evidence of elevated androgens
C) Clinical symptoms of androgen excess such as hirsuitism
D) Polycystic ovaries on ultrasound
E) All of the above

Answer and Discussion

The answer is E. Although there are several proposed diagnostic criteria for PCOS, a summary report from a 2012 National Institutes of Health Workshop suggests that the Rotterdam 2003 criteria be used for now. Using these criteria, two out of three of the following are required to make the diagnosis of PCOS:

- Oligo- and/or anovulation
- Clinical and/or biochemical signs of hyperandrogenism
- Polycystic ovaries (by ultrasound)

In addition, other conditions that mimic PCOS must be excluded (e.g., disorders that cause oligo/anovulation and/or hyperandrogenism, such as thyroid disease, nonclassic congenital adrenal hyperplasia, hyperprolactinemia, and androgen-secreting tumors).

Additional testing is usually recommended to determine whether another condition is the cause of these signs and/or symptoms. Blood tests for pregnancy, prolactin level, TSH, and FSH may be recommended. Insulin levels are not used to diagnose PCOS partly because insulin levels are high in people who are above normal body weight and because there is no level of insulin that is "diagnostic" for PCOS.

If PCOS is confirmed, blood glucose and cholesterol testing are usually performed. An oral glucose tolerance test is the best way to diagnose prediabetes and/or diabetes. A fasting glucose level is often normal even when prediabetes or diabetes is present. Many clinicians who treat PCOS patients also recommend screening for sleep apnea with questionnaires or overnight sleep studies in a sleep laboratory. In women with moderate to severe hirsutism (excess hair growth), blood tests for testosterone and Dehydroepiandrosterone sulfate DHEA-S may be recommended.

> **Additional Reading:** Diagnosis of polycystic ovary syndrome in adults. In: Basow DS, ed. *UpToDate.* Waltham, MA: UpToDate; 2013.

> **Category:** Endocrine system

120. Which of the following is the best test for Chlamydia infection using a urine specimen rather than urethral or cervical swabs?
A) Nucleic Acid Amplification Test (NAAT)
B) Nucleic acid hybridization tests
C) Cell culture
D) Direct immunofluorescence
E) Enzyme immunoassay (EIA)

Answer and Discussion

The answer is A. Culture, nucleic acid hybridization tests, direct immunofluorescence, enzyme immunoassay, and NAATs are all available for the detection of *C. trachomatis*. Culture and hybridization tests require urethral swab specimens, whereas NAATs can be performed on urine specimens. Because of their higher sensitivity, NAATs are preferred for the detection of *C. trachomatis*. Three types of NAAT are commercially available: PCR, transcription-mediated amplification, and strand-displacement amplification.

Additional Reading: Chlamydial infections. *CDC Sexually Transmitted Disease Treatment Guidelines;* 2010.

Category: Reproductive system

121. Which of the following medications is used in PCOS to restore menstrual cyclicity and induce ovulation?
A) Bromocriptine
B) Misoprostol
C) Rosiglitazone
D) Metformin (Glucophage)
E) Bupropion (Wellbutrin)

Answer and Discussion

The answer is D. Metformin, a biguanide and insulin-sensitizing agent, has been used to restore menstrual cyclicity and induce ovulation in PCOS without the use of additional fertility drugs. Use of this agent is associated with reductions in serum levels of bioavailable androgen, LH, and atherogenic lipids. Metformin is presently classified as a category "B" risk in pregnancy, which indicates that there are no apparent fetal defects associated with its use in the late trimester of pregnancy, on the basis of animal studies. Because the human effects of first-trimester use are unknown, discontinuation of therapy at the onset of pregnancy confirmation has been standard. However, a recent prospective study of women with PCOS who continued metformin therapy through the first trimester of pregnancy showed no evidence of fetal harm, calling into question this recommendation. Metformin therapy is associated with a slight risk of lactic acidosis and is not used in patients with impaired liver or renal function.

> **Additional Reading:** Treatment of polycystic ovary syndrome in adults. In: Basow DS, ed. *UpToDate.* Waltham, MA: UpToDate; 2013.

Category: Reproductive system

122. Which of the following statements concerning oral contraceptive use is true?
A) Oral contraceptives may decrease the risk of cervical cancer.
B) Oral contraceptives increase the risk of cholelithiasis.
C) Women who use oral contraceptives have a higher incidence of ectopic pregnancy.
D) The use of oral contraceptives is associated with a higher incidence of PID.
E) Women who use oral contraceptives have a higher incidence of endometrial carcinoma.

Answer and Discussion

The answer is B. The use of oral contraceptives for birth control is widely accepted and prescribed. Properly used, the pill approaches 100% effectiveness in preventing pregnancy. Its mechanism of action involves the prevention of ovulation by the regulation of hormones (suppression of FSH and LH) during the menstrual cycle, induction of atrophic changes to the endometrium that are not conducive to implantation, and the alteration of cervical mucus. Basically, there are two types: combination pills that include estrogen and progestin components and pills that contain only progestin. Pills that contain only progestin are best suited for women older than 35 years, smokers, or those who cannot tolerate estrogen. Additionally, oral contraceptives are divided into monophasic (fixed combination of estrogen and progestin component) and multiphasic (varying amount of progestin during each of the 3 weeks of medication with a fixed amount of estrogen). Overall, the multiphasic oral contraceptives are highly effective and may provide a lower dose of estrogen and progestin. Absolute contraindications to oral contraceptives include pregnancy, active liver disease, uncontrolled hypertension, significant hyperlipidemia, diabetes with vascular changes, previous DVT, coronary artery disease, stroke, or estrogen-dependent cancers. Relative contraindications include migraine headaches, hypertension, smoking, diabetes, major surgery within 1 month, sickle cell disease, gallbladder disease, immobilization of the lower extremities, undiagnosed vaginal bleeding, and age older than 40 years with cardiovascular risk factors. Complications associated with oral contraceptive use include increased blood pressure, midcycle bleeding between periods, headaches, weight gain, hirsutism, acne, increased risk of cholelithiasis, melasma, increased risk for myocardial infarction in smokers older than 35 years, and, rarely, benign hepatic lipomas. Women who use oral contraceptives are at decreased risk for ovarian cancer, endometrial cancer, PID, and ectopic pregnancy. No consistent association has been found between breast cancer and oral contraceptive use, except for the possibility of a slightly elevated risk in users of oral contraceptives for more than 3 years before 25 years of age. Women who are taking antiepileptic medication have an increased risk for oral contraceptive failure because of the enzyme-inducing action of the antiseizure medication. Antibiotic use may also decrease the effectiveness of oral contraceptives.

> **Additional Reading:** Hatcher RA, et al. Oral contraceptives. *Contraceptive Technology,* 20th ed. New York, NY: Ardent Media; 2011.

Category: Reproductive system

123. Which of the following is a contraindication for external cephalic version?
A) 36 weeks' gestation
B) Maternal age of 35
C) Polyhydramnios
D) Maternal diabetes
E) Obesity

Answer and Discussion

The answer is A. External cephalic version can be attempted on fetuses that are detected before the onset of labor and after 37 weeks' gestation. A tocolytic medication is delivered, and abdominal manipulation is performed under ultrasound guidance. Version before 37 weeks is not recommended because of the risk that the fetus may revert to a breech presentation before delivery and the risk of delivery of a premature infant. The success rate is approximately 75%. The procedure should be performed in the hospital so that cesarean section can be done if complications arise. The most common complications are placental abruption and cord compression. Contraindications for external cephalic version include uteroplacental insufficiency, hypertension, intrauterine growth retardation, oligohydramnios, or history of prior uterine surgery.

> **Additional Reading:** External cephalic version. *Williams Obstetrics,* 23rd ed. New York, NY: McGraw-Hill; 2010.

Category: Reproductive system

124. Which of the following is not considered appropriate tocolysis for preterm labor at 32 weeks' gestation?
A) Magnesium sulfate intravenously for 48 hours
B) Magnesium sulfate intravenously until 34 weeks' gestational age
C) Ritodrine for 48 hours
D) Indomethacin for 48 hours
E) Nifedipine for 48 hours

Answer and Discussion

The answer is B. Corticosteroids are recommended for all pregnant women between 24 and 34 weeks of gestation who are at risk of pre-term delivery within 7 days. Evidence supports the use of tocolytic treatment with any of a variety of agents including magnesium sul-fate, beta-adrenergic agonist (e.g., ritodrine) calcium-channel block-ers (e.g., nifedipine) or nonsteroidal anti-inflammatory drugs (e.g., indomethacin) only for short-term prolongation of pregnancy (up to 48 hours) to allow for the administration of antenatal steroids. There is accumulated evidence that magnesium sulfate ($MgSO_4$) reduces the severity and risk of cerebral palsy in surviving infants if adminis-tered when birth is anticipated before 32 weeks' gestational age, and hospitals that elect to use $MgSO_4$ are expected to develop specific guidelines for this indication. Maintenance therapy with tocolytics (i.e., beyond 48 hours of use) is ineffective for preventing preterm birth and improving neonatal outcome and is not recommended for this purpose. Antibiotics should not be used to prolong gestation or improve neonatal outcomes in women with preterm labor and intact membranes.

Additional Reading: Management of preterm labor. *ACOG Practice Bulletin* no. 127, 2012. From: http://www.acog.org/ Resources_And_Publications/Committee_Opinions_List

Category: Reproductive system

125. Which of the following statements is NOT true regarding IUDs?
A) The risk of unintended pregnancy in the 1st year of IU use is <1% and 1 year continuation rates for IUD use are near 80%.
B) IUDs can be placed at any time during the menstrual cycle, as long as pregnancy can be reasonably excluded.
C) The copper IUD is an effective method of emergency contraception when inserted within 5 days of unprotected intercourse.
D) Women with mucopurulent cervical discharge or known gonor-rhea or chlamydial infection should be treated before placement of an IUD.
E) The detection of actinomyces on a cervical Pap of a woman with an IUD in place necessitates IUD removal.

Answer and Discussion

The answer is E. The 1-year continuation rate for the copper IUD is 78%, and 80% for the levonorgestrel-containing IUD, and both types of IUDs have 1-year pregnancy rates of <1%. IUDs may be in-serted anytime during the menstrual cycle. Documentation of a nega-tive pregnancy test, preferably at least 2 weeks after last unprotected intercourse, is recommended. Insertion may be performed during menstruation to provide additional reassurance that the woman is not pregnant. The copper IUD is a more effective method of emer-gency contraception than oral emergency contraceptives and reduces the chance of pregnancy by 99% when taken within 5 days of un-protected intercourse. The effectiveness of levonorgestrel-containing IUD for emergency contraception has not been studied and is not recommended. The IUD should not be placed in a patient with documented chlamydial, gonococcal, or nonspecific mucopurulent cervicitis until treatment has been given. Routine screening for sexu-ally transmitted infections is recommended before IUD placement in high-risk women, but not in low-risk women. Screening may be performed on the same day as the IUD placement. Expectant man-agement is appropriate if actinomyces is detected on cervical cytol-ogy in asymptomatic patients with an IUD. This includes education regarding the small risk of actinomycosis.

Additional Reading: Guidelines for the use of long-acting revers-ible contraceptives. *Am Fam Physician.* 2012;85(4):403–404.

Category: Reproductive system

126. Which of the following is *not* an acceptable treatment for un-complicated gonoccocal infections of the cervix?
A) Cefixime 400 mg PO + azithromycin 1 g PO
B) Ceftriaxone 250 mg IM + azithromycin 1 g PO
C) Cefoxitin 2 g IM with probenecid 1 g PO + azithromycin 1 g PO
D) Ceftizoxime 500 mg IM + azithromycin 1 g PO
E) Cefotazime 500 mg IM + azithromycin 1 g PO

Answer and Discussion

The answer is A. Treatment for gonorrhea is challenging due to the ability of *N. Gonorrhea* to develop resistance to antibiotics. Quinolone-resistant *N. gonorrhoeae* strains are now widely dissemi-nated throughout the United States and the world. As of April 2007, quinolones are no longer recommended in the United States for the treatment of gonorrhea and associated conditions, such as PID. Cur-rently only single-dose injectable cephalosporins are recommended for the treatment of gonorrhea. Ceftriaxone 250 mg IM, as a single dose injection, provides high bactericidal levels in the blood, curing 99.2% of uncomplicated urogenital and anorectal and 98.9% of pha-ryngeal infections in published clinical trials. A 400-mg oral dose of cefixime does not provide as high, nor as sustained, a bactericidal level as that provided by the 250-mg dose of ceftriaxone and, as of 2012, are no longer recommended for treatment of gonorrhea. Single-dose injectable cephalosporin regimens (other than ceftriaxone 250 mg IM) that are safe and highly effective against uncomplicated urogenital and anorectal gonococcal infections include Cefoxitin 2 g IM (given with probenecid 1 g PO), Cefotazime 500 mg IM, and Ceftizoxime 500 mg IM. Patients infected with *N. gonorrhoeae* frequently are coinfected with *C. trachomatis*; this finding has led to the recommendation that patients treated for gonococcal infection also be treated routinely with a regimen that is effective against uncomplicated genital *C. trachomatis* infection. Because most gonococci in the United States are susceptible to doxycycline and azithromycin, routine cotreatment might also hin-der the development of antimicrobial-resistant *N. gonorrhoeae*.

Additional Reading: Gonococcal infections. Update to CDC's *Sexually Transmitted Diseases Treatment Guidelines,* 2010: oral cephalosporins no longer a recommended treatment for gono-coccal infections. *MMWR.* 2012;61(31):590–594.

Category: Reproductive system

127. Which of the following oral contraceptives is approved by the FDA for the treatment of acne vulgaris in women and adolescent girls?
A) Ethinyl estradiol–norelgestromin (OrthoEvra patch)
B) Ethinyl estradiol–levonorgestrel (Preven)
C) Norethindrone (Micronor)
D) Ethinyl estradiol–desogestrel (Desogen)
E) Ethinyl estradiol–norgestimate (Ortho Tri-Cyclen)

Answer and Discussion

The answer is E. Oral contraceptives may be a useful adjunctive therapy for all types of acne in women and adolescent girls. Sebum production is controlled by androgens, and oral contraceptives are known to decrease androgen levels by increasing sex-hormone-binding globulin levels, thus reducing the availability of biologically active free testosterone. The third-generation progestin norgesti-mate has lower intrinsic androgenicity than other progestins and is effective in treating moderate inflammatory acne. Ortho Tri-Cyclen is a triphasic combination of norgestimate and ethinyl estradiol that has been labeled by the FDA for the treatment of acne vulgaris in women and adolescent girls. Other contraceptive agents that contain norgestimate (Ortho-Cyclen) or desogestrel (Desogen) are also reasonable choices but are not FDA-approved for this indication. Two other FDA-approved OCPs for use in acne treatment are Estrostep (ethinyl estradiol and norethindrone) and YAZ (drospirenone/ethinyl estradiol). Two to 4 months of therapy may be required before improvement is noted, and relapses are common if medication is stopped.

Additional Reading: Oral contraceptive pills for acne: an overlooked option? *Pract Dermatol.* 2009;47–50.

Category: Reproductive system

128. When considering treatment for osteoporosis, which of the following is true?
A) Impaired eyesight is not a factor to consider in the decision to start medication.
B) Less than 30% of White women have an osteoporotic fracture at some point in their lifetime.
C) BMD testing is recommended in all women ages 65 and older, regardless of additional risk factors.
D) BMD testing should be performed only in postmenopausal women below age 65 who have two or more additional risk factors for osteoporosis (in addition to menopause).
E) Weight-bearing exercise should be avoided in postmenopausal women.

Answer and Discussion
The answer is C.

- BMD testing is recommended for all women ages 65 and older, regardless of additional risk factors. All women should be counseled about the risk factors for osteoporosis. Risk factors for osteoporotic fracture include personal history of fracture as an adult, history of fracture in a first-degree relative, white race, advanced age, female sex, dementia, poor health/frailty, cigarette smoking, low body weight (<127 lb [58 kg]), estrogen deficiency, lifelong low calcium intake, alcoholism, impaired eyesight despite adequate correction, recurrent falls, and inadequate physical activity.
- All postmenopausal women with a fracture be evaluated for osteoporosis using BMD testing to determine if the woman has osteoporosis and to determine disease severity. A measurement of the hip is the best predictor of hip fractures, and hip measurement can predict fractures at other sites as well.
- BMD testing should be considered in women below age 65 who have one or more additional risk factors for osteoporosis (in addition to menopause).
- All adults should be advised to consume an adequate intake of dietary calcium (1,200 mg/day, including supplements if necessary) and vitamin D (400 to 800 IU/day for persons at risk of deficiency).
- All patients should be counseled to avoid smoking and to limit alcohol intake to moderate levels. All patients should be encouraged to participate in regular weight-bearing and muscle-strengthening exercise to reduce the risk of falls and fractures.
- Physicians should consider osteoporosis treatment for all postmenopausal women who present with vertebral fractures or hip fractures.
- Bone mineral tests provide physicians with a T score expressed in standard deviation; the more negative the number, the greater the risk of fracture. Each standard deviation represents a 10% to 12% bone loss, and a T score of −2.5 indicates osteoporosis.

Additional Reading: Screening for osteoporosis. *The U.S. Preventive Services Task Force (USPSTF) recommendations on screening for osteoporosis; 2011.* From: http://www.uspreventiveservicestaskforce.org/uspstf/uspsoste.htm

Category: Reproductive system

129. Gestational hypertension is associated with
A) Systolic blood pressure >140 mm Hg and diastolic blood pressure >90 mm Hg
B) Proteinuria
C) Thrombocytopenia
D) Decreased urine output
E) Seizures

Answer and Discussion
The answer is A. Gestational hypertension is defined as systolic blood pressure that is greater than 140 mm Hg or diastolic blood pressure >90 mm Hg. Unlike preeclampsia, no proteinuria is noted and preeclampsia labs such as platelet count, hematocrit, creatinine, and liver transaminases should remain within normal limits. Edema is no longer one of the criteria for preeclampsia and can be present in either normal pregnancies or pregnancies with superimposed hypertensive disorders. Patients with mild gestational hypertension can be managed expectantly with rest and frequent visits for blood pressure and urine protein monitoring. Progression to preeclampsia can occur in 50% or more of patients with gestational hypertension, and gestational hypertension may become more severe, even in the absence of proteinuria. Consideration should be given to induction of labor with the development of preeclampsia or more severe range gestational hypertension, depending on gestational age of the fetus. Seizures are not generally seen in gestational hypertension with no superimposed preeclampsia.

Additional Reading: Hypertensive disorders of pregnancy. *Am Fam Physician.* 2008;78(1):93–100.

Category: Cardiovascular system

130. The treatment of choice for BV is
A) Metronidazole
B) Doxycycline
C) Ceftriaxone
D) Nystatin vaginal tablets
E) Vinegar douche

Answer and Discussion
The answer is A. BV is a condition that is caused by replacement of the normal hydrogen peroxide producing *Lactobacillus* sp. in the vagina by an overgrowth of anaerobic bacteria including *Prevotella* sp., *Mobiluncus* sp., *G. vaginalis*, *Ureaplasma*, and *Mycoplasma*. BV is associated with having multiple male or female partners, a new sex partner, douching, lack of condom use, and lack of vaginal lactobacilli; women who have never been sexually active can also be affected. The cause of the microbial alteration that characterizes BV is not fully understood, nor is whether BV results from acquisition of a sexually transmitted pathogen. The condition accounts for as many as 50% of all cases of vaginitis and is characterized by a gray, often frothy, foul-smelling vaginal discharge. When 10% to 20% potassium hydroxide is applied, the discharge gives off a characteristic amine-like fishy odor. Patients often report vaginal irritation and a foul-smelling discharge, though a majority of patients with BV are asymptomatic. Microscopic examination of the discharge shows "clue cells" (epithelial cells that are covered with coccobacilli on the cell walls). The vaginal secretion pH is >4.5. Treatment of choice is oral

or vaginal metronidazole. Topical 2% clindamycin cream can also be used. Cultures are not helpful because *Gardnerella* may be a normal inhabitant of the vagina. Women with BV are at increased risk for the acquisition of some STDs (e.g., HIV, *N. gonorrhoeae*, *C. trachomatis*, and HSV-2), complications after gynecologic surgery, pregnancy complications, and recurrence of BV. Treatment of male sex partners has not been beneficial in preventing the recurrence of BV.

> **Additional Reading:** Vaginitis: diagnosis and treatment. *Am Fam Physician.* 2011;83(7):807–815.

Category: Reproductive system

131. Which of the following statements about sexual intercourse and uncomplicated pregnancy is true?
A) Intercourse should be avoided until 36 weeks' gestation because of the risk of premature labor.
B) Intercourse should be avoided 2 weeks before the estimated date of confinement because of the risk of infection.
C) Intercourse is safe during pregnancy; however, orgasm should be avoided because of the risk of preterm labor.
D) Intercourse is not considered dangerous during normal pregnancy.
E) Intercourse should be avoided during pregnancy because of the risk for placental abruption.

Answer and Discussion
The answer is D. Sexual intercourse during pregnancy is generally considered safe as long as the mother has not had complications during pregnancy that would put the infant at risk (e.g., preterm labor, abnormal vaginal bleeding, PROM). Orgasm with uterine contractions does not induce labor; however, milk ejection may occur and is a normal response. In many cases, the woman has an increased desire for intercourse during pregnancy; however, other women may have a decrease in desire. Both responses are considered normal. Abstention from sexual intercourse was formerly recommended during the final months of pregnancy; however, it is no longer considered a risk in normal pregnancies.

> **Additional Reading:** Prenatal care: common concerns. *Williams Obstetrics,* 23rd ed. New York, NY: McGraw-Hill; 2010.

Category: Reproductive system

132. The vaginal ring contraceptive can be left in place for
A) 3 days
B) 1 week
C) 3 weeks
D) 3 months
E) 1 year

Answer and Discussion
The answer is C. After 3 weeks, the contraceptive vaginal ring is removed for 1 week, and a new ring is inserted. Withdrawal bleeding occurs during the ring-free week.

> **Additional Reading:** New contraceptive options. *Am Fam Physician.* 2004;69:853–860.

Category: Reproductive system

133. How long can the vaginal ring be out of the vagina before an additional form of contraception is necessary?
A) 30 minutes
B) 1 hour
C) 3 hours
D) 24 hours
E) 1 week

Answer and Discussion
The answer is C. If the ring is removed from the vagina for more than 3 hours, additional back-up contraception should be used until the ring has been back in place for 7 days.

> **Additional Reading:** Preventing gaps when switching contraceptives. *Am Fam Physician.* 2011;83(5):567–570.

Category: Reproductive system

> If a vaginal ring is removed from the vagina for more than 3 hours, additional back-up contraception should be used until the ring has been back in place for 7 days.

134. A hypertensive woman uses enalapril for her blood pressure management. She has excellent control. Which of the following oral contraceptives when used with enalapril can lead to hyperkalemia?
A) Ethinyl estradiol–norelgestromin
B) Ethinyl estradiol–levonorgestrel
C) Norethindrone
D) Ethinyl estradiol–drospirenone
E) Ethinyl estradiol–norgestimate

Answer and Discussion
The answer is D. Drospirenone has antimineralocorticoid activity and has been shown to decrease the water retention, negative affect, and appetite changes that are commonly associated with menstrual cycle changes. Serum potassium levels should be monitored when using this OCP in conjunction with other medicines that also raise potassium levels, because of the risk of developing hyperkalemia.

> **Additional Reading:** Contraception choices in women with underlying medical conditions. *Am Fam Physician.* 2010;82(6): 621–628.

Category: Cardiovascular system

135. The oral contraceptive levonorgestrel–ethinyl estradiol (Seasonale) is different from 28-day oral contraceptives due to having
A) Once-a-month dosing
B) Increased effectiveness
C) Higher adherence to correct usage
D) More days of active pills and fewer days of nonhormonal pills

Answer and Discussion
The answer is D. The extended-cycle levonorgestrel–ethinyl estradiol OCP regimen consists of 84 days of active pills and 7 days of nonhormonal pills, prescribed as a 91-day extended-cycle pack (e.g., Seasonale, Seasonique, and Lo-Seasonique). These OCPs may be especially desirable for women who do not want monthly periods, as this regimen results in only 4 menses per year. Fewer withdrawal bleeds per year, with fewer hormone-free intervals may benefit women with estrogen withdrawal symptoms, dysmenorrheal, or endometriosis. No differences in effectiveness, safety, and adherence have been shown between extended cycle versus 28-day cycle. Lybrel is a continuous-cycle levonorgestrel–ethinyl estradiol pill taken daily throughout the year with no hormone-free interval to induce a scheduled withdrawal bleed. Women on Lybrel often have initial unscheduled spotting, then ultimately amenorrhea.

> **Additional Reading:** The new extended-cycle levonorgestrel-ethinyl estradiol oral contraceptives. *Clin Med Insights: Reprod Health.* 2011;549–554.

Category: Reproductive system

136. A 15-year-old girl presents to the office complaining that she has not had a period in 3 months. The young girl emphatically states that she is not pregnant, and her mother assures you she is not pregnant. The most appropriate initial test would be

A) Urine pregnancy test
B) Thyroid function test
C) Serum prolactin level
D) Progesterone challenge test
E) Serum cortisol level

Answer and Discussion

The answer is A. Abnormal menses are normal in the immediate pubertal period. Lack of menses for 3 to 4 months presents no concern if there is no possibility that the girl is pregnant. However, the history given by young, sexually active girls often cannot be trusted. The first step in the evaluation of amenorrhea is to determine if the patient is pregnant. Other tests for the workup of amenorrhea include a serum prolactin level and sensitive thyroid-stimulating hormone. If these tests are normal and the pregnancy test is negative, a progesterone challenge test can be performed. In this test, medroxyprogesterone acetate is given for 7 to 10 days, and withdrawal bleeding is usually induced after administration. If withdrawal bleeding occurs (positive test), the diagnosis of anovulation can be made. If no withdrawal bleeding occurs (negative test), the differential diagnosis includes PCOS or an adrenal enzyme deficiency that leads to an excess of progesterone. If amenorrhea continues on a regular basis and the patient is diagnosed with anovulation, a daily dose of medroxyprogesterone can be prescribed for the first 10 days of alternative months. Pathologic amenorrhea is divided into primary amenorrhea (absence of menses before the age of 16) and secondary amenorrhea (absence of menses for 3 months or more in patients who have had previous periods).

Additional Reading: Rakel R. Amenorrhea. *Textbook of Family Medicine,* 6th ed. Philadelphia, PA: Saunders/Elsevier; 2007.

Category: Reproductive system

137. Which of the following statements about postpartum depression is true?

A) Postpartum depression usually occurs 9 to 12 months after delivery.
B) Social support has little impact on the development of postpartum depression.
C) Those with obstetric complications are at increased risk.
D) Those affected are at increased risk for postpartum depression with subsequent pregnancies.
E) Patients who have postpartum depression have no higher risk of developing depression in later years when compared with the general population.

Answer and Discussion

The answer is D. Mild postpartum depression (also referred to as the "baby blues") is usually seen within the first few days after delivery. The incidence ranges up to 25%, and those with poor social support are more commonly affected. There appears to be no relationship with obstetric complications. Symptoms vary but are usually mild and self-limited. In most cases, reassurance that these feelings are common is all that is needed. In more severe cases, in which the mother's symptoms last for extended periods or if the mother shows a lack of interest in the newborn, has suicidal or homicidal thoughts or gestures, or shows psychotic behavior, further therapy (including medication and psychotherapy) may be needed. Women who are affected with severe postpartum depression are at risk for development of further depressive episodes and recurrent postpartum depression with subsequent pregnancies.

Additional Reading: Postpartum major depression. *Am Fam Physician.* 2010;82(8):926–933.

Category: Psychogenic

138. Prenatal vitamins are important during pregnancy because they help to reduce the incidence of neural tube defects. Which of the following is responsible for this protective effect?

A) Calcium
B) Iron
C) Folic acid
D) Vitamin C
E) Vitamin B_{12}

Answer and Discussion

The answer is C. Prenatal vitamins are recommended for pregnant women when dietary intake does not satisfy nutritional needs (multiple gestations, drug abusers, vegetarians, epileptics, and women with hemoglobinopathies) and in those who are planning pregnancy. The supplementation of iron during pregnancy is needed to prevent severe anemia and is usually accomplished by the use of prenatal vitamins. The following are the recommended requirements for pregnant women:

- Calcium 1,200 to 1,500 mg/day
- Iron 30 mg/day
- Folic acid at least 0.4 mg/day

The use of prenatal vitamins before pregnancy can supply adequate folic acid, which has been shown to help prevent neural tube defects. Excessive use of vitamin A supplements should be avoided because of a small number of case reports that suggest a link to birth defects. Furthermore, if the infant is breast-fed, the use of prenatal vitamins for the mother is usually encouraged.

Additional Reading: Recommendations for preconception care. *Am Fam Physician.* 2007;76(3):397–400.

Category: Reproductive system

139. Which of the following statements is true regarding BV during pregnancy?

A) Studies have shown that BV is associated with adverse pregnancy outcomes.
B) Symptomatic women should be treated.
C) Routine screening is recommended for all pregnant patients.
D) Oral metronidazole should be avoided in pregnancy due to potential teratogenic effects.
E) Vaginal clindamycin or vaginal metronidazole are both good choices for treatment of BV in pregnancy.

Answer and Discussion

The answer is B. Treatment is recommended for all pregnancy women with symptomatic BV. Although BV in pregnancy is associated with a variety of adverse peripartum outcomes such as preterm rupture of membranes, preterm labor, preterm delivery, intra-amniotic infection, and postpartum endometritis, the only proven benefit of treatment is a reduction in signs/symptoms of vaginal infection. Efforts have been made to assess the benefits of screening for BV in women at high risk for preterm delivery and whether the treatment of asymptomatic BV in pregnancy women who are at low risk for preterm delivery reduces adverse pregnancy events, but neither intervention has consistently been shown to yield improved outcomes. Recommended antibiotic regimens for treating symptomatic pregnant women with BV include

1. metronidazole 500 mg orally twice a day for 7 days
2. metronidazole 250 mg orally three times a day for 7 days
3. clindamycin 300 mg orally twice a day for 7 days

Regardless of the antimicrobial agent used to treat pregnant women, oral therapy is preferred because of the possibility of subclinical upper genital tract infection. Providers should also be aware that intravaginal clindamycin cream might be associated with adverse outcomes if used in the latter half of pregnancy. Multiple studies have shown no documented increase in teratogenic effects in newborns with a history of maternal metronidazole use in pregnancy.

Additional Reading: Diseases characterized by vaginal discharge. *CDC Sexually Transmitted Disease Treatment Guidelines*; 2010.

Category: Reproductive system

140. A 65-year-old woman presents to your office concerning about uterine prolapse. During her examination, you note the cervix is visible outside of the vaginal introitus. The uterus is not visible. Based on your findings, you classify her as having _____.
A) First-degree prolapse
B) Second-degree prolapse
C) Third-degree prolapse
D) No prolapse

Answer and Discussion
The answer is B. Uterine prolapse is classified by degree. In first-degree uterine prolapse, the cervix is visible when the perineum is depressed. In second-degree prolapse, the cervix is visible outside of the vaginal introitus while the uterine fundus remains inside. In third-degree prolapse, or *procidentia*, the entire uterus is outside of the vaginal introitus. Uterine prolapse is associated with urinary incontinence, vaginitis, cystitis, and, possibly, uterine malignancy.

Additional Reading: Pelvic organ prolapse. *Am Fam Physician.* 2010;81(9):1111–1117.

Category: Reproductive system

141. The most common cause of first-trimester spontaneous abortion is
A) Incompetent cervix
B) Chromosomal abnormalities
C) Increased maternal age
D) Inadequate levels of progesterone during the luteal phase
E) Lupus anticoagulant

Answer and Discussion
The answer is B. Up to 15% of recognized pregnancies end in miscarriage, and as many as 80% of miscarriages occur in the first trimester, with chromosomal abnormalities (usually autosomal trisomies which are incompatible with life) as the leading cause. Other factors that may contribute to spontaneous abortion include maternal smoking, increased maternal age, maternal illness, incompetent cervix, lupus anticoagulant, and inadequate levels of progesterone during the luteal phase of the menstrual cycle. In general, no interventions have been proven to prevent miscarriage; occasionally, women can modify their risk factors or receive treatment for relevant medical conditions. Patients with miscarriage usually report vaginal bleeding and uterine cramps. Unless products of conception are seen during pelvic exam, the diagnosis of miscarriage is made with ultrasonography and, when ultrasonography is not available or is nondiagnostic, with measurement of β-hCG levels. Management options for early pregnancy loss

include expectant management, medical management with misoprostol, and uterine aspiration with a manual vacuum device. Expectant management is highly effective for the treatment of incomplete abortion, whereas misoprostol and uterine aspiration are more effective for the management of anembryonic gestation and embryonic demise. Misoprostol in a dose of 800 mcg administered vaginally is effective and well tolerated. Compared with dilation and curettage in the operating room, uterine aspiration is the preferred procedure for early pregnancy loss; aspiration is equally safe, quicker to perform, more cost-effective, and amenable to use in the primary care setting. All management options are equally safe; thus, patient preference should guide treatment choice.

Additional Reading: Office management of early pregnancy loss. *Am Fam Physician.* 2011;84(1):75–82.

Category: Reproductive system

142. The presence of sterile pyuria in a sexually active individual is most commonly associated with
A) Gonorrhea
B) Syphilis
C) Chlamydia
D) Herpes genitalis
E) HPV

Answer and Discussion
The answer is C. Chlamydia is an STD that is caused by *Chlamydia trachomatis*. Approximately 50% of nongonococcal urethritis and most cases of cervicitis are caused by chlamydia. Men usually report discomfort associated with the urethra, dysuria, or a clear to mucopurulent discharge that occurs 1 to 3 weeks after exposure. Most women are asymptomatic, although they may report dysuria, pelvic discomfort with dyspareunia, and vaginal discharge that may have a clear to yellow mucopurulent appearance. Diagnosis is made with immunologic studies performed on urine; vaginal, penile, or cervical secretions; or culture. The presence of sterile pyuria in a sexually active individual should raise the suspicion of chlamydia. The presence of gonorrhea must be ruled out and patients should be treated for gonorrhea if chlamydia is found, and vice versa. Single-dose therapy with azithromycin 1 g orally is as effective as a 7-day course of doxycycline, and both are the primary recommended regimens for treatment of chlamydia infection. Doxycycline is less expensive, but azithromycin may be cost-beneficial and associated with higher compliance because it provides single-dose, directly observed therapy. Erythromycin and quinolones, including levofloxin or ofloxacin, are alternative regiments used to treat *C. trachomatis*. Erythromycin is less efficacious than azithromycin and doxycycline, and its adverse gastrointestinal effects may decrease patient compliance. Ofloxacin and levofloxin are as effective as the recommended regimens but offer no dosing or cost advantages. Doxycycline and fluoroquinolones are contraindicated in pregnant women.

Additional Reading: Chlamydial infections. *CDC Sexually Transmitted Disease Treatment Guidelines;* 2010.

Category: Reproductive system

143. Treatment for vaginismus includes which of the following?
A) Desensitization therapy with continued regular intercourse until it becomes comfortable
B) Treatment with muscle relaxants
C) Kegel exercises
D) Dilation with vaginal probes
E) Transcutaneous electrical nerve-stimulation treatment

Answer and Discussion

The answer is D. Vaginismus is a condition that is characterized by involuntary spasm of the lower vaginal muscles, resulting in an unconscious effort to prevent penile penetration. Causes include psychiatric factors, local trauma, infection, or mechanical factors, including vaginal stenosis or dryness. Women with vaginismus frequently have a history of sexual abuse or other sexual trauma in their past. Women report extreme discomfort with attempts at penetration. Treatment involves correction of reversible causes, psychological and sexual counseling, and gradual and repeated attempts at vaginal dilation with vaginal or (shorter) rectal probes. Treatment can be continued by the patient at home in a private environment after the appropriate technique is learned. Intercourse can be attempted once the patient is able to tolerate larger dilators without discomfort. Communication with the patient's partner often is helpful in overcoming the patient's fears.

> **Additional Reading:** Vaginismus. In: Domino F, ed. *The 5-Minute Clinical Consult.* Philadelphia, PA: Lippincott Williams and Wilkins; 2014.

Category: Reproductive system

144. Which of the following is *not* useful in treating premenstrual syndrome (PMS)?
A) Vitamin B$_6$
B) Selective serotonin reuptake inhibitors
C) Calcium and Vitamin D supplementation
D) Decreased intake of caffeine, salt, and refined sugar

Answer and Discussion

The answer is D. Premenstrual syndrome is defined as recurrent moderate psychological and physical symptoms that occur during the luteal phase of menses and resolve with menstruation. It affects 20% to 32% of premenopausal women. Women with premenstrual dysphoric disorder (PMDD) experience affective or somatic symptoms that cause severe dysfunction in social or occupational realms. The disorder affects 3% to 8% of premenopausal women. Proposed etiologies include increased sensitivity to normal cycling levels of estrogen and progesterone, increased aldosterone and plasma renin activity, and neurotransmitter abnormalities, particularly serotonin. The Daily Record of Severity of Problems is one tool with which women may self-report the presence and severity of premenstrual symptoms that correlate with the criteria for premenstrual dysphoric disorder. Symptom relief is the goal for treatment of premenstrual syndrome and premenstrual dysphoric disorder. There is limited evidence to support the use of chasteberry, calcium, vitamin D, vitamin B$_6$, supplementation, and insufficient evidence to support cognitive behavior therapy or other oral supplements such as ginkgo, saffron, St. John's wort, soy, or vitamin E. Serotonergic antidepressants (citalopram, escitalopram, fluoxetine, sertraline, venlafaxine) are first-line pharmacologic therapy and can be used daily, with consideration for an increased dose during the luteal phase.

> **Additional Reading:** Premenstrual syndrome and premenstrual dysphoric disorder. *Am Fam Physician.* 2011;84 (8):918–924.

Category: Psychogenic

145. Which of the following statements is true regarding postcoital emergency contraception?
A) Birth defects often occur if the method is unsuccessful.
B) Emergency contraception is 95% effective.
C) Emergency contraception is most effective if administered within 72 hours.
D) Ulipristal acetate (Ella®) is less effective than levonorgestrel taken as a single 1.5-mg pill (Plan B One-Step™).

Answer and Discussion

The answer is C. Women should be offered the option to use emergency contraception to prevent pregnancy after known or suspected failure of birth control or after unprotected intercourse. Emergency contraception has been an off-label use of OCPs since the 1960s. Products including the Yuzpe regimen (Preven) and levonorgestrel (Plan B) were marketed in the United States after 1998, but had been available in Europe for years before that. The first Plan B option consists of two tablets, each containing 0.75 mg of levonorgestrel. (This amount differs from the 0.075 mg dose of norgestrel in certain progestin-only pills.) Consensus emerged that the levonorgestrel-containing emergency contraception should be given in preference to the Yuzpe regimen where available because it was shown to be more effective and have fewer side effects. Plan B One-Step™ simplified the original Plan B two-tablet regimen to administer a single 1.5-mg dose of levonorgestrel, which was shown to be equally effective emergency contraception without causing an increase in side effects. A third approved method of emergency contraception is the insertion of a copper-containing IUD. Emergency contraception is about 75% to 85% effective. It is most effective when initiated within 72 hours after unprotected intercourse. The mechanism of action may vary, depending on the day of the menstrual cycle on which treatment is started. Ulipristal acetate, a selective progesterone receptor modulator, when taken as a single 30-mg dose, is a new, safe, and effective emergency contraceptive that can be used from the first day and up to 5 days following unprotected intercourse. During clinical development, ulipristal acetate has been shown to be more effective than levonorgestrel in delaying or inhibiting ovulation. A recent meta-analysis of two randomized clinical trials showed ulipristal acetate to have a pregnancy risk 42% lower than levonorgestrel up to 72 hours and 65% lower in the first 24 hours following unprotected intercourse. Moreover, when taken beyond 72 hours, significantly more pregnancies were prevented with ulipristal acetate than with levonorgestrel. Side effects are mild and similar to those seen with levonorgestrel. Despite the large number of women who have received emergency contraception, there have been no reports of major adverse outcomes. If a woman becomes pregnant after using emergency contraception, she may be reassured about the lack of negative effects emergency contraception has on fetal development.

> **Additional Reading:** Update on emergency contraception. *Adv Ther.* 2011;28(2):87–90.

Category: Reproductive system

146. Oligohydramnios (in the absence of ruptured membranes) is NOT correlated with an increased risk for
A) Intrauterine growth restriction
B) Fetal gastrointestinal abnormalities
C) Induction of labor
D) Meconium-stained amniotic fluid
E) Abnormal FHR patterns

Answer and Discussion

The answer is B. *Oligohydramnios* is defined as an amount of amniotic fluid that is less than what is expected (i.e., <5th percentile) for gestational age. Amniotic fluid is usually quantified with ultrasound determination, by measuring and adding together four-quadrant vertical fluid pocket measurements to obtain the amniotic fluid index (AFI). An AFI of <5 at any gestational age is also commonly used as a definition for oligohydramnios, though there is some evidence that using gestational age-specific calculations are more closely associated with perinatal morbidity. Oligohydramnios seen early in pregnancy is a poor prognostic sign. Pregnancies that have oligohydramnios from an early gestational age have an increased risk of limb contractures and pulmonary hypoplasia due to restriction in movement of the developing fetus. Oligohydramnios at all gestational ages are associated with underlying renal congenital abnormalities of the fetus that result in a lack of adequate amniotic fluid. Fetal gastrointestinal abnormalities that result in the inability of the fetus to swallow amniotic fluid more often result in polyhydramnios, rather than oligohydramnios. Oligohydramnios is more common in postterm pregnancies and also in association with growth-restricted fetuses and is a frequent indication for induction of labor. Meconium-stained fluid and abnormalities of the fetal heart tracing due to either cord compression or utero-placental insufficiency are also seen more often in patients with oligohydramnios.

Additional Reading: Assessing the optimal definition of oligohydramnios associated with adverse neonatal outcomes. *J Ultrasound Med.* 2011;30(3):303–307.

Category: Reproductive system

147. A 22-year-old woman is diagnosed with primary syphilis. She has no allergies and is otherwise healthy. The drug of choice is
A) Oral penicillin
B) Oral azithromycin
C) Intramuscular ceftriaxone
D) Parenteral penicillin G
E) Oral ciprofloxacin

Answer and Discussion

The answer is D. Syphilis is a systemic disease caused by the sexual transmission of *Treponema pallidum*. It can occur as primary, secondary, or tertiary disease. Primary disease presents with one or more painless ulcers or chancres at the inoculation site. Secondary disease manifestations include rash and adenopathy. Cardiac, neurologic, ophthalmic, auditory, or gummatous lesions characterize tertiary infections. Latent disease may be detected by serologic testing, without the presence of signs and symptoms. Early latent disease is defined as disease acquired within the preceding year. All other cases of latent syphilis are considered late latent disease or disease of unknown duration. Penicillin G, administered parenterally, is the preferred drug for treating all stages of syphilis. The preparation used (i.e., benzathine, aqueous procaine, or aqueous crystalline), the dosage, and the length of treatment depend on the stage and clinical manifestations of the disease. For primary, secondary, and early latent syphilis, benzathine penicillin G 2.4 million units IM in a single dose is the treatment of choice. Selection of the appropriate penicillin preparation is important because *T. pallidum* can reside in sequestered sites (e.g., the CNS and aqueous humor) that are poorly accessed by some forms of penicillin. Combinations of benzathine penicillin, procaine penicillin, and oral penicillin preparations are not considered appropriate for the treatment of syphilis. Pregnant patients with syphilis who are allergic to penicillin should be desensitized and treated with penicillin as well.

Additional Reading: Diseases characterized by genital, anal, or perianal ulcers. *CDC Sexually Transmitted Disease Treatment Guidelines;* 2010.

Category: Reproductive system

148. Rubella infection during pregnancy
A) Rarely affects the fetus
B) Has its most devastating effects during the third trimester
C) Is associated with cataracts, cardiac defects, and cleft palate
D) Is associated with neural tube defects
E) Can be prevented with immunization during the pregnancy

Answer and Discussion

The answer is C. Rubella infection ("German measles") during pregnancy can have devastating effects on the fetus. They are most severe for those fetuses that are affected during the first trimester. Clinical findings of congenital rubella include cataracts, blindness, and cardiac abnormalities (including patent ductus arteriosus, pulmonary valve stenosis, and ventricular septal defect). Other findings include pigmented birthmarks, hemolytic anemia, cleft palate, deafness, mental retardation, cerebral palsy, and fetal death. Treatment is aimed at prevention by immunizing all prospective mothers. The vaccine should be given at least 3 months before conception because of the live attenuated vaccine.

Additional Reading: Rubella (German measles) vaccination. From: http://www.cdc.gov/vaccines/vpd-vac/rubella/default.htm#clinical

Category: Reproductive system

149. The most frequently reported symptom in women with vulvar cancer is
A) Bleeding
B) Dyspareunia
C) Vaginal dryness
D) Itching
E) Vaginal discharge

Answer and Discussion

The answer is A. The most frequently reported symptom of vulvar cancer is vaginal bleeding. Other common presenting symptoms include vulvar itching, discharge, dysuria, and pain. The most common presenting sign of vulvar cancer is a vulvar lump or mass. Rarely, patients present with a large, fungating mass.

Additional Reading: Vulvar malignancy. In: Domino F, ed. *The 5-Minute Clinical Consult*. Philadelphia, PA: Lippincott Williams and Wilkins; 2014.

Category: Reproductive system

150. A 70-year-old woman presents with severe vulvar itching of several months duration. She has been unable to have intercourse due to vulvar discomfort. On exam, the surface of her vulvar area appears thin and whitened, with attenuation of the labia minor and narrowing of the introitus. A vulvar punch biopsy shows lichen sclerosus. Appropriate treatment at this point includes
A) Testosterone cream
B) Oral estrogen-replacement therapy
C) Topical estrogen cream
D) 1% hydrocortisone cream
E) High-potency corticosteroid ointment

Answer and Discussion

The answer is E. Lichen sclerosus is a type of vulvar nonneoplastic epithelial disorder (VNED) that is characterized by intense vulvar itching and can affect men and women of all ages, but it manifests most commonly in postmenopausal women. Initially, the skin may appear white, thickened, and excoriated, with edema and resorption of the labia minora. As the disease progresses, the skin loses pigmentation and becomes very thin and wrinkled, classically referred to as a "cigarette paper" appearance. With further progression, anatomic features may become severely distorted as the clitoris becomes buried under the clitoral hood, the labia minora disappear, and the introitus narrows. This architectural distortion can be partly responsible for dyspareunia and dysuria. Definitive diagnosis of lichen sclerosus depends on the histology of biopsied tissue. Moreover, it is important to identify and biopsy any thickened areas of epithelium in patients with lichen sclerosus because such acanthotic epidermal areas can be suggestive of squamous cell hyperplasia. Patients with lichen sclerosus—especially those with squamous cell hyperplasia—have an increased risk of vulvar malignancy and should be monitored accordingly. The increased risk of developing squamous cell carcinoma is approximately 5% in patients with lichen sclerosus. Lichen sclerosus is treated with potent topical steroids to alleviate symptoms, prevent architectural damage, and reverse histologic changes. The recommended regimen for lichen sclerosus begins with a high-potency corticosteroid, (e.g., clobetasol propionate 0.05% ointment [Temovate]) used daily until all active lesions have resolved (usually in 2 to 3 months), then tapered to once or twice per week. In the past, topical testosterone and progesterone were accepted therapies for lichen sclerosus, but recent clinical trials have shown that clobetasol is more effective than testosterone and that 2% testosterone is no more effective than petrolatum ointment.

> **Additional Reading:** Non-neoplastic epithelial disorders of the vulva. *Am Fam Physician.* 2008;77(3):321–326.

> Category: Integumentary

151. A major risk factor for shoulder dystocia includes which of the following?
A) Young maternal age
B) Gestational diabetes
C) Precipitous delivery
D) Preterm delivery
E) Thin body habitus

Answer and Discussion

The answer is B. Shoulder dystocia occurs in 1 of 300 deliveries. Risk factors include diabetes, postterm pregnancy, obesity, previous shoulder dystocia, prolonged second stage of labor, advanced maternal age, and multiparity.

Risk of shoulder dystocia is related to the size of the fetus:

- Less than 3,000 g = 0%
- 3,001 to 3,500 g = 0.3%
- 3,501 to 4,000 g = 1.0%
- 4,001 to 4,500 g = 5.4%
- Greater than 4,500 g = 19%

Warning signs for shoulder dystocia include a prolonged second stage of labor and retraction of the fetal head tightly against the vaginal introitus after delivery of the head. Complications include a fractured clavicle or humerus, brachial plexus injuries, anoxic brain injuries, and even death of the fetus.

> **Additional Reading:** Shoulder dystocia. *Williams Obstetrics,* 23rd ed. New York, NY: McGraw-Hill; 2010.

> Category: Reproductive system

152. Which of the following tumor markers can be used to follow the effectiveness of ovarian cancer treatment?
A) α-Fetoprotein
B) Carcinoembryonic antigen
C) CA 125
D) β-hCG
E) None of the above

Answer and Discussion

The answer is C. Ovarian carcinoma usually affects women in their 50s. It is the fifth most common cancer that affects women, and approximately 25,000 new cases are diagnosed yearly in the United States. Because of the difficulty in diagnosis, most cases have metastasized outside the pelvis at the time of diagnosis; therefore, prognosis is usually poor. Risk factors include a positive family history, *BRCA1* gene mutation on chromosome 17, white race, high-fat diet, asbestos or talc exposure, and nulliparity or low parity. The use of oral contraceptives may be protective. Any ovarian mass ≥ 5 cm deserves careful follow-up. Postmenopausal women usually have atrophic ovaries that are not palpable; thus, any palpable ovary in a postmenopausal woman deserves further investigation. The types of tumors are divided histologically into those that arise from the ovarian epithelium:

- Serous cystadenocarcinomas (most common)
- Clear cell carcinomas
- Mucinous cystadenocarcinomas
- Endometrioid tumors
- Celioblastomas (Brenner tumors)
- Tumors not classified

In addition, tumors arise from germ cells and stroma, such as

- Sertoli–Leydig cell tumors
- Malignant teratomas
- Dysgerminomas
- Granulosa-theca cell tumors

Patients may report lower abdominal fullness or discomfort, gastrointestinal complaints, abnormal vaginal bleeding, or pelvic pain. Diagnosis is usually aided with ultrasound or CT examination. Treatment of ovarian carcinoma depends on the staging and cell type but involves surgical excision and in some cases chemotherapy or radiation. Metastasis is usually to lung or bone. The blood test CA 125 can be used to follow patients for recurrence of tumor after surgery or the response to chemotherapy but is not a suitable screening test. Benign masses that affect the ovary include functional cysts, which usually resolve within 2 months, and benign cystic teratoma (dermoid tumor), which may contain hair follicles or tooth formations. Another condition that may be seen with ovarian masses is Meigs' syndrome, which is associated with ascites, right hydrothorax, and benign fibroma or thecoma.

> **Additional Reading:** Serum biomarkers for evaluation of an adnexal mass for epithelial carcinoma of the ovary, fallopian tube, or peritoneum. In: Basow DS, ed. *UpToDate.* Waltham, MA: UpToDate; 2013.

> Category: Reproductive system

153. Which laboratory test would best support lung maturity in a fetus whose mother has shown signs of premature labor?
A) Lecithin–sphingomyelin (L/S) ratio of 1.75
B) L/S ratio of 1.5
C) Absence of phosphatidylinositol
D) Absence of phosphatidylglycerol (PG)
E) L/S ratio of 2.2 with a positive PG level

Answer and Discussion

The answer is E. Premature birth can result in severe lung-related problems (i.e., RDS) secondary to inadequate lung development. A number of different medications have been advocated to improve lung maturation. Currently, the use of antenatal corticosteroids reduces mortality and the incidence of RDS and intraventricular hemorrhage in new preterm infants. They are typically administered between 24 and 34 weeks. The benefits usually peak at 24 hours and continue for 7 days. Treatment consists of betamethasone given in two intramuscular doses 24 hours apart. Antenatal steroids should be administered unless immediate delivery is anticipated. Tests for lung maturity include the lecithin/sphingomyelin (L:S) ratio, lamellar body count (LBC), and detection of PG. The levels are measured by obtaining amniotic fluid via amniocentesis. RDS is rare if the L/S ratio is >2 and PG is present. If the L/S ratio is <2 but PG is present, RDS develops in <5% of infants. LBCs are a direct measurement of surfactant production by the fetal lungs, and testing for these is less labor intensive and therefore faster than the L:S ratio, which is often done simultaneously with PG testing. LBCs that are less than 30,000/mL are considered to represent underlying fetal lung immaturity, whereas LBCs greater than 50,000/mL are associated with positive fetal lung maturity. LBCs in the range of 30,000 to 50,000/mL are inconclusive, so some centers do LBCs as an initial screen, and if results are very high or very low, a diagnosis of fetal lung maturity or immaturity is made, and if the LBC is indeterminant due to falling in the middle range, the lengthier L:S and PG testing is then done.

Additional Reading: Assessment of fetal lung maturity. In: Basow DS, ed. *UpToDate*. Waltham, MA: UpToDate; 2013.

Category: Reproductive system

> RDS is rare if the lecithin–sphingomyelin ratio (L/S ratio) is greater than 2 and PG is present.

154. Which of the following is true regarding ovarian cancer?
A) Symptoms often involve a combination of gastrointestinal and genitourinary symptoms.
B) It is often diagnosed at an early and treatable stage.
C) Effective screening strategies exist.
D) Transvaginal ultrasound and CA-125 measurements are of little diagnostic value.

Answer and Discussion

The answer is A. No effective screening test exists for ovarian cancer. Ovarian cancer is often detected at an advanced stage, with 5-year survival of 20% to 30%. The symptoms most commonly reported in patients with ovarian cancer include bloating, increased abdominal size, abdominal or pelvic pain, and urinary tract symptoms, although these are also common in women with benign masses. Symptoms tend to be more severe, more frequent, and of shorter duration in women with malignant masses than in women with benign masses. Women with ovarian cancer also are more likely to present with a combination of symptoms. Women with persistent and progressive symptoms should be evaluated with physical exam (including pelvic exam), transvaginal ultrasound, and CA-125 level. CA-125 levels can be elevated from a variety of nonmalignant conditions, including leimyomas and endometriosis, and CA-125 levels can be normal in early-stage ovarian cancer, but a very elevated CA-125 level in conjunction with a solid mass by ultrasound is highly suggestive of ovarian cancer, particularly in postmenopausal women.

Additional Reading: The role of the obstetrician-gynecologist in the early detection of epithelial ovarian cancer. *ACOG Committee Opinion* no. 477, 2011. From: http://www.acog.org/Resources_And_Publications/Committee_Opinions_List

Category: Reproductive system

155. A 61-year-old woman is found to have a new 2.5-cm unilocular ovarian cyst (confirmed by ultrasound) during her routine well-woman examination. Her CA-125 level is normal. Appropriate management at this time includes
A) Serial ultrasounds and CA-125 levels
B) Laparoscopic surgical removal
C) Hysteroscopic evaluation and biopsy
D) Cone radiation ablation
E) No further monitoring is necessary

Answer and Discussion

The answer is A. In postmenopausal women, most ovarian cysts <50 mm in diameter are benign and can be managed safely by regular monitoring of cyst size and serum CA-125 level.

Additional Reading: Evaluation of ovarian cysts. *Am Fam Physician*. 2011;84(3).

Category: Reproductive system

156. Which of the following statements about striae distensae (stretch marks) is true?
A) They usually respond to topical corticosteroids.
B) They rarely fade after pregnancy.
C) They may be related to excessive corticosteroids that are produced during pregnancy.
D) The condition is secondary to excessive weight gain (>40 lb) during pregnancy.
E) None of the above.

Answer and Discussion

The answer is C. Striae distensae, also known as striae gravidarum (stretch marks), are abnormal skin findings that are noted with varying degree during pregnancy. They affect up to 50% of pregnant women. Typically they are initially erythematous, pink or purple, and slightly raised to form ridges. They can occur in different areas but are usually found associated with the abdomen, breast, or hips. The cause of stretch marks was once believed to be excessive stretching of the skin; however, more recently it has been thought that they are secondary to excessive corticosteroids produced endogenously during pregnancy, combined with the body changes that occur with pregnancy. Excessive weight gain is not the reason for striae development. Unfortunately, there is no effective treatment for stretch marks. They usually fade after pregnancy and are barely noticeable.

Additional Reading: Common skin conditions during pregnancy. *Am Fam Physician*. 2007;75(2):211–218.

Category: Integumentary

157. At what month during pregnancy does the mother's appendix move upward to a level above the iliac crest?

A) Third month
B) Sixth month
C) Ninth month
D) The appendix does not change location.
E) When the fetal head engages in the pelvis

Answer and Discussion

The answer is B. Because of the normal changes during pregnancy, such as leukocytosis, nausea, vomiting, anorexia, and abdominal discomfort, the diagnosis of appendicitis may be difficult. The condition occurs with equal frequency during each trimester of pregnancy. As the sixth month approaches, the appendix moves upward, above the iliac crest. The risk for perforation is particularly increased in the third trimester. With perforation, the perinatal risk is increased. Complications of appendectomy include premature labor and wound infection. The differential diagnosis includes placental abruption, round ligament pain, acute pyelonephritis, renal colic, and cholecystitis.

> **Additional Reading:** Acute appendicitis in pregnancy. In: Basow DS, ed. *UpToDate.* Waltham, MA: UpToDate; 2013.

> **Category:** Gastroenterology system

158. An increase in blood pressure that is seen with oral contraceptive use is

A) Rarely a problem in patients with underlying hypertension
B) More common in women with a positive family history for hypertension
C) Not associated with increased age of the patient
D) Related to a permanent increase in blood pressure despite discontinuation of the drug
E) An indication to begin antihypertensive therapy

Answer and Discussion

The answer is B. A slight increase in blood pressure (systolic, 5 to 6 mm Hg; diastolic, 1 to 2 mm Hg) is expected in some women who take oral contraceptives. In fact, hypertension is five to six times more likely to develop in women who use oral contraceptives than in those who do not use them. Women who are older or who have a positive family history for hypertension and those using oral contraceptives for longer durations are at increased risk. Blood pressure increases may occur within weeks; however, it may not be noted for months or even years after starting medication. Discontinuation of oral contraceptives in most patients allows the blood pressure to decrease to normal levels, and most patients will not require antihypertensive therapy. Patients should be seen for a blood pressure check within 3 months after the initiation of the contraceptive. If significant increases occur, oral contraception medication should be discontinued. Underlying preexisting hypertension is a relative contraindication for oral contraceptive use.

> **Additional Reading:** Contraception choices in women with underlying medical conditions. *Am Fam Physician.* 2010;82(6): 621–628.

> **Category:** Cardiovascular system

159. Which of the following is an independent risk factor for the development of vulvar cancer?

A) Diabetes
B) Hypertension
C) Obesity
D) Syphilis
E) HPV

Answer and Discussion

The answer is E. Vulvar intraepithelial neoplasia (VIN) is clearly a premalignant finding and is associated with HPV infection, particularly subtypes 16 and 18. Hypertension, diabetes mellitus, and obesity have been found to coexist in up to 25% of patients, although they are not considered independent risk factors. In the past, syphilis and other granulomatous diseases have been associated with vulvar cancer.

> **Additional Reading:** Vulvar malignancy. In: Domino F, ed. *The 5-Minute Clinical Consult.* Philadelphia, PA: Lippincott Williams and Wilkins; 2014.

> **Category:** Reproductive system

160. Which of the following is the most important risk factor in the transmission of HIV from an infected mother to her newborn?

A) Preterm delivery (<34 weeks' gestation)
B) Low birth weight
C) Low maternal CD4 count
D) Prolonged rupture of membranes (>4 hours)
E) Intravenous drug use during pregnancy

Answer and Discussion

The answer is D. HIV infection types 1 and 2 are diagnosed by the enzyme-linked immunosorbent assay (ELISA) test initially. If the ELISA is positive, the ELISA test should be repeated first, and then, if still positive, the results should be confirmed with the Western blot test. Antibodies to HIV generally appear in the circulation 2 to 12 weeks after infection. Detection in the newborn is more difficult when the mother is infected with HIV because the child will be positive for the ELISA and the Western blot as a result of maternal transmission of the antibody transplacentally. Because of this, the HIV DNA PCR testing is the preferred test in developed countries. Almost 40% of infected newborns have positive tests in the first 2 days of life, with more than 90% testing positive by 2 weeks of age. Reported rates of transmission from mother to child have varied; most large studies in the United States and Europe have documented transmission rates in untreated women of between 12% and 30%. Rates are reported to be higher in Africa and Haiti. Perinatal treatment of HIV-infected mothers with antiretroviral drugs has dramatically decreased these rates to <2%. Several risk factors increase the rate of vertical transmission:

- Preterm delivery (<34 weeks' gestation)
- Low birth weight
- Low maternal antenatal CD4 count (<29%)
- Intravenous drug use during pregnancy
- Prolonged rupture of membranes (>4 hours), which is the most important variable that increases risk

Cesarean section combined with prenatal, intrapartum, and neonatal zidovudine therapy decreases the transmission rate by 87%. HIV can be transmitted via breast milk and colostrum. Homosexuals who practice the insertive role in intercourse are eight times more likely to get hepatitis B than HIV. Practicing the receptive role in intercourse increases the risk of HIV transmission. If a patient has either virus, he or she is at risk for contracting the other. Needle-stick injuries result in the transmission of HIV in approximately 0.3% of cases.

> **Additional Reading:** Mother-to-child (Perinatal) HIV transmission and prevention 2012. From: http://www.cdc.gov/hiv/topics/perinatal/resources/factsheets/pdf/perinatal.pdf

> **Category:** Patient/population-based care

161. Which of the following HPV subtypes are most associated with the development of cervical and other anogenital cancers?
A) Types 43 and 54
B) Types 7 and 9
C) Types 16 and 18
D) Types 24 and 28
E) Types 33 and 40

Answer and Discussion

The answer is C. A preponderance of evidence suggests a causal link between HPV infection and cervical neoplasia. Virtually, all cervical cancers are caused by HPV, with just two subtypes 16 and 18 responsible for about 70% of all cases. HPV 16 is responsible for approximately 85% of anal cancers, and HPV types 16 and 18 have been found to cause close to half of vulvar, vaginal, and penile cancers.

> **Additional Reading:** National Cancer Institute HPV and Cancer Fact Sheet 2012. From: http://www.cancer.gov/cancertopics/factsheet/Risk/HPV

> **Category:** Reproductive system

162. Female children of women who are exposed to diethylstilbestrol during their pregnancy are at increased risk for which of the following?
A) Early menopause
B) Clear cell carcinoma of the vagina
C) Ovarian carcinoma
D) Severe limb defects in their offspring
E) Mental retardation

Answer and Discussion

DES

The answer is B. Diethylstilbestrol was widely used from the 1940s to the early 1970s to help prevent spontaneous abortion in diabetic pregnant women. Approximately 2 to 3 million fetuses were exposed to the medication. Unfortunately, later studies showed that girls who were born to mothers who took the medication while they were pregnant were at increased risk of developing clear cell carcinoma of the vagina as well as cervical and vaginal intraepithelial neoplasia. These patients are also at risk for vaginal adenosis (most common anomaly associated with exposure), septated vagina, cervical collar, hypoplasia of the cervix, and uterine abnormalities. In addition to lower genital tract anomalies, upper genital tract anomalies occur in 50% of patients. The most common is a T-shaped uterus and small uterine cavity. Daughters of women who took this drug may have difficulty in conceiving, higher rates of ectopic pregnancy, spontaneous abortion, and premature births as well as a slightly increased risk for breast cancer. All exposed women are encouraged to undergo thorough vaginal examinations, including colposcopy, starting at menarche or age 14, whichever comes first. Male children of women who took the medication may show testicular or epididymal abnormalities and low sperm counts.

> **Additional Reading:** Outcome and follow-up of diethylstilbestrol (DES) exposed individuals. In: Basow DS, ed. *UpToDate.* Waltham, MA: UpToDate; 2013.

> **Category:** Reproductive system

163. Which of the following is an absolute contraindication for trial of labor after cesarean section (TOLAC).
A) Twin gestation
B) Two prior low cervical transverse cesarean sections
C) Previous cesarean section with unknown scar
D) History of classical (vertical) uterine incision during prior cesarean section

Answer and Discussion

The answer is D. All pregnant women who have had prior lower cervical transverse cesarean section should be counseled regarding the availability of a TOLAC and the benefits of successful vaginal delivery after cesarean (VBAC). These benefits include a decrease maternal morbidity as well as a decreased risk of complications in future pregnancies. Risks of TOLAC with a focus on the risk of uterine rupture during labor need to be reviewed, and this risk is related to the type of uterine incision that women have had in their prior cesarean sections. Women who have had a previous cesarean section via a classic vertical incision should undergo repeat cesarean section for delivery because of the increased risk of uterine rupture. Preferably, candidates for TOLAC have documentation of one prior lower cervical transverse cesarean; however, women who have unknown uterine scars can be allowed to attempt TOLAC if there is not felt to be high risk of a previous classical incision, on the basis of the history obtained from the patient of the circumstances of her previous cesarean. There are limited data on TOLAC in women who have had two prior cesarean sections; however, these women can be allowed a TOLAC after appropriate counseling regarding risks and benefits. Women who attempt TOLAC after adequate antepartum counseling are quite successful (approximately 60% to 80%) in vaginal deliveries with subsequent births. Women who are unsuccessful during a trial of labor and require repeat cesarean section at that time have higher complication rates then women who undergo elective repeat cesareans. Women with previous cesarean sections (low transverse incision) can also receive oxytocin during labor, but the contractions and the fetus should be closely monitored. Misoprostol as a cervical ripening agent is contraindicated in women with prior cesarean section.

> **Additional Reading:** Vaginal birth after previous cesarean delivery. *ACOG Practice Bulletin* no. 115, 2013. From: http://www.acog.org/Resources_And_Publications/Committee_Opinions_List

> **Category:** Reproductive system

164. Which of the following is associated with oral contraceptive use?
A) Increased risk of endometrial cancer
B) Increased risk of ovarian cancer
C) Decreased risk of cervical cancer
D) Decreased risk of liver cancer
E) Fewer ectopic pregnancies

↳ ↓ protection against PID?

Answer and Discussion

The answer is E. The neoplastic effects of oral contraceptives have been extensively studied, and recent meta-analyses indicate that there is a reduction in the risk of endometrial and ovarian cancer, a possible small increase in the risk for breast and cervical cancer, and an increased risk of liver cancer. Benefits include reduction in menstrual-related symptoms, fewer ectopic pregnancies, a possible increase in bone density, and possible protection against PID.

> **Additional Reading:** Safety concerns and health benefits associated with oral contraception. *Am J Obstet Gynecol.* 2004;190(suppl 4):S5–S22.

> **Category:** Reproductive system

165. Which of the following is the most common cause of hair loss in women?
A) Androgenetic alopecia
B) Alopecia areata
C) Telogen effluvium
D) Cicatricial alopecia
E) Traumatic alopecia

Answer and Discussion

The answer is A. Alopecia can be divided into disorders in which the hair follicle is normal but the cycling of hair growth is abnormal, and disorders in which the hair follicle is damaged. Androgenetic alopecia is the most common cause of hair loss in women. Other disorders include alopecia areata (smooth hairless patches, which often spontaneously resolve), telogen effluvium (sudden loss of hair, which usually regrows once the precipitating cause is addressed), cicatricial alopecia (permanent hair loss from destruction of the hair follicles by inflammatory or autoimmune diseases), and traumatic alopecias.

> **Additional Reading:** Diagnosing and treating hair loss. *Am Fam Physician.* 2009;80(4):356–362.

> **Category:** Reproductive system

166. What is the preferred management for a 32-year-old woman whose Pap smear results indicate a low-grade squamous intraepithelial lesion (LGSIL) and negative high-risk HPV?

A) Immediate colposcopy
B) Repeat co-testing with Pap smear cytology and high-risk HPV testing in 1 year
C) Repeat Pap smear (cytology only) in 6 months
D) Cryotherapy

Answer and Discussion

The answer is B. According to the American Society for Colposcopy and Cervical Pathology, the preferred management for a patient in this age group with a LGSIL Pap smear and negative testing for high-risk HPV is to repeat her Pap smear and high-risk HPV testing in 1 year. Immediate colposcopy is an acceptable alternative and would be the preferred management if the patient had a LGSIL Pap with no HPV co-test.

> **Additional Reading:** 2012 updated consensus guidelines for the management of abnormal cervical cancer screening tests and cancer precursors. *J Low Genit Tract Dis.* 2013;17(5):1–27.

> **Category:** Reproductive system

167. Which of the following statements about diaphragm contraception is true?

A) The diaphragm should be left in place for no more than 4 hours after intercourse.
B) The diaphragm should not be used with contraceptive jelly because of the risk of slippage.
C) The diaphragm is associated with an increase in vaginal and urinary infections.
D) The diaphragm can be prescribed on the basis of patient's height and weight.
E) Diaphragm use is associated with an increased risk of cervical cancer.

Answer and Discussion

The answer is C. The diaphragm is a contraceptive device. It is a round, dome-shaped piece of rubber that has a spring incorporated on the outer edge. The device is placed in the vagina and positioned so that it covers the cervix. The diaphragm should be placed in the vagina before intercourse and left in place for 8 hours after intercourse. Contraceptive foam or jelly should always be used with the diaphragm to improve its effectiveness. When used properly, pregnancy rates are approximately 3% but can be as high as 15% with improper use. The diaphragm is associated with an increased risk of vaginal and urinary infections. Patients who desire to use a diaphragm should have it fitted by a physician, and they should demonstrate proper diaphragm positioning to the physician before leaving the office to ensure proper use.

> **Additional Reading:** Diaphragm fitting. *Am Fam Physician.* 2004;69(1):97–100.

> **Category:** Reproductive system

Mental Health/ Community Health

QUESTIONS

Each of the following questions or incomplete statements is followed by suggested answers or completions. Select the ONE BEST ANSWER in each case.

1. Cognitive therapy involves
A) Repetition of negative thoughts that eventually dissipate
B) Changing a thought that involves a situation that leads to a change of mood, behavior, or reaction
C) Repeated acts of fearful situations that allow adaptation
D) Negative reinforcement of harmful activities
E) None of the above

Answer and Discussion

The answer is B. Cognitive therapy is a psychological treatment method that helps patients correct false self-beliefs that contribute to certain moods and behaviors. The basic principle behind cognitive therapy is that a thought precedes a mood and that both are interrelated with a person's environment, physical reaction, and subsequent behavior. Therefore, changing a thought that arises in a given situation changes mood, behavior, and physical reaction. Although it is unclear who benefits most from cognitive therapy, motivated patients who have an internal center of control and the capacity for introspection likely would benefit most.

> Additional Reading: Stern TA, Rosenbaum JF, Fava F, et al., eds. *Massachusetts General Hospital Comprehensive Clinical Psychiatry*, 1st ed. Philadelphia, PA: Mosby/Elsevier; 2008:189–191.

Category: Psychogenic

The basic principle behind cognitive therapy is that a thought precedes an emotion and that both are interrelated with a person's environment, physical reaction, and subsequent behavior.

2. The most common side effect of high-dose St. John's wort is
A) Transient photosensitivity
B) Hoarseness
C) Myalgias
D) Hypertension
E) Tremor

Answer and Discussion

The answer is A. Transient photosensitivity is generally the most common side effect of St. John's wort and occurs more commonly at higher dosages. Other side effects include gastrointestinal (GI) upset, increased anxiety, minor palpitations, fatigue, restlessness, dry mouth, headache, and increased depression.

> Additional Reading: Stern TA, Rosenbaum JF, Fava F, et al., eds. *Massachusetts General Hospital Comprehensive Clinical Psychiatry*, 1st ed. Philadelphia, PA: Mosby/Elsevier; 2008:702–703.

Category: Integumentary

3. Which of the following medications can be affected by the concurrent use of St. John's wort?
A) Amoxicillin
B) Gabapentin
C) Oral contraceptives
D) Glipizide
E) Hydrochlorothiazide

Answer and Discussion

The answer is C. Due to the induction of CYP 3A4, concurrent use of St. John's wort may reduce the effectiveness of oral contraceptives. There are case reports of breakthrough bleeding and undesired pregnancy in women taking oral contraceptive pills, presumably due to lowering of ethinylestradiol concentrations. Women using oral contraceptives should be counseled regarding possible breakthrough bleeding and might consider a barrier method of contraception when taking St. John's wort.

> Additional Reading: Mills E, Montori VM, Wu P, et al. Interaction of St John's wort with conventional drugs: systematic review of clinical trials. *BMJ*. 2004;329(7456):27.

Category: Reproductive

4. Which of the following is the definition of *adjustment disorder with depressed mood*?
A) Tearfulness related to the death of a loved one 1 year ago.
B) Development of low mood, tearfulness or hopelessness, or behavioral symptoms in response to an identifiable stressor that occurs within 3 months of the onset of the stressor.
C) Thoughts of death and morbid preoccupation with worthlessness with no prior triggering event.
D) Lifetime obsession with morbid thoughts.
E) Transient, normal depressive responses or mood changes to stress.

Answer and Discussion

The answer is B. *Adjustment disorder with depressed mood* is defined as development of emotional or behavioral symptoms in response to an identifiable stressor that occurs within 3 months of the stressor. Symptoms include depressed mood, tearfulness, and hopelessness and occur out of proportion to the severity or intensity of what would usually be expected from exposure to the stressor and cause significant impairment in social and occupational/academic functioning. Once the stressor (or its consequences) has terminated, the symptoms resolve within 6 months.

> **Additional Reading:** American Psychiatric Association. *Diagnostic and statistical manual of mental disorders,* 5th ed. Arlington, VA: American Psychiatric Publishing; 2013.

> Category: Psychogenic

5. Which of the following medications is limited by potentially life-threatening rashes?
A) Phenytoin
B) Lamotrigine (Lamictal)
C) Carbamazepine (Tegretol)
D) Gabapentin
E) Tramadol (Ultram)

Answer and Discussion

The answer is B. Lamotrigine is efficacious for treating bipolar depression. Many rapid cycling bipolar patients with major depression do not respond to a first-line treatment with quetiapine, and for these patients treatment with lamotrigine is indicated. Evidence for the efficacy of lamotrigine includes a meta-analysis of five randomized trials (1,072 patients with bipolar major depression) that compared lamotrigine (100 to 400 mg per day) with placebo. Lamotrigine has also been proved to be modestly effective in patients with trigeminal neuralgia, neuropathy associated with human immunodeficiency virus (HIV) infection, and poststroke pain. The drug is ineffective in patients with unspecified refractory neuropathic pain. However, the use of lamotrigine is limited by potentially life-threatening rashes, which may develop in up to 10% of patients during the initial 1 to 2 months of therapy and necessitates discontinuation of the drug. The risk of developing a life-threatening rash such as Stevens-Johnson syndrome, toxic epidermal necrolysis, or angioedema is approximately 1 in 1,000 adults.

> **Additional Reading:** Stovall J, Keck P, Solomon D. Bipolar disorder in adults: pharmacotherapy for acute depression. UpToDate. Accessed September 2013.

> Category: Integumentary

6. Which of the following means is the most common for suicide completion among men?
A) Firearms
B) Prescription medication overdose
C) Illicit drug overdose
D) Carbon monoxide poisoning
E) Hanging

Answer and Discussion

The answer is A. Access to means to attempt suicide is an important precipitating cause. This is true even after controlling for other risk factors such as depression or substance use. Firearms are the most common means for suicide completion among men. Other means include medications, illicit drugs, toxic chemicals, carbon monoxide, hanging, and cutting. Poisoning is the most common means among women. Almost anything can be used as a means to attempt suicide, but access to the most lethal means often is preventable. Men die by suicide four times as often as women; however, women attempt suicide two to three times as often as men.

> **Additional Reading:** Centers for Disease Control and Prevention, National Center for Injury Prevention and Control. Web-based Injury Statistics Query and Reporting System (WISQARS) [online]. (2010).

> Category: Patient/Population-based care

7. Which of the following statements is true regarding the use of haloperidol?
A) The drug has been approved for intravenous (IV) use.
B) Haloperidol is considered safe in those with a known seizure disorder.
C) The drug can cause prolongation of the QT interval.
D) Electrocardiogram (ECG) monitoring is not necessary when the drug is given intravenously.
E) None of the above.

Answer and Discussion

The answer is C. Although haloperidol has not been FDA approved for IV use, it is commonly used intravenously and is generally thought to be safe. Haloperidol may alter cardiac conduction and prolong the QT interval leading to life-threatening arrhythmias. It should be used with caution or avoided in patients with electrolyte abnormalities. Electrocardiographic monitoring is necessary. Haloperidol should be avoided if possible in patients with a known seizure disorder.

> **Additional Reading:** Berul CI, Seslar SP, Zimetbaum PJ, et al. Acquired long QT syndrome. UpToDate, version 17.2. Accessed November 17, 2009.

> Category: Psychogenic

8. Which of the following is true regarding Intimate partner violence (IPV)
A) Is higher among Caucasian women as compared with other ethnic classes
B) Affects men and women equally
C) Rarely affects the elderly
D) Increases during pregnancy
E) Is rarely associated with a spouse

Answer and Discussion

The answer is D. Studies show that women are much more likely than men to be the victims of IPV. The Centers for Disease Control and Prevention's (CDC) report on the National Intimate Partner and Sexual Violence Survey (NISVS) of 2010 estimates that more than 1 in 3 women (35.6%) have experienced IPV in their lifetime. Pregnancy may be one of the only times women, especially of lower socioeconomic status, are connected with health care. Screening for IPV during pregnancy is therefore incredibly important. In January 2013, the U.S. Preventive Services Task Force (USPSTF) released updated recommendations on screening for IPV. The USPSTF now recommends that clinicians screen women of childbearing age for IPV and provide or refer women who screen positive to intervention services (B recommendation). This recommendation applies to women who do not have signs or symptoms of abuse. The USPSTF concludes that the current evidence is insufficient to assess the balance of benefits and harms of screening all elderly or vulnerable adults (physically or mentally dysfunctional) for abuse and neglect. IPV among gay and lesbian relationships appears to be as common as in heterosexual relationships and is also a significant problem among the elderly. Elder abuse is associated with an increase in reports of chronic pain, depression, number of health conditions, and an increased mortality. The abuser is most commonly a relative (usually the spouse). Domestic violence often begins or, if already present, increases during pregnancy and the postpartum period. IPV is much more common among black, Hispanic, and native American women as compared with Caucasian women.

> Additional Reading: U.S. Department of Health and Human Services, Health Resources and Services Administration, Maternal and Child Health Bureau. *A comprehensive approach for community-based programs to address intimate partner violence and perinatal depression.* Rockville, MD: U.S. Department of Health and Human Services, 2013; and *Annals of Internal Medicine* (the USPSTF original source article, January 22, 2013, if that reference is preferred).

Category: Patient/Population-based care

Screening for IPV among women who do not have any signs or symptoms of abuse is a USPSTF B recommendation. Although elder abuse is also common, there is insufficient data to recommend routine screening.

9. When considering light therapy for seasonal affective disorder (SAD), which of the following is *not* a factor that predicts a positive result?
A) Hypersomnia
B) High number of vegetative symptoms
C) Increased intake of sweet foods in the afternoon
D) History of reactivity to ambient light
E) Positive family history of SAD

Answer and Discussion

The answer is E. Light therapy involves exposure to minimum 2,500 lux of visible light. 10,000 lux for 30 minutes/day has been shown to be effective. Factors that have predicted a positive response to light therapy include hypersomnia, high rate of vegetative symptoms, an increased intake of sweet foods in the afternoon, and a history of reactivity to ambient light. A positive family history does not necessarily increase a positive response to light therapy.

> Additional Reading: Saeed SA, Bruce TJ. Seasonal affective disorder. UpToDate, version 17.2. Accessed November 17, 2009.

Category: Psychogenic

10. Risk factors for smoking include all of the following *except*
A) Exposure to secondhand smoke
B) Presence of a smoker in the family
C) Poor academic performance
D) Single parent at home
E) Lack of concern over weight and body image, particularly in women

Answer and Discussion

The answer is E. Risk factors for smoking include exposure to secondhand smoke, presence of a smoker in the household, comorbid psychiatric disorders, strained relationship with parent and/or single parent at home, low level of expressed self-esteem and self-worth, poor academic performance, increased adolescent perception of parental approval of smoking, affiliation with smoking peers, and

availability of cigarettes. An additional risk factor for boys is high levels of aggression and rebelliousness; among girls, preoccupation with weight and body image is a separate risk factor.

> Additional Reading: Rennard RI, Rigotti NA, Daughton DM. Management of smoking cessation. UpToDate, version 17.2. Accessed November 17, 2009.

Category: Patient/Population-based care

11. Smoking is associated with an increased risk of all of the following *except*
A) Infertility
B) Spontaneous abortion
C) Ectopic pregnancy
D) Premature menopause
E) Multiple births

Answer and Discussion

The answer is E. Smoking is associated with infertility, spontaneous abortion, ectopic pregnancy, and premature menopause.

> Additional Reading: Rennard RI, Rigotti NA, Daughton DM. Management of smoking cessation. UpToDate, version 17.2. Accessed November 17, 2009.

Category: Patient/Population-based care

12. Which of the following has been shown to be beneficial in smoking cessation?
A) Fluoxetine
B) Venlafaxine
C) Bupropion
D) Sertraline
E) Doxepin

Answer and Discussion

The answer is C. Bupropion (also marketed as Wellbutrin) has been available for use as an antidepressant in the United States since 1989 and is thought to act by enhancing central nervous system noradrenergic and dopaminergic function. A sustained-release formulation of the drug (Zyban) is licensed as an aid to smoking cessation.

> Additional Reading: Rennard RI, Rigotti NA, Daughton DM. Management of smoking cessation. UpToDate, version 17.2. Accessed November 17, 2009.

Category: Patient/Population-based care

13. Urges or impulses for repetitive intentional behavior performed in a stereotyped manner in an attempt to relieve anxiety is termed
A) Adaptation
B) Congruence
C) Compulsion
D) Obsession
E) Transference

Answer and Discussion

The answer is C. *Obsessions* are persistent thoughts, urges, or images that are experienced at some time during the disturbance as intrusive and unwanted and that in most individuals cause marked anxiety or distress. The person tries to suppress such thoughts, urges, or images or to neutralize them with some other thoughts or action (e.g., compulsion). In many cases, these obsessions have a theme that an insignificant oversight will result in tremendous catastrophe. Other common themes are contamination, a need for ordering things, aggressive impulses, and sexual imagery. *Compulsions* are

(1) repetitive behaviors or mental acts (e.g., hand washing, ordering, checking) that the individual feels driven to perform in response to an obsession or according to rules that must be rigidly applied and (2) the behaviors or mental acts that are aimed at preventing or reducing anxiety or distress or preventing some dreaded situation (even though they are not connected in any realistic way with what they are designed to neutralize or prevent, or are clearly excessive).

> **Additional Reading:** American Psychiatric Association. *Diagnostic and statistical manual of mental disorders,* 5th ed. Arlington, VA: American Psychiatric Publishing; 2013.

Category: Psychogenic

14. Which of the following medications is used in the classic treatment of bipolar disorder?
A) Lithium
B) Sertraline
C) Amitriptyline
D) Phenytoin
E) Alprazolam

Answer and Discussion

The answer is A. Lithium is considered a first-line medication for bipolar disorder and has been more widely studied than any other maintenance treatment for bipolar disorder and is consistently supported across multiple randomized trials. Bipolar disorder is most commonly diagnosed in persons between 18 and 24 years of age, with the mean age of onset for a first manic, hypomanic, or depressive episode at 18. The clinical presentations of this disorder are diverse and include mania, hypomania, and psychosis. Frequently associated conditions include substance abuse, attention-deficit/hyperactivity disorder (ADHD), and anxiety disorders and other mood disorders. Patients with acute mania must be evaluated urgently. Treatment involves the use of mood stabilizers such as lithium, valproic acid, and carbamazepine.

> **Additional Reading:** Smith LA, Cornelius V, Warnock A, et al. Effectiveness of mood stabilizers and antipsychotics in the maintenance phase of bipolar disorder: a systematic review of randomized controlled trials. *Bipolar Disord.* 2007;9(4):394.

Category: Psychogenic

15. A 21-year-old presents with complaints of an inflated self-esteem, decreased need for sleep, and distractibility. The most likely diagnosis is
A) Depression
B) Hypothymia
C) Borderline personality
D) Mania
E) Antisocial personality

Answer and Discussion

The answer is D. The diagnosis of mania consists of a distinct period of abnormally and persistently elevated, expansive or irritable mood and abnormally and persistently increased goal-directed activity or energy, lasting at least 1 week and present most of the day, nearly every day. During the period of mood disturbance and increased energy or activity, three or more of the following are present in sufficient degree and represent a noticeable change from usual behavior:

1. Inflated self-esteem or grandiosity
2. Decreased need for sleep (e.g., feels rested after only 3 hours of sleep)
3. More talkative than usual, or pressure to keep talking
4. Flight of ideas, or subjective experience that thoughts are racing

5. Distractibility (i.e., attention too easily drawn to unimportant or irrelevant external stimuli)
6. Increase in goal-directed activity (either socially, at work or school, or sexually) or psychomotor agitation
7. Excessive involvement in pleasurable activities that have a high potential for painful consequences (e.g., engaging in unrestrained buying sprees, sexual indiscretions, foolish business investments)

> **Additional Reading:** American Psychiatric Association. *Diagnostic and statistical manual of mental disorders,* 5th ed. Arlington, VA: American Psychiatric Publishing; 2013.

Category: Psychogenic

16. Which of the following is the greatest risk factor for suicide?
A) Unemployment
B) Single status
C) Low income status
D) Resident of urban area
E) History of admission to a psychiatric hospital

Answer and Discussion

The answer is E. Each year, about 30,000 people in the United States die by suicide. Suicide rates were higher in residents of urban areas compared with nonurban residents. The risk of suicide was also increased with unemployment, single status (never married), low income, and receipt of pension or social security benefit. One of the strongest risk factors, however, is psychiatric illness, and the severity of psychiatric illness is associated with risk of suicide. One meta-analysis found that the lifetime risk of suicide is 8.6% in patients who have had a psychiatric inpatient admission involving suicidal ideation, 4% in patients who have had a psychiatric admission for an affective disorder without suicidality, 2.2% in psychiatric outpatients, and less than 0.5% in the general population. More specifically, admission to a psychiatric hospital is a significant risk factor for suicide. Almost one-half of the persons who committed suicide had a history of admission to psychiatric facilities. Regardless of diagnosis, the greatest risk was during hospital admission and in the first week following discharge. Finally, the strongest single factor predictive of suicide is prior history of attempted suicide.

> **Additional Reading:** Centers for Disease Control and Prevention, National Center for Injury Prevention and Control. Web-based Injury Statistics Query and Reporting System (WISQARS) [online]; 2010.

Category: Psychogenic

> The risk of suicide is increased with unemployment, single status, low income, and receipt of pension or social security benefit. The strongest risk factor of those in the question is admission to a psychiatric hospital; however, previous suicide attempt is the single strongest predictor.

17. In a dying patient, which of the following is used to detect depression?
A) Pervasive hopelessness
B) Weight loss
C) Crying
D) Dependency
E) Concern over being a burden

Answer and Discussion

The answer is A. Serious and progressive illness evokes distress in patients, families, and clinicians, engendering fear, anxiety, anger, dread, sadness, helplessness, and uncertainty. Hope permits patients, their families, and loved ones to cope with these difficult emotions and helps them endure the stresses of treatment. A person who is grieving maintains a sense of hope. Hope may change from the hope for a cure to the hope for prolonging life to the hope to live comfortably and without pain for the duration of life, but it is not lost in persons who are dying. Grief is an adaptive, universal, and highly personalized response to the multiple losses that occur at the end of life. The symptoms of grief may overlap with those of major depression or a terminal illness or its treatment; however, grief is a distinct entity. Feelings of pervasive hopelessness, helplessness, worthlessness, guilt, lack of pleasure, and suicidal ideation are present in patients with depression, but not in those experiencing grief. Pervasive hopelessness, however, is a hallmark of depression.

> **Additional Reading:** Widera EW, Susan D. Managing grief and depression at the end of life. *Am Fam Physician.* 2012;86(3):259–264.

Category: Psychogenic

18. Which of the following electrolyte abnormalities is associated with bulimic patients?
A) Metabolic acidosis
B) Respiratory acidosis
C) Metabolic alkalosis
D) Respiratory alkalosis
E) Normal electrolytes

Answer and Discussion

The answer is C. Symptoms and signs of bulimia include reflux esophagitis, abdominal cramping, diarrhea, and rectal bleeding. Electrolyte abnormalities and metabolic alkalosis signal extreme purging habits in a bulimic patient. Patients with anorexia generally have laboratory test results within normal limits until the very late stage of the condition.

> **Additional Reading:** Willimans P, Goodie J, Motsinger C. Treating eating disorders in primary care. *Am Fam Physician.* 2008;77(2):187–195.

Category: Psychogenic

19. A 42-year-old man is seen in your office. He has recently seen a psychiatrist and is being treated for severe depression. The patient cannot recall the medication that he is taking, but he remembers that the psychiatrist told him not to eat cheeses or aged meats. Which of the following agents is this patient most likely taking?
A) Tricyclic antidepressant (TCA)
B) Selective serotonin release inhibitor
C) Monoamine oxidase inhibitor (MAOI)
D) Neuroleptic
E) Anxiolytic

Answer and Discussion

The answer is C. Antidepressant medications fall into three basic categories:

1. *TCAs:* These include amitriptyline, imipramine, nortriptyline, and desipramine. TCAs have been commonly used in the treatment of depression since the mid-1980s. These medications may require 2 to 6 weeks before full therapeutic effect is noted. Many have anticholinergic side effects. Amitriptyline has the most anticholinergic properties, including dry mouth, blurred vision, constipation, ileus, urinary retention, and even delirium. In most cases, these side effects improve with time. Drug selection should depend on the symptoms and the side-effect profile of the medication.

2. *Selective serotonin reuptake inhibitors (SSRIs):* These include fluoxetine, paroxetine, citalopram, escitalopram, and sertraline. SSRIs are popular mainly because of their reduced side-effect profile and once-a-day dosing. These medications are very effective in the treatment of depression and are associated with a lower incidence of side effects compared with TCAs. The risk of death from overdose is very low with these medications. They are activating and should be given during the day.
   - *Serotonin modulators:* The medications block primarily the 5-HT2 receptor and inhibit reuptake of 5-HT and norepinephrine. The group includes nefazodone, trazadone, and mirtazapine.
   - *Serotonin–norepinephrine reuptake inhibitors:* This group includes venlafaxine and duloxetine. They have dual 5-HT and norepinephrine mechanism of action.
   - *Dopamine–norepinephrine reuptake inhibitors:* The only drug in this class is bupropion.

3. *MAOIs:* These include phenelzine and tranylcypromine. MAOIs are not used as frequently for the treatment of depression because of the potential for severe side effects. Interactions with sympathomimetic medications or tyramine-containing foods (e.g., cheeses, wines, beers, aged meats and fruits, beans, liver, yeast extracts) can lead to a hypertensive crisis. Orthostatic hypotension, nausea, insomnia, and sexual dysfunction are also common.

> **Additional Reading:** Beers MH, Porter RS, Jones TV, et al., eds. *The Merck Manual of Diagnosis and Therapy,* 18th ed. Whitehouse Station, NJ: Merck Research Laboratories; 2006:1708–1709.

Category: Psychogenic

20. A 30-year-old woman presents with fatigue, difficulty with concentration, weight loss, and insomnia. She is an avid equestrian, but recently has not been interested in riding. The most likely diagnosis is
A) Somatoform disorder
B) Depression
C) Anorexia nervosa
D) Bulimia
E) Cyclothymia

Answer and Discussion

The answer is B. Common symptoms that are associated with clinical depression include depressed mood, diminished interest or pleasure, significant appetite or weight change, sleep disturbances, agitation, fatigue, feelings of worthlessness or guilt, difficulty with concentration, or suicidal thoughts. Symptoms must be present for at least 2 weeks before the diagnosis is made. In addition, symptoms must be present almost daily and must represent a change from the patient's previous level of functioning. Other contributing causes must be ruled out. Either a depressed mood or anhedonia (a loss of pleasure in previously enjoyable activities) must be present for the diagnosis.

> **Additional Reading:** American Psychiatric Association. *Diagnostic and statistical manual of mental disorders,* 5th ed. Arlington, VA: American Psychiatric Publishing; 2013.

Category: Psychogenic

21. In young women with an eating disorder, at what point would you expect her menstrual periods to resume?
A) 75% of ideal body weight
B) 80% of ideal body weight
C) 90% of ideal body weight
D) 100% of body weight
E) It is unusual for menstrual cycles to resume with any weight gain.

Answer and Discussion

The answer is C. Menstruation usually resumes in women affected with anorexia when the patient approaches 90% of ideal body weight.

> **Additional Reading:** Mehler PS. Diagnosis and care of patients with anorexia nervosa in the primary care setting. *Ann Intern Med.* 2001;134:1048–1059.

Category: Psychogenic

22. Which of the following behaviors is associated with bulimia?
A) Mood disorders
B) Anxiety
C) Substance abuse
D) Poor impulse control
E) All of the above

Answer and Discussion

The answer is E. Young women with bulimia characteristically have psychiatric comorbidities, across a wide range of mental disorders. There is increased frequency of depressive symptoms, low self-esteem, and bipolar and depressive disorders. There is also an increased frequency of anxiety disorders as well as substance use disorder, especially alcohol and stimulant use. Poor impulse control is associated with bulimia nervosa, which might result in patients engaging in risky behaviors such as unprotected sexual activity, self-mutilation, and suicide attempts.

> **Additional Reading:** American Psychiatric Association. *Diagnostic and statistical manual of mental disorders,* 5th ed. Arlington, VA: American Psychiatric Publishing, 2013.

Category: Psychogenic

23. Which of the following statements regarding obsessive–compulsive disorder (OCD) is true?
A) Obsessions are repetitive behaviors.
B) Most affected patients have obsessions as well as compulsions.
C) Compulsions are thoughts or ideas that recur.
D) Anxiety is a central feature.
E) Patients are usually unaware of their actions and thoughts and are resistant to them.

Answer and Discussion

The answer is D. OCD is characterized by the presence of obsessions and/or compulsions (i.e., recurrent actions or ideas that interfere with normal daily activities). The patient is usually aware of the actions and thoughts and feels a strong inner resistance toward them. *Obsessions* are defined as thoughts or ideas that recur, and the patient tries to repress them. Common obsessions include fear of dirt, germs, or contamination; disgust with bodily waste or secretions; fear of harming a family member or friend; concern with order, symmetry (balance), and exactness; worry that a task has been done poorly, even when the person knows this is not true; fear of thinking evil or sinful thoughts; constantly thinking about certain sounds, images, words, or numbers; or a constant need for reassurance. Compulsions are repetitive behaviors that are performed in response to the obsessions. Common compulsions include cleaning and grooming rituals, such as excessive hand washing, showering, and tooth-brushing; checking rituals involving drawers, door locks, and appliances to be sure they are shut, locked, or turned off; repeating rituals, such as going in and out of a door, sitting down and getting up from a chair, and touching certain objects several times; putting items in a certain order or arrangement; counting over and over to a certain number; saving newspapers, mail, or containers when they are no longer needed; or seeking reassurance and approval. Obsessions and compulsions can have an aggressive or sexual attachment. Fewer than 10% of patients have both obsessions and compulsions; however, individuals may exhibit multiple obsessions or multiple compulsions. Anxiety is a central feature of this disorder, but it is generated by internal thoughts as opposed to external circumstances. The neurosis affects men and women equally and is usually found in those of a higher socioeconomic class with above-average intelligence. The condition usually becomes apparent in childhood. Until recently, OCD has been a difficult illness to treat. However, we now have better medicines. Clomipramine (Anafranil) helps many people with OCD and usually decreases symptoms to mild levels. Side effects from this drug, such as dry mouth, constipation and drowsiness, and sometimes an inability to achieve orgasm, are common. Fluoxetine, sertraline, paroxetine, and fluvoxamine (Luvox) can also help some patients with OCD.

> **Additional Reading:** American Psychiatric Association. *Diagnostic and statistical manual of mental disorders,* 5th ed. Arlington, VA: American Psychiatric Publishing; 2013.

Category: Psychogenic

24. High fever, tachycardia, tachypnea, diaphoresis, hypertension, and seizures develop in a psychiatric patient who is receiving haloperidol. The most likely diagnosis is
A) Malignant hyperthermia
B) Rhabdomyolysis
C) Neuroleptic malignant syndrome
D) Sepsis
E) Serotonin syndrome

Answer and Discussion

The answer is C. Neuroleptic malignant syndrome is an uncommon idiosyncratic condition that is associated with the use of dopamine antagonist (i.e., antipsychotic medications). Usually associated with the more potent medications, such as haloperidol and piperazine phenothiazines, the symptoms include high fever (102°F to 104°F), tachycardia, tachypnea, diaphoresis, autonomic dysfunction, mental status changes, hypertension and hypotension, tremors, seizures, muscle rigidity, and leukocytosis. Significant elevations of serum creatinine kinase may signal rhabdomyolysis. Other complications include respiratory failure, myocardial infarction, and renal and hepatic failure. Disseminated intravascular coagulopathy may also occur. The treatment involves stopping the antipsychotic, supportive care, and the use of IV dantrolene. Bromocriptine, amantadine, and benzodiazepines can also be used. Mortality approaches 30%.

> **Additional Reading:** Beers MH, Porter RS, Jones TV, et al., eds. *The Merck Manual of Diagnosis and Therapy*, 18th ed. Whitehouse Station, NJ: Merck Research Laboratories; 2006:1671.

Category: Neurologic

25. *Panic disorder* is defined as recurrent, unexpected attacks that may involve which of the following symptoms?
A) Flight of ideas
B) Hallucinations
C) Feelings of envy
D) Impulsivity
E) Feeling of Choking

Answer and Discussion

The answer is E. As much as 33% of the population may have a panic attack during the year, but far fewer are affected with panic disorder. According to the *Diagnostic and Statistical Manual of Mental Disorders (DSM),* 5th ed., the definition of *panic attack* is a sudden surge of intense fear or intense discomfort that reaches a peak within minutes, and during which time four (or more) of the following symptoms develop:

1. Palpitation, pounding heart, or accelerated heat rate
2. Sweating
3. Trembling or shaking
4. Sensations of shortness of breath or smothering
5. Feelings of choking
6. Chest pain or discomfort
7. Nausea or abdominal distress
8. Feeling dizzy, lightheaded, unsteady, or faint
9. Chills or heat sensations
10. Paresthesias
11. Derealization
12. Fear of losing control or going crazy
13. Fear of dying

Panic disorder further requires recurrent unexpected attacks and that at least one of the attacks has been followed by 1 month (or more) of one or both the following:

- Persistent concern or worry about additional attacks or its consequences.
- Significant maladaptive change in behavior related to the attacks.

The panic attacks cannot be due to the direct physiologic effects of a substance (drug abuse, medication) and are not better accounted for by another mental disorder. Treatment for panic disorders involves counseling, antidepressants (paroxetine), buspirone, and benzodiazepines (alprazolam).

Additional Reading: American Psychiatric Association. *Diagnostic and statistical manual of mental disorders,* 5th ed. Arlington, VA: American Psychiatric Publishing; 2013.

Category: Psychogenic

> Panic attacks are a sudden surge of intense fear or intense discomfort that reaches a peak within minutes is not due to the direct physiologic effects of a substance (drug abuse, medication).

26. Which of the following medications is best indicated in a patient with Parkinson's disease who experiences psychosis?
A) Haloperidol (Haldol)
B) Olanzapine (Zyprexa)
C) Quetiapine (Seroquel)
D) Risperidone (Risperdal)
E) Thioridazine (Mellaril)

Answer and Discussion

The answer is C. Psychosis is a frequent complication of Parkinson's disease, and it is characterized mainly by visual hallucinations and delusions, which are often paranoid in flavor. Hallucinations are the most common manifestation, and they affect up to 40% of patients with Parkinson's disease, particularly those at an advanced stage of illness. Quetiapine (Seroquel) has shown promise in the treatment of psychosis in elderly patients with Alzheimer's disease and Parkinson's

disease. It improves psychosis in patients with Parkinson's disease without exacerbating movement disorders. This feature has led some experts to recommend it as the first-line agent for treatment of psychosis in patients with Parkinson's disease. Haloperidol and thioridazine can cause drug-induced parkinsonism, akathisia, acute dystonia, and tardive dyskinesia (TD). Risperidone exacerbates movement disorders in patients with Parkinson's disease. In patients with Parkinson's disease, olanzapine was found to increase motor symptoms.

Additional Reading: Juncos JL, Roberts VJ, Evatt ML, et al. Quetiapine improves psychotic symptoms and cognition in Parkinson's disease. *Mood Disord.* 2004;19(1):29.

Category: Neurologic

27. Which of the following is a potential side effect of quetiapine?
A) Agranulocytosis
B) Cataract formation
C) Hepatotoxicity
D) QT interval prolongation
E) Thrombocytopenia

Answer and Discussion

The answer is B. Immediate-release quetiapine should be initiated at 50 mg once daily at bedtime on day 1; increase to 100 mg once daily on day 2, further increase by 100 mg daily each day until 300 mg once daily is reached by day 4. Usual dose for treating depression is 300 mg once daily; maximum dose: 300 mg once daily. For bipolar disorder, the recommended dosage is higher. Common side effects include sedation, headache, and orthostatic hypotension. Cataract formation was noticed in premarketing studies, but a causal relationship has not been found. Screening for cataract formation is recommended at the initiation of therapy and at 6-month intervals thereafter.

Additional Reading: Quetiapin: drug information. UpToDate. Accessed September 2013.

Category: Special sensory

28. Which of the following statements about fluoxetine is true?
A) Side effects often include dry mouth, urinary retention, and blurred vision.
B) The treatment of panic disorder typically requires higher doses than the recommended starting dose for depression.
C) The mechanism of action involves the reuptake of dopamine at the postsynaptic junction.
D) The drug has significant anticholinergic activity.
E) Treatment of bulimia typically requires higher doses than the recommended starting dose for depression.

Answer and Discussion

The answer is E. Fluoxetine is U.S. Food and Drug Administration (FDA) approved for the treatment of depression, OCD, premenstrual dysphoric disorder (PDD), panic disorder, and bulimia nervosa. Other uses include the treatment of dysthymic disorder, posttraumatic stress disorder (PTSD), social phobia, and bipolar disorder depression in combination with other medication, fibromyalgia, and Raynaud's phenomena. The medication is an SSRI and has advantages when compared with the older TCAs. SSRIs have very little anticholinergic activity (which can cause blurred vision, urinary retention, and dry mouth); thus, they are better tolerated. The starting dose of fluoxetine is usually 10 to 20 mg/day, which can then tittered up to achieve a clinical response; 80 mg/day is the maximum dosage. The full therapeutic response may take up to 4 weeks. Higher doses (e.g., 60 mg/day or more) is recommended for the treatment of bulimia and OCD. The treatment of panic disorder often requires smaller initial doses. Initial doses of 20 mg often precipitate panic attacks and lead to a high discontinuation rate, so starting at 10 mg/day for patients with panic disorder can be helpful. Side effects include headaches, anxiety, nervousness, excessive sweating, insomnia, anorexia, weight loss, nausea, diarrhea, and rash. Depressed patients should be monitored closely for suicidal thoughts or gestures, especially once their depression starts to improve. In most cases, medication for depression is complemented with counseling and is more effective than medication alone.

Additional Reading: Fluoxetine: drug information. UpToDate. 2013.

Category: Psychogenic

29. The treatment of choice for SAD is
A) TCAs
B) Electroconvulsive shock treatment
C) Psychotherapy
D) Intense white light therapy
E) MAOIs

Answer and Discussion

The answer is D. SAD is a pattern of major depressive episodes that occur and remit with changes in seasons. Two patterns have been identified. The most often recognized is the fall-onset type, also known as *winter depression,* in which major depressive episodes begin in the late fall to early winter months and remit during the summer months. Atypical signs and symptoms of depression predominate in cases of winter depression and include the following:

- Increased rather than decreased sleep
- Increased rather than decreased appetite and food intake with carbohydrate craving
- Marked increase in weight
- Irritability
- Interpersonal difficulties (especially rejection sensitivity)
- Leaden paralysis (a heavy, leaden feeling in the arms or legs)

A spring-onset pattern (summer depression) also has been described in which the severe depressive episode begins in late spring to early summer and is characterized by typical vegetative symptoms of depression, such as decreased sleep, weight loss, and poor appetite. Patients with winter depression usually reside in the more northern regions, and symptoms tend to develop when the days become shorter and nighttime is more prolonged. Treatment with intense white light has proved to be successful in controlling symptoms. Light therapy is initiated with a 10,000-lux light box directed toward the patient at a downward slant. The patient's eyes should remain open throughout the treatment session, although staring directly into the light source is unnecessary and is not advised. The patient should start with a single 10-to-15-minute session per day, gradually increasing the session's duration to 30 to 45 minutes. Sessions should be increased to twice a day if symptoms worsen. Ninety minutes a day is the conventional daily maximum duration of therapy, although there is no reason to limit the duration of sessions if side effects are not severe.

Additional Reading: Stern TA, Rosenbaum JF, Fava F, et al., eds. *Massachusetts General Hospital Comprehensive Clinical Psychiatry,* 1st ed. Philadelphia, PA: Mosby/Elsevier; 2008:393.

Category: Psychogenic

30. Which of the following is a characteristic of antisocial personality disorder?
A) Those who are affected suppress their conflicts
B) Symptoms include severe agoraphobia
C) Schizophrenia may coexist
D) Many have a record of stealing, fighting, rape, or arson
E) Adolescents under the age of 18 are commonly affected

Answer and Discussion

The answer is D. Patients with antisocial personality disorder are often impulsive, reckless, and immoral. They often had previous problems concerning truancy, cruelty to animals and other individuals, and initiation of fights and use of weapons with fighting. They usually have a record of stealing, possible rape, arson, and falsifying the truth since childhood. Although DSM diagnostic criteria state that someone must be above 18 years of age, the definition also requires that a pattern of irresponsible behavior must be present since the age of 15, with school suspension, employment problems, poor parenting, lack of monogamy (no monogamous relationship lasting more than 1 year), and failed financial obligations in the absence of schizophrenia or manic episodes. People with antisocial personality disorder act out their conflicts or go against the rules of social normalcy and, in many cases, those affected lack regard for other people's rights.

Additional Reading: American Psychiatric Association. *Diagnostic and Statistical Manual of Mental Disorders,* 5th ed. Washington, DC: American Psychiatric Association; 2013.

Category: Psychogenic

31. Which of the following is *not* classified as an SSRI?
A) Sertraline (Zoloft)
B) Mirtazapine (Remeron)
C) Escitalopram (Lexapro)
D) Paroxetine (Paxil)
E) Fluoxetine (Prozac)

Answer and Discussion

The answer is B. Mirtazapine (Remeron) is a tetracyclic antidepressant unrelated to TCAs and SSRIs. It is unique in its action among the currently available antidepressants. It is referred to as a *serotonin modulator.* Mirtazapine is a presynaptic α_2-adrenergic receptor antagonist plus a potent antagonist of postsynaptic 5-HT$_2$ and 5-HT$_3$ receptors. The net outcome of these effects is stimulation of the release of norepinephrine and serotonin. The drug has antidepressant and anxiolytic effects. It can cause sedation and weight gain, but does not cause sexual dysfunction.

Additional Reading: Beers MH, Porter RS, Jones TV, et al., eds. *The Merck Manual of Diagnosis and Therapy,* 18th ed. Whitehouse Station, NJ: Merck Research Laboratories; 2006:1709.

Category: Psychogenic

32. Which of the following is most likely to cause withdrawal symptoms with abrupt discontinuation?
A) Fluoxetine (Prozac)
B) Sertraline (Zoloft)
C) Paroxetine (Paxil)
D) Citalopram (Celexa)
E) None of the SSRIs cause withdrawal symptoms.

Answer and Discussion

The answer is C. Studies have shown that when comparing fluoxetine, sertraline, paroxetine, and citalopram, withdrawal from paroxetine was shown to cause more severe symptoms that may occur more quickly, even after the second missed dose. Withdrawal symptoms can include dysphoric mood, irritability, agitation, dizziness, sensory disturbances (e.g., electric shock-like sensations), anxiety, confusion, headache, lethargy, emotional lability, insomnia, hypomania, tinnitus, and seizures. Because of its long half-life, fluoxetine may have the least severe symptoms. Methods to prevent antidepressant discontinuation syndrome include tapering the drug and educating the patient to avoid sudden cessation of the medication. Reintroduction of the medication will usually reverse severe symptoms within 24 hours.

Additional Reading: Michelson D, Fava M, Amsterdam J, et al. Interruption of selective serotonin reuptake inhibitor treatment: double-blind, placebo-controlled trial. *Br J Psychiatry.* 2000;176:363–368.

Category: Psychogenic

> Studies have shown that when comparing fluoxetine, sertraline, paroxetine, and citalopram, withdrawal from paroxetine was shown to cause more severe symptoms.

33. A 20-year-old college student presents to her dentist. Her vital signs are normal, and her weight is 120 lb. On examination, extensive upper dental erosion is noted. The most likely diagnosis is
A) OCD
B) Anorexia nervosa
C) Hypothyroidism
D) Bulimia nervosa
E) Crohn's disease

Answer and Discussion

The answer is D. The core features of bulimia nervosa are binge eating (i.e., eating an amount of food that is definitely larger than most people would eat under similar circumstances), inappropriate compensatory behavior to prevent weight gain, and excessive concern about body weight and shape. The prototypic sequence of behavior in bulimia nervosa consists of caloric restriction, followed by binge eating, and then self-induced vomiting. Other manifestations of compensatory behaviors include excessive exercise and the misuse of diuretics, laxatives, or enemas. Although the etiology of this disorder is unknown, genetic and neurochemical factors have been implicated. Bulimia nervosa is more common in women than men by a ratio of 3:1, and the median age of onset is 20. The condition usually becomes symptomatic between the ages of 13 and 20 years, and it has a chronic, sometimes episodic, course. Unlike anorexia nervosa, those affected with bulimia are usually within 15% of their desirable weight. Common physical signs in bulimia nervosa include hypotension, tachycardia, and dry skin. In addition, menstrual irregularities are seen in approximately one-third to one-half of female patients. Regular vomiting can cause dehydration, hypokalemia, hypochloremia, metabolic alkalosis, and dental enamel erosion (particularly the upper dentition; the lower dentition is protected by the tongue during vomiting), as well as hypertrophy of the parotid glands and "puffy" cheeks. Severe cases may also result in gastric dilation, esophagitis, electrolyte abnormalities, aspiration, or pancreatitis. Treatment involves psychotherapy with behavior modification and the use of antidepressants (SSRIs, especially fluoxetine). Many patients relapse and require long-term therapy.

Additional Reading: Williams P, Goodies J, Motsinger C. Treating eating disorders in primary care. *Am Fam Physician.* 2008;77(2): 187–195.

Category: Special sensory

34. Which of the following factors is associated with dysthymic disorder (now called *persistent depressive disorder* in DSM 5)?
A) Substance abuse
B) Sleep disturbances
C) Mania
D) Myasthenia gravis
E) Flight of ideas

Answer and Discussion

The answer is B. Dysthymia is known as a condition characterized by depressed mood for at least 2 years with concomitant impairment in some areas of functioning. The DSM 5 consolidated major depressive disorder and dysthymia into a diagnosis called persistent depressive disorder. Persistent depressive disorder is characterized by depressed mood for most of the day, more days than not, for at least 2 years. While depressed, two or more of the following must also be present:

- Appetite changes
- Sleep disturbances
- Low energy or fatigue
- Low self-esteem
- Poor concentration/difficulty making decisions
- Feelings of hopelessness

In this new diagnosis, criteria for major depressive disorder can be present continuously but the symptoms must not have another medical cause or explained by the use of substances. The patient cannot have a history of mania, hypomania, or cyclothymia.

Additional Reading: American Psychiatric Association. *Diagnostic and Statistical Manual of Mental Disorders,* 5th ed. Washington, DC: American Psychiatric Association; 2013.

Category: Psychogenic

35. Children who exhibit symptoms of school avoidance with nausea, vomiting, and abdominal pain may benefit from
A) Antidepressant medication
B) Methylphenidate
C) Psychotherapy
D) Benzodiazepines
E) Mood stabilizers

Answer and Discussion

The answer is C. Separation anxiety disorder affects children below the age of 18 years and consists of developmentally inappropriate and excessive anxiety concerning separation from home or a major attachment figure that lasts for at least 4 weeks. Periods of exacerbations and remissions are typical. These children (in many cases, school-aged children with school avoidance) often have no siblings and come from an extremely close family. Boys and girls are equally affected. It is a normal developmental response for children to cry when their parents leave the room beginning at approximately 8 months of age and continuing up to 2 years of age. The response varies with each child. Many first-time parents overreact and fear that the child is emotionally harmed by the separation. Reassuring the parents that this is a normal response is appropriate for treatment. However, occasionally, a child exhibits symptoms of nausea, vomiting, and abdominal pain, with separation from a major attachment figure, which signals an abnormal response. Psychotherapy (family therapy) may be necessary for these children. Medication is not recommended.

> **Additional Reading:** American Psychiatric Association. *Diagnostic and Statistical Manual of Mental Disorders,* 5th ed. Washington, DC: American Psychiatric Association; 2013.

Category: Psychogenic

36. Which of the following medications is least likely to cause sexual side effects?

A) Fluoxetine
B) Sertraline
C) Venlafaxine (Effexor)
D) Citalopram
E) Bupropion

Answer and Discussion

The answer is E. Sexual side effects, usually delayed ejaculation or anorgasmia, may occur in both men and women who are taking SSRIs and venlafaxine. Treatment consists of several options: reducing the dosage, switching to another agent, or adding another agent to overcome the sexual side effects. Sexual dysfunction typically resolves within 1 to 3 days after discontinuation of the antidepressant and returns on reintroduction. Recovery after withdrawal from fluoxetine may occur within 1 to 3 weeks. Studies suggest that bupropion does not cause sexual side effects. Uncontrolled studies and case reports suggest that the addition of bupropion (Wellbutrin), cyproheptadine (Periactin), nefazodone, or mirtazapine may decrease sexual side effects. In patients with antidepressant-induced erectile dysfunction, sildenafil (Viagra) may be useful if the patient has no history of angina and is not taking nitrates.

> **Additional Reading:** Ables AZ, Baughman OL. 3rd. Antidepressants: update on new agents and indications. *Am Fam Physician.* 2003;67:547–554.

Category: Reproductive

37. After discontinuing fluoxetine, how long should a clinician wait before prescribing an MAOI?

A) 1 day
B) 3 days
C) 1 week
D) 5 weeks
E) No delay is necessary.

Answer and Discussion

The answer is D. Because of its long half-life, patients should allow at least 5 weeks between discontinuation of fluoxetine and commencement of MAOI therapy. Since the combination of MAOIs and other antidepressants can result in severe toxicity (e.g., hypertensive crisis, serotonin syndrome), it is recommended that 2 weeks elapse between discontinuing an MAOI and starting a different antidepressant. Two weeks should also elapse between discontinuing a TCA, SSRI (other than fluoxetine), venlafaxine, duloxetine, or mirtazapine and starting an MAOI. When switching between MAOIs, we recommend that 2 weeks elapse between discontinuing the first MAOI and starting the second.

> **Additional Reading:** Hirsch M, Bimbaum RJ, Roy-Byrne PP, Solomon D. Antidepressant medication in adults: switching and discontinuing medication. UpToDate. 2013.

Category: Psychogenic

38. Which of the following statements is associated with adjustment disorder?

A) The patient has an expected reaction to a known stressor.
B) The condition is usually chronic, lasting for several years or more.
C) Depression and anxiety are commonly associated.
D) Medication is usually indicated for treatment.
E) Support groups are rarely of any benefit.

Answer and Discussion

The answer is C. An *adjustment disorder* is defined as an excessive maladaptive reaction to an identifiable psychosocial stressor (e.g., death of a loved one, loss of a job, marital discord, divorce) that has occurred within the previous 3 months. The reaction may affect social relationships or the ability to function effectively at work or school. The disturbance cannot last for more than 6 months, and other mental disorders must be ruled out. In most cases, depression and anxiety are major manifestations. The best treatment is psychosocial support to help enhance the patient's ability to cope and adapt to stressful conditions. In most cases, medication is not necessary; rather, psychotherapy (individual, family, behavioral, and self-help groups) is used in treatment.

> **Additional Reading:** Stern TA, Rosenbaum JF, Fava F, et al., eds. *Massachusetts General Hospital Comprehensive Clinical Psychiatry,* 1st ed. Philadelphia, PA: Mosby/Elsevier; 2008:522–523.

Category: Psychogenic

39. Which of the following is true about somatization disorder, now called *somatic symptom disorder* in DSM 5?

A) Men are more commonly affected than women.
B) Patients exhibit multiple physical complaints that usually have an identifiable physiologic basis.
C) The condition usually develops after age 50.
D) Symptoms rarely affect the patient's interpersonal relationships.
E) Treatment involves frequent office visits and reassurance to the patient.

Answer and Discussion

The answer is E. Somatic symptom disorder (previously called *somatization disorder* in DSM-IV-TR) is a condition characterized by one or more somatic complaints that are distressing and result in disruption of daily life. Excessive thoughts, feelings, or behaviors related to the somatic symptoms are manifested as one or more of the following: disproportionate and persistent thoughts about the seriousness of one's symptoms; persistent high levels of anxiety about health or symptoms; and excessive time and energy devoted to these symptoms or health concerns. The condition generally develops in the teen years and almost always before 30 years of age. Women are more commonly affected than men, and there is usually a positive family history. The symptoms generally interrupt one's job and interpersonal relationships. Because there is an increased association with depressive disorders, there is also a corresponding increased suicide risk. Diagnosis should specify if pain is a predominant symptom, if the symptoms are persistent or episodic, and level of severity (mild, moderate, or severe). With regard to treatment, reassurance with frequent office visits and sensitivity to the patient's needs is usually beneficial. Costly tests and repeated subspecialty consultations are discouraged unless there are questions with the diagnosis.

> **Additional Reading:** American Psychiatric Association. *Diagnostic and Statistical Manual of Mental Disorders,* 5th ed. Washington, DC: American Psychiatric Association; 2013.

Category: Psychogenic

40. Which of the following statements about the use of buspirone (Buspar) is true?

A) The drug is used in the treatment of acute anxiety.

B) The drug may cause displacement of tightly bound drugs, such as phenytoin and warfarin, leading to toxicity.

C) Side effects include dizziness, fatigue, nervousness, and headache.

D) The medication is commonly associated with abuse.

E) The drug can be used in combination with MAOIs to treat resistant depression.

Answer and Discussion

The answer is C. Buspirone is an antianxiety medication that is used for chronic anxiety. It is not associated with abuse, drowsiness, or functional limitations. Buspirone is not useful in the treatment of acute anxiety because it often takes several days to weeks (depending on the patient) to produce its therapeutic effect. The drug's mechanism of action involves serotonin, norepinephrine, and dopamine receptors, and it indirectly affects gamma-aminobutyric acid (GABA) receptors. The medication does not affect other tightly bound drugs, such as warfarin, propranolol, or phenytoin, but may affect less tightly bound drugs, such as digoxin. Patients receiving MAOIs should not use buspirone because of the risk of elevated blood pressure and hypertensive crisis. Side effects reported with the use of buspirone include dizziness, fatigue, nervousness, headache, decreased concentration, palpitations, nausea, and abdominal complaints.

Additional Reading: Stern TA, Rosenbaum JF, Fava F, et al., eds. *Massachusetts General Hospital Comprehensive Clinical Psychiatry*, 1st ed. Philadelphia, PA: Mosby/Elsevier; 2008:606.

Category: Psychogenic

41. Which of the following is rated the greatest problem in children 8 to 15 years of age by children of that age?

A) Racism

B) Pressure to have sex

C) Pressure to drink alcohol

D) Pressure to do drugs

E) Bullying

Answer and Discussion

The answer is E. Childhood bullying has been viewed as an inevitable part of growing up. However, recent survey data show that American children 8 to 15 years of age rate bullying as a greater problem than racism or pressure to have sex or use alcohol and other drugs.

Additional Reading: Lyznicki JM, McCaffree MA, Robinowitz CB. Childhood bullying: implications for physicians. *Am Fam Physician*. 2004;70:1723–1730.

Category: Patient/Population-based care

42. A 42-year-old woman presents to your office. Her life appears chaotic and she transfers many of her dysfunctional feelings and conflicts to you, her physician. She is at times paranoid, depressed, and angry. She has a history of multiple unstable interpersonal relationships. The most likely diagnosis is

A) Borderline personality disorder

B) Antisocial behavior

C) Narcissistic disorder

D) Histrionic disorder

E) None of the above

Answer and Discussion

The answer is A. Borderline personality disorder is a pattern of instability in interpersonal relationships, self-image, and affects, and marked impulsivity beginning in early adulthood and present in a variety of contexts. Treating borderline personality disorder can be difficult and challenging because of their instability; patients can present with a wide range of symptoms, including depression, anger, paranoia, extreme dependency, self-mutilation, and alternating idealization and devaluation of the physician. Their lives tend to be chaotic. They transfer many of their dysfunctional feelings and conflicts to the treating physician and the medical encounter. There are a number of common co-occurring disorders with borderline personality disorder, including mood disorders, substance use disorders, bulimia nervosa, PTSD, and ADHD. A detached professional stance and clear limit setting in terms of availability, appointment frequency, appropriate behavior, and medication use are necessary to manage these patients successfully. It is important to monitor one's own feelings and to refrain from responding inappropriately to verbal attacks and manipulation. The development of a formal behavioral treatment plan and insistence on participation in behavioral health/psychiatric care may be helpful to establish an effective working relationship.

Additional Reading: Ward RK. Assessment and management of personality disorders. *Am Fam Physician*. 2004;70:1505–1512.

Category: Psychogenic

When treating borderline personality disorder, a detached professional stance and clear limit setting in terms of availability, appointment frequency, appropriate behavior, and medication use are necessary to manage these patients successfully.

43. A 17-year-old girl is brought to your office by her parents. She has been having hallucinations over the past year and recently experienced a psychotic episode that lasted for 2 weeks. She has been out of school for 3 years and has not been able to hold a job. Her mother reports that the girl often remains in her room. The most likely diagnosis is

A) Agoraphobia

B) Panic attacks

C) Schizophrenia

D) School avoidance

E) Major depression

Answer and Discussion

The answer is C. Schizophrenia is a common psychiatric disorder and usually has a strong family history. Typically, patients are in the late teens or early 20s when the condition is identified. The definition describes a condition in which there is chronic impairment of functioning that involves disturbances of thinking, feeling, and behavior, with continuous signs of the symptoms for at least 6 months. Specific criteria involve two or more of the following: (1) delusions; (2) hallucinations; (3) disorganized speech; (4) grossly disorganized or catatonic behavior; or (5) negative symptoms (diminished emotional expression or avolition)—at least one of these must be (1), (2), or (3). Signs must be present for a significant portion of time during a 1-month period and must impair level of functioning. Often patients experience social isolation, difficulties with social functioning or job requirements, peculiar behavior, impaired hygiene, abnormal thought processes, inappropriate affect, and lack of energy or interest.

Treatment involves the use of antipsychotics and psychotherapy. The prognosis in patients with schizophrenia is worsened the longer the duration of psychosis before institution of effective antipsychotic therapy and the greater the number of psychotic relapses. Use of traditional antipsychotic medications has been limited by their side effects and failure to achieve long-term control of symptoms in some cases. New "atypical" antipsychotic drugs (clozapine, risperidone, and olanzapine) are used for the treatment of resistant cases of schizophrenia and improvement in patient tolerance and compliance. These medications have been more successful than traditional antipsychotic drugs in treating the negative symptoms of schizophrenia, such as social withdrawal and apathy. The atypical antipsychotic drugs produce fewer extrapyramidal side effects and no TD or dystonia. However, they are associated with neuroleptic malignant syndrome, metabolic syndrome, and clozapine can produce fatal agranulocytosis. Use of these medications in selected patients who do not benefit from, or cannot tolerate, traditional agents is an important step in improving the lives of individuals with schizophrenia. Despite advancement in medication, relapses are common.

Additional Reading: Beers MH, Porter RS, Jones TV, et al., eds. *The Merck Manual of Diagnosis and Therapy*, 18th ed. Whitehouse Station, NJ: Merck Research Laboratories; 2006:1722–1728.

Category: Psychogenic

44. A 7-year-old boy is brought to your office. The parents report that the child has had problems in school for the last 6 months. His teacher reports lack of concentration and excessive fidgeting. The child typically interrupts others and often loses objects. After further assessment and a diagnosis of ADHD, the most appropriate treatment is
A) Reassurance
B) Stimulant medication
C) Antidepressant medication
D) Short-acting benzodiazepines
E) Strict discipline

Answer and Discussion

The answer is B. ADHD is a condition characterized by a persistent patterns of inattention and/or hyperactivity-impulsivity that interferes with functioning or developments and is characterized by (1) a short attention span and/or (2) distractibility that persists for longer than 6 months. Other symptoms include failure to attend to details, making careless mistakes, not listening when spoken to, inability to follow through on tasks, difficulty with organization, loses things often, forgetful in daily activities, fidgeting or squirming in one's seat, restlessness, inability to remain seated when required to do so, difficulty in awaiting one's turn, excessive talking, blurting out answers to questions before they are completed, interrupting others, and engaging in dangerous activities without consideration of the consequences. Boys are more commonly affected, and the onset typically occurs before 7 years of age but must be present by age 12. Symptoms must occur in 2 or more settings. The clinical history is usually all that is needed to determine the diagnosis, although psychological and educational testing may help to support the diagnosis. Treatment is often accomplished with stimulants, such as methylphenidate and dextroamphetamine, which have a paradoxical calming effect on young patients. Atomoxetine (Strattera) is a selective norepinephrine reuptake inhibitor that is approved for use in children above age 6. Most children show improvement with medication; drug holidays (at least 2 weeks/year) are important during chronic therapy to see if further medication is necessary. Behavior modification for the child and family counseling may also be helpful.

Additional Reading: American Psychiatric Association. *Diagnostic and Statistical Manual of Mental Disorders*, 5th ed. Washington, DC: American Psychiatric Association; 2013.

Category: Patient/Population-based care

45. Which of the following statements about suicide is true?
A) Men make more suicide attempts
B) Women are more successful
C) Anxiety is the most common contributing factor
D) Most suicides occur during December
E) Married people have the lowest risk for suicide

Answer and Discussion

The answer is E. Suicide is an ever-increasing problem in the United States. Men tend to be more successful at suicide attempts, whereas women make more attempts. Underlying depression is the most common contributing factor. Persons in the 40-to-50-year age range are at particular risk, as are those with chronic diseases (e.g., acquired immunodeficiency syndrome, cancer, and respiratory illnesses, and patients who require hemodialysis). Groups that are particularly affected include those who feel overwhelmed with their personal problems, those who attempt to control others with their actions, those with severe depression who are overwhelmed by a stressful situation or accusation, and those with underlying psychotic illness. Other risk factors include drug abuse, family history of suicide, previous suicide attempts, lack of social support system, and recent loss of a loved one, particularly in older patients. The number of suicides increases slightly in the spring and summer; however, contrary to popular belief, suicides do not increase in December and holiday periods. Married people have the lowest suicide rates.

Additional Reading: Stern TA, Rosenbaum JF, Fava F, et al., eds. *Massachusetts General Hospital Comprehensive Clinical Psychiatry*, 1st ed. Philadelphia, PA: Mosby/Elsevier; 2008:733.

Category: Psychogenic

46. A 31-year-old woman you are treating is emotional and seductive in her behavior. She is very focused on her appearance to others and wants to be the center of attention. You note she has a difficult time making decisions. The most likely diagnosis is
A) Borderline personality disorder
B) Antisocial behavior
C) Narcissistic disorder
D) Histrionic disorder
E) None of the above

Answer and Discussion

The answer is D. The essential feature of histrionic personality disorder is pervasive and excessive emotionality and attention-seeking behavior in a variety of contexts. Histrionic patients are often not satisfied if they are not the center of attention. They tend to be emotional and seductive, suggestible, and use their appearance to attract the attention of others. As a result, the implications of illness and aging may have a profound impact on their psychological functioning. When faced with these patients, the physician should maintain an awareness of the patients' interpersonal style and be empathetic to their issues, while avoiding inappropriate emotional or seductive behaviors. Additionally, these patients have difficulties in dealing with facts, details, and decision making. As a result, they may require extra assistance in processing medical information.

Additional Reading: Ward RK. Assessment and management of personality disorders. *Am Fam Physician*. 2004;70:1505–1512.

Category: Psychogenic

47. Before the diagnosis of PTSD is made, symptoms should be present for at least
A) 1 year
B) 6 months
C) 3 months
D) 1 month
E) 1 week

Answer and Discussion

The answer is D. PTSD can occur after any major traumatic event (exposure to actual or threatened death, serious injury, or sexual violence). Exposure can be from direct experience, witnessing the event, learning that the traumatic event occurred, or experiencing extreme repeated or extreme exposure to aversive details of the traumatic event. Symptoms include intrusive symptoms such as disturbing thoughts and nightmares about the traumatic event, dissociative reactions (flashbacks), reactions to cues/triggers that symbolize the event; avoidance symptoms such as avoiding memories or external reminders; negative alterations in cognitions and mood; and marked arousal and reactivity. To fulfill the DSM 5 criteria for PTSD, an individual must have been exposed to a traumatic event; have at least one intrusion symptoms; one avoidance symptom; two negative cognition/mood symptoms; and two arousal symptoms. The symptoms must be present for at least 1 month; and the symptoms must cause clinically important distress or reduced day-to-day functioning. Acute stress disorder occurs immediately after a trauma and last at least 3 days but up to 1 month after a major traumatic event. Different types of trauma lead to a similar clinical presentation of PTSD, and there is a lot of evidence that PTSD is associated with numerous health conditions and poor health outcomes. Treatments for PTSD can include SSRI medication, cognitive processing therapy, prolong exposure therapy, and other medications to manage symptoms. However, benzodiazapines should be avoided in patients with PTSD.

Additional Reading: American Psychiatric Association. *Diagnostic and Statistical Manual of Mental Disorders,* 5th ed. Washington, DC: American Psychiatric Association; 2013.

Category: Psychogenic

48. Which of the following agents is the most appropriate treatment for a patient with bipolar disorder?
A) Haloperidol
B) Chlorpromazine (Thorazine)
C) Diazepam (Valium)
D) Lithium (Eskalith)
E) Fluoxetine

Answer and Discussion

The answer is D. Bipolar disorder is characterized by one or more episodes of mania (i.e., a distinct period during which there is an abnormal, persistently elevated, expansive, or irritable mood and persistently increased activity or energy that is present for most of the day, nearly every day, for a period of at least 1 week). Manic episodes may involve flight of ideas, excessive spending, aggressive and grandiose behavior, little sleep, and activities that are later regretted. In bipolar I, there are typically episodes of major depression as well (e.g., anhedonia, inability to concentrate, withdrawal from activities, chronic fatigue, loss of sexual drive, insomnia, anorexia with weight loss). The mean age of onset for the first manic, hypomanic, or depressive episode among patients with bipolar I disorder is 18 years. Differentiating true mania from mania that results from secondary causes

can be challenging. Initially, during the manic phase, these behaviors may attract other people; however, in the long term, they lead to significant interpersonal difficulties and conflicts. The episodes, which begin abruptly and are often precipitated by life stresses, may last for up to several months; however, they are often shorter in duration. Women are more likely to have rapid cycling and mixed states. The lifetime risk of suicide among patients with bipolar is estimated to be at least 15 times greater than the general population. Co-occurring mental disorders are common. Bipolar II disorder is characterized by meeting criteria for a current or past hypomanic episode and a current or past episode of major depression. Bipolar II is typically brought to medical attention when the patient is depressed. A careful history usually illuminates the diagnosis revealing episodes of hypomania. Some depressed patients will develop hypomania when given antidepressants. Lithium is a first-line treatment for bipolar disorder. It is important to remember that lithium levels need to be followed, and abnormalities associated with the kidneys and thyroid can be induced with medication. Valproic acid (Depakene) can also be used to treat the manic symptoms. If the patient is psychotic, a neuroleptic medication may also be given. Long-acting benzodiazepines can be used for treating agitation. However, in patients with a substance abuse history, benzodiazepines should be used with caution because of the addictive potential of these agents. When the patient with bipolar disorder becomes depressed, an SSRI or bupropion is recommended. The use of TCAs should be avoided because of the possibility of inducing rapid cycling of symptoms.

Additional Reading: Malhi GS, Adams D, Cahill CM, et al. The management of individuals with bipolar disorder: a review of the evidence and its integration into clinical practice. *Drugs.* 2009;69(15):2063.

Category: Psychogenic

49. Tardive Dyskinesia (TD) is associated with
A) Use of lithium
B) Chronic blockade of dopaminergic receptors
C) Use of serotonin reuptake inhibitors
D) Short-term use of phenothiazine neuroleptics
E) Anti-Parkinson's medications

Answer and Discussion

The answer is B. TD is a condition characterized by repetitive, involuntary, and purposeless choreiform movements of the extremities and buccal, oral, and lingual structures. Although often considered an extrapyramidal symptom, TD is a separate, mechanistically distinct phenomenon. The condition is thought to be secondary to chronic blockage of dopamine receptors in the brain. It is usually associated with side effects of long-term use of phenothiazine neuroleptics and anticholinergic medication. Older patients and those with previous brain injury have a higher incidence of TD. In most cases, the symptoms do not resolve when the medication is discontinued. A systematic review was completed with limited studies to determine whether the following interventions were effective and safe for people with neuroleptic-induced TD: botulin toxin, endorphin, essential fatty acid, EX11582A, ganglioside, insulin, lithium, naloxone, oestrogen, periactin, phenylalanine, piracetam, stepholidine, tryptophan, neurosurgery, or electroconvulsive therapy (ECT). Studies were selected if they focused on people with schizophrenia or other chronic mental illnesses with neuroleptic-induced TD and compared the use of the interventions listed above versus placebo or no intervention. There is no strong evidence to support the everyday use of any of the agents noted above. Prevention of TD and the early detection and treatment of potentially reversible cases of TD are therefore of paramount importance. The only certain method of TD prevention is to avoid treatment with antipsychotic drugs. However, sometimes the benefits outweigh the risks. Patients on antipsychotic drugs, particularly for longer than 3 months, require careful and continuous evaluation.

Additional Reading: Soares-Weiser K, Irving CB, Rathbone J. Miscellaneous treatments for neuroleptic-induced tardive dyskinesia. *Cochrane Database Syst Rev.* 2003;2:CD000208.

Category: Neurologic

50. Laboratory findings seen in anorexia nervosa include
A) Hyperkalemia
B) Leukocytosis
C) Prolonged QT interval on electrocardiogram
D) Metabolic acidosis
E) Elevated sedimentation rate

Answer and Discussion

The answer is C. Anorexia nervosa is a psychiatric problem that centers on restriction of energy intake that leads to a significantly low body weight, intense fear of gaining weight or becoming fat, and persistent behavior that interferes with weight gain, as well as disturbance in the way one's body weight and shape are experienced, undue influence of body weight or shape on self-evaluation, and persistent lack of recognition of the seriousness of the low body weight. Among women, the lifetime prevalence of anorexia nervosa is 0.5% to 3.7%. Symptoms can include binge eating and self-induced vomiting or extreme restriction through dieting, exercise, and fasting. Women account for 95% of those affected. Onset is usually during adolescence but can occur earlier. Severe cases can be fatal. Most patients are described as being compulsive, intelligent, and meticulous; they are usually high achievers. Physical findings include cachexia (>15% less than ideal weight), amenorrhea, loss of sexual desire, low body temperature, cold intolerance, bradycardia, dental erosions, hypotension, hypothermia, edema, and hirsutism. Depression may also be present. Laboratory findings include electrolyte disorders (e.g., hypokalemia), metabolic alkalosis, increased blood urea nitrogen secondary to dehydration, thrombocytopenia, leukopenia, low or normal erythrocyte sedimentation rate, and prolonged QT interval on electrocardiogram. Short-term treatment involves active intervention to restore weight (which may require hospitalization), correction of electrolytes, and preservation of vital functions; long-term treatment involves psychiatric and psychological treatment including family therapy to restore a healthy body image and to treat possible underlying depression. The goals of treatment for anorexia nervosa are to restore patients to a healthy weight, treat the physical complications, enhance the patient's motivation to cooperate with treatment, and provide education about healthy nutrition and eating habits. Other goals of treatment include correcting maladaptive thoughts, attitudes, and feelings related to the eating disorder; treating associated psychiatric conditions; enlisting family support; and attempting to prevent relapse. Medication should be considered in the treatment of anorexia but should not be the sole or primary treatment.

Additional Reading: Williams P, Goodie J, Motsinger C. Treating eating disorders in primary care. *Am Family Physician.* 2008;77(2):187–195.

Category: Cardiovascular system

51. An 80-year-old man is hospitalized secondary to pneumonia. On day 2 of his hospitalization, the nurse calls and tells you he is confused and calling out from his room. He has made multiple attempts to leave his room. You suspect delirium. He has no history of drug or alcohol abuse. Appropriate medication would include
A) Diazepam
B) Lorazepam (Ativan)
C) Haloperidol
D) Mirtazapine
E) Fluoxetine

Answer and Discussion

The answer is C. The management of delirium involves identifying and correcting the underlying medical problem and symptomatically managing any behavioral or psychiatric symptoms. Low doses of antipsychotic drugs can help to control agitation. The use of benzodiazepines should be avoided except in cases of alcohol or sedative–hypnotic withdrawal. Environmental interventions, including frequent reorientation of patients by nursing staff and education of patients and families, should be instituted in all cases.

Additional Reading: Gleason OC. Delirium. *Am Fam Physician.* 2003;67:1027–1034.

Category: Neurologic

The management of delirium involves identifying and correcting the underlying medical problem and symptomatically managing any behavioral or psychiatric symptoms.

52. Among patients with severe alcohol use disorders, which of the following is not true with regard to the risk of relapse?
A) Level of alcohol consumption predicts later relapse.
B) Older men are less likely to relapse than younger men after recovery.
C) Patients who try to use controlled drinking tend to relapse more often than patients who choose abstinence.
D) Current evidence does not support the effectiveness of Alcoholics Anonymous (AA) for preventing relapse.
E) Women are more likely to relapse than men.

Answer and Discussion

The answer is E. The abstinence-based method is most commonly used to treat alcohol/drug addiction. However, advocates for harm reduction may acknowledge that abstinence is the best outcome, but that not every individual achieves this end, and that controlled drinking for some individuals is an achievable aim, which reduces risk to patients. Common interventions for alcohol-related disorders include motivational enhancement therapy, psychotherapy, cognitive behavior techniques, and referral to 12-step recovery programs, such as AA and Narcotics Anonymous (NA). AA is the best known peer-support program for substance use disorders. It is an international organization of recovering alcoholics that offers emotional support and a model of abstinence for people recovering from alcohol dependence using a 12-step approach. Abstinence is encouraged on a "one day at a time" basis. Members attend meetings (either open to all or restricted to participants with alcoholism) in which experiences related to drinking and recovery are shared and steps in the Twelve Steps to Recovery are discussed. The Twelve Step program entails acknowledgment that alcohol has led to loss of control, that recovery is a spiritual journey through belief in a higher power, and through personal exploration and acceptance. Despite the long history and popularity of AA, no experimental studies unequivocally demonstrated the effectiveness of AA or 12-step programs for reducing alcohol dependence or problems. Alcohol dependence is a chronic illness, so with all treatment approaches relapse is fairly common. Factors associated with higher rates of relapse include male gender, younger age, fewer social supports, greater alcohol consumption before treatment, and poor compliance with drug therapy. Abstinence represents the most stable form of remission for most recovering alcoholics. Physicians who continue to be supportive encourage AA participation and treat comorbid anxiety or depression may help reduce the incidence of relapse.

Additional Reading: Ferri M, Amato L, Davoli M. Alcoholics anonymous and other 12-step programmes for alcohol dependence. *Cochrane Database Syst Rev.* 2006;3:CD005032; and Dawson DA, Goldstein RB, Grant BF. Rates and correlates of relapse among individuals in remission from DSM-IV alcohol dependence: a 3-year follow-up. *Alcohol Clin Exp Res.* 2007;31(12):2036.

Category: Patient/Population-based care

53. Which of the following is considered the "date rape" drug?
A) 3,4-Methylenedioxymethamphetamine (MDMA)
B) Flunitrazepam (Rohypnol)
C) Ketamine (Ketalar)
D) Cocaine
E) Cannabis

Answer and Discussion

The answer is B. The most widely used club drugs are MDMA, also known as ecstasy; gamma-hydroxybutyrate (GHB); flunitrazepam; and ketamine. These drugs are popular because they are inexpensive and are conveniently dispensed as small pills, powders, or liquids. Club drugs usually are taken orally and may be taken in combination with each other, with alcohol, or with other drugs. Adverse effects of MDMA ingestion result from sympathetic overload and include tachycardia, mydriasis, diaphoresis, tremor, hypertension, arrhythmias, parkinsonism, esophoria (tendency for eyes to turn inward), and urinary retention. However, the most dangerous potential outcome of MDMA ingestion is hyperthermia and the associated "serotonin syndrome." Serotonin syndrome is manifested by grossly elevated core body temperature, rigidity, myoclonus, and autonomic instability; it can result in end-organ damage, rhabdomyolysis and acute renal failure, hepatic failure, adult respiratory distress syndrome, and coagulopathy. GHB produces euphoria, progressing with higher doses to dizziness, hypersalivation, hypotonia, and amnesia. Overdose may result in Cheyne–Stokes respiration, seizures, coma, and death. Coma may be interrupted by agitation, with flailing activity described similar to a drowning swimmer fighting for air. Bradycardia and hypothermia are present in about one-third of patients admitted to a hospital for using GHB and appear to be correlated with the level of consciousness. Chronic use of GHB may produce dependence and a withdrawal syndrome that includes anxiety, insomnia, tremor, and in severe cases, treatment-resistant psychoses. In the United States, imported Rohypnol came to prominence in the 1990s as an inexpensive recreational sedative and the "date rape" drug. Effects of Rohypnol occur about 30 minutes after ingestion, peak at 2 hours, and may last up to 8 to 12 hours. The effects are much greater with the concurrent ingestion of alcohol or other sedating drugs. Some users experience hypotension, dizziness, confusion,

visual disturbances, urinary retention, or aggressive behavior. Ketamine is difficult to develop; therefore, most of the illegal supply is obtained from human and veterinary anesthesia products. Ketamine is distributed in a liquid form that can be ingested or injected. In clubs, it is usually smoked in a powder mixture of marijuana or tobacco, or is taken intranasally. A typical method uses a nasal inhaler, called a "bullet" or "bumper"; an inhalation is called a "bump." Ketamine is often taken in "trail mixes" of methamphetamine, cocaine, sildenafil citrate (Viagra), or heroin. Effects of ketamine ingestion appear rapidly and last about 30 to 45 minutes, with sensations of floating outside the body, visual hallucinations, and a dream-like state. Along with these "desired" effects, users also commonly experience confusion, anterograde amnesia, and delirium. They also may experience tachycardia, palpitations, hypertension, and respiratory depression with apnea. "Flashbacks" or visual disturbances can be experienced days or weeks after ingestion. Some chronic users become addicted and exhibit severe withdrawal symptoms that require detoxification.

Additional Reading: Gahlinger PM. Club drugs: MDMA, gamma-hydroxybutyrate (GHB), rohypnol, and ketamine. *Am Fam Physician.* 2004;69:2619–2627.

Category: Patient/Population-based care

54. Galactorrhea is associated with which of the following medications?
A) Benzodiazepines
B) TCAs
C) MAOIs
D) Antipsychotic medication
E) Dopamine agonist

Answer and Discussion

The answer is D. Antipsychotic (neuroleptic) medications are dopamine receptor antagonist(s) and include the following:

- Phenothiazines—chlorpromazine, thioridazine, mesoridazine (Serentil), perphenazine (Trilafon), trifluoperazine (Stelazine), and fluphenazine (Prolixin)
- Thioxanthenes—thiothixene (Navane)
- Butyrophenones—haloperidol
- Dihydroindolones—molindone (Moban)
- Dibenzoxazepine—loxapine (Loxitane)

Side effects of these medications are extensive and include anticholinergic effects such as dry mouth, blurred vision, urinary retention, delayed gastric emptying, acute glaucoma in patients with narrow anterior chamber angles, orthostatic hypotension, sexual dysfunction, cardiac arrhythmias, and endocrine abnormalities (hyperglycemia and hyperprolactinemia with galactorrhea). Extrapyramidal symptoms include akathisias (the desire to be in constant motion), acute dystonias (bizarre muscle spasms of the head, neck, and tongue), drug-induced parkinsonism (pill-rolling tremor, rigidity, and bradykinesia), and TD (abnormal repetitive movements of the face, tongue, trunk, or limbs). The medications are indicated in the treatment of schizophrenia, psychoses, and mania. The risk for TD increases with age and the length of administration of the medication. Neuroleptic malignant syndrome is a severe life-threatening side effect of antipsychotics that requires prompt recognition and treatment. Newer atypical antipsychotics have fewer side effects and are dopamine–serotonin antagonists.

Additional Reading: Stern TA, Rosenbaum JF, Fava F, et al., eds. *Massachusetts General Hospital Comprehensive Clinical Psychiatry,* 1st ed. Philadelphia, PA: Mosby/Elsevier; 2008:537,581–582.

Category: Neurologic

55. An effective parenting strategy is?
A) Bargaining
B) Redirecting
C) Dependence
D) Variability
E) Inconsistency

Answer and Discussion

The answer is B. Since discipline plays an important role in the social and emotional development of children, physicians should be trained to discuss this issue with parents during routine well-child examinations and counsel parents about safe, effective methods of discipline. Discipline should be instructive and age-appropriate and should include positive reinforcement for good behavior and redirecting undesirable behavior. Commonly, children misbehave when they are tired, bored, or hungry. Children may also misbehave when they are deprived of adult attention, and when misbehavior elicits adult attention, this can unintentionally reinforce the undesired behavior. Parental attention is a powerful form of positive reinforcement, and parents should attempt to use attention and other positive reinforcers when they are pleased with their child's behavior. Consistency, reliable standards, and expectations are all helpful parenting practices as well. One good method for infants and toddlers is *redirecting*. When one redirects a child, one replaces an unwanted (bad) behavior with an acceptable (good) behavior. For example, if throwing a ball inside the house is not allowed, a parent can take the child outside to throw the ball. Time-out is a commonly practiced parenting technique to try to eliminate unacceptable behavior and can be effective when implemented correctly. Time-out involves removing the child from the problem situation to a neutral, boring, nonfrightening, and safe setting for a specified and brief period of time. Time-out works well for children from 18 months up to 5 or 6 years of age.

> **Additional Reading:** Banks JB. Childhood discipline: challenges for clinicians and parents. *Am Fam Physician.* 2002;66(8):1447–1453.

> Category: Psychogenic

56. Which of the following is a recognized symptom of depression?
A) Sense of entitlement
B) Changes in appetite or eating habits
C) Hallucination
D) Flight of ideas
E) Depersonalization

Answer and Discussion

The answer is B. Depression is one of the most common problems seen by family physicians. Women are more affected than men, and the most common age range is 20 to 50 years. DSM 5 requires that at least five of the following symptoms are present for at least 2 weeks. The patient must show either anhedonia or depressed mood and

- Depressed or irritable mood, or both (most of the day)
- Diminished interest or pleasure, or both, in most activity
- Significant change in weight or appetite, or both, with no effort
- Insomnia; hypersomnia
- Psychomotor retardation or agitation
- Fatigue; decreased activity
- Feelings of worthlessness or inappropriate guilt
- Poor concentration; indecisiveness
- Recurrent thoughts of death or suicide, or both

The patient must have no evidence of previous psychiatric diagnosis, no organic contributing cause, and no recent emotional loss. Many patients have a family history of depression and substance abuse. Evaluation should be performed to rule out causative factors such as anemia, infections, hypothyroidism, medication-related side effects, and alcohol or illegal drug abuse. Psychotherapy and antidepressant medication are the mainstays of treatment. Electroconvulsive therapy is reserved for severe cases. Hospitalization is indicated if a patient is suicidal.

> **Additional Reading:** American Psychiatric Association. *Diagnostic and Statistical Manual of Mental Disorders,* 5th ed. Washington, DC: American Psychiatric Association; 2013.

> Category: Psychogenic

57. Which of the following statements is true regarding inhalant abuse?
A) Twenty percent of children in middle school and high school have experimented with inhalants.
B) Inhalant use is not addictive.
C) A comprehensive drug screen can help identify the inhalant used.
D) Reversing agents can assist with recovery from an inhalant toxicity.
E) Hepatic damage is not associated with inhalant abuse because of the lack of enterohepatic circulation of the substance.

Answer and Discussion

The answer is A. Inhalant abuse is prevalent in adolescents. Studies show that roughly 20% of children in middle school and high school have experimented with inhalants. The method of delivery is inhalation of a solvent from its container, a soaked rag, or a bag. Solvents include household cleaning agents or propellants, paint thinners, glue, and lighter fluid. Inhalant abuse typically can cause a euphoric feeling and can become addictive. Acute effects include sudden sniffing death syndrome, asphyxia, and serious injuries (e.g., falls, burns, frostbite). Chronic inhalant abuse can cause cardiac, renal, hepatic, and neurologic damage. Inhalant abuse during pregnancy can lead to fetal abnormalities. Diagnosis of inhalant abuse is difficult and relies almost entirely on a thorough history and a high index of suspicion. No specific laboratory tests confirm solvent inhalation. There are no reversal agents for inhalant intoxication.

> **Additional Reading:** Anderson CE, Loomis GA. Recognition and prevention of inhalant abuse. *Am Fam Physician.* 2003;68:869–874, 876.

> Category: Patient/Population-based care

58. Which of the following is true regarding ADHD?
A) The condition is more common in women.
B) Combining psychosocial therapy with medication has proven to be superior to medication alone.
C) ADHD is best diagnosed using rating scales from parents and teachers and the DSM 5 diagnostic criteria.
D) Symptoms tend to increase over time.
E) Other psychiatric comorbidities are rare.

Answer and Discussion

The answer is C. ADHD presents as some combination of inappropriate hyperactivity, impulsivity, and inattention. ADHD cannot be easily diagnosed by a specific test or biologic marker. Based on study results, the pooled prevalence of ADHD is between 6.8% and 10.3%, with boys having a threefold higher rate. Psychiatric comorbidities, including oppositional-defiant disorder, conduct disorder, depressive disorder, and anxiety disorders are common. There are several ADHD-specific checklists with high sensitivity for identification of children with the disorder several checklists when completed by multiple adults with knowledge of the child's behavior in different settings (e.g., Vanderbilt Rating Scales; Conners' ADHD Index and symptom scales). Reviews of the pharmacologic management of ADHD with methylphenidate hydrochloride, dextroamphetamine sulfate, and pemoline show these drugs to be effective. Nonpharmacologic treatments that have some beneficial effect on behavior and academic performance are behavioral modification and intensive contingency management therapy. Combining drug therapy with psychosocial therapy shows no clear advantage when compared with drug therapy alone. However, the addition of behavioral therapies to medication may have some benefit, including reduction of anxiety and improvement in social skills. Other psychiatric comorbidities are common and should be identified and properly managed. The symptoms of ADHD tend to decrease over the long term but may continue into adolescence and adulthood. The most common treatment is stimulant medication.

Additional Reading: Wolraich M, Brown L, Brown RT, et al. ADHD: clinical practice guideline for the diagnosis, evaluation, and treatment of attention-deficit/hyperactivity disorder in children and adolescents. Subcommittee on attention-deficit/hyperactivity disorder, steering committee on quality improvement and management. *Pediatrics.* 2011;128(5):1007.

Category: Psychogenic

59. Chronic alcohol abuse is associated with which of the following?
A) Hyperuricemia
B) Alanine aminotransferase-aspartate aminotransferase ratio of 2:1
C) Decreased mean corpuscular volume
D) Decreased γ-glutamyl transferase
E) Decreased triglycerides

Answer and Discussion

The answer is A. Alcohol use disorder is a problematic pattern of alcohol use leading to clinically significant impairment or distress. It may or may not include symptoms of tolerance or withdrawal. Symptoms include repeatedly consuming more alcohol than intended, desire or unsuccessful efforts to cut down, excessive time spent obtaining, using, or recovering from alcohol use, cravings, alcohol use despite consequences and failing to fulfill role obligations, use in physically hazardous situations, and continued drinking despite interpersonal and social impacts. Many patients with alcohol use disorders have chronic anxiety or tension, insomnia, depression, headaches, legal and marital problems, GI discomfort, frequent falls, and minor injuries. Complications include gastritis, peptic ulcer disease, cirrhosis, sexual dysfunction, nutritional deficiencies, neuropathy, and pancreatitis. Laboratory findings may include mild elevations of liver function tests. The aspartate aminotransferase–alanine aminotransferase ratio is often 2:1. A macrocytosis with an elevated mean corpuscular volume is usually the result of folate deficiency. Hypertriglyceridemia, hyperuricemia, and elevations in γ-glutamyl transferase are also seen. Treatment has historically been aimed at abstinence of alcohol and participation in rehabilitation programs such as AA. However, harm-reduction models of treatment to reduce the negative consequences of alcohol use and focus on safety are more common and just as relevant in primary care settings. Close monitoring, including hospitalization, may be necessary if withdrawal symptoms are anticipated.

Additional Reading: Ferri F. *Ferri's Clinical Advisor 2010, Instant Diagnosis and Treatment.* Philadelphia, PA: Elsevier/Mosby; 2010:36–38.

Category: Psychogenic

60. A patient whose spouse recently died presents to your office complaining of anxiety, insomnia, depressed mood, and anorexia. She reports that she continues to work and remains active playing bridge. The most appropriate treatment is
A) Antidepressant medications
B) Major tranquilizers
C) Frequent office visits to receive biofeedback
D) Inpatient psychiatric counseling
E) Normalization of symptoms, reassurance, and emotional support

Answer and Discussion

The answer is E. Grief or bereavement reaction occurs in response to significant loss or separation. Situations such as the death of a loved one, marital separation, loss of a girlfriend or boyfriend, or a move to a different and unfamiliar location can give rise to the condition. The reaction is a normal process that usually improves with time. Symptoms include anxiety, insomnia, depressed mood, anorexia, and mood swings. Treatment involves frequent, short office visits to allow patients to express their grief or referral to a behavioral health provider. Patients should be encouraged to maintain regular patterns of activity, sleep, exercise, and nutrition as much as possible, as these activities appear to enhance adaptation during bereavement. The use of major tranquilizers and antidepressants is unnecessary and may interfere with the normal grieving process. Sleep disruption is a common symptom of grief. Short-term prescription of a sleep hypnotic may be effective in promoting sleep. For individuals who experience high levels of anxiety, a time-limited prescription of an anxiolytic can be useful as a crisis measure. However, these medications generally should not be prescribed at high doses or for long periods since their use has the potential to retard and inhibit the grieving process. It is common for grief to intensify during the holidays or special events. Patient reassurance is usually all that is needed. In severe cases, in which there is significant functional impairment over a longer period of time or psychomotor retardation, antidepressants may become necessary.

Additional Reading: Block S, Roy-Byrne P, Schmader K. Grief and bereavement. UpToDate, version 21.8. Accessed September 2013.

Category: Psychogenic

> The use of major tranquilizers and antidepressants during a significant loss is unnecessary and may interfere with the normal grieving process.

61. A 28-year-old man is noted to have impairment in social situations and job-related problems because of a pervasive pattern of grandiosity, lack of empathy, and extreme sensitivity to criticism. Coworkers report he frequently takes advantage of others for self-promotion. The most likely diagnosis is
A) Borderline personality disorder
B) Bipolar disorder
C) Narcissistic personality disorder
D) Paranoid personality disorder
E) Antisocial personality disorder

Answer and Discussion

The answer is C. Patients who are affected with narcissistic personality disorder fulfill the following DSM 5 criteria and exhibit impairment in social or job situations with a pervasive pattern of grandiosity, need for admiration, lack of empathy, and extreme sensitivity to the evaluation and judgment of others. They must exhibit at least five of the following behaviors:

1. Shows arrogant, haughty behaviors or attitudes
2. Interpersonally explosive (takes advantage of others for self-promotion)
3. Requires constant attention and admiration of others
4. Lacks empathy toward others
5. Obsessed with feelings of envy
6. Possesses a sense of entitlement
7. Possesses a grandiose sense of self-importance
8. Remains preoccupied with fantasies of unlimited success
9. Believes he or she is unique and can only be understood by other special people

Many highly successful people exhibit traits that are considered narcissistic; however, only when these traits are inflexible, maladaptive, and persist despite impairment and distress are they clinically significant. Patients with narcissistic personality disorder often experience depression and severe bouts of envy toward others. Occasionally, those who are affected become delusional in their thoughts. Criticism may leave patients with narcissistic personality disorder feeling degraded and humiliated, and they may react with disdain, rage, or defiance. The course of this disease is chronic; however, narcissistic symptoms tend to diminish after the age of 40, when pessimism usually develops.

> Additional Reading: Stern TA, Rosenbaum JF, Fava F, et al., eds. *Massachusetts General Hospital Comprehensive Clinical Psychiatry,* 1st ed. Philadelphia, PA: Mosby/Elsevier; 2008:533.

Category: Psychogenic

62. Traditionally, what cutoff score is used to suggest significant cognitive impairment on the Mini–Mental Status Examination (MMSE)?
A) 15
B) 18
C) 24
D) 27
E) 30

Answer and Discussion

The answer is C. Primary care physicians often do not recognize cognitive impairment in the brief time available for an office visit. Studies have found between 29% and 76% of cases of dementia or probable dementia are not diagnosed by primary care physicians. The USPSTF found that the published evidence did not demonstrate a clear benefit to screening all asymptomatic older individuals, nor did it rule out the possibility of a benefit. However, the task force emphasized the necessity of carefully assessing older adults presenting with cognitive or cognitive-related functional complaints. Whether or not clinicians screen all older individuals, every physician who provides care for adults will encounter patients with memory complaints, and therefore they must be able to assess them for dementing illnesses. The MMSE is probably the best known and most widely used measure of cognition in clinical practice worldwide. The MMSE includes items that cover most cognitive domains, particularly those abilities most relevant to dementia of the Alzheimer's type (AD). This scale can be easily administered by clinicians or researchers with minimal training, takes around 10 minute, and assesses cognitive function in the areas of orientation, memory, attention and calculation, language, and visual construction. Patients score between 0 and 30 points, and cutoffs of 23/24 have typically been used to show significant cognitive impairment. Using a cutoff of 24 points, the MMSE had a sensitivity of 87% and a specificity of 82% in a large population-based sample. However, the test is not sensitive for mild dementia, and scores may be influenced by age and education, as well as language, motor, and visual impairments. The MMSE is unfortunately sometimes misunderstood as a diagnostic test, when it is in fact a screening test with relatively modest sensitivity. The MMSE can also show a ceiling effect allowing many individuals, especially those with a higher level of education, even those with cognitive impairment, to have a perfect score of 30/30. This ceiling effect may limit the sensitivity of the MMSE, especially for individuals with mild cognitive impairment or mild dementia. It also has limited sensitivity to change. Other screening tools for dementia in primary care are useful including the clock drawing as a single task that covers multiple cognitive domains and screens for cognitive problems. Clock drawings are helpful in 1- to 3-minute forms, but must be scored appropriately, and sensitivity to mild forms of impairment can be low. The Montreal Cognitive Assessment (MOCA) is another tool that was originally developed to help screen for mild cognitive impairment. It takes minimal training and can be used in about 10 minute by any clinician. It assesses attention/concentration, executive functions, conceptual thinking, memory, language, calculation, and orientation. A score of 25 or lower (from maximum of 30) is considered significant cognitive impairment. It performs at least as well as MMSE, including in screening for dementia. It has been widely translated. As it assesses executive function, it is particularly useful for patients with vascular impairment, including vascular dementia.

> Additional Reading: Holsinger T, Deveau J, Boustani M, et al. Does this patient have dementia? *JAMA.* 2007;297(21):2391–2404.

Category: Neurologic

63. Which of the following statements is true regarding Tourette's syndrome?
A) Only 1% of the population is affected.
B) Tourette's syndrome is a familial disorder.
C) Patients with tic disorders rarely have other associated psychological conditions.
D) TCAs are the treatment of choice.
E) The long-term prognosis for treatment is poor.

Answer and Discussion

The answer is B. Tic disorders are rather common in the general population. Once thought to be rare, Tourette's syndrome is now known to be a more common disorder that represents the most complex and severe manifestation of the spectrum of tic disorders. Tourette's syndrome is a chronic familial disorder with a fluctuating course; the long-term outcome is generally favorable. It is more common among men than women. Although the exact underlying pathology has yet to be determined, evidence indicates a disorder localized to the frontal-subcortical neural pathways. Tourette's syndrome is associated with ADHD, OCD, behavior problems, and learning disabilities. These associated conditions can make the management of Tourette's syndrome more difficult. Use of antipsychotic medications (resperidone, pimozide, olanzapine, and haloperidol) and clonidine can be effective but may be associated with significant side effects.

> Additional Reading: Kurlan R. Clinical practice. Tourette's Syndrome. *N Engl J Med.* 2010;363(24):2332.

Category: Neurologic

64. Which of the following would be the drug of first choice for the treatment of mild Tourette's syndrome?
A) Carbamazepine
B) Phenobarbital
C) Primidone
D) Phenytoin
E) Lorazepam

Answer and Discussion

The answer is E. Tourette's syndrome is a genetically transmitted disorder that begins in childhood as a simple tic, progressing to multiple tics as the patient ages. Tics may begin as grunts or barks and progress to involuntary compulsive utterances called *coprolalia*. These outbursts may become severe and significantly disable the patient from a physical or social standpoint. Tics tend to be more complex than myoclonus but less flowing than choreic movements, from which they must be differentiated. The patient may voluntarily suppress them for seconds or minutes. Simple tics may respond to benzodiazepines. For simple and complex tics, clonidine is effective in some patients. Long-term use of clonidine does not cause TD; its limiting adverse effect is hypotension. Intermediate-acting benzodiazepines (e.g., lorazepam) may be useful as adjuvant treatment. For more severe cases, antipsychotics, such as haloperidol, olanzapine, resperidone, or pimozide, may be required. Side effects of dysphoria, parkinsonism, akathisia, and TD may limit their use. Antipsychotics should be started cautiously, and patients should be told about potential adverse outcomes.

> **Additional Reading:** Kurlan R. Clinical practice. Tourette's Syndrome. *N Engl J Med.* 2010;363(24):2332.

> **Category:** Neurologic

65. Which of the following statements about conversion disorder is true?
A) Neurological or other medical conditions rarely coexist with conversion disorder.
B) Symptoms have a definitive physiologic or pathophysiologic explanation.
C) Men are more commonly affected.
D) Treatment usually involves pharmacotherapy.
E) Those who are affected often subject themselves to unnecessary medical testing.

Answer and Discussion

The answer is E. Conversion disorder, also known as functional neurological symptom disorder, involves one or more symptoms of altered voluntary motor or sensory function in which clinical findings are incompatible between the symptom and recognized neurological or medical conditions. Motor symptoms include weakness or paralysis; abnormal movements such as tremor or dystonic movements; gait abnormalities; and abnormal limb posturing. Sensory symptoms include alerted, reduced or absent skin sensation, vision, or hearing. Episodes of psychogenic or nonepileptic seizures are also common. Although the diagnosis requires that the symptom is not explained by neurological disease, it should not be made simply because results from investigations are normal or because the symptom is "bizarre." The diagnosis of conversion disorder should be based on the overall clinical picture and not on a single finding. The phenomenon of *la belle indifference* (i.e., lack of concern about the nature or implications of the symptom) has been associated conversion disorder but it is not specific for conversion disorder and should not be used to make the diagnosis. Conversion disorder is 2 to 3 times more prevalent in women, and onset has been reported throughout the lifespan. Onset may be associated with stress or trauma (psychological or physical) but is not exclusive to the occurrence. The diagnosis may be difficult initially because the patient believes that the symptoms stem from a physical disorder and other neurological or medical conditions commonly coexist with conversion disorder. Also, physicians are taught almost exclusively to consider (and exclude) physical disorders as the cause of physical symptoms. Commonly, the diagnosis is considered only after extensive physical examinations and laboratory tests fail to reveal a disorder that can fully account for the symptom and its effects. Although ruling out a possible underlying physical disorder is crucial, early consideration of conversion may avoid tests that increase the costs and risks to the patient and that may unduly delay diagnosis. The best clue is that conversion symptoms rarely conform fully to known anatomic and physiologic mechanisms. Many patients, because of their complaints, subject themselves to unnecessary medical tests. Treatment usually involves psychotherapy. Medication is generally not warranted.

> **Additional Reading:** American Psychiatric Association. *Diagnostic and Statistical Manual of Mental Disorders*, 5th ed. Washington, DC: American Psychiatric Association; 2013.

> **Category:** Psychogenic

66. Which of the following medications should be monitored in the blood of newborns when treating a mother who is breast-feeding for postpartum depression?
A) Fluoxetine
B) Sertraline
C) Bupropion
D) Paroxetine
E) Mirtazapine

Answer and Discussion

The answer is A. Because of the long elimination half-life of fluoxetine, if a woman who was taking this drug during pregnancy wishes to breast-feed while continuing fluoxetine treatment, she should have the infant's blood tested after about 6 weeks of breast-feeding to rule out drug accumulation. In infants exposed to any antidepressant through breast milk, plasma concentrations of the drug should be determined if they are exhibiting persistent unexplained irritability.

> **Additional Reading:** Davanzo R, Copertino M, De Cunto A, et al. Antidepressant drugs and breastfeeding: a review of the literature. *Breastfeed Med.* 2011;6(2):89–98.

> **Category:** Psychogenic

67. Which of the following should be used initially in conjunction with benzodiazepines in the treatment of serotonin syndrome?
A) Diphenhydramine
B) Prednisone
C) Cyproheptadine
D) Dantrolene
E) Nitroprusside

Answer and Discussion

The answer is C. The initial pharmacologic treatment of serotonin syndrome is with benzodiazepines and cyproheptadine (an antihistamine with serotonin antagonist properties). Other medications may include dantrolene and methysergide. If muscular rigidity and hyperthermia do not respond to these interventions, neuromuscular paralysis with endotracheal intubation is appropriate.

Additional Reading: Boyer EW, Shannon M. The serotonin syndrome. *N Engl J Med.* 2005;352:1112.

Category: Psychogenic

68. Which of the following statements is true regarding lithium administration?
A) Hepatotoxicity can develop after 4 weeks of therapy.
B) The drug may affect thyroid function.
C) Renal function can be improved with the use of lithium.
D) Peripheral neuropathy is a possible side effect.
E) Drug levels remain constant and rarely need monitoring.

Answer and Discussion

The answer is B. Lithium is used in the treatment of bipolar disorder. In most cases, it takes 1 week before the effects are noted. Side effects of the medication include tremor, polydipsia, polyuria, GI irritation, and diarrhea. Hypothyroidism and renal toxicity are other complications of lithium administration. Toxicity is characterized by lethargy, seizures, nephropathy, and coma. Blood levels should be monitored carefully and adjusted as necessary. In addition, serum creatinine and thyroid function tests should be evaluated periodically. Drugs that decrease renal clearance, such as nonsteroidal anti-inflammatory agents, should be used cautiously in patients receiving lithium.

Additional Reading: Stern TA, Rosenbaum JF, Fava F, et al., eds. *Massachusetts General Hospital Comprehensive Clinical Psychiatry,* 1st ed. Philadelphia, PA: Mosby/Elsevier; 2008:194–196, 399.

Category: Endocrine

69. A 30-year-old woman makes frequent visits to your office with vague somatic complaints that are out of proportion to any organic findings. In addition, she has frequent mood swings and unstable interpersonal relationships. In the past, she has had problems with alcohol. She is very interested in your personal life and thinks you are a "wonderful doctor." The most likely diagnosis is
A) Borderline personality disorder
B) Bipolar disorder
C) Schizophrenia
D) Dysthymic disorder
E) Narcissistic personality disorder

Answer and Discussion

The answer is A. Patients with borderline personality disorder are often encountered in the family physician's office. Characteristics of this disorder include impulsiveness, unstable and intense interpersonal relationships, substance abuse, and self-destructive behavior with accident proneness. Those who are affected lack self-control, lack self-fulfillment, and have identity problems. Their behaviors include aggressive and suicidal actions with frequent mood swings. In many cases, they present with vague, unexplainable somatic complaints; do not follow therapeutic recommendations; and can be very frustrating to their physicians. Most affected persons present during adolescence. Treatment involves adequate communication, supportive limit setting, frequent office visits, and occasionally medication. Acute crisis may require hospitalization. Patients with this disorder have high comorbidity with other psychiatric disorders and high rates of suicidal ideation, and they cause particular treatment difficulties, including hostility toward caregivers and low rates of treatment compliance. The central feature of patients with borderline personality disorder is a morbid fear of abandonment, with consequential pathologic responses to perceived rejection. Such patients may demand inappropriate amounts of time or support from a primary care physician, and they may become hostile and demanding or suicidal if these needs are not met. The family practitioner should be alert to the following "red flags": a history of doctor shopping; a history of legal suits against physicians or other professionals; a history of suicide attempts; a history of several brief marriages or intimate relationships; an immediate idealization of you as a "wonderful doctor," especially if the patient compares you with disappointing caregivers of the past; and excessive interest in your personal life, eventually leading to invitations to socialize with you. Behavior of this type implies boundary violations, and its purpose is to cement a relationship with the physician, allaying the patient's ever-present fear of abandonment.

Additional Reading: Beers MH, Porter RS, Jones TV, et al., eds. *The Merck Manual of Diagnosis and Therapy*, 18th ed. Whitehouse Station, NJ: Merck Research Laboratories; 2006:1719.

Category: Psychogenic

70. Which of the following drugs has been shown to be beneficial in the treatment of Premenstrual dysphoric disorder (PDD)?
A) Haloperidol
B) Progesterone
C) Fluoxetine
D) Furosemide
E) Lithium

Answer and Discussion

The answer is C. PDD is associated with mood-related symptoms leading to functional impairment that distinguish it from premenstrual syndrome (PMS). Women with premenstrual syndrome experience a wide variety of cyclic and recurrent physical, emotional, behavioral, and cognitive symptoms that begin in the luteal phase (second half) of the menstrual cycle and resolve shortly after the onset of menses (the follicular phase). However, the core symptoms include affective symptoms such as depression, angry outbursts, irritability, and anxiety, and somatic symptoms such as breast pain, bloating and swelling, and headache. The core feature is the recurrent expression of symptoms during the end of the luteal phase of the menstrual cycle with a symptom-free period shortly after the onset of menses. According to DSM-5, patients with PDD. Patients must have a symptom-free postmenopausal week, and they typically experience the symptom of being overwhelmed or out of control during the most affected time. At least one of the following must be present to make the diagnosis: mood swings; marked irritability or anger; marked depressed mood or hopelessness; marked anxiety or tension. The time of greatest well-being is just before ovulation. The average age of presentation is 36. Many report that their symptoms began when they were in their 20s and worsened over time. Those who are affected are at higher risk for development of a major depressive disorder. Fluoxetine (Sarafem, Prozac) was found to be beneficial in treating symptoms, as was sertraline.

Additional Reading: Yonkers KA, Casper RF, Barbieri RL, et al. Clinical manifestations and diagnosis of premenstrual syndrome and premenstrual dysphoric disorder. UpToDate, version 21.8. Accessed September 2013.

Category: Reproductive

> PDD is associated with mood-related symptoms leading to functional impairment that distinguish it from premenstrual syndrome.

71. Which of the following is most commonly associated with TCA toxicity?
A) Third-degree atrioventricular (AV) block
B) Prolongation of the PR interval
C) Prolongation of the QT interval
D) Widened QRS interval
E) T-wave elevation

Answer and Discussion

The answer is C. The TCAs are used less frequently as first-line agents with the development of the SSRIs and other newer antidepressants. This is mainly due to the less benign side-effect profile of the cyclic antidepressants. These drugs interact with a wide variety of brain-receptor types that result in their antidepressant efficacy and side-effect profiles. Most serious is the toxicity of the cyclic antidepressants in overdose. In comparison with the SSRIs, the cyclic antidepressants can be fatal in doses as little as five times the therapeutic dose. The toxicity is usually due to prolongation of the QT interval, leading to arrhythmias.

> **Additional Reading:** Ray WA, Meredith S, Thapa PB, et al. Cyclic antidepressants and the risk of sudden cardiac death. *Clin Pharmacol Ther.* 2004;75:234.

Category: Cardiovascular system

72. Which of the following has the least amount of sexual side effects?
A) Fluoxetine
B) Sertraline
C) Bupropion
D) Paroxetine
E) Citalopram

Answer and Discussion

The answer is C. Bupropion appears to have no or only a limited effect on sexual function.

> **Additional Reading:** Zajecka J. Strategies for the treatment of antidepressant-related sexual dysfunction. *J Clin Psychiatry.* 2001;62(suppl 3):35.

Category: Reproductive

73. A 41-year-old presents with feelings of being "choked up." The symptoms are rather constant and are not made worse with swallowing. He denies that food is stuck in the throat, and he has had no recent weight change. Eating and drinking help to relieve symptoms. The most likely diagnosis is
A) Globus hystericus
B) Panic attacks
C) Barrett's esophagus
D) Reflux esophagitis
E) Zenker's diverticulum

Answer and Discussion

The answer is A. *Globus hystericus* is defined as the subjective sensation of a lump or mass in the throat. No specific cause or mechanism has been determined, although there is some evidence to suggest that increased cricopharyngeal (upper esophageal sphincter) pressures or abnormal hypopharyngeal motility exist during the time of symptoms. The sensation may result from gastroesophageal reflux or from frequent swallowing and drying of the throat associated with anxiety or other emotional states. Although not related to a specific psychiatric disorder, globus may be a symptom of certain mood states. Suppression of sadness is most often implicated. Symptoms resemble the normal sensation of being "choked up." With globus, symptoms do not become worse during swallowing, food does not stick in the throat, and eating or drinking often provides relief. No pain or weight loss occurs. Chronic symptoms may be experienced during grief reactions and may be relieved by crying. The diagnosis is based on the history and physical examination and is a diagnosis of exclusion. The treatment involves treating the underlying psychological condition.

> **Additional Reading:** Beers MH, Porter RS, Jones TV, et al., eds. *The Merck Manual of Diagnosis and Therapy*, 18th ed. Whitehouse Station, NJ: Merck Research Laboratories; 2006:69–70.

Category: Gastroenterology

74. A 7-year-old is brought to your office by his parents at the request of his teachers. The child appears to have understanding of spoken language but has a reading disorder that involves single-word decoding. The parents report that the father has similar problems that were detected during his schooling. The most likely diagnosis is
A) Attention-deficit disorder
B) Autism
C) Dyslexia
D) Congenital hearing loss
E) Mental retardation

Answer and Discussion

The answer is C. Dyslexia is a specific learning disability that is neurological in origin. It is characterized by difficulties with accurate and/or fluent word recognition and by poor spelling and decoding abilities. These difficulties typically result from a deficit in the phonologic component of language that is often unexpected in relation to other cognitive abilities and the provision of effective classroom instruction. Secondary consequences may include problems in reading comprehension and reduced reading experience that can impede the growth of vocabulary and background knowledge. According to the DSM 5, dyslexia fits within the category of a specific learning disorder with impairment in reading and is one of the most common manifestations of a specific learning disorder. The inability to learn derivational rules of printed language is often considered part of dyslexia. Affected children may have difficulty in determining root words or word stems and determining which letters in words follow others and form specific sound–symbol associations, such as vowel patterns, affixes, syllables, and word endings. The cause of dyslexia is unknown, but a strong genetic link has been established. Cerebrovascular accidents, prematurity, and intrauterine complications have been linked to dyslexia. Most experts agree that dyslexia is left hemisphere related and is associated with deficiencies or dysfunctions in the areas of the brain that are responsible for language association (Wernicke's area) and sound and speech production (Broca's area) and in the interconnection of these areas. Most dyslexics are not identified until kindergarten or first grade, when symbolic learning is taught. However, dyslexia in preschool children may manifest itself as delayed language production, speech articulation problems, and difficulties in remembering the names of letters, numbers, and colors, particularly in children with a family history of reading or learning problems. Many dyslexics confuse letters and words with similar configurations or have difficulty in visually selecting or identifying letter patterns and clusters (sound–symbol association) in words. Reversals or visual confusions tend to be seen frequently during the early school years. Most reading and writing reversals occur because dyslexics forget or confuse the names of letters and words that have similar structures; subsequently, *d* becomes *b*, *m* becomes *w*, *h* becomes *n*, *was* becomes *saw*, and *on* becomes *no*, for example. Students with a history of delayed language acquisition use or who are not accelerating in word learning by the middle or end of first grade, or who are not reading at the level expected for their verbal or intellectual abilities at any grade level, should be evaluated. Many dyslexics develop functional reading skills with direct instruction, although dyslexia is a lifelong problem, and many dyslexics never reach full literacy. Compensatory approaches, such as taped texts, readers, and scribes, are used to assist the dyslexic with higher-order learning.

> **Additional Reading:** Vellutino FR, Fletcher JM, Snowling MJ, et al. Specific reading disability (dyslexia): what have we learned in the past four decades? *J Child Psychol Psychiatry.* 2004;45(1):2.

Category: Neurologic

75. Medication for the treatment of premature ejaculation includes
A) Finasteride (Proscar)
B) Tamsulosin (Flomax)
C) Sildenafil (Viagra)
D) Sertraline (Zoloft)
E) Progesterone (Provera)

Answer and Discussion

The answer is D. *Premature ejaculation* is best defined as persistent or recurrent ejaculation with minimal stimulation before, on, or shortly after penetration and before the sexual partner wishes it. Premature ejaculation is thought to be the most common form of male sexual dysfunction, with an estimated prevalence of up to 40%. Treatment of ejaculatory dysfunction centers on relationship counseling, behavioral therapy, and pharmacologic interventions. Behavioral therapy has been considered the gold standard of treatment. Techniques include the Semen's pause maneuver, the Masters and Johnson pause–squeeze technique, and the Kaplan stop–start method. These techniques are directed at the induction of male sexual arousal to the point of ejaculation followed by relaxation before orgasm is allowed to occur. The methods can be self-applied, although with suboptimal outcomes; hence, involvement of the sexual partner is essential. Because of the limitations of behavioral therapy, pharmacologic interventions are often used to treat premature ejaculation. Anorgasmia and delayed ejaculatory response are well-known side effects of TCAs (clomipramine) and SSRIs. Recent studies have shown that these drugs modify the ejaculatory response in men with premature ejaculation. Results appear better with clomipramine, but sertraline was better tolerated and had a better safety profile.

> **Additional Reading:** Montague DK, Jarow J, Broderick GA, et al. Erectile dysfunction guideline update panel. AUA guideline on the pharmacologic management of premature ejaculation. *J Urol.* 2004;172(1):290.

Category: Reproductive

76. When initiating antidepressants in children and adolescents, the risk of suicide is maximum during
A) The first hours of medication administration
B) During the first few weeks
C) During the first few months
D) Usually a year or more after starting therapy
E) The risk of suicide is not increased

Answer and Discussion

The answer is B. The U.S. Food and Drug Administration advisory panel concluded there is a small, but real, increased risk of suicidal thoughts or behavior in children taking antidepressants compared with placebo. The risk appears to be greatest in the first few weeks after initiation of therapy. Careful monitoring of symptoms can be helpful when the benefits of pharmacotherapy for depression in children and adolescents outweigh the risks.

> **Additional Reading:** Jick H, Kaye JA, Jick SS. Antidepressants and the risk of suicidal behaviors. *JAMA.* 2004;292:338.

Category: Psychogenic

77. Which of the following has the best side-effect profile?
A) Amitriptyline
B) Nortriptyline
C) Desipramine
D) Clomipramine
E) Fluoxetine

Answer and Discussion

The answer is E. The TCAs are used less frequently as first-line agents with the development of the SSRIs and other newer antidepressants. This is mainly due to the less benign side-effect profile of the cyclic antidepressants.

> **Additional Reading:** Ray WA, Meredith S, Thapa PB, et al. Cyclic antidepressants and the risk of sudden cardiac death. *Clin Pharmacol Ther.* 2004;75:234.

Category: Psychogenic

78. Which of the following factors may contribute to an increased risk of domestic violence?
A) More than three children in the home
B) Power differential in the relationship
C) Women with depression
D) Prior divorce
E) One spouse undergoing schooling

Answer and Discussion

The answer is B. Studies have not identified any consistent psychiatric diagnoses among abusers, but abusive men share some common characteristics such as rigid sex role stereotypes, low self-esteem, depression, a high need for power and control, a tendency to minimize and deny their problems or the extent of their violence, a tendency to blame others for their behavior, violence in the family of origin (particularly witnessing parental violence), and drug and alcohol abuse (which are not causative but are often associated). Men who have alcoholism combined with a major depressive disorder or antisocial personality disorder are more likely to commit domestic violence than are men with either of these conditions alone. Most researchers believe that abusive behavior is the result of multiple factors, including individual characteristics, a family history of violence, and the culturally rooted belief that violence is an acceptable means of solving problems and that violence toward women is acceptable or tolerated. Factors that specifically relate to partner abuse include the following:

- A power differential in the relationship in which one partner is financially or emotionally dependent on the other.
- A temporary or permanent disability (including pregnancy).
- A force orientation—a belief on the part of the perpetrator that violence is an acceptable solution to conflicts and problems.
- A personal or family history of abuse.

Signs that often indicate a need to further assess the risk of abuse include excessive work loss, sleep disturbances, substance abuse, anxiety, sexual dysfunction, depression, frequent injuries, or being "accident prone." It is imperative to discuss events noted in these records with the patient and to assess any discrepancy between an injury and its reported causative mechanism because injuries that are related to battering are often attributed to falling on the stairs or some other household accident. In such cases, the patient should be asked to describe the accident in more detail, or the physician should ask about precipitating factors (e.g., "Were you pushed?"). Ancillary tests should be obtained as indicated for the specific injury or infection. The physician should be especially alert for pregnancy complications and sexually transmitted infections, including human immunodeficiency virus infection.

Additional Reading: U.S. Department of Health and Human Services, Health Resources and Services Administration, Maternal and Child Health Bureau. *A comprehensive approach for community-based programs to address intimate partner violence and perinatal depression*. Rockville, Maryland: U.S. Department of Health and Human Services, 2013; and *Annals of Internal Medicine* (the USPSTF original source article, January 22, 2013, depending on which source is preferable).

Category: Patient/Population-based care

79. Which of the following statements regarding the use of psychotropic agents in a nursing home setting is true?
A) Phenobarbital does not require monitoring.
B) Sedative–hypnotics should be used to sedate patients who are at risk for falls.
C) Periodic dose reductions should be performed.
D) The physician is ultimately responsible for drug monitoring.
E) Tranquilizers, regardless of their effectiveness in patients before admission to the nursing home, should not be used.

Answer and Discussion

The answer is C. All psychotropic drugs (antidepressants, anxiolytics, sedative–hypnotics, and antipsychotics) are subject to the "unnecessary drug" regulation of the Omnibus Budget Reconciliation Act (OBRA). According to the federal government guidelines, "nursing home residents must be free of unnecessary drugs," which are defined as those that are duplicative, excessive in dose or duration, or used in the presence of adverse effects or without adequate monitoring or indication. Medical, environmental, and psychosocial causes of behavioral problems must be ruled out, and nonpharmacologic management must be attempted before psychotropic drugs are prescribed to nursing home residents. Because treatment with psychotropic medications is indicated only to maintain or improve functional status, diagnoses and specific target symptoms or behaviors must be documented, and the effectiveness of drug therapy must be monitored. Specific dosage limits must be observed, and periodic dosage reductions or drug discontinuations must be undertaken. Side effects (of antipsychotics in particular) must be monitored. Barbiturates and certain other older tranquilizers may not be prescribed unless they were being used successfully before a patient was admitted to a long-term care facility. Phenobarbital can be used only to control seizures. OBRA restricts the use of antipsychotic drugs only in patients with dementia. None of the OBRA dosage restrictions or monitoring requirements applies in patients with psychotic disorders (e.g., schizophrenia). Each nursing home is surveyed annually. Because facilities that do not meet the federal government's requirements may be denied Medicare reimbursement, physicians who prescribe medications for nursing home residents must document the medical necessity of noncompliance with regulations (e.g., drug

prescriptions in excess of OBRA-mandated dosages). In most cases, a local consultant pharmacist reviews all charts monthly and assists with compliance. According to the OBRA strategy, the long-term care facility, rather than the prescribing physician, is accountable for monitoring drug use. Regardless of where final responsibility lies, physicians need to be aware of the federal government's interpretive guidelines for the fulfillment of OBRA requirements.

Additional Reading: Gurvich T, Cunningham JA. Appropriate use of psychotropic drugs in nursing homes. *Am Fam Physician*. 2000;61:1437–1446.

Category: Patient/Population-based care

80. Which of the following antidepressant medications has the lowest risk of drug interactions?
A) Fluoxetine
B) Paroxetine
C) Sertraline
D) Citalopram
E) Amitriptyline

Answer and Discussion

The answer is D. Most SSRIs are associated with significant drug interactions. The SSRIs may inhibit hepatic cytochrome P450 enzymes that metabolize other medications, thereby causing drug–drug interactions. Fluoxetine, paroxetine, and, to a lesser extent, sertraline inhibit the metabolism of warfarin (Coumadin), cisapride (Propulsid), benzodiazepines, quinidine, TCAs, theophylline, and some statins. In patients who are at risk for these interactions, citalopram may offer an advantage. Studies have shown that compared with other SSRIs, citalopram and escitalopram have less of an inhibitory effect on the cytochrome P450 system. They are as effective as fluoxetine and sertraline in the treatment of depression and thus good choices for situations in which drug–drug interactions are a concern.

Additional Reading: Hirsch M, Birnbaum RJ, Roy-Byrne PP, et al. Unipolar depression in adults and selective serotonin reuptake inhibitors (SSRIs): pharmacology, administration, and side effects. UpToDate, version 21.8. Accessed September 2013.

Category: Psychogenic

> Compared with other SSRIs, citalopram has less of an inhibitory effect on the cytochrome P450 system and therefore lower risk for drug interactions.

81. A 47-year-old man complains of a depressed mood over the last 3 years. He complains of low energy and low self-esteem. The condition has not prevented him from working nor has it seemed to interfere with his family life. You explain to him he has the diagnosis of
A) Major depression
B) Persistent depressive disorder (dysthymia)
C) Dissociation disorder
D) Attention-deficit disorder
E) Introvert personality disorder

Answer and Discussion

The answer is B. Persistent depressive disorder (previously called dysthymia in DSM-IV-TR) is a more chronic, low-intensity mood disorder. By definition, symptoms must be present for more than 2 years consecutively. It is characterized by anhedonia, low self-esteem, and low energy. It may have a more psychological than biologic explanation and tends to respond to medication and psychotherapy equally. Long-term psychotherapy is frequently able to establish a permanent change in dysthymic individuals.

Additional Reading: American Psychiatric Association. *Diagnostic and Statistical Manual of Mental Disorders,* 5th ed. Washington, DC: American Psychiatric Association; 2013.

Category: Psychogenic

82. SSRIs are
A) Associated with GI bleeding in patients taking nonsteroidal anti-inflammatory drugs (NSAIDs)
B) Contraindicated in diabetics
C) Not associated with withdrawal symptoms
D) Cardiotoxic in doses that approach therapeutic range
E) Contraindicated in patients with a history of suicidal attempts

Answer and Discussion

The answer is A. Studies have suggested that SSRIs may increase the risk of abnormal bleeding. Observed complications include stroke, upper GI bleeding, and intraoperative bleeding, as well as more minor problems such as easy bruising, petechiae and purpura, epistaxis, and hematomas. There is no indication that any specific SSRI is more strongly associated with abnormal bleeding. In addition, the risk of bleeding may be amplified in patients who are taking other medications that can cause bleeding, such as nonsteroidal anti-inflammatory drugs (e.g., aspirin, ibuprofen, or naproxen).

Additional Reading: de Abajo FJ, García-Rodríguez LA. Risk of upper gastrointestinal tract bleeding associated with selective serotonin reuptake inhibitors and venlafaxine therapy: interaction with nonsteroidal anti-inflammatory drugs and effect of acid-suppressing agents. *Arch Gen Psychiatry.* 2008;65(7):795.

Category: Gastroenterology

83. Bupropion is structurally related to
A) Anxiolytics
B) Stimulants
C) Barbiturates
D) Alcohol
E) Antibiotics

Answer and Discussion

The answer is B. Bupropion is a monocyclic aminoketone that is structurally related to amphetamine. Some authorities classify the drug as a dopamine–norepinephrine reuptake inhibitor because it inhibits presynaptic reuptake of dopamine and norepinephrine (with a greater effect upon dopamine). The drug has little effect upon other neurotransmitters, and little to no affinity for postsynaptic receptors. Bupropion is used to treat major depression, SAD, ADHD, tobacco dependence, hypoactive sexual disorder, and obesity. Contraindications include bulimia nervosa, anorexia nervosa, use of MAOIs in the past 2 weeks, seizure disorders, and abrupt withdrawal from alcohol, benzodiazepines, or other sedatives. The most common adverse reactions include tremor, headaches, rash, and urticaria. Other adverse effects include insomnia and dry mouth. Bedtime administration should be avoided.

Additional Reading: Labbate LA, Fava M, Rosenbaum JF, et al. Drugs for the treatment of depression. In: *Handbook of Psychiatric Drug Therapy*, 6th ed. Philadelphia, PA: Lippincott Williams & Wilkins; 2010:54.

Category: Psychogenic

84. Children whose parents are divorcing are at increased risk for
A) Academic difficulties
B) Externalizing behaviors and acting out
C) Relationship problems
D) Increased somatic symptoms
E) All of the above

Answer and Discussion

The answer is E. Exposure to high levels of parental conflict is predictive of poor emotional adjustment by the child regardless of the parents' marital status. Still, up to half of children show a symptomatic response during the first year after their parents divorce. Risk factors for continuing childhood difficulty include ongoing parental discord, maternal depression, psychiatric disorders in either parent, and poverty. The clinical manifestations of divorce in children depend on many variables, including the child's age; the predivorce level of the family's psychosocial functioning; the parents' ability in the midst of their own anger, loss, and discomfort to focus on their child's feelings and needs; and the child's temperament and temperamental fit of parents with their children.

- Infants and children younger than 3 years may reflect their caregivers' distress, grief, and preoccupation; they often show irritability, increased crying, fearfulness, separation anxiety, sleep and GI problems, aggression, and developmental regression.
- At 4 to 5 years of age, children often blame themselves for the breakup and parental unhappiness, become more clingy, show externalizing behavior (acting out), misperceive the events of the divorce situation, fear that they will be abandoned, and have more nightmares and fantasies.
- School-aged children may be moody or preoccupied; show more aggression, temper, and acting-out behavior; seem uncomfortable with gender identity; and feel rejected and deceived by the absent parent. School performance may decrease, and they may agonize about their divided loyalties and feel that they should be punished.
- Adolescents may feel decreased self-esteem and may develop premature emotional autonomy to deal with negative feelings about the divorce and their deidealization of each parent. Their anger and confusion often lead to relationship problems, substance abuse, decreased school performance, inappropriate sexual behavior, depression, and aggressive and delinquent behavior.
- At all ages, children frequently have psychosomatic symptoms as a response to anger, loss, grief, feeling unloved, and other stressors.

Although divorce may be associated with a variety of negative reactions in all members of the family, protective and risk factors have been identified. Factors that lead to better outcomes include positive child temperament and an optimistic view of the future, consistent parental discipline, parental acceptance and warmth, and maintenance of as normal a routine as possible. Some children have long-lasting emotional and adjustment problems associated with their parents' divorce; however, most adjust and function well over time, particularly those who have supportive relationships and a positive temperament and receive professional counseling.

Additional Reading: George C. Helping children and families deal with divorce and separation. Committee on psychosocial aspects of child and family health. *Pediatrics.* 2002;110(5):1019–1023.

Category: Psychogenic

85. Which of the following is considered tertiary prevention?
A) Pneumococcal (Pneumovax) immunization
B) Purified protein derivative determination in a patient who is affected with tuberculosis
C) Smoking cessation counseling in a patient who is known to have chronic obstructive pulmonary disease
D) Administration of erythromycin eye drops to neonates
E) Hepatitis A vaccination for travelers

Answer and Discussion

The answer is C. The following are three types of prevention:

1. *Primary prevention:* These types of treatments prevent the development of disease. Examples include tetanus, influenza, or pneumococcal polyvalent vaccination (Pneumovax) vaccination and intraocular administration of erythromycin to prevent neonatal chlamydia or gonorrhea.
2. *Secondary prevention:* These are steps taken in the early course of illness and help identify those who are affected. Examples include purified protein derivative determination in patients affected with tuberculosis or Venereal Disease Research Laboratory (VDRL) determination in those with syphilis.
3. *Tertiary prevention:* These are steps that are taken after the development of a condition to help rehabilitate the patient. Examples include counseling a patient with emphysema or chronic bronchitis to stop smoking.

Additional Reading: Rakel R. Key concepts in evidenced based prevention. *Textbook of Family Medicine,* 6th ed. Philadelphia, PA: Saunders/Elsevier; 2007.

Category: Patient/population-based care

86. Which of the following is the primary treatment of schizophrenia?
A) Cognitive therapy
B) Behavioral therapy
C) Interpersonal therapy
D) Psychodynamic psychotherapy
E) Pharmacotherapy

Answer and Discussion

The answer is E. Schizophrenia is a psychiatric disorder involving chronic or recurrent psychosis. It is commonly associated with impairments in social and occupational functioning and is the most disabling and economically catastrophic medical disorders, ranked by the World Health Organization as one of the top 10 illnesses contributing to the global burden of disease.

Pharmacotherapy is the primary treatment for schizophrenia and other psychotic disorders, specifically antipsychotic medications. They have been shown in clinical trials to be effective in treating symptoms and behaviors associated with the disorder. Antipsychotic medications have significant side effects; assessment and management of these adverse effects are an important part of treatment. Evidence-based psychosocial interventions in conjunction with pharmacotherapy can also help patients achieve recovery.

Additional Reading: Stroup TS, Marder S, Stein MB, et al. Pharmacotherapy for schizophrenia: acute and maintenance phase treatment. UpToDate, version 21.8. Accessed September 2013.

Category: Psychogenic

87. Which of the following foods is safe to eat if the patient is taking an MAOI?
A) Fermented cheese
B) Soy sauce
C) Bananas
D) Smoked sausage
E) Wheat bread

Answer and Discussion

The answer is E. MAOIs are often avoided because of their potential to precipitate enhanced sympathetic activity and severe hypertension with the concomitant ingestion of tyramine-containing foods (e.g., fermented cheeses; imported beer; Chianti, champagne, and some other wines; soy sauce; avocados; bananas; overripe or spoiled food; and any fermented, smoked, or aged fish or meat).

Additional Reading: Katon W, Ciechenowski P. Initial treatment of depression in adults. UpToDate, version 17.2. Accessed November 17, 2009.

Category: Psychogenic

88. Which of the following drugs used in the treatment of ADHD is not a first-line agent?
A) Methylphenidate (Ritalin)
B) Dextroamphetamine (Dexedrine)
C) Pemoline (Cylert)
D) Amphetamines

Answer and Discussion

The answer is C. ADHD is the most common pediatric psychiatric disorder. Diagnosis of ADHD requires a detailed history from the family and use of rating scales to collect observations from two or more settings. Effective treatment, including behavior management, appropriate educational placement, and stimulant medication, improves academic performance and behavior in most patients. Children in whom initial management fails or for whom the diagnosis is unclear or complicated should be referred to appropriate mental health professionals. Stimulants are the first-line agent in the treatment of ADHD. Although these medicines have a stimulating effect in most, they have a calming effect in children and adults with ADHD. In most systematic reviews, methylphenidate, dexmethylphenidate, and amphetamines appear to be equally effective and to have similar adverse-effect profiles. The preferences of the patient and family must be taken into consideration when choosing among these agents. Other medications include atomoxetine, clonidine, desipramine, imipramine, and bupropion. Side effects include headaches, GI symptoms, anorexia and weight loss, insomnia, and palpitations. Pemoline has been associated with hepatotoxicity and is no longer used. Other medications (e.g., alpha-2-adrenergic agonists) are usually used when children respond poorly to a trial of stimulants or atomoxetine, have unacceptable side effects, or have significant coexisting conditions. The choice of the initial medication depends upon a number of factors, including

- The duration of desired coverage
- The ability of the child to swallow pills or capsules
- The time of day when the target symptoms occur
- The desire to avoid administration at school
- Coexisting tic disorder (avoidance of stimulants or use of alpha-2 adrenergic agonists may be warranted)
- Coexisting emotional or behavioral condition (an alpha-2-adrenergic agonist may be useful for patients who are overaroused, easily frustrated, highly active, or aggressive)
- Potential adverse effects

- History of substance abuse in patient or household member: avoid stimulants or use stimulants with less potential for abuse
- Preference of the child/adolescent and his or her parent/guardian
- Expense

Dosing of medications should be 30 to 45 minutes before meals (breakfast and lunch). Lunchtime doses can be given at school for some children. An alternative is the use of longer-acting preparations. The long-acting form of these medications should not be crushed, broken, or chewed before swallowing. The long-acting forms are dosed (usually) once a day, before breakfast.

Additional Reading: Wolraich M, Brown L, Brown RT, et al. ADHD: clinical practice guideline for the diagnosis, evaluation, and treatment of attention-deficit/hyperactivity disorder in children and adolescents. Subcommittee on Attention-Deficit/Hyperactivity Disorder, Steering Committee on Quality Improvement and Management. *Pediatrics*. 2011;128(5):1007.

Category: Psychogenic

89. Kava is included in an herbal remedy that is used in the treatment of
A) Depression
B) Impotence
C) Anxiety
D) Memory loss
E) Attention-deficit disorder

Answer and Discussion

The answer is C. The term *kava* refers to a Pacific island plant (*Piper methysticum*) and the beverage that is prepared from it. The drug may be beneficial in the management of anxiety and tension of nonpsychotic origin and does not adversely affect cognitive function, mental acuity, or coordination. Long-term use of high doses has been associated with scaling of the skin on the extremities. Kava may potentiate the action of other centrally mediated agents and interact with alcohol. Kava has been associated with liver toxicity as well.

Additional Reading: Beers MH, Porter RS, Jones TV, et al., eds. *The Merck Manual of Diagnosis and Therapy*, 18th ed. Whitehouse Station, NJ: Merck Research Laboratories; 2006:2732.

Category: Psychogenic

> Kava may be beneficial in the management of anxiety and tension of nonpsychotic origin and does not adversely affect cognitive function, mental acuity, or coordination.

90. Which of the following conditions is commonly seen in patients with mental retardation?
A) Hyperthyroidism
B) Hyperparathyroidism
C) Diabetes mellitus
D) Osteoporosis
E) Pernicious anemia

Answer and Discussion

The answer is D. Osteoporosis is a common condition seen in patients with mental retardation, particularly among non-weight-bearing patients. It has been estimated that as many as 50% of adults with mental retardation have osteoporosis or osteopenia. Conditions associated with an increased risk of osteoporosis include cerebral palsy, Down's syndrome, use of antiepileptics, special diets (e.g., ketogenic diet for seizure control), and hypogonadism. Aggressive evaluation of traumatic injuries with radiographic studies may be justified even when there are few physical findings. Furthermore, osteoporosis and use of antiepileptics may predispose patients to degenerative disk disease with spinal cord compromise, leading to functional decline.

Additional Reading: Prater CD, Zylstra RG. Medical care of adults with mental retardation. *Am Fam Physician*. 2006;73:2175–2184.

Category: Psychogenic

91. Which of the following medications is more likely to have a paradoxical reaction in patients affected with mental retardation?
A) Haloperidol
B) Lorazepam
C) Phenobarbitol
D) Phenytoin
E) Buspirone

Answer and Discussion

The answer is B. In patients affected with mental retardation, many of the most challenging behaviors are caused by the same neuropsychiatric disorders that affect the general population and most respond to the same treatments. One notable exception is benzodiazepine therapy, which can precipitate paradoxical reactions of increased irritability and aggression in 10% to 15% of patients with mental retardation.

Additional Reading: Kalachnik JE, Hanzel TE, Sevenich R, et al. Benzodiazepine behavioral side effects: review and implications for individuals with mental retardation. *Am J Ment Retard*. 2002;107:376–410.

Category: Endocrine

92. Valerian is an herbal remedy that is used for the treatment of
A) Sleep disorders
B) Mania
C) Depression
D) Menstrual disorders
E) Bulimia

Answer and Discussion

The answer is A. Valerian is derived from the perennial herb *Valerian officinalis*. The herb is used in the treatment of anxiety and sleep disorders. It interacts with the inhibitory neurotransmitter GABA. Valerian may potentiate the effects of other central nervous system depressants. The incidence of adverse side effects with its use appears to be low; however, more research is needed.

Additional Reading: Beers MH, Porter RS, Jones TV, et al., eds. *The Merck Manual of Diagnosis and Therapy*, 18th ed. Whitehouse Station, NJ: Merck Research Laboratories; 2006:2733.

Category: Psychogenic

93. Patients with which of the following conditions should use ginkgo biloba with caution?
A) Peptic ulcer disease
B) Peripheral neuropathy
C) Cardiac conduction defects
D) Renal insufficiency
E) Prior deep venous thrombosis

Answer and Discussion

The answer is A. Numerous clinical trials have been performed using ginkgo biloba for a variety of central nervous system and vascular conditions. It is thought that there are two main groups of active constituents responsible for ginkgo biloba's medicinal effects: terpene lactones and ginkgo flavone glycosides, which are present in varying concentrations in the leaf of the ginkgo tree. Caution should be exercised when using ginkgo combined with anticoagulant treatment including aspirin when there is risk of bleeding as in peptic ulcer disease and subdural hematoma. Safety in pregnancy and in lactation has not been determined. The most common adverse affect is headache. Isolated reports of seizure associated with ginkgo use have been published but whether ginkgo lowers seizure threshold is uncertain. Use of ginkgo in patients with seizure disorders should therefore be done with caution. An extract of the dried leaves of the *Ginkgo biloba* tree is used in Europe to alleviate symptoms that are associated with a range of cognitive problems and has been approved in Germany for the treatment of dementia. Ginkgo is thought to have antioxidant properties, although its exact mechanism of action is unclear. Le Bars and colleagues conducted a randomized, double-blind, placebo-controlled trial to test the efficacy of ginkgo in the management of patients with Alzheimer's disease and multi-infarct dementia. Adverse events were not significantly different between the treatment and placebo groups and were considered to be mild to moderate in intensity. The authors conclude that treatment with extract of *Ginkgo biloba* is safe for up to 1 year in patients with dementia and can improve cognitive performance and functioning. The improvement was significant enough to be identified by the patient's caregiver.

> **Additional Reading:** Bent S, Goldberg H, Padula A, et al. Spontaneous bleeding associated with ginkgo biloba: a case report and systematic review of the literature. *J Gen Intern Med.* 2005;20(7):657.

Category: Neurologic

94. Yohimbine has been associated with which of the following?
A) Colon polyps
B) Priapism
C) Cataract formation
D) Skin pigmentation
E) Hypertensive complications

Answer and Discussion

The answer is E. Yohimbine is an indole alkaloid that is obtained from the bark of a West African tree (*Pausinystalia yohimba*). The product is an α-adrenergic receptor antagonist that is marketed for the treatment of impotence. Results of studies have shown consistent ability of the drug to enhance erectile functioning. Yohimbine increases sympathetically mediated plasma norepinephrine, which in turn produces a pressor response. Therefore, yohimbine should be administered with caution to patients with high blood pressure or those who are undergoing concomitant treatment with TCAs or other drugs that interfere with neuronal uptake or metabolism of norepinephrine. The drug may induce panic attacks in patients with anxiety disorders.

> **Additional Reading:** Rakel R. *Textbook of Family Medicine,* 6th ed. Philadelphia, PA: Saunders/Elsevier; 2007:1341.

Category: Gastroenterology

95. *Cognitive therapy* is defined as
A) Repeated exposure to one's fears to overcome associated anxiety
B) A treatment that helps patients reverse unhelpful beliefs that lead to distressing moods and behaviors
C) A confrontation with the patient that exposes certain inadequacies in social interaction
D) An exhaustive review of past events that outlines previous failures
E) An introspective review of past behaviors that highlights poor judgment

Answer and Discussion

The answer is B. Cognitive therapy is defined as a treatment process that helps patients identify and change unhelpful beliefs that lead to problematic moods and behaviors. The basic principle behind cognitive therapy is that a thought comes before an emotion and that both are associated with a person's environment, physical reaction, and subsequent behavior. As a result, changing a thought that arises in a given situation can alter one's emotions, behavior, and physical reactions. Motivated patients who have an internal locus of control and the capacity for introspection tend to benefit most. During cognitive therapy, the therapist assists the patient with several steps. First, the patient accepts that some of his or her perceptions and interpretations of reality may not be entirely true (because of past experience or hereditary or biologic reasons) and that these interpretations lead to negative thoughts. Next, the patient learns to recognize the negative (surface or "automatic") thoughts and discovers alternative thoughts that reflect reality more closely. The patient then decides internally whether the evidence supports the negative thought or the alternative thought. Ideally, the patient will recognize distorted thinking and "reframe" the situation. As cognitive therapy progresses, it focuses more on reframing deeply held or "core" beliefs about self and the world. In cognitive behavior therapy (CBT) for depression, behavioral principles are used to overcome a patient's reluctance at the beginning of therapy and to reinforce positive activities. An important part of cognitive behavior therapy for depression is having the patient participate in pleasurable activities, especially with others, that usually give positive reinforcement.

> **Additional Reading:** Rupke SJ, Blecke D, Renfrow M. Cognitive therapy for depression. *Am Fam Physician.* 2006;73:83–86, 93.

Category: Cardiovascular system

96. Which of the following medications is preferred in the treatment of alcohol withdrawal syndrome?
A) Haloperidol
B) Lorazepam
C) Phenytoin
D) Phenobarbitol
E) Carbamazepine

Answer and Discussion

The answer is B. Pharmacologic treatment of alcohol withdrawal syndrome involves the use of medications that are cross-tolerant with alcohol. Benzodiazepines have been shown to be safe and effective, particularly for preventing or treating seizures and delirium, and are the preferred agents for treating the symptoms of alcohol withdrawal syndrome.

> **Additional Reading:** Bayard M, McIntyre J, Hill KR, et al. Alcohol withdrawal syndrome. *Am Fam Physician.* 2004;69:1443–1450.

Category: Psychogenic

97. Which of the following medications is least likely to cause problems with libido?
A) Risperidone
B) Cimetidine
C) Bupropion
D) Fluoxetine
E) Citalopram

Answer and Discussion

The answer is C. Consistent evidence shows that, with the exception of bupropion, mirtazipine, and trazadone, most antidepressant medications may cause a decline in libido or sexual functioning despite improvement of depression. Up to one-half of patients surveyed before and after starting therapy with the SSRIs fluoxetine, paroxetine, fluvoxamine, citalopram, and sertraline reported a decline in libido with medication use. Even when patients report improvements in depression with treatment, some continue to experience a lowered libido. Sexual dysfunction, including low sexual desire, in men and women may be the consequence of psychological or emotional factors, hormonal abnormalities, autonomic neuropathy, vascular insufficiency, or drug side effects. The loss of libido is a common problem that is addressed by family physicians, even in the absence of depression. Several antipsychotic agents, including haloperidol, thioridazine, and risperidone, can decrease libido. Cimetidine, in contrast to ranitidine, has been found to lower libido and cause erectile dysfunction. Perimenopausal women who take oral contraceptives and postmenopausal women who are given estrogen replacement therapy may experience an improvement of depressive symptoms but a lowering of libido as a result of estrogen-induced deficiency of free testosterone. Testosterone testing and supplementation should be considered in women who experience a decline in libido after starting estrogen therapy. Testosterone testing should also be considered in men who have a gradual loss of libido and no improvement despite adequate treatment for depression. Psychological and interpersonal factors commonly affect sexual desire. These factors include stressful life events (loss of job or family trauma), life milestones (children leaving home), fatigue, lack of privacy, and ongoing relationship problems. Alcohol and narcotics are known to decrease libido, arousal, and orgasm.

> **Additional Reading:** Phillips RL, Slaughter JR. Depression and sexual desire. *Am Fam Physician.* 2000;62:782–786.

> **Category:** Psychogenic

98. Adenosylmethionine (S-adenosyl methionine [SAMe]) is thought to affect levels of the neurotransmitter
A) Acetylcholine
B) GABA
C) Serotonin
D) Norepinephrine

Answer and Discussion

The answer is C. SAMe is an alternative medication that is used for the treatment of depression. SAMe is a metabolite of folate that facilitates the synthesis of neurotransmitters (including dopamine, norepinephrine, and serotonin) and may be effective and well tolerated for treatment-resistant depression. Oral and IV SAMe supplementation has been shown to increase SAMe levels significantly in cerebrospinal fluid, indicating SAMe's crossover through the blood–brain barrier. This has been associated with increased levels of serotonin metabolites in cerebrospinal fluid. Depressed patients may have low serotonin levels associated with low levels of SAMe. A few randomized trials have compared adjunctive SAMe with placebo among patients with unipolar major depression and found it effective with lower rates of discontinuation due to side effects. However, because no studies have yet validated the long-term safety or efficacy of SAMe, further large long-term studies should be conducted before it receives widespread recommendation.

> **Additional Reading:** Nelson JC. S-adenosyl methionine (SAMe) augmentation in major depressive disorder. *Am J Psychiatry.* 2010;167(8):889.

> **Category:** Reproductive

99. Puerperal psychosis typically develops
A) During the first month after delivery
B) 3 to 4 months after delivery
C) 6 to 12 months after delivery
D) After the child has reached the age of 1 year

Answer and Discussion

The answer is A. When trying to determine if the presence of a symptom is a sign of depression or a normal postpartum reaction, the physician should consider the circumstances. Loss of energy and diminished concentration are frequently the result of sleep deprivation. However, for a postpartum woman to have no energy or to have such difficulty in concentrating that she frequently loses her train of thought or has considerable difficulty in making decisions is cause for concern. Determining how much time has elapsed since delivery helps the physician to distinguish Psychotic Major Depression (PMD) from subclinical mood fluctuations, which occur with such frequency during the first 2 weeks after delivery that they are considered part of the normal postpartum experience. Postpartum blues refer to a transient condition characterized by mild, and often rapid, mood swings from elation to sadness, irritability, anxiety, decreased concentration, insomnia, tearfulness, and crying spells. Forty percent to 80% of postpartum women develop these mood changes, generally within 2 to 3 days of delivery, with symptom peak on the fifth postpartum day and resolution of symptoms within 2 weeks. Women who experience them have an increased risk for PMD later in the postpartum period, especially if the blues symptoms were severe. Subclinical mood swings in either direction (high vs. low) after delivery are an indication for more intensive follow-up later in the postpartum period, and clinician are encouraged to screen for PMD and related symptoms at the first postpartum follow-up visit or at least by 6 weeks postpartum. Finally, PMD must be distinguished from puerperal psychosis. Most puerperal psychoses have their onset within the first month of delivery and are related to mania. An inability to sleep for several nights, agitation, expansive or irritable mood, and avoidance of the infant are early warning signs that herald the onset of puerperal psychosis. Because the woman is at risk of harming herself or her baby (or both), postpartum psychosis is a medical emergency. Most patients with puerperal psychosis are treated in a hospital with neuroleptic agents and mood stabilizers. Before a definitive diagnosis of PMD is made, depression caused by a medical condition such as thyroid dysfunction or anemia must be ruled out.

> **Additional Reading:** Wisner KL, Parry BL, Piontek CM. Postpartum depression. *N Engl J Med.* 2002;347:194–199.

> **Category:** Psychogenic

Many women experience the "baby blues," characterized mild, and often rapid, mood swings from elation to sadness, irritability, anxiety, decreased concentration, insomnia, tearfulness, and crying spells. These symptoms usually resolve within 2 weeks after birth.

100. Alcohol affects which of the following neurotransmitters?
A) GABA
B) Dopamine
C) Norepinephrine
D) Acetylcholine
E) None of the above

Answer and Discussion

The answer is A. Alcohol enhances the effect of GABA on GABA-A neuroreceptors, resulting in decreased overall brain excitability. Chronic exposure to alcohol results in a compensatory decrease of GABA-A neuroreceptor response to GABA, evidenced by increasing tolerance of the effects of alcohol.

Additional Reading: Bayard M, McIntyre J, Hill KR, et al. Alcohol withdrawal syndrome. *Am Fam Physician.* 2004;69:1443–1450.

Category: Psychogenic

101. A 56-year-old business executive with a history of alcoholism and associated liver disease presents to your office and would like to stop drinking. In order to prevent alcohol withdrawal, you select which of the following medications?
A) Lorazepam
B) Clonazepam
C) Diazepam
D) Flurazepam
E) Buspirone

Answer and Discussion

The answer is A. An evidence-based guideline from the American Society of Addiction Medicine recommends benzodiazepines as a first-line agent for the treatment of alcohol withdrawal. The guideline notes that although agents with a longer duration of action may provide fewer breakthrough symptoms, those with a shorter duration of action, such as lorazepam, may be preferred when there is concern about prolonged sedation (e.g., in patients with significant comorbidities or liver disease).

Additional Reading: Ntais C, Pakos E, Kyzas P. Benzodiazepines for alcohol withdrawal. *Cochrane Database Syst Rev.* 2005;3:CD005063.

Category: Psychogenic

102. An 18-year-old high school student presents with her mother to your office. Mom reports her daughter is binge eating and purging in order to lose weight. You suspect bulimia. Of the medications listed, which would be best indicated in treatment of the condition?
A) Sertraline (Zoloft)
B) Paroxetine (Paxil)
C) Fluoxitene (Prozac)
D) Venlafaxine (Effexor)
E) Buproprion (Wellbutrin)

Answer and Discussion

The answer is C. Persons affected by bulimia nervosa are often normal weight and are not easily detected by physiological and medical markers. This disorder is characterized by these key features: binge eating; compensatory behaviors to prevent weight gain (e.g., purging); excessive concern about body weight and shape; as well as self-evaluation being unduly influenced by body weight and shape. Bulimia is most common in late adolescent girls. Associations with other psychiatric disorders is also common. Pharmacotherapy is efficacious for bulimia nervosa and may be used alone or added to other first-line treatments, which consists of nutritional rehabilitation plus psychotherapy. Nutritional rehabilitation aims to restore a structured and consistent meal pattern, typically three meals and two snacks per day. Cognitive-behavioral therapy and interpersonal psychotherapy can effectively facilitate nutritional rehabilitation. Disturbances in serotonergic systems have been suggested as contributing to bulimia. The SSRI fluoxetine has been approved by the U.S. Food and Drug Administration for treatment of bulimia. Fluoxetine is first-line treatment because of its efficacy for the behavioral and cognitive symptoms of bulimia nervosa, as well as its tolerability. Fluoxetine has been more widely studied for bulimia nervosa than any other medication with evidence of decreased bingeing and purging episodes as well as improved dietary restraint, food preoccupation, and excessive concern and dissatisfaction with body weight and shape. Multiple randomized trials have established that the target dose for fluoxetine in bulimia nervosa is 60 mg per day, which is higher than the standard dose for major depression. Clinicians should prescribe an initial dose of 20 mg once per day and titrate up by increments of 20 mg per day each week, depending upon the therapeutic response, tolerability, and clinical urgency. However, it is feasible to start at a dose of 60 mg per day, rather than escalating the dose. Most bulimics purge by vomiting, although abuse of laxatives or diuretics can also occur. The number of times a bulimic patient purges can vary widely, from as seldom as once or twice weekly to as often as 10 times per day (at least once a week for 3 months is required for DSM 5 diagnosis). Repeatedly induced vomiting can lead to the loss of dental enamel, increased dental caries, swollen salivary glands, Mallory–Weiss esophageal tears, and gastroesophageal reflux. Laxative abusers can develop constipation on withdrawal of laxatives. The typical electrolyte abnormalities associated with bulimia are hypokalemia and metabolic acidosis. Although severe hypokalemia in an otherwise healthy young woman suggests bulimia, most patients who purge do not develop electrolyte abnormalities. As a result, screening for hypokalemia or other electrolyte disturbances is not a sensitive means for detecting bulimia. Treatment of the complications associated with bulimia is usually possible, but the underlying disorder can be challenging to treat. Fluoridated mouthwash and toothpaste can help prevent dental caries, and the use of sour candies may decrease salivary gland swelling. Antacid medications help reduce gastroesophageal reflux symptoms, and nonstimulant laxatives may be used to decrease constipation in those with stimulant laxative abuse. Oral replacement of potassium is typically accomplished with 40 to 80 mEq/day of supplementary potassium, until a normal serum potassium level is achieved. Patients with severe hypokalemia and metabolic alkalosis need volume repletion with IV normal saline to allow normalization of potassium levels. Cognitive-behavioral therapy has demonstrated efficacy in the treatment of bulimia, but relapse is common.

Additional Reading: Broft A, Berner LA, Walsh BT. Pharmacotherapy for bulimia nervosa. In: Grilo CM, Mitchell JE, eds. *The Treatment of Eating Disorders: A Clinical Handbook.* New York, NY: The Guilford Press; 2010:388.

Category: Psychogenic

103. Which of the following is *not* associated with anorexia nervosa in adolescent girls?
A) Bradycardia
B) Low blood pressure
C) Low bone density
D) Low estradiol levels
E) Precocious puberty

Answer and Discussion

The answer is E. Adolescent girls with anorexia nervosa have an increased risk for hematologic, metabolic (low estradiol levels), hemodynamic, and skeletal abnormalities (low bone density), including bradycardia, low blood pressure, and pubertal delay, compared with healthy girls.

Additional Reading: Misra M, Aggarwal A, Miller KK. Effects of anorexia nervosa on clinical, hematologic, biochemical, and bone density parameters in community-dwelling adolescent girls. *Pediatrics.* 2004;114:1574–1583.

Category: Psychogenic

104. When distinguishing delirium from preexisting psychiatric disorders, which of the following is a characteristic of delirium?
A) Slow onset with a variable course
B) Slowing on electroencephalography (EEG) recordings
C) Auditory hallucinations
D) Memory impairment
E) Feelings of hopelessness

Answer and Discussion

The answer is B. Specific signs and symptoms can assist physicians in distinguishing between delirium and a preexisting psychiatric disorder. Visual hallucinations are an indicator of an underlying metabolic disturbance or adverse effect of medication or substance abuse. Although visual hallucinations can occur in patients with primary psychiatric illnesses such as schizophrenia, they are much less common than auditory hallucinations. In primary psychiatric disorders, visual hallucinations are associated with other, more characteristic signs and symptoms of the disorders. Visual hallucinations that occur in patients with delirium can be formed (e.g., people, animals) or unformed (e.g., spots, flashes of light). EEG can be useful in differentiating delirium from other conditions. In patients with delirium, the EEG displays a diffuse slowing of the background rhythm. An exception is patients with delirium tremens, where the EEG shows fast activity. EEGs are also useful in detecting ictal and postictal seizure activity, as well as nonconvulsive status epilepticus, all of which can present as delirium. Abnormal EEG readings would not be expected in patients with psychotic disorders or depression. However, slowing may occur in patients with dementia. Additionally, the acute onset and fluctuating nature of delirium are hallmark features in distinguishing it from primary psychiatric disorders. Patients are often unable to provide an adequate history. It is important to interview family members and caregivers to determine the time of onset of symptoms and other pertinent medical and psychiatric information, including a review of medications and a history of substance abuse. It is also important to know how patients are currently different from their normal cognitive state. Psychiatric symptoms that arise in persons 50 years and older without a prior psychiatric history or the development of new symptoms in patients with preexisting psychiatric illness should undergo a thorough medical work-up.

Additional Reading: Gleason OC. Delirium. *Am Fam Physician.* 2003;67:1027–1034.

Category: Reproductive

> The acute onset and fluctuating nature of delirium are hallmark features in distinguishing it from primary psychiatric disorders.

105. OCD is characterized by recurrent obsessions and compulsive behaviors such as repeated hand washing and checking routines. Which of the following statements regarding the disorder is true?
A) Patients affected rarely know they are affected.
B) Serotonin reuptake inhibitors are often first-line therapy.
C) Cognitive-behavioral therapy is rarely helpful in treatment.
D) Structural changes are not found in the brain.
E) Successful treatment leads to symptom resolution.

Answer and Discussion

The answer is B. OCD typically appears during the young adult years and has a chronic variable course. Although treatment can lessen the severity of the disorder, patients typically have some residual symptoms. It is often many years before affected patients are properly diagnosed and treated. OCD appears to have a genetic basis. Although some neurologic findings have been associated with OCD, such as increased gray matter and decreased white matter on brain imaging, the diagnosis remains a clinical one. Patients with OCD are plagued by recurrent obsessions and often perform compulsive washing and checking rituals in an attempt to deal with the anxiety provoked by their obsessions. Those affected by OCD usually are aware that their behavior is irrational and may spend a lot of effort to hide their symptoms from others. Cognitive-behavioral therapy is helpful in the treatment of OCD. In most patients, combining medication with behavioral therapy produces the best results. SSRIs should be utilized first, with other psychotropic agents added if initial therapy fails. The optimal SSRI dosage for OCD tends to be higher than the dosage used to treat depression, and an adequate trial of medication may take up to 12 weeks.

Additional Reading: Jenike MA. Obsessive–compulsive disorder. *N Engl J Med.* 2004;350:259–265.

Category: Neurologic

Emergent and Surgical Care

QUESTIONS

Each of the following questions or incomplete statements is followed by suggested answers or completions. Select the ONE BEST ANSWER in each case.

1. A 42-year-old carpenter presents with wrist pain and grip weakness. On exam, he is found to have pain over the radial aspect of the wrist that is aggravated by flexing the thumb and applying ulnar flexion. The most likely diagnosis is
A) Carpal tunnel syndrome
B) Scaphoid fracture
C) de Quervain's tenosynovitis
D) Boxer's fracture
E) Hamate fracture

Answer and Discussion

The answer is C. The combination of wrist pain and grip weakness is characteristic of de Quervain's tenosynovitis. Local tenderness is present over the distal portion of the radial styloid adjacent to abductor pocillis longus tendon. The pain is generally reproduced with direct palpation of the involved tendons. Pain is aggravated by passively stretching the thumb tendons over the radial styloid in thumb flexion (the Finkelstein maneuver).

Carpal tunnel syndrome will present with parathesia and/or weakness primarily in the distribution of the median nerves—thumb and index finger. A scaphoid fracture presents with mild, dull pain, deep in the radial wrist that is worsened when making a grip. On exam, there is tenderness to palpation in the anatomical "snuff box"—this is a sensitive, but not specific test. A boxer's fracture refers to a fracture of the midshaft of the 5th metacarpal (typically following a blow with a closed fist). A hamate fracture presents with pain along the ulnar side of the hand and is frequently seen in sports that require swinging of bats or racquets.

Additional Reading: de Quervain's tenosynovitis. In: Basow DS, ed. *UpToDate*. Waltham, MA: UpToDate; 2013.

Category: Musculoskeletal system

> The combination of wrist pain and grip weakness is characteristic of de Quervain's tenosynovitis.

2. Which of the following statements is true regarding corneal injuries?
A) Patients should have the affected eye patched for 24 hours.
B) Topical antibiotics are recommended to prevent superinfection.
C) Foreign bodies should not be removed because of potential further injury to the cornea.
D) Topical anesthetics should be given to treat the discomfort.
E) None of the above.

Answer and Discussion

The answer is B. Controlled studies have not found patching to improve the rate of healing or comfort in patients with traumatic or foreign body abrasions. Patients should be treated with topical antibiotics to prevent superinfection. Antibiotics ointment is better than drops.

If a corneal foreign body is detected, an attempt can be made to remove it by irrigation. The topical anesthetics administration is controversial. Animal studies showed that it can delay corneal epithelial healing. In humans, some studies showed that dilute solutions of proparacaine 0.05% provide analgesia without impairing healing after several days of treatment.

Additional Reading: Evaluation and management of corneal abrasions. *Am Fam Physician*. 2013;87(2):114–120.

Category: Special sensory

3. Which finger is most likely to be affected with disruption of the flexor digitorum profundus tendon (also known as a *jersey finger*)?
A) Thumb
B) Index finger
C) Third finger
D) Ring finger
E) Fifth finger ("pinky")

Answer and Discussion

The answer is D. Disruption of the flexor digitorum profundus tendon, also known as jersey finger, commonly occurs when an athlete's finger catches on another player's clothing, usually while playing a tackling sport such as football or rugby. The injury causes forced extension of the distal interphalangeal (DIP) joint during active flexion. The ring finger is the weakest finger and accounts for 75% of jersey finger cases. Acute pain and swelling over the volar aspect of the DIP joint and distal phalanx is characteristic. The characteristic finding of jersey finger is the inability to actively flex the DIP joint.

Additional Reading: Acute finger injuries: Part I. Tendons and ligaments. *Am Fam Physician.* 2006;73:810–816, 823.

Category: Musculoskeletal system

> The pathognomonic finding of jersey finger is the inability to actively flex the DIP joint.

4. Injury to the extensor tendon at the DIP joint is also known as
A) Boutonnière deformity
B) Jersey finger
C) Mallet finger
D) Swan necking
E) "Jammed" finger

Answer and Discussion
The answer is C. Injury to the extensor tendon at the DIP joint is also known as mallet finger. The condition is the most common closed tendon injury of the finger. Mallet finger is usually caused by an object (e.g., a ball) striking the finger, creating a forced flexion of an extended DIP. The extensor tendon may be strained, partially torn, or completely ruptured or separated by a distal phalanx avulsion fracture. Those affected with mallet finger complain of pain at the dorsal DIP joint; inability to actively extend the joint; and, often, with a characteristic flexion deformity. It is critical to isolate the DIP joint during the evaluation to ensure extension is from the extensor tendon and not the central slip. The absence of full passive extension may indicate bony or soft tissue entrapment requiring surgical intervention. Mallet finger most often involves the middle finger and the next.

Additional Reading: Common finger fractures and dislocations. *Am Fam Physician.* 2012;85(8):805–810.

Category: Musculoskeletal system

5. Where are most Morton's neuromas found?
A) In the tarsal tunnel of the 3rd toe
B) At the first metatarsal phalangeal joint
C) Between the second and third toes
D) At the attachment of the plantar fascia
E) At the head of the fifth metatarsal

Answer and Discussion
The answer is C. Morton's neuromas are typically found between the metatarsal of the third and fourth toes or at the bifurcation of the four plantar digital nerve. The second and third common digital branches of the medial plantar nerve are the most frequent sites for development of interdigital neuromas. Morton's neuromas develop as a result of chronic trauma and repetitive stress, as occurs in persons wearing tight-fitting or high-heeled shoes. Pain and paresthesias are usually mild at onset and are located in the interdigital space of the affected nerve. In some cases, the interdigital space between the affected toes may be widened as a result of an associated ganglion or synovial cyst. Pain is noted in the affected interdigital space when the metatarsal heads of the foot are squeezed together. Injection with 1% lidocaine can assist in confirming the diagnosis.

Additional Reading: Busconi BD, Stevenson JH. Approach to the athlete with Morton's neuroma. *Sports Medicine Consult: A Problem-Based Approach to Sports Medicine for the Primary Care Physician.* Philadelphia, PA: Lippincott, Williams & Wilkins; 2009.

Category: Musculoskeletal system

6. Which of the following tests is the most sensitive and specific for the detection of renal stones?
A) KUB plain film
B) Ultrasound
C) Intravenous pyelography
D) Noncontrast helical computed tomography (CT)

Answer and Discussion
The answer is D. A noncontrast helical CT can detect both stones and urinary tract obstruction and has become the gold standard for the diagnosis of the stone disease. The specificity of helical CT is nearly 100%. Ultrasonography is the procedure of choice for patients who should avoid radiation, including pregnant women and possibly women of childbearing age. It is sensitive for the diagnosis of urinary tract obstruction and can detect radiolucent stones mixed on KUB. Intravenous pyelogram (IVP) has a higher sensitivity and specificity than an abdominal pain film for the detection of stones and provides data about the degree of obstruction.

Additional Reading: Treatment and prevention of kidney stones: an update. *Am Fam Physician.* 2011;84(11):1234–1242.

Category: Nephrologic system

7. Which of the following statements regarding cholecystectomy is *false*?
A) Between 5% and 26% of patients undergoing elective laparoscopic cholecystectomy require conversion to an open procedure.
B) A common reason for conversion to an open procedure is failure to identify the anatomy.
C) Laparoscopic cholecystectomy is safer than an open procedure.
D) Laparoscopic cholecystectomy has a lower rate of common bile duct injury.
E) Common bile duct injuries are extremely difficult to repair.

Answer and Discussion
The answer is D. The overall incidence of laparoscopic cholecystectomy bile duct injuries range from 1.7% in the first case to 0.17% at the 50th case (0.4 to 0.6). The incidence is four times higher that an open cholecystectomy. Between 5% and 26% of patients undergoing elective laparoscopic cholecystectomy require conversion to an open procedure. A common reason for conversion is the inability to clearly identify the biliary anatomy.

Additional Reading: Cholelithiasis. In: Domino F, ed. *The 5-Minute Clinical Consult.* Philadelphia, PA: Lippincott Williams and Wilkins; 2014.

Category: Gastroenterology system

> Laparoscopic cholecystectomy is considered the gold standard for the surgical treatment of gallstone disease.

8. A 31-year-old is seen in the emergency room for lateral foot pain that occurred when he fell playing basketball. X-rays of the foot confirm a displaced fracture of the proximal fifth metatarsal. Appropriate management consists of
A) Nonsteroidal anti-inflammatory drugs (NSAIDs) and limited weight bearing with a gradual return to usual activities in 2 to 4 weeks
B) Crutches with no weight bearing for 4 to 6 weeks
C) Short leg walking cast for 6 to 8 weeks
D) External reduction followed by casting for 6 to 8 weeks with limited weight bearing
E) Orthopedic referral

Answer and Discussion

The answer is E. Fractures of the proximal portion of the fifth metatarsal may be classified as avulsions of the tuberosity or fractures of the shaft within 1.5 cm of the tuberosity. The tuberosity, or styloid, is the most proximal portion of the fifth metatarsal. It protrudes in the lateral and plantar planes. Fracture of the tuberosity are among the most common lower extremities fractures. Tuberosity avulsion fractures cause pain and tenderness at the base of the fifth metatarsal. Bruising, swelling, and other injuries may be present. Nondisplaced tuberosity fractures are usually treated conservatively and heal without difficulty; however, orthopedic referral is indicated for (a) fractures that are comminuted or displaced, (b) fractures that involve more than 30% of the cubometatarsal articulation surface, and (c) fractures with delayed union. Management and prognosis of acute (Jones fracture) and stress fracture of the fifth metatarsal within 1.5 cm of the tuberosity depend on the type of fracture, on the basis of classification. Simple fractures are generally treated conservatively with a non–weight-bearing short leg cast for 6 to 8 weeks. Fractures with delayed union may also be treated conservatively or may be managed surgically, depending on patient preference and other factors. All displaced fractures and nonunion fractures should be managed surgically. Although most fractures of the proximal portion of the fifth metatarsal respond well to appropriate management, delayed union, muscle atrophy, and chronic pain may be long-term complications.

> **Additional Reading:** Proximal fifth metatarsal fractures. In: Basow DS, ed. *UpToDate*. Waltham, MA: UpToDate; 2013.

> **Category:** Musculoskeletal system

9. A 47-year-old man presents with a skin lesion that has been changing in size and shape. On examination, she is found to have a 7-mm, asymmetric, darkly pigmented lesion with some color variegation and irregular borders. Which one of the following skin biopsy techniques is most appropriate for confirming the diagnosis?
A) A shave biopsy
B) Electrodesiccation and curettage
C) Elliptical excision
D) Mohs' surgery

Answer and Discussion

The answer is C. This lesion is suspicious for melanoma, on the basis of the asymmetry, irregular border, color variegation, and size larger than 6 mm. In addition, a history of evolution of the lesion, with changes in size, shape, or color, has been shown in some studies to be the most specific clinical finding for melanoma. The preferred method of biopsy for any lesion suspicious for melanoma is complete elliptical excision with a small margin of normal-appearing skin. The depth of the lesion is crucial to staging and prognosis, so shave biopsies are inadequate. A punch biopsy of the most suspicious-appearing area is appropriate if the location or size of the lesion makes full excision inappropriate or impractical, but a single punch biopsy is unlikely to capture the entire malignant portion in larger lesions. Electrodesiccation and curettage is not an appropriate treatment for melanoma. Mohs' surgery is sometimes used to treat melanomas, but is not used for the initial diagnosis.

> **Additional Reading:** Cutaneous malignant melanoma: a primary care perspective. *Am Fam Physician*. 2012;85(2):161.

> **Category:** Integumentary

10. Which of the following is *not* a contraindication for breast conservative therapy?
A) Estrogen/progesterone receptor positive tumor
B) Two tumors are located in different quadrants
C) Diffuse microcalcifications that appear malignant
D) History of prior therapeutic radiotherapy that included a portion of the affected breast
E) Negative resection surgical margins

Answer and Discussion

The answer is E. When there are two or more primary tumors located in different quadrants of the breast or there are associated diffuse microcalcifications that appear malignant, breast-conserving therapy is not considered appropriate. Additionally, a woman with previous breast irradiation is also not a candidate for breast conservation treatment. Breast irradiation cannot be given during pregnancy, but it may be possible to perform breast-conserving surgery in the third trimester and administer irradiation after delivery. Positive surgical margins are also an absolute contraindication.

> **Additional Reading:** Treatment of breast cancer. *Am Fam Physician*. 2010;81(11):1339–1346.

> **Category:** Integumentary

11. Which of the following antibiotics given alone is adequate for prophylaxis when performing an appendectomy?
A) Cephalexin
B) Ceftriaxone
C) Cefotaxime
D) Metronidazole
E) Cefoxitin

Answer and Discussion

The answer is E. Antibiotic prophylaxis is warranted in the setting of uncomplicated appendicitis. Reasonable regimens include a cephalosporin with anaerobic activity: Cefoxitin or cefotetan. Complicated appendicitis consists of perforated or gangrenous appendicitis, including peritonitis or abscess formation.

> **Additional Reading:** Clinical practice guidelines for antimicrobial prophylaxis in surgery. *Surg Infect*. 2013;14(1):73.

> **Category:** Gastroenterology system

12. Which of the following may have an antiplatelet activity and should be stopped before surgery?
A) Ephedra
B) Ginseng
C) Valerian
D) St. John's wort
E) Kava

Answer and Discussion

The answer is B. Ginseng is touted to protect the body against stress. Pharmacologically, ginseng lowers blood glucose levels (even in patients without diabetes mellitus) and, therefore, may cause intraoperative complications, especially in patients who fasted before surgery. Ginseng may also have a platelet inhibitory effect, and this effect may be irreversible. It should be discontinued at least 7 days before surgery.

Additional Reading: Asian ginseng. *National Center for Complementary and Alternative Medicine (NCCAM)*. From: http://nccam .nih.gov/health/asianginseng/ataglance.htm.

Category: Nonspecific system

13. After hip surgery, deep vein thrombosis (DVT) prophylaxis should be maintained for at least
A) 24 hours
B) 3 days
C) 10 days
D) 1 month
E) Indefinitely

Answer and Discussion

The answer is C. The 2012 ACCP anticoagulation guidelines recommend starting low-molecular-weight heparin either 12 hours or more preoperatively or 12 hours or more postoperatively. Thromboembolic prophylaxis should be continued for at least 10 to 14 days postoperatively and until the patient is full ambulatory. Patient at high risk for DVT may require a longer course of anticoagulation. Patients at increased risk include those who experience prolonged immobility post-repair, patient in whom surgery was delayed, or prior history of thromboembolism.

> Additional Reading: Prevention of VTE in orthopedic surgery patients: antithrombotic therapy and prevention of thrombosis, 9th ed. American College of Chest Physician Evidence-Based Clinical Practice Guidelines. *Chest.* 2012;141(suppl 2): e278S.

Category: Cardiovascular system

14. A general surgeon contacts you regarding preoperative clearance for an otherwise healthy 42-year-old scheduled for an appendectomy. The patient has no history of excessive bleeding, no family history of bleeding disorders, and is on no medications. He inquires about the need for coagulation studies, which have not been performed. A correct response is
A) A prothrombin time (PT)/partial thromboplastin time (PTT) must be performed before surgery.
B) A bleeding time is sufficient for assessing the risk of bleeding.
C) A prior normal PT/PTT test performed within the last year is sufficient to clear this patient for surgery.
D) No further testing is necessary to clear this patient for surgery.

Answer and Discussion

The answer is D. Coagulation times are not routinely indicated in patients undergoing surgery. Studies have shown that the yield is very low and that abnormal results are expected or do not significantly affect management. Coagulation studies would be indicated if the patient is receiving anticoagulant therapy, has a family or personal history that suggests a bleeding disorder, or has evidence of liver disease.

> Additional Reading: Practice advisory for preanesthesia evaluation: an updated report by the American Society of Anesthesiologist Task Force of Preanesthesia Evaluation. *Anesthesiol.* 2012;116(3):522–538.

Category: Hematologic system

15. A 2-year-old child is seen in the emergency room and diagnosed with multiple contusions in various stages of healing and a spiral-type fracture of the left radius secondary to falling down the stairs at home. The most appropriate initial treatment is
A) Splinting of the fracture with orthopedic referral
B) Hospitalization
C) Social service consultation
D) Immediate reduction of the fracture and safety counseling for the child's parents
E) Open reduction and internal fixation and follow-up in 3 days

Answer and Discussion

The answer is B. Child abuse is a difficult problem that must be identified as quickly as possible. Most children who die of child abuse are younger than 5 years. Most child abuse takes place in the home and is instituted by persons known to and trusted by the child. Although widely publicized, abuse in day care and foster-care settings accounts for only a minority of confirmed cases of child abuse. Child abuse is 15 times more likely to occur in families in which spousal abuse occurs. Children are three times more likely to be abused by their fathers than by their mothers. Once a health care worker has any suspicion of child abuse, he or she is legally required to report the case for investigation. Protection of the child is the most important goal. The child should be hospitalized in a safe environment while further investigation by social workers is performed. Children younger than 3 years are the most commonly abused. Clinical findings include multiple fractures (especially spiral-type fractures), multiple bruises in different stages of healing, intestinal trauma injuries, burns, poor nutrition, poor development, and bizarre accidents reported by parents. More than 50% of fractures in children younger than 1 year are secondary to abuse. Before discharge from the hospital, the child's home environment must be determined to be safe by the appropriate protection agency. Further counseling for the child and family should be initiated after discharge. Unfortunately, therapy for child-abusing adults fails in approximately 33% of cases. As adults, children who were abused have a higher incidence of depression and drug abuse.

> Additional Reading: Abused and neglected children. *Nelson Textbook of Pediatrics*, 19th ed. Philadelphia, PA: Elsevier/Saunders; 2011.

Category: Patient/population-based care

16. You receive a call from the newborn nursery and are told that there is a breast-fed newborn who is vomiting bile-stained emesis. The most appropriate management is
A) Decrease feeding frequency
B) Upper gastrointestinal (GI) contrast series
C) Administration of rectal promethazine
D) Barium enema
E) Nasogastric feedings

Answer and Discussion

The answer is B. The diagnosis of intestinal malrotation should be suspected in any infant who presents with bilious emesis, acute duodenal obstruction, or abdominal tenderness associated with hemodynamic deterioration. Intestinal malrotation is a condition that results during development of the fetus. As the bowel develops outside the abdomen, it returns to the body cavity with a counterclockwise rotation. When malrotation occurs, the bowel returns in a clockwise rotation, and intestinal obstruction can result. Presenting symptoms that include vomiting of bile-stained material, abdominal distention, and dehydration soon after birth. Barium enema may be misleading in the diagnosis of malrotation and is used only as an adjunct to the upper GI series. Barium enema can be helpful in the diagnosis of volvulus if it shows complete obstruction of the transverse colon, particularly if the head of the barium column has a beaked appearance.

Additional Reading: Schaider JJ. Malrotation. *Rosen and Barkin's 5-Minute Emergency Medicine Consult.* Philadelphia, PA: Lippincott Williams and Wilkins; 2010.

Category: Gastroenterology system

17. Which of the following statements about lumbar disc disease is true?
A) It usually involves the L5-S1 interspace.
B) It typically involves anterior herniation of the nucleus pulposus.
C) It usually requires surgical intervention.
D) Treatment involves strict bed rest for 1 to 2 weeks.
E) Forward flexion of the trunk often helps relieve symptoms.

Answer and Discussion

The answer is A. Lumbar disc disease usually results from posterior herniation of the nucleus pulposus that impinges on the spinal cord. The most common site is the L5-S1 interspace, which affects the first sacral nerve root. Patients typically recall a precipitating event such as lifting a heavy object. Symptoms include severe back pain that radiates to the legs and is aggravated by coughing, sneezing, or forward flexion of the trunk. The condition is the most common cause of sciatica. Examination may show decreased sensation in a dermatome pattern, weakness, decreased reflexes, and a positive straight leg-raising test. In severe cases, patients may experience bowel or bladder incontinence. Radiographs and laboratory tests are generally unnecessary, except in the few patients in whom a serious cause is suspected on the basis of a comprehensive history and physical examination. Surgical evaluation is indicated in patients with worsening neurologic deficits or intractable pain that is resistant to conservative treatment. Bed rest should not be recommended for patients with nonspecific acute low back pain. Moderate quality evidence suggests that bed rest is less effective at reducing pain and improving function at 3 to 12 weeks than advice to stay active. Prolonged bed rest can also cause adverse effects such as joint stiffness, muscle wasting, loss of bone mineral density, pressure ulcers, and venous thromboembolism (VTE). The treatment plan should be reassessed in patients who do not return to normal activity within 4 to 6 weeks. Most mild cases can be treated with the limitation of aggravating activity, anti-inflammatory agents, and muscle relaxants.

Additional Reading: Diagnosis and treatment of acute low back pain. *Am Fam Physician.* 2012;85(4):343–350.

Category: Musculoskeletal system

18. Which of the following is *not* an indication for referral for Mohs' micrographic surgery?
A) Lesion in close proximity to nose
B) Lesion size > 2 cm
C) Lesion with indistinct margin
D) Recurrent lesions
E) Lesion is identified as an actinic keratosis

Answer and Discussion

The answer is E. Patients with nonmelanoma skin cancer measuring >2 cm, lesions with indistinct margins, recurrent lesions, and those close to important structures, including the eyes, nose, and mouth, or for more invasive histologic subtypes (micronodular, infiltrative, and morpheaform), or for tumors with high risk of recurrence should be considered for referral for complete excision via Mohs' micrographic surgery. The Mohs' surgeon can confirm the complete removal of the lesion by immediately reviewing the pathology during a staged excision, which, in these high-risk settings, can require removal of much more tissue than might have been clinically apparent initially. The recurrence rate for tumors treated with Mohs' micrographic surgery is approximately 1% at 5 years, whereas standard surgical excision has an approximately 5% of recurrence rate at 5 years.

Additional Reading: Diagnosis and treatment of basal cell and squamous cell carcinoma. *Am Fam Physician.* 2012;86(2):161–168.

Category: Integumentary

> Treatment of basal cell carcinoma with Mohs' micrographic surgery has the lowest recurrence rate.

19. A newborn who develops aspiration pneumonia should be evaluated for
A) Tracheoesophageal fistula
B) Hypothyroidism
C) Cystic fibrosis
D) Human immunodeficiency virus
E) Tetralogy of Fallot

Answer and Discussion

The answer is A. Tracheoesophageal fistula is a congenital defect seen in newborns. The incidence is 1 in 3,500 live births. Boys and girls are equally affected. The condition is commonly associated with esophageal atresia. Polyhydramnios occurs in approximately two-thirds of pregnancies. Symptoms include excessive secretions with coughing and aspiration after feedings. Complications include the development of cyanosis and aspiration pneumonia. Diagnosis can be established by the inability to pass a red-rubber catheter or nasogastric tube further than approximately 10 to 15 cm into the stomach. Antero-posterior radiographs confirm catheter curled in the upper esophageal pouch. If gas is noted below the diaphragm, then an associated fistula is present. If not, the patient most likely is affected with esophageal atresia alone. Care must be taken to avoid aspiration of dye during diagnostic tests.

Additional Reading: Schwartz MW. Tracheoesophageal fistula and esophageal atresia, Pediatric. *The 5-Minute Pediatric Consult.* Philadelphia, PA: Lippincott Williams and Wilkins; 2012.

Category: Gastroenterology system

20. Extracorporeal shock-wave therapy for renal stones
A) Requires stones to be present in the renal pelvis
B) Rarely requires repeated treatment regardless of stone size
C) Is more effective for stones <2 cm in diameter
D) Requires less energy for calcium oxalate and cystine stones
E) Rarely achieves optimal results

Answer and Discussion

The answer is C. Lithotripsy has been used to fragment and remove renal and ureteral stones. The procedure involves placing the patient on a lithotripsy gantry so the calculus overlies a circular window in the table containing the water bath and is focused on the calculus. The procedure is more effective for stones <2 cm in diameter. Calcium oxalate and cystine stones are usually dense and require increased energy. Alternative modes of stones should be considered for large or hard calculi, stones in a calyceal diverticulum, or in patients with complex renal anatomy. Percutaneous nephrolithotomy and extracorporeal shock-wave lithotripsy may reduce the need for further invasive surgery, but the risks and benefits should be weighed carefully in asymptomatic persons.

Additional Reading: Treatment and prevention of kidney stones: an update. *Am Fam Physician.* 2011;84(11):1234–1242; and Clinical evidence kidney stones. *Am Fam Physician.* 2013;87(6):441–443.

Category: Nonspecific system

21. Topical lidocaine is used with _____ to treat chronic anal fissures.
A) Nifedipine
B) Cocaine
C) Sildenafil
D) Nystatin
E) Mupirocin

Answer and Discussion

The answer is A. Topical nifedipine in addition to lidocaine gel is effective and well tolerated in the treatment of chronic anal fissures.

Additional Reading: Hemorrhoids. *Am Fam Physician.* 2011; 84(2):204–210.

Category: Gastroenterology system

22. A 24-year-old woman presents to your office. She is quite concerned that she is bleeding internally, because her stools have been dark, tarry black. Further questioning reveals that she has been having episodes of diarrhea, which have resolved with the use of Pepto-Bismol. She denies abdominal pain, light-headedness, nausea, vomiting, or fevers. The most likely cause of her dark stools is
A) Upper GI bleeding source
B) Lower GI bleeding source
C) Rectal outlet bleeding
D) Bismuth ingestion
E) None of the above

Answer and Discussion

The answer is D. Melena is the passage of black tarry stools, which is secondary to GI bleeding. In most cases, the source is located in the upper GI tract; however, a source in the distal right colon or small intestine can also cause melena. Approximately 100 to 200 mL of blood loss is needed to cause melena. Other causes for black stools that are often confused with melena include iron, bismuth, licorice, blueberries, and lead. Beets and tomatoes can sometimes make stools appear reddish.

Additional Reading: Diagnosis and management of upper gastrointestinal bleeding. *Am Fam Physician.* 2012;85(5):469–476.

Category: Gastroenterology system

23. Which of the following local anesthetics has the longest duration of action?
A) Procaine (Novocaine)
B) Bupivacaine (Marcaine)
C) Mepivacaine (Carbocaine)
D) Lidocaine (Xylocaine)
E) All are about the same

Answer and Discussion

The answer is B. The following local anesthetics *without epinephrine* have the following durations of action:

- Procaine: 15 to 30 minutes
- Bupivacaine: 120 to 240 minutes, the longest-acting anesthetic; good for nerve blocks
- Mepivacaine: 30 to 120 minutes
- Lidocaine: 30 to 120 minutes

The use of epinephrine should be avoided in areas such as the fingers, nose, penis, and toes or other distal appendages. The vasoconstrictive effect can lead to ischemic necrosis. The most common reason for inadequate anesthesia is not allowing enough time for the anesthetic to take effect. In most cases, the surgeon should wait at least 5 minutes after injection before starting a procedure.

The following local anesthetics *with epinephrine* have the following durations of action:

- Bupivacaine 240 to 280 minutes
- Lidocaine 60 to 400 minutes
- Mepivacaine 180 to 360 minutes
- Proacaine 60 to 400 minutes

Additional Reading: Infiltration of local anesthetics. In: Basow DS, ed. *UpToDate.* Waltham, MA: UpToDate; 2013.

Category: Integumentary

24. Blunt objects in the esophagus (with the exception of button batteries) may be observed for _____ before performing endoscopy for removal.
A) 4 hours
B) 24 hours
C) 3 days
D) 1 week
E) 10 days

Answer and Discussion

The answer is B. Most blunt objects (with the exception of button batteries) in the esophagus may be observed for up to 24 hours. If the object fails to pass into the stomach, it should be removed or possibly pushed into the stomach. Objects that have been lodged in the esophagus for >24 hours or for an unknown duration should be removed endoscopically. If the object has been lodged in the esophagus for >2 weeks, there is significant risk of erosion into surrounding structures, and surgical consultation should be obtained before attempting removal. Early intervention is indicated for patients who have swallowed button or disc batteries because of the potential for voltage burns and direct corrosive effects. Burns can occur as early as 4 hours after ingestion.

Additional Reading: Body ingestion in children. *Am Fam Physician.* 2005;72(2):287–291.

Category: Gastroenterology system

25. Which of the following statements regarding preoperative evaluations is correct?
A) A patient with a previous coronary bypass graph 2 years earlier should undergo cardiac stress testing before clearance, regardless of the presence of cardiac symptoms.
B) Urine pregnancy testing should be considered for women of childbearing age.
C) Coagulation studies should be included in your laboratory assessment of all surgical candidates.
D) Patients who have had angioplasty within 6 months are not required to have further cardiology assessment.
E) A baseline renal function study should be assessed for all surgical candidates.

Answer and Discussion

The answer is B. Before elective surgery, a review of the patient's history is necessary. Routine pre-op labs (complete blood count [CBC], hemoglobin, platelets, electrolytes, glucose, coagulation, and liver test) have not been shown to improve outcomes for otherwise healthy patients. Hemoglobin measurement for patients >65 years old who are undergoing major surgery and for younger patients undergoing surgery that is expected to result in significant blood loss should be considered. Creatinine is indicated for patient >50 undergoing intermediate or high-risk surgery and younger patients suspected of having renal disease, when hypotension is likely during surgery or when nephrotoxic medications will be used. A urine pregnancy test should be considered for women of childbearing age. Coagulation studies would be indicated if the patient is receiving anticoagulant therapy, has a family or personal history that suggests a bleeding disorder, or has evidence of liver disease. An electrocardiogram (ECG) is indicated for vascular surgical procedures, for patients with preexisting cardiovascular disease who are undergoing intermediate-risk surgery, and in severely obese patient with poor effort tolerance or at least one additional cardiovascular risk. Chest X-rays or pulmonary function test are not ordered for the healthy patient, but is indicated for those with cardiopulmonary disease and those >50 who are undergoing abdominal aortic aneurysm (AAA) surgery or upper abdominal/thoracic surgery. In general, patients in whom cardiac stress testing was normal within the previous 2 years or who have had coronary bypass surgery within the previous 5 years and are without symptoms require no further assessment. Clinically stable patients who have undergone angioplasty between 6 months and 5 years previously require no further assessment. However, patients who have had angioplasty within the previous 6 months may require cardiac reevaluation and/or consultation with a cardiologist before surgery. Patients at high risk for complications usually warrant cardiology consultation and possibly angiography. Cardiac stress testing should be performed in patients at intermediate risk and with poor functional capacity or who are undergoing high-risk procedures such as vascular surgery. For patients with minor clinical predictors, only patients who have poor functional capacity and are undergoing a high-risk procedure requires stress testing. Patients with positive stress test results warrant cardiology consultation before proceeding with surgery. Assessment of left ventricular function is not routinely indicated for preoperative evaluation whether or not the patient has cardiac disease. The preoperative assessment guideline from the American College of Physicians notes that radionuclide or echocardiographic assessment of left ventricular function does not appear to improve the risk prediction provided by the clinical examination alone. In summary, recommendations do not call for preoperative cardiac testing in all patients. The need for further cardiac evaluation before surgery is determined by the clinical risk predictors identified from the patient's history, physical examination, ECG, and functional status, along with the risk associated with the operation itself. Pulmonary function testing may be helpful in diagnosing and assessing disease severity. Baseline chest radiographs may be helpful in at-risk patients. Preoperative guidelines do not define the degree of pulmonary function impairment that would prohibit surgery other than that for lung resection.

Additional Reading: Preoperative testing before noncardiac surgery: guidelines and recommendations. *Am Fam Physician.* 2013;87(6):414–418.

Category: Nonspecific system

26. A 65-year-old retired secretary presents with a painful bump that is associated with the medial first metatarsal joint. She reports that the bump has slowly developed over the past few years. The most likely diagnosis is
A) Hallux valgus
B) Morton's neuroma
C) Chronic gout
D) Metatarsalgia
E) Bunionette

Answer and Discussion

The answer is A. Hallux valgus (bunions) is more common in women than in men. Symptoms include a painless or painful bump (exostosis) that forms on the medial aspect of the first metatarsal joint. Contributing physical factors include hyperelasticity syndromes, metatarsus varus, short first metatarsal joint, and pes valgus. Other factors include a family history of bunions and the prolonged use of narrow high-heeled shoes. Conservative treatment is usually all that is needed and includes wide shoes, the use of bunion pads, ice, rest, and anti-inflammatory agents for acute pain. Most cases referred for surgery have intermetatarsal angles greater than 10 degrees or fail to improve with conservative measures. Absolute contraindications for surgery include peripheral vascular disease and local tissue infections, whereas relative contraindications include narcissistic personality disorders, painless cosmetic bunions, and age 65 years or older. A bunionette is a bony prominence on the lateral aspect of the fifth metatarsal head.

Additional Reading: Hallux valgus deformity. In: Basow DS, ed. *UpToDate.* Waltham, MA: UpToDate; 2013.

Category: Musculoskeletal system

27. When injecting a local anesthetic with epinephrine, which of the following locations should be avoided?
A) Lip
B) Ear lobe
C) Forehead
D) Back
E) Scalp

Answer and Discussion

The answer is B. Epinephrine administration should be avoided in the following areas: nose, ear lobes, or tip of the penis. It is also avoided near the terminal arterial branches in the digits. Epinephrine is contraindicated in digital anesthesia in patients with peripheral artery disease and in patients with periorbital infiltration with narrow-angle glaucoma and in large wounds in patients with underlying conditions (e.g., hyperthyroidism, pheochromocytoma, severe hypertension, coronary artery disease) that may be exacerbated by epinephrine effect.

Epinephrine infiltration with local anesthetics should be avoided in patients receiving beta blockers, monoamine oxidase inhibitors, phenothiazines, or tricyclic antidepressants and patients with catecholamine sensitivity.

Additional Reading: Myth of not using lidocaine with epinephrine in the digits. *Am Fam Physician.* 2010;81(10):1188.

Category: Integumentary

28. Which of the following is the standard prophylaxis treatment for subacute bacterial endocarditis (SBE) for dental procedures in low-risk adult patients?
A) Amoxicillin: 1 g given intravenously at the time of the procedure
B) Amoxicillin: 2 g given orally 1 hour before the procedure
C) Ampicillin: 2 g given intravenously plus gentamicin (1.5 mg/kg intravenously) 30 minutes before the procedure; dose repeated 8 hours after the procedure
D) Ampicillin: 500 mg given orally 1 hour before the procedure and 250 mg given 6 hours after the procedure
E) None

Answer and Discussion

The answer is E. Antibiotic prophylaxis (amoxicillin 2 g orally 30 to 60 minutes before the procedure) is recommended for patients who have high-risk cardiac conditions, which include

- prosthetic cardiac valve
- history of infective endocarditis
- unrepaired cyanotic congenital heart disease; or a completely repaired congenital heart defect with prosthetic material, during the first 6 months after the procedure; or a repaired congenital heart defect with residual defects at the site or adjacent to the site of a prosthetic patch or prosthetic device (which inhibits endothelialization)
- cardiac transplantation recipients with cardiac valvular disease

The guidelines suggest preventive treatment for high-risk cardiac patients, not for all dental procedures but only for those that involve manipulation of gingival tissue (around bone and teeth) or the periapical region of teeth (tip of the tooth root). The guidelines do not recommend antibiotics for routine anesthetic injections through noninfected tissue, placement or adjustment of orthodontic appliances, shedding of baby teeth, or bleeding from trauma to the lips or inside of the mouth.

Further the American Heart Association (AHA) guideline no longer consider any GI (colonoscopy or esophagogastroduodenoscopy) or genitourinary procedures high risk and therefore do not recommend routine use of endocarditis prophylaxis even in patient with the highest risk cardiac conditions.

Vaginal or cesarean delivery is not an indication for routine antibiotic prophylaxis.

Additional Reading: Prevention of infective endocarditis: guidelines from the American Heart Association. *Circulation.* 2007;116(15):1736.

Category: Cardiovascular system

> The 2007 AHA guideline for the prevention of infective endocarditis recommends prophylaxis only for patients at highest risk.

29. A 5-year-old boy is brought to the emergency room with inspiratory and expiratory stridor, high fever, and drooling. Initial treatment consists of
A) Oxygen therapy
B) Airway management by trained personnel
C) Inhaled bronchodilators
D) Lying the child in the supine position
E) Administration of epinephrine

Answer and Discussion

The answer is B. Epiglottitis is a severe, life-threatening condition usually seen in children between 3 and 10 years of age. The condition was usually the result of a *Haemophilus influenzae* type B (Hib) infection. In recent years, the occurrence of epiglottitis has been reduced dramatically by the widespread use of the Hib vaccine. Other causes include bacterial infections by *Streptococcus* and *Staphylococcus* species. Manifestations include stridor with inspiration and expiration, high fever, dysphagia, drooling, and toxic appearance. Children may lean forward with their neck outstretched to minimize airway obstruction. Laboratory findings include an elevated white blood cell (WBC) count and positive blood cultures. Arterial blood gases may show hypoxia. Lateral neck radiographs show a swollen epiglottis with obstruction of the airway (positive thumb sign). Treatment involves securing the

child's airway, but this should be accomplished only by trained personnel. Before intubation, the child should not be moved nor placed in a supine position. Oxygen should also be avoided because of the risk of aggravating the child and possible complete obstruction of the airway. Intravenous antibiotics should be started immediately, and the child should be monitored in an intensive care setting.

Additional reading: Acute inflammatory upper airway obstruction: acute epiglottitis. *Nelson Textbook of Pediatrics,* 19th ed. Philadelphia, PA: Elsevier/Saunders; 2011.

Category: Respiratory system

30. Of the following, which local anesthetic has the fastest onset of action?
A) Lidocaine
B) Mepivicaine
C) Bupivicaine
D) Procaine
E) Tetracaine

Answer and Discussion

The answer is A. Lidocaine has the fastest onset of action.

- Lidocaine onset <2 min
- Bupivicaine onset 5 min
- Procaine onset 2 to 5 min

Additional Reading: Infiltration of local anesthetics. In: Basow DS, ed. *UpToDate.* Waltham, MA: UpToDate; 2013.

Category: Integumentary

31. Which of the following sutures is *not* absorbable?
A) Catgut
B) Vicryl
C) Polypropylene
D) Dexon
E) Chromic catgut

Answer and Discussion

The answer is C. The goal of suturing is to approximate the skin and eliminate unnecessary dead space. Tension at the wound site should be minimized. To achieve maximal cosmetic result, a suture is chosen based on the clinical situation. Monofilament sutures have significantly lowered the incidence of infection compared with multifilament sutures that can harbor bacteria. Nonabsorbable sutures (i.e., nylon, silk, polypropylene [prolene], braided polyester [Mersilene/Surgidac, ethibond/Ti-cron], and polybutester) are usually used to close the superficial layer of skin.

Absorbable sutures (i.e., catgut, chromic catgut, Dexon II [polycaprolate], Maxon, and Vicryl [Polyglactin 10], Poliglecaprone [PDSII], and Caprosyn) are used to close deep layers of skin.

Additional Reading: Essentials of skin laceration repair. *Am Fam Physician.* 2008;78(8):945–951.

Category: Nonspecific system

32. A 38-year-old woman presents with complaints of left eye redness with pain. She denies any recent trauma or injury. Which one of the following should be done initially?
A) Irrigation
B) Funduscopic examination
C) Visual acuity testing
D) Fluorescein staining
E) Application of a local anesthetic

Answer and Discussion

The answer is C. Almost all patients with ocular problems should have visual acuity testing before anything else is done. If this is difficult, a local anesthetic may be applied. The main exception to this rule is a chemical burn of the eye, which should be irrigated for 30 minutes before further evaluation or treatment is undertaken.

Additional Reading: Ocular emergencies. *Am Fam Physician.* 2007;76(6):829–836.

Category: Special sensory

33. A 34-year-old woman complains of abdominal pain and requests a surgical evaluation. She has a history of unexplained physical symptoms that began in her late teenage years. She is vague concerning past medical evaluations, but a review of her rather extensive medical record reveals numerous normal lab and imaging tests, and several surgical procedures that have failed to alleviate her symptoms; along with frequent requests for refills of narcotics. This history is most compatible with which one of the following?
A) Hypochondriasis
B) Malingering
C) Panic disorder
D) Generalized anxiety disorder
E) Somatization disorder

Answer and Discussion

The answer is E. Somatization disorder usually begins in the teens or twenties and is characterized by multiple unexplained physical symptoms, insistence on surgical procedures, and an imprecise or inaccurate medical history. Abuse of alcohol, narcotics, or other drugs is also commonly seen.

Hypochondriacs are overly concerned with bodily functions and often provide extensive, detailed medical histories. Malingering is an intentional pretense of illness to obtain personal gain. Patients with panic disorder have episodes of intense, short-lived attacks of cardiovascular, neurologic, or GI symptoms. Generalized anxiety disorder is characterized by unrealistic worry about life circumstances accompanied by symptoms of motor tension, autonomic hyperactivity, or vigilance and scanning.

Additional Reading: *Kaplan & Sadock's Comprehensive Textbook of Psychiatry.* Philadelphia, PA: Lippincott Williams & Wilkins; 2009, pp. 1927–1935.

Category: Psychogenic

34. A 32-year-old woman is brought to the emergency room by ambulance. She was involved in a motor vehicle accident. Close observation shows that her chest expands with expiration and contracts with inspiration. The most likely diagnosis is
A) Ruptured thoracic aorta
B) Pneumothorax
C) Ruptured esophagus
D) Flail chest
E) Cardiac contusion

Answer and Discussion

The answer is D. In cases of severe blunt trauma to the chest, multiple rib fractures may lead to flail chest. By definition, a flail chest occurs in the presence of two or more fractures in three or more consecutive ribs, causing instability of the chest wall; however, the condition can also occur after costochondral separation. The diagnosis is made by noting paradoxical chest wall motion in which the chest wall depresses with inspiration and expands with expiration.

There may be coexisting intrathoracic or intra-abdominal injuries. Initial management of flail chest consists of oxygen and close monitoring of early signs of respiratory compromise, ideally using both pulse oxymetry and capnography. Noninvasive positive airway pressure by mask may obviate the need for endotracheal intubation in alert patients. Patients with severe injuries, respiratory distress, or progressively worsening respiratory function require endothracheal intubation in alert patients.

Additional Reading: Schaider JJ. Flail chest. *Rosen and Barkin's 5-Minute Emergency Medicine Consult.* Philadelphia, PA: Lippincott Williams and Wilkins; 2010.

Category: Respiratory system

35. Which of the following can be added to lidocaine to reduce the burning sensation when it is administered?
A) Sodium bicarbonate
B) Epinephrine
C) Normal saline
D) Lactated Ringer's solution
E) Aluminum hydroxide

Answer and Discussion

The answer is A. Sodium bicarbonate may be added to neutralize the acidic local anesthetic and to reduce the burning sensation associated with anesthetic administration. Addition of a 1 cc of a 1 mEq/mL solution of bicarbonate for every 9 cc of local anesthetic can alleviate this burning and improve patient comfort.

Additional Reading: Infiltration of local anesthetics. In: Basow DS, ed. *UpToDate.* Waltham, MA: UpToDate; 2013.

Category: Integumentary

36. Which of the following statements about total parenteral nutrition (TPN) is true?
A) Lipid emulsions can lead to fatty emboli and are not added to TPN solutions.
B) Electrolytes should be monitored closely until stable.
C) In most cases, TPN is administered through peripheral access.
D) Equivalent amounts of calories can be delivered via a central or peripheral access.
E) Because glucose is delivered in standard amounts at predetermined rates, there is little need to follow glucose on a regular basis.

Answer and Discussion

The answer is B. TPN is indicated for those patients who require nutritional support but cannot meet their nutritional needs through oral intake and for whom enteral feedings is contraindicated or not tolerated. Central venous access is usually required. TPN requires water (30 to 40 mL/kg/day), carbohydrate as dextrose (70% 3.4 kcal/g), amino acids 10% (4 kcal/g), and fat 20% (9 kcal/g), depending on the degree of catabolism. Indications include malnourished patients scheduled for surgery, chemotherapy, or radiation. Patients with severe burns, anorexia, coma, Crohn's disease, ulcerative colitis, or pancreatitis may benefit from TPN. The following should be monitored daily: weight, plasma urea and glucose (several times daily until stable), complete blood cell count, blood gases, accurate fluid balance, 24-hour urine, and electrolytes. When the patient becomes stable, the frequency of these tests can be reduced. Liver function tests should be performed, and plasma proteins, PT, plasma and urine osmolality, and calcium, magnesium, and phosphate should be measured.

Additional Reading: Nutrition support in critically ill patients: parenteral nutrition. In: Basow DS, ed. *UpToDate*. Waltham, MA: UpToDate; 2013.

Category: Nonspecific system

37. Which of the following factors makes appendicitis during pregnancy difficult to diagnose?
A) Location of the appendix
B) Presence of fever
C) Rectal tenderness
D) Rebound tenderness
E) Presence of pyuria

Answer and Discussion

The answer is A. Appendicitis during pregnancy may be difficult to diagnose. The WBC count is mildly elevated during a normal pregnancy, making it difficult to distinguish the leukocytosis seen with infection. In addition, as pregnancy progresses, the position of the appendix migrates superiorly (usually above the iliac crest in patients at more than 5 months' gestation). Therefore, there is a greater risk for perforation in those with appendicitis as pregnancy progresses. In addition, there is a greater risk of perinatal mortality when the appendix is perforated. The complications involved with appendectomy include premature labor and infection. The differential diagnosis of abdominal pain during pregnancy is extensive and includes gastroenteritis, inflammatory bowel disease, cholecystitis, intestinal obstruction, pancreatitis, pyelonephritis, nephrolithiasis, spontaneous abortion, round ligament pain, ectopic pregnancy, uterine contractions, placental abruption, and pelvic infections.

Additional Reading: Evaluation of acute pelvic pain in women. *Am Fam Physician*. 2010;82(2):141–147.

Category: Gastroenterology system

38. When diagnosing an acute appendicitis, which of the following tests has the highest accuracy rate?
A) Plain films of the abdomen
B) Barium enema
C) CT of the abdomen
D) HIDA scan
E) Abdominal ultrasound

Answer and Discussion

The answer is C. Acute appendicitis is the most common reason leading to emergent abdominal surgery. The overall diagnostic accuracy achieved by traditional history, physical examination, and laboratory tests has been approximately 80%. The accuracy of diagnosis varies and is more difficult in women of childbearing age, children, and elderly persons. If the diagnosis of acute appendicitis is clear from the history and physical examination, prompt surgical referral is warranted. In atypical presentations, ultrasonography and CT may help lower the rate of false-negative appendicitis diagnoses, reduce morbidity from perforation, and lower medical expenses. Ultrasonography is safe and readily available, with sensitivity of 86% and specificity of 81%; however, CT scan has better specificity (91% to 98%) and sensitivity (95% to 100%). Disadvantages of CT include radiation exposure, cost, and possible complications from contrast media.

Additional Reading: Appendicitis acute. In: Domino F, ed. *The 5-Minute Clinical Consult*. Philadelphia, PA: Lippincott Williams and Wilkins; 2014.

Category: Gastroenterology system

39. Pain over the anatomic "snuff box" may indicate
A) Colles' fracture
B) Cuboid fracture
C) Scaphoid fracture
D) Hook of the hamate fracture
E) Boxer's fracture

Answer and Discussion

The answer is C. Scaphoid fractures account for approximately 60% of carpal bone fractures and are often missed on the initial radiograph. They frequently occur following a fall onto an outstretched hand. Symptoms include pain over the anatomic "snuff box" (area between the extensor pollicis brevis and the extensor pollicis longus tendons) and pain with radial deviation of the wrist. Reduction is seldom necessary; however, the arm, wrist, and thumb should be immobilized with a thumb spica cast for at least 6 weeks. If pain persists for longer than 4 months, there is an increased risk of nonunion or avascular necrosis with development of arthritis. Surgery may be indicated for this condition. If clinically suspected, radiographs (including scaphoid views) should be performed initially. Plain wrist films usually do not detect these fractures. In some cases, a bone scan or tomograms may be necessary to confirm the diagnosis. Bony electrical stimulation has also been shown to be effective in the healing of scaphoid fractures. Displaced fractures require open reduction with screw fixation.

Additional Reading: Diagnosis and management of scaphoid fractures. *Am Fam Physician*. 2004;70(5):879–884.

Category: Musculoskeletal system

40. Relief of hip pain after hip replacement occurs
A) Almost immediately
B) After 3 months
C) After 6 months
D) Usually after 1 year
E) Rarely; hip replacement mostly improves functionality

Answer and Discussion

The answer is A. Hip arthroplasty is usually reserved for elderly patients with severe degenerative or rheumatoid arthritis. Indications include intractable pain or severe limitation of motion that interferes with the patient's activity level. Those patients with rheumatoid arthritis have longer and more lasting improvement than those with osteoarthritis. Complications include bleeding, infection, and the major immediate complication of thromboembolism. Bone resorption is a major complication that may affect the life of the prosthesis. Long-term complications include loosening of the prosthesis, which may require further surgery. In most cases, relief is immediate after hip replacement, and 90% of hip replacements are never revised.

Additional Reading: Osteoarthritis of the hip. *Am Fam Physician*. 2010;81(4):444–445.

Category: Musculoskeletal system

41. A felon is a
A) Prominence of the distal fifth toe
B) Herpetic infection associated with a phalanx
C) Neuroma associated with the flexor tendon
D) Asymmetric nevus
E) Infection of the distal pulp space of a phalanx

Answer and Discussion

The answer is E. A felon is an infection of the pulp space of a phalanx. A felon usually is caused by inoculation of bacteria into the fingertip through a penetrating trauma. The most commonly affected digits are the thumb and index finger. Predisposing causes include splinters, bits of glass, abrasions, and minor trauma. A felon also may arise when an untreated paronychia spreads into the pad of the fingertip. The most common site is the distal pulp, which may be involved centrally, laterally, and apically. The septa between pulp spaces ordinarily limit the spread of infection, resulting in an abscess, which creates pressure and necrosis of adjacent tissues. The underlying bone, joint, or flexor tendons may become infected, and intense throbbing pain and a swollen pulp are present. If diagnosed in the early stages of cellulitis, a felon may be treated with elevation, oral antibiotics, and warm-water or saline soaks. Radiographs should be obtained to evaluate for osteomyelitis or a foreign body. Tetanus prophylaxis should be administered when necessary. If fluctuance is present, incision and drainage are appropriate along with administration of appropriate antibiotics (usually a cephalosporin or anti-staphylococcal penicillin).

Additional Reading: Common acute hand infections. *Am Fam Physician.* 2003;68:2167–2176.

Category: Integumentary

42. You are asked to consult on a 69-year-old man who has just had knee-replacement surgery. His diabetes is treated with pioglitazone (Actos), 30 mg daily, and metformin (Glucophage), 1,000 mg twice daily. He is now awake and has been able to eat his dinner. His exam is normal except for mild obesity and edema of his right leg. A complete blood count and chemistry profile were normal except for a serum glucose level of 200 mg/dL. A hemoglobin A1c done during his pre-op evaluation was 6.7%. Which one of the following would be the best management for his diabetes at this time?
A) Stop her usual medications and begin a sliding-scale insulin regimen.
B) Stop the metformin only.
C) Initiate an insulin drip to maintain glucose levels of 80 to 120 mg/dL.
D) Decrease the dosage of pioglitazone.
E) Continue with her usual medication regimen.

Answer and Discussion

The answer is E. Use of a "sliding-scale" insulin regimen to control glucose in hospitalized diabetics is inadequate, and while post-op patients using an insulin drip to maintain control have a decreased risk of sepsis, there is no mortality benefit. Metformin should be stopped if the serum creatinine level is >1.5 mg/dL in men or >1.4 mg/dL in women, or if an imaging procedure requiring contrast is needed. In patients who have not had their hemoglobin A1c measured in the past 30 days, this could be done to provide a better indication of glucose control. If adequate control has been demonstrated and no contraindications are noted, the patient's usual medication regimen should be continued.

Additional Reading: Glycemic control in hospitalized patients not in intensive care: beyond sliding-scale insulin. *Am Fam Physician.* 2010;81(9):1130–1135.

Category: Endocrine system

43. A pipe smoker is found to have a white elevated plaque on his buccal mucosa during a general medical examination. The area cannot be wiped away with sterile gauze. The most likely diagnosis is
A) Squamous cell carcinoma
B) Thrush
C) Gingivitis
D) Leukoplakia
E) Periodontitis

Answer and Discussion

The answer is D. Leukoplakia is a precancerous lesion that appears as a white, elevated, plaque-like growth that usually has asymmetric borders and usually affects the oral mucosa. It cannot be wiped off. The lesions tend to occur on the lip, mouth, buccal mucosa, or vaginal mucosa. Those at risk are cigarette smokers, pipe smokers, smokeless tobacco users, and heavy alcohol users. Others at risk include those with chronic oral infections, chronic malocclusion, or chronic ultraviolet light exposure. If suspected, these lesions should be biopsied to rule out malignancy. Approximately 10% may show malignant transformation. *Candida* infections can resemble leukoplakia, but *Candida* can be removed using a cotton swab.

Additional Reading: Common oral lesions: Part II. Masses and neoplasia. *Am Fam Physician.* 2007;75(4):509–512.

Category: Integumentary

44. A 2-year-old child is brought into your office. Mom reports the boy fell off his bed and has been limping for the last 3 days. He did hit his head, but had no loss of consciousness and has been acting normally since his fall. You note retinal hemorrhages and several areas of bruising on the head, legs, thighs, and arms in varying stages of healing. The most likely cause is
A) Autism
B) Abuse
C) Hemophilia
D) Leukemia
E) Poor coordination

Answer and Discussion

The answer is B. Determining whether head injuries in children are accidental or a result of physical abuse is very important. Children with head injuries related to abuse tend to be younger than those with accidental injuries. Boys are more frequently affected. Subdural hematoma (SDH), subarachnoid hemorrhage, and retinal hemorrhage are more common in abused children. Child abuse should be strongly suspected when such injuries are present in a child without a history of a fall or with a history of a fall from a relatively low height. Multiple injuries in various stages of healing should also alert the clinician to the possibility of abuse. A skeletal survey for children younger than 3 years should be performed when inflicted head injuries are suspected.

Additional Reading: Child abuse: approach and management. *Am Fam Physician.* 2007;75(2):221–228.

Category: Nonspecific system

45. A 65-year-old man presents to your office complaining of abdominal pain. His vital signs are stable. Examination reveals a pulsatile mass in the midabdomen. The most appropriate test is
A) Magnetic resonance imaging (MRI) of the abdomen
B) Laboratory tests, including complete blood count, electrolytes, and erythrocyte sedimentation rate
C) Ultrasound examination of the abdomen
D) Upper GI series
E) Barium enema

Answer and Discussion

The answer is C. Aortic abdominal aneurysm is defined as dilated aorta with a diameter at least 1.5 times the diameter measured at the level of renal arteries. AAAs result from a weakening in the wall of the aorta. Most cases occur inferior to the renal arteries and are asymptomatic; however, back pain or abdominal pain may precede rupture.

Most aneurysms are the result of atherosclerotic disease that results in weakening of the vessel. Strong evidence suggests a genetic susceptibility to AAAs. Patients with these aneurysms have a 20% chance of having a first-degree relative with the same condition. Male siblings are at particular risk. Approximately 75% of AAAs are asymptomatic and are detected during routine physical examination or during an unrelated radiologic or surgical procedure. Symptoms of an AAA may result from expansion or rupture of the aneurysm, pressure on adjacent structures, embolization, or thrombosis. The most commonly reported symptom is any type of abdominal, flank, or back pain. Pressure on adjacent viscera may result in compression of the bowel. Patients may present with early satiety and, occasionally, nausea and vomiting. Rarely, ureteral compression may result in a partial ureteral obstruction. Thrombus and atheromatous material, which line nearly all AAAs, may occasionally result in distal arterial embolization and, rarely, aneurysm thrombosis. The abrupt onset of severe, constant pain in the abdomen, flank, or back, unrelieved by positional changes, is characteristic of expansion or rupture of the aneurysm. Physical examination often reveals a pulsating abdominal mass. Obesity, uncooperativeness, ascites, tortuosity of the aorta, and excessive lumbar lordosis are conditions that may make diagnosis by palpation difficult. Examination of the abdominal aorta is facilitated by having the patient lie on the examination table with the knees slightly flexed. The aorta is palpated during exhalation. A pulsatile abdominal mass left of midline—between the xiphoid process and the umbilicus—is highly suggestive of an AAA. Diagnosis is made with ultrasound or CT examination. B-mode ultrasound is the screening method of choice for asymptomatic AAAs. It is available in most hospitals, is inexpensive, does not require ionizing radiation, reveals details of the vessel wall and associated atherosclerotic plaques, and allows accurate measurement of the aneurysm in longitudinal and transverse dimensions. Typically, aneurysms >5.5 to 6 cm are treated surgically, whereas smaller aneurysms are observed for any changes. If they grow 1 cm/year, larger surgery is recommended. Endovascular repair is safer, results in shorter hospital stays and quicker recovery, and translates into significant cost savings when compared with conventional surgery. The operative mortality rate is usually <5%. The mortality rate of patients with aneurysms >6 cm is approximately 50% in 1 year; patients with aneurysms between 4 and 6 cm have a mortality rate of 25% in 1 year.

Additional Reading: Abdominal aortic aneurysm. *Am Fam Physician.* 2006;73(7):1198–1204.

Category: Cardiovascular system

46. Which of the following can impede the healing of decubitus ulcers?
A) Wet-to-dry dressing changes
B) Doughnut cushions
C) Frequent position changes
D) Air-fluidized mattresses
E) Debridement of nonviable tissue

Answer and Discussion

The answer is B. Decubitus ulcers occur when there is prolonged pressure of skin against an external object such as a bed or a wheelchair. It occurs most often in patients who are debilitated and have impaired sensory function. The sacrum, ischia, greater trochanters, external malleoli, and heels are at particular risk for tissue breakdown. There are four stages in the development of a decubitus ulcer:

- *Stage 1*—nonblanchable erythema of intact skin
- *Stage 2*—partial-thickness dermal or epidermal loss causing a blister, shallow crater, or abrasion

- *Stage 3*—full-thickness necrosis causing a deep crater down to fascia
- *Stage 4*—full-thickness destruction of muscle, bone, or supporting structures

Intrinsic and extrinsic factors play a role in the development of pressure ulcers. Intrinsic factors include loss of pain and pressure sensations (which ordinarily prompt the patient to shift position and relieve the pressure) and minimal fat and muscle padding between bony weight-bearing prominences and skin. Disuse atrophy, malnutrition, anemia, and infection also contribute. In a paralyzed patient, loss of vasomotor control leads to lowered tone in the vascular bed and lowered circulatory rate. Spasticity, especially in patients with spinal cord injuries, can place a shearing force on the blood vessels to further compromise circulation. Extrinsic factors include pressure due to infrequent shifting of the patient's position; friction, irritation, and pulling of the skin from ill-adjusted supports or wrinkled bedding or clothing also contribute. In an immobilized patient, severe pressure can impair local circulation in less than 3 hours, causing local tissue anoxia that, if unrelieved, progresses to necrosis of the skin and subcutaneous tissues. Moisture (e.g., from perspiration or incontinence) leads to tissue maceration and predisposes to pressure sores. The treatment of decubitus ulcers includes wet-to-dry dressing changes and the use of air-fluidized beds, particularly for large ulcers. Ulcers that have not advanced beyond stage 3 may heal spontaneously if the pressure is removed and the area is small. New hydrophilic gels and hydrocolloid dressings speed healing. Stage 4 ulcers require debridement or more extensive surgery. When the ulcers are filled with pus or necrotic debris, dextranomer beads or newer hydrophilic polymers may hasten debridement without surgery. Conservative debridement of necrotic tissue with forceps and scissors should be instituted. Some ulcers may be debrided by cleansing them with hydrogen peroxide. Whirlpool baths may also assist debridement. The use of egg-crate mattresses, sheepskins, and doughnut cushions is not adequate to prevent ulcers; doughnut cushions can actually decrease the blood flow to the area of the body in the center of the cushion, thereby impeding the healing process. The use of antibiotics is unnecessary unless cellulitis, osteomyelitis, or systemic infection is present. The use of topical antiseptics and antibiotics may also impede the healing process by damaging fibroblasts, which are needed for healing. Compared with standard hospital mattresses, pressure-reducing devices decrease the incidence of pressure ulcers.

Additional Reading: Pressure ulcers. Prevention, evaluation and management. *Am Fam Physician.* 2008;78(10):1186–1194.

Category: Integumentary

47. Of the following measurements, which would be considered the threshold for surgical intervention in treating a man with an AAA?
A) 4.0 cm
B) 5.5 cm
C) 6.5 cm
D) 7.0 cm
E) 8.0 cm

Answer and Discussion

The answer is B. Aneurysm diameter is one of the strongest predictors of aneurysm rupture, with risk increasing markedly at diameters greater than 5.5 cm. Since it is uncommon for AAAs smaller than 5 cm to rupture, many vascular surgeons adopted this measurement as an indication for elective repair.

Additional Reading: Abdominal aortic aneurysm. *Am Fam Physician.* 2006;73(7):1198–1204.

Category: Cardiovascular system

In patients with AAAs with a diameter >5.5 cm, the risk of rupture is increased markedly and surgical repair is indicated if the patient can tolerate the intervention.

48. A 51-year-old woman presents to the office with a 2-day history of right-upper-quadrant, colicky abdominal pain, as well as nausea and vomiting. Examination shows significant pain with palpation in the right upper quadrant. Laboratory findings include an elevated WBC count, alkaline phosphatase, and bilirubin level. The most likely diagnosis is

A) Viral gastroenteritis
B) Dissecting abdominal aneurysm
C) Acute pancreatitis
D) Acute cholecystitis
E) Perforated duodenal ulcer

Answer and Discussion

The answer is D. Cholecystitis is an acute inflammation of the gallbladder wall. The condition usually results from an obstruction of the bile ducts as a result of biliary stones (most commonly cholesterol). Risk factors for cholesterol gallstone formation include age, obesity, rapid weight loss, pregnancy, female gender, use of exogenous estrogens, diabetes, certain GI conditions, and certain medications. Symptoms include colicky right-upper-quadrant abdominal pain that starts out mild and crescendos into more severe pain that may last several hours before resolving spontaneously. Patients may also report nausea and vomiting and low-grade fevers. Physical examination usually shows marked right-upper-quadrant tenderness with a positive Murphy's sign (marked abdominal pain and inspiratory arrest with palpation of the right upper quadrant). A palpable gallbladder is present in as many as 30% to 40% of patients. Jaundice is present in 15% of patients. Laboratory findings include an elevated WBC count, increased serum transaminases, alkaline phosphatase, bilirubin levels, and, in some cases, amylase levels. The diagnosis is usually made with ultrasound, which has 84% sensitivity and 99% specificity; however, cholescintigraphy (HIDA scan) is the most sensitive test to document obstruction in the biliary system, with 97% sensitivity and 90% specificity. Oral cholecystograms are rarely used for diagnosing acute cholecystitis. CT scans are not superior to ultrasound and are more expensive. Up to one-half of stones in the common bile duct are not detected on ultrasonography. In the gallbladder, stones <2 mm in diameter may be missed or misdiagnosed as sludge. Endoscopic retrograde cholangiopancreatography is the test of choice to detect stones in the common bile duct.

Additional Reading: Schaider JJ. *Rosen and Barkin's 5-Minute Emergency Medicine Consult.* Philadelphia, PA: Lippincott Williams and Wilkins; 2010.

Category: Gastroenterology system

49. A 65-year-old woman asks if she should be screened for carotid artery stenosis, as it is being offered for free at her church and she has a family history of stroke. She has well-controlled hypertension and hypercholesterolemia. No bruits are heard on exam and she is asymptomatic. Which one of the following is consistent with U.S. Preventive Services Task Force (USPSTF) and AHA recommendations regarding carotid artery ultrasonography for this patient?

A) She does not need screening ultrasonography at this time.
B) She should have one-time screening ultrasonography now.
C) She should have routine screening ultrasonography now and every 5 years.
D) She should have routine screening ultrasonography now and every 10 years.

Answer and Discussion

The answer is A. The USPSTF and the AHA/American Stroke Association recommend not performing carotid artery screening with ultrasonography or other screening tests in patients without neurologic symptoms because the harms outweigh the benefits. In the general population, screening tests for carotid artery stenosis would result in more false-positive results than true-positive results. This would lead to surgical procedures that are not indicated or to confirmatory angiography. As a result of these procedures, some patients would suffer serious harms such as death, stroke, or myocardial infarction, which outweigh the potential benefit surgical treatment may have in preventing stroke.

Additional Reading: Screening for carotid artery stenosis. 2007 update. *US Preventive Service Task Force.* From: http://www.uspreventiveservicestaskforce.org/uspstf07/cas/casart2.htm.

Category: Neurologic

50. A 25-year-old patient arrives in the emergency room after being involved in a high-speed motor vehicle accident. The patient is conscious, hypotensive, and complains of abdominal pain. The most appropriate management includes

A) Flat and upright abdominal series
B) Diagnostic peritoneal lavage
C) Abdominal ultrasound
D) Emergent abdominal CT scan
E) Exploratory laparotomy

Answer and Discussion

The answer is B. Patients who have experienced significant abdominal trauma, have abdominal pain, or are unstable and the diagnosis remains unclear should undergo diagnostic peritoneal lavage once they arrive in the emergency room. The procedure involves making a small incision between the umbilicus and pubis after local anesthesia is administered. A small 1-cm incision is then made in the peritoneal fascia, and a peritoneal dialysis catheter is placed. The catheter is directed to the posterior sacral area and 1,000 mL of normal saline is infused into the peritoneal cavity and allowed to return by gravity. A return of at least 10 mL of gross blood; a bloody lavage effluent; a red blood cell (RBC) count greater than 100,000/mm^3; a WBC count greater than 500/mm^3; an amylase greater than 175 IU/dL; or the detection of bile, bacteria, or food fibers in the aspirated fluid is considered a positive response and requires immediate laparotomy to look for an internal bleeding site. Patients who are clinically stable may undergo CT or ultrasound to further evaluate the abdomen when blunt trauma has occurred. Diagnostic peritoneal lavage is highly sensitive for the presence of intraperitoneal blood; however, specificity is low.

Additional Reading: Initial evaluation and management of blunt abdominal trauma in adults. In: Basow DS, ed. *UpToDate.* Waltham, MA: UpToDate; 2013.

Category: Nonspecific system

51. A 33-year-old homeless person presents to the emergency room. While scavenging in garbage cans, the patient cut his left hand. He does not recall if he has ever had immunization for tetanus before. The most appropriate immunization is

A) Adult diphtheria tetanus toxoid (dT)
B) Diphtheria–pertussis–tetanus vaccine (DPT)
C) dT and tetanus immunoglobulin (TIG)
D) Observation

Answer and Discussion

The answer is C. Tetanus immunization should be administered to those who have completed only the primary series of immunization or who received a booster immunization more than 5 years previously. Tetanus toxoid (0.5 mL IM) and tetanus immune globulin (250 units IM) should be given with wounds who have received less than three doses of tetanus toxoid or whose immunization status is uncertain.

> **Additional Reading:** Tetanus. In: Domino F, ed. *The 5-Minute Clinical Consult.* Philadelphia, PA: Lippincott Williams and Wilkins; 2014.

> Category: Nonspecific system

52. Which of the following statements is true regarding hip fractures?
A) Most hip fractures do not require surgery for repair.
B) Avascular necrosis of the femoral head is a serious complication.
C) Nonunion or malunion does not occur with hip fractures.
D) Location of the fracture has no bearing on the outcome.
E) None of the above.

Answer and Discussion

The answer is B. The distinction between intracapsular and extracapsular hip fracture has prognostic value for the patient's outcome. Early detection of intracapsular fractures is especially important because these fractures are prone to complications for two primary reasons. First, interruption of the blood supply to the femoral head frequently occurs and can lead to avascular necrosis. Second, the head fragment of the fracture is often a shell containing fragile cancellous bone that provides poor attachment for a fixation device, a situation that often increases the possibility of nonunion or malunion. Asymptomatic lesions of the femoral head that involve less than 15% of the femoral head may resolve without surgical intervention and may, therefore, be treated nonoperatively. Asymptomatic avascular necrosis that involves more than 30% of the femoral head are likely to collapse despite surgical interventions; thus these patients may also be nonoperatively managed at the outset with anticipation of eventual total hip arthorplasty.

> **Additional Reading:** Management of hip fracture: the family physician's role. *Am Fam Physician.* 2006;73(12):2195–2200.

> Category: Musculoskeletal system

53. Which of the following types of polyps is associated with the greatest risk of malignant transformation?
A) Distal hyperplastic polyp
B) Tubular adenoma
C) Villous adenoma
D) Mixed tubulovillous adenoma
E) All have equal risk

Answer and Discussion

The answer is C. The development of colon polyps has been associated with a high-fat, low-fiber diet. They also occur more frequently in patients with a positive family history (two to four times more common than in the healthy population). Villous histology, increasing polyps size, and high-grade dysplasia are risk factors for focal cancer within and individual adenoma. Ademomatous polyps >1 cm in diameter are a risk factor for containing colorectal cancer (CRC) and are also a risk factor for metachronus cancer development. There is up to fourfold increase in cancer risk during follow-up with polyps >1 cm in size. Adenomatous polyps with >25%

villous histology are a risk factor for developing metachronous CRC. High-grade dysplasia often coexist with areas of invasive cancer in the polyps. Older age is also associated with high-grade dysplasia within an adenoma, independent of size or histology. The number of adenomas, particularly three or more, was the sole risk factor for development of metachronic adenomas with advanced pathologic features. Polyps are divided into differing histologic types, including the following:

1. Hyperplasic polyps: Distal small hyperplastic polyps rarely develop into cancer.
2. Tubular adenoma: 5% chance of cancer development
3. Villous adenoma: 40% chance of cancer development
4. Mixed tubulovillous adenoma: 22% chance of cancer development

> **Additional Reading:** Colonic polyps. In: Domino F, ed. *The 5-Minute Clinical Consult.* Philadelphia, PA: Lippincott Williams and Wilkins; 2014.

> Category: Gastroenterology system

54. A 40-year-old woman is found to have chronic cholestasis. The most serious complication is the development of
A) Intractable hiccups
B) Primary biliary cirrhosis
C) Cholelithiasis
D) Hypercholesterolemia
E) Chronic urticaria

Answer and Discussion

The answer is B. Primary biliary cirrhosis is a condition that is characterized by chronic cholestasis, which can damage the liver and ultimately result in the development of cirrhosis. The cause is unknown but may be associated with an underlying autoimmune disorder. The condition typically affects women between 35 and 70 years of age; the condition can occur in men. The disease usually involves four stages:

1. Bile duct inflammation
2. Periportal fibrosis
3. Progressive scarring
4. Cirrhosis

Symptoms include itching secondary to elevations of bilirubin, fatigue, and jaundice. Physical findings include hepatosplenomegaly, skin xanthomas (especially around the eyelids and involving the tendons), clubbing, and jaundice. Laboratory tests show elevated alkaline phosphatase, bilirubin, γ-glutamyl transferase, aspartate aminotransferase (AST), and alanine aminotransferase. Serum cholesterol is also usually elevated. Diagnostic procedures include ultrasound, endoscopic retrograde cholangiopancreatography, and liver biopsy. Unfortunately, no specific treatment is available; however, those affected may be candidates for liver transplantation if they develop cirrhosis with hepatic failure. Cholestyramine may be beneficial for the pruritus. Those affected have a variable prognosis, depending on the severity of the disease. Those with slow progression may be minimally affected. Chronic urticaria may be associated with underlying urticarial vasculitis and is diagnosed by skin biopsy.

> **Additional Reading:** Clinical manifestations, diagnosis, and natural history of primary biliary cirrhosis. In: Basow DS, ed. *UpToDate.* Waltham, MA: UpToDate; 2013.

> Category: Gastroenterology system

55. A 54-year-old man with no prior history of DVT presents with unilateral swelling of the right lower extremity after a recent prolonged plane flight. The patient is found to have a below-the-knee DVT associated with the calf. He has no contraindication for anticoagulation therapy. What is the appropriate therapy?
A) Heparin therapy followed by oral anticoagulation for 12 weeks.
B) No anticoagulation and monitor for proximal extension with duplex ultrasound two times per week for 2 weeks.
C) No anticoagulation and monitor for proximal for proximal extension with duplex ultrasound once a week for 4 weeks.
D) No anticoagulation and application of compressive stockings.
E) No anticoagulation and elevation of the extremity and early mobilization.

Answer and Discussion

The answer is A. In general all symptomatic Patients with DVT, whether proximal or distal, should be treated with low-molecular-weight (LMW) heparin, fondaparinux, unfractionated intravenous heparin or adjusted dose subcutaneous insulin. When unfractional heparin is used, the dose should be sufficient to prolonged the activated PTT (aPTT) to 1.5 to 2.5 times the mean of the control value or the upper limit of the normal activated PTT range. Treatment with low-molecular-weight heparin, fondaparinux, or unfractionated heparin should be continued for at least 5 days, and oral anticoagulation with a vitamin K antagonist should be overlapped with low-molecular-weight heparin, fondaparinux, or unfractionated heparin for at least 4 to 5 days. No such overlap is required if rivaroxaban is chosen. For most patients, warfarin should be initiated simultaneously with heparin, at an initial dose of 5 mg/day. The heparin product can be discontinued on day 5 or 6 if the international normalized ratio (INR) has been therapeutic for two consecutive days. Inferior vena cava filter is recommended when there is a contraindication to, or a failure of, anticoagulant therapy in an individual with, or at high risk for, proximal vein thrombosis or pulmonary embolism (PE). It is also recommended in patients with recurrent thromboembolism despite adequate anticoagulation, for chronic recurrent embolism with pulmonary hypertension, and with the concurrent performance of surgical pulmonary embolectomy or pulmonary thromboendarterectomy.

Patients with a first thromboembolic even in the context of reversible or time-limited risk factor (e.g., trauma, surgery) should be treated for 3 months. Patients with a first idiopathic thromboembolism event should be treated with a minimum of 3 months. Following this, all patients should be evaluated for the risk–benefit ratio of long-term therapy. Indefinite therapy is preferred in patients with a first unprovoked episode of proximal DVT who have a greater concern about recurrent venous thromboembolism and a relative lower concern about the burdens of long-term anticoagulation therapy. Most patients with advance malignancy should be treated indefinitely or until the cancer resolves.

Additional Reading: Antithrombotic therapy for VTE disease: antithrombotic therapy and prevention of thrombosis, 9th ed. American College of Chest Physician Evidence-Based Clinical Practice Guidelines. *Chest.* 2012;141(suppl 2):e419S.

Category: Cardiovascular system

56. A 45-year-old woman complains of rectal discomfort and bleeding aggravated by bowel movements. The patient reports a long history of constipation. On examination, there is a small fissure at the lateral 9 o'clock position. Which of the following statements is true?
A) Rectal spasms increase blood flow and accelerate healing.
B) A cause other than passage of hard stool should be considered.

C) Bowel movements help relieve symptoms.
D) Exercise often leads to development of fissures.
E) Corticosteroid creams should be avoided because of the risk of bacterial overgrowth.

Answer and Discussion

The answer is B. Anal fissures are small tears in the mucosa of the anal canal. They often produce pain disproportionate to the size of the lesion. The cause is thought to be secondary to traumatic tearing of the mucosa with the passage of large, hard stools. Other causes include proctitis as a result of previous rectal surgery, hemorrhoids, or rectal cancer. Because of its location in the area of the rectal sphincter, spasms may keep the area from healing. Fissures are most commonly located anterior or posterior to the anus. When fissures are found laterally, syphilis, tuberculosis, occult abscesses, leukemic infiltrates, carcinoma, herpes, acquired immunodeficiency syndrome, or inflammatory bowel disease should be considered as causes. Symptoms include rectal pain and bleeding, which is aggravated with bowel movements. Treatment involves the use of stool softeners and laxatives, hydrocortisone creams, benzocaine ointments, and warm sits baths, as well as increased oral fluids and adequate exercise or nifedipine injected botulinum toxin is also used. Another nonsurgical treatment for anal fissure is nitroglycerin ointment 2% diluted to 0.2% qid. Calcium channel blockers, oral or topical, are not better than nitrates but have fewer side effects. Surgery is indicated for severe cases that are refractive.

Additional Reading: Anal fissure. In: Domino F, ed. *The 5-Minute Clinical Consult.* Philadelphia, PA: Lippincott Williams and Wilkins; 2014.

Category: Gastroenterology system

57. Which of the following is true regarding patient-controlled analgesia (PCA)?
A) The administration is labor intensive.
B) Oversedation can usually be avoided.
C) The delivery system can usually increase the time interval between patient demand and delivery of the medication.
D) Basal infusion rates should be routinely delivered.
E) Patient response is not a good indicator of PCA effectiveness.

Answer and Discussion

The answer is B. Patient-controlled analgesia (PCA) is the preferred mode of administering opioids for moderate to severe postoperative pain. The benefits include easier patient access to pain medication, reduced chance or medication error, and ready titration. Morphine, hydromorphine, and fentanyl can be administered via PCA pump. The pump is discontinued when the patient is able to tolerate oral analgesics. A fentanyl PCA may be used for patients with allergies or intolerances to morphine and hydromorphine, but is less desirable in most patients because of its short duration of action. Fentanyl may be easier to titrate in patients with renal and hepatic insufficiency. Alternatively hydromorphone can be used in patient with renal insufficiency.

PCA pumps avoid the lag period between when the patient senses pain and initiates the call for medication and actual delivery by the nurse. It can also reduce the amount of work of drawing up and delivering multiple doses of medication by the nursing staff. PCA pumps can also deliver a constant rate of medication per hour whether or not the patient hits the demand button.

Compared with conventional parenteral analgesia, PCA provide better pain control and result in greater patient satisfaction in spite of a higher incidence of pruritus.

Additional Reading: Management of postoperative pain. In: Basow DS, ed. *UpToDate*. Waltham, MA: UpToDate; 2013.

Category: Nonspecific system

58. A 39-year-old white woman complains of several episodes of right-upper-quadrant pain during the past year. The episodes typically last 2 to 4 hours and are associated with nausea and vomiting. Her most recent episode occurred 2 weeks ago, and they seem to be happening more often. Which one of the following is most likely to provide an explanation for the patient's symptoms?
A) A bilirubin level
B) An AST (SGOT) level
C) A plain film of the abdomen
D) An HIDA scan
E) Abdominal ultrasonography

Answer and Discussion

The answer is E. Cholecystitis (inflammation of the gallbladder) usually results as a complication of cholelithiasis (gallstones) and obstruction of the biliary duct by gallstones. The condition is seen more commonly in women than in men. The incidence increases with age. Symptoms include rapid onset of intermittent cramping abdominal pain in the upper-right quadrant, which gradually becomes worse and lasts several hours; fever, nausea, and vomiting may be present in some cases. Physical findings include right-upper-quadrant pain, guarding, and a positive Murphy's sign (significant tenderness with palpation in the right upper quadrant with inspiration). Chronic cholelithiasis follows a more indolent course with less severe symptoms that are shorter in duration and are recurrent.

In a patient with a typical history for gallstones, an abdominal ultrasonography is likely to show stones and support the diagnosis. Serum bilirubin and AST levels are usually normal except at the time of an attack. Patients with chronic cholecystitis rarely have abnormal laboratory studies. An HIDA scan may be useful if performed during an attack, since the scan assesses the patency of the cystic duct. A plain abdominal film will detect only 10% to 15% of cases of cholelithiasis.

Laparoscopic cholecystectomy is the procedure of choice for uncomplicated acute and chronic cholecystitis. Stones can be composed of cholesterol (most common), pigment, and mixed stones. Oral cholecystography is no longer commonly used in the diagnosis of cholecystitis. Prophylactic cholecystectomy for asymptomatic cholelithiasis is generally not recommended.

Additional Reading: Cholelithiasis. In: Domino F, ed. *The 5-Minute Clinical Consult*. Philadelphia, PA: Lippincott Williams and Wilkins; 2014.

Category: Gastroenterology system

Prophylactic cholecystectomy for asymptomatic cholelithiasis is generally not recommended.

59. What is the annual risk of major hemorrhage when treating a DVT?
A) 2%
B) 25%
C) 50%
D) 75%
E) 98%

Answer and Discussion

The answer is A. Risk factors for increased bleeding with warfarin include increased age, female sex, diabetes mellitus, presence of malignancy, hypertension >180/100, acute or chronic alcoholism, liver disease, severe chronic kidney disease, anemia, poor drug compliance or clinic attendance, prior stroke or intracerebral hemorrhage, presence of bleeding lesion, bleeding disorder, concomitant use of aspirin, NSAIDs, antiplatelet agents, antibiotics, amiodarone, statins, fibrates, instability of INR control, INR >3, pretreatment INR >1.2, and previous severe hemorrhage during treatment with warfarin with an INR in the therapeutic range. Typical bleeding rated reported in randomized trials are in the range of 1% to 3% per person per year.

Additional Reading: Antithrombotic therapy for VTE disease: antithrombotic therapy and prevention of thrombosis, 9th ed. American College of Chest Physician Evidence-Based Clinical Practice Guidelines. *Chest*. 2012;141(suppl 2):e419S.

Category: Cardiovascular system

60. Which of the following statements about an abnormal breast lesion is true?
A) Cystic lesions are usually benign.
B) A risk factor for breast cancer is early menopause.
C) Mammograms can be used to determine whether the lesion is cystic or solid.
D) Baseline mammogram screening should begin at 35 years of age.
E) Mammograms have less than a 5% false-negative rate.

Answer and Discussion

The answer is A. The development of a breast mass requires a thorough evaluation to rule out a possible malignancy. Risk factors for breast cancer include increased age, early menarche, late menopause, *BRCA* gene mutation, being nulliparous, having a first-degree relative with breast cancer, or having cancer in the contralateral breast. A palpable mass can be evaluated with fine-needle or excisional biopsy. It is important to remember that mammograms have a 10% to 15% false-negative rate; therefore, a palpable solid mass should, in most cases, be biopsied despite a negative mammogram. In addition, a solid lesion is more worrisome for malignancy than a cystic lesion, and ultrasound may be used to differentiate between the two. If the mass is cystic, it can be watched closely with serial ultrasounds or aspirated. The screening guidelines for the diagnosis of breast cancer are continually changing. The USPSTF and the American College of Physicians recommend beginning routine screening at age 50; however, many other organizations recommend starting at age 40. These include the American Cancer Society, American College of Radiology, American Medical Association, the National Cancer Institute, the American College of Obstetricians and Gynecologist, and the National Comprehensive Cancer Network.

Additional Reading: Screening for breast cancer, 2009. *US preventive service task force*. From: http://www.uspreventiveservicestaskforce.org/uspstf09/breastcancer/brcanrs.htm#recommendations.

Category: Integumentary

61. A 71-year-old hospitalized patient who previously underwent bowel resection and is now receiving TPN is noted to have a mild elevation in his liver function test. The most appropriate action is
A) Observation
B) Ultrasound examination of the liver, pancreas, and gallbladder
C) Exploratory laparoscopy
D) Discontinuation of parenteral nutrition
E) Liver biopsy

Answer and Discussion

The answer is A. TPN is the intravenous administration of a patient's daily nutritional requirements. Generally, the concentrated solution is given through central vein access. Patients who may be candidates for

TPN include burn victims, malnourished patients in the perioperative period, or patients who have severe trauma or are in a comatose state. Formulations include daily nutritional requirements, including vitamin supplementation. Patients should be monitored closely with laboratory tests, daily weights, and accurate intakes and outputs. Complications involve metabolic, nutritional deficiencies and administration complications (e.g., infection of intravenous sites) and refeeding syndrome. Laboratory abnormalities may include elevated liver function tests, hepatosplenomegaly, thrombocytopenia, or hyperlipidemia. Hepatic dysfunction is a common manifestation of long-term TPN support. Steatosis is associated with mild elevations of the transaminases, alkaline phosphate, and bilirubin. Cirrhosis is the end result. Cholecystitis, particularly the acalculus type, may occur in patient who receive TPN for extended periods.

> **Additional Reading:** Nutrition support in critically ill patients: parenteral nutrition. In: Basow DS, ed. *UpToDate*. Waltham, MA: UpToDate; 2013.

Category: Nonspecific system

62. Which of the following statements is true regarding vasectomies?
A) Early failure rate is approximately 1 in 300.
B) Development of sperm antibodies occurs in <1%.
C) Sperm antibodies are related to the future development of coronary artery disease.
D) The incidence of testicular cancer increases after vasectomy.
E) Patients may resume unprotected intercourse after one sperm-free semen analysis.

Answer and Discussion

The answer is A. Vasectomies are performed to provide sterilization for men. Complications include bleeding, hematoma, infection, sperm granuloma (15% to 40%), and postvasectomy pain syndrome. The patient should have at least 20 ejaculates since the time of vasectomy. If motile sperm are confirmed on two samples 1 month apart, it is likely the vasectomy has failed. The patient should be advice to have a second procedure and use alternative contraception. As many as 60% to 80% of patients develop sperm antibodies after vasectomy. There is no association between antisperm antibodies and other immune-mediated diseases, such as lupus erythematous, scleroderma, or rheumatoid arthritis. There is a twofold increase of risk association between vasectomy and kidney stones in men younger than age 46 (RR 1.9, 95% CI 1.2–3.1). Studies have found no increased risk of cardiovascular disease, prostate cancer, or testicular cancer with vasectomy. Vasectomy failure can be due to technical errors, recanalization, or unprotected intercourse before azoospermia is documented. Vasectomy failure range from 0.02% to 29.7%. Intraluminal needle cautery <1%, cautery both ends and fascial interruption <1.2%, cautery only and fascial interruption 0.02% to 2.4%, cautery of both ends and excision of a segment 4.8% or less. Ligation and excision of segment 1.5% to 29%.

> **Additional Reading:** Vasectomy: an update. *Am Fam Physician.* 2006;74(12):2069–2074.

Category: Reproductive system

63. Which of the following deters healing of anal fissures?
A) Sitz baths
B) Internal sphincter spasms
C) Poor blood supply to the dentate line
D) External hemorrhoids
E) Rectal rugae

Answer and Discussion

The answer is B. Fissures of the anal canal are usually due to traumatic lacerations as a result of chronic constipation with perhaps an underlying infection of the lesion. Other associated conditions include chronic proctitis, rectal carcinoma, hemorrhoids, or previous rectal surgery. The lesion is often associated with the internal sphincter and can cause spasms that can deter healing. Symptoms include a sudden onset, feeling of passing "shards of glass" occurring during bowel movement, with small amount of bright red blood in stool. Physical examination usually shows evidence of a linear fissure located in the midline. Treatment involves the use of stool softeners, fiber supplements, sitz baths, and hydrocortisone- or benzocaine-containing cream, which may aid in decreasing any associated pain or inflammation and promote healing. Other options include topical nitroglycerine 0.2% ointment on a botulinum toxin A (Botox), topical calcium channel blocker, and topical bethanecol. Surgery is reserved for cases that fail to respond to medical therapy.

> **Additional Reading:** Evaluation and management of common anorectal conditions. *Am Fam Physician.* 2012;85(6):624–630.

Category: Gastroenterology system

64. A 16-year-old gymnast suffers a fall onto an outstretched hand. On exam, she appears to have an unstable distal radioulnar joint. Which of the following injuries is most likely?
A) Greenstick fracture of the radius
B) de Quervain's tenosynovitis
C) Colles' fracture
D) Injury to the triangular fibrocartilage complex (TFCC)
E) Scaphoid fracture

Answer and Discussion

The answer is D. Ulnar wrist pain and weakness caused by a fall onto an outstretched hand may suggest injury to the triangular fibrocartilage complex, which is the primary stabilizer of the distal radioulnar joint. Triangular fibrocartilage complex injury is common in gymnasts and in racquetball, tennis, and hockey players.

The greenstick fracture is an incomplete fracture that occurs most often during infancy and childhood when bones are soft and tends to take place in the middle, slower growing parts of bone. A Colles fracture is one of the most common distal radius fractures in which the broken fragment of the radius tilts upward. A scaphoid fracture frequently occur following a fall onto an outstretched hand; however, symptoms include pain over the anatomic "snuff box" (area between the extensor pollicis brevis and the extensor pollicis longus tendons) and pain with radial deviation of the wrist.

The combination of wrist pain and grip weakness is characteristic of de Quervain's tenosynovitis. Local tenderness is present over the distal portion of the radial styloid, and the pain is generally reproduced with direct palpation of the involved tendons. Pain is aggravated by passively stretching the thumb tendons over the radial styloid in thumb flexion (the Finkelstein maneuver).

> **Additional Reading:** Busconi BD, Stevenson JH. Approach to the patient with triangular fibrocartilage complex tears. *Sports Medicine Consult: A Problem-Based Approach to Sports Medicine for the Primary Care Physician.* Philadelphia, PA: Lippincott, Williams & Wilkins; 2009.

Category: Musculoskeletal system

65. Which of the following blood types is considered the universal donor?
A) AB positive
B) O positive
C) AB negative
D) O negative
E) B negative

Answer and Discussion

The answer is D. In trauma settings, the use of intravenous fluid is important to maintain adequate perfusion to vital tissues and organs. The use of blood for fluid replacement requires typing and proper storing, making it impractical to use in emergent settings in which time is extremely valuable. Because of this, a trauma patient should receive two large-bore (16-gauge or larger) intravenous lines and normal saline or lactated Ringer's solution until proper blood can be given in a controlled setting. For adults, 1,000 mL of crystalloid solution should be given as an initial bolus—children should receive 20 mL/kg. In some emergent situations, O-negative blood, the universal donor blood, can be given until appropriately typed blood arrives.

Additional Reading: Initial evaluation and management of shock in adult trauma. In: Basow DS, ed. *UpToDate*. Waltham, MA: UpToDate; 2013.

Category: Nonspecific system

> In some emergent situations, O-negative blood (the universal donor blood) can be given until appropriately typed blood arrives.

66. A 3-year-old is brought into the emergency room by her parents. The child has had a high fever, sore throat, and now has stridor. The child is sitting on a stretcher leaning forward with her neck extended. The most likely diagnosis is
A) Strep throat
B) Herpangina
C) Meningitis
D) Epiglottitis
E) Herpes stomatitis

Answer and Discussion

The answer is D. Epiglottitis is a rapidly progressive and potentially fatal infection that causes swelling of the epiglottis and may lead to compromise of the child's airway. In the past, it was most commonly caused by *H. influenzae*. The highest incidence occurs in children between 2 and 5 years of age. In recent years, the occurrence of epiglottitis has been reduced dramatically by the widespread use of the Hib vaccine. Symptoms include a sore throat, high fever, hoarseness, and dysphagia with drooling and stridor. Children affected usually lean forward and hyperextend the neck to open the compromised airway. Bacteremia is common. Because of the rapid course of the infection, the child should be immediately hospitalized and the airway secured. Inspection of the pharynx can precipitate a complete obstruction of the airway and should not be performed unless there are qualified personnel present who can simultaneously intubate the child during the inspection procedure if necessary. Lateral and anteroposterior soft tissue radiographs should be taken and can confirm the diagnosis. The characteristic "thumb sign" is noted on the lateral radiograph. In addition to securing an airway, parenteral antibiotics should be administered and the child monitored closely in an intensive care setting.

Additional Reading: Acute inflammatory upper airway obstruction (croup, epiglottitis, laryngitis, and bacterial tracheitis). *Nelson Textbook of Pediatrics,* 19th ed. Philadelphia, PA: Elsevier/Saunders; 2011.

Category: Respiratory system

67. When treating anaphylaxis, which of the following, in addition to intravenous fluid, is considered the mainstay of treatment?
A) Diphenhydramine
B) Prednisone
C) Propanolol
D) Epinephrine
E) Naproxen

Answer and Discussion

The answer is D. Anaphylaxis is a life-threatening reaction with respiratory, cardiovascular, cutaneous, GI, and neurological manifestations that results from an exposure to an allergen, and response is usually immunoglobulin E-mediated, which leads to mast cell and basophil activation. Dermatologic and respiratory symptoms are most common, occurring in 90% and 70% of episodes, respectively. The risk of anaphylaxis is doubled in patients with mild asthma and tripled in those with severe disease. The most common triggers are food (egg, fish, food additives, milk, peanuts, sesame, shellfish, tree nuts), latex, insect stings (bee, wasp, fire ants, hymenoptera), medications (allopurinol, angiotensin-converting enzyme inhibitors, beta-lactams, aspirin, biological modifiers, nonsteroidal inflammatory drugs, opioids), radiocontrast media, and animal dander. The diagnosis of anaphylaxis is typically made when symptoms occur within 1 hour of exposure to a specific antigen. Confirmatory testing using serum histamine and tryptase levels is difficult because blood samples must be drawn with strict time consideration. Allergen skin testing and in vitro assay for serum immunoglobulin E or specific allergens do not reliably predict who will develop anaphylaxis. Administration of intramuscular epinephrine (1:1,000 dilution dosed at 0.01 mg per kg [maximal dose of 0.3 mg in children and 0.5 mg in adults], along with appropriate management of airway, breathing, and circulation, is the first and most important therapeutic option to epinephrine. Histamine H1 receptors antagonist and corticosteroids may be useful adjuncts.

Additional Reading: Anaphylaxis: recognition and management. *Am Fam Physician*. 2011;84(10):111–118.

Category: Nonspecific system

68. The first step in the management of a lower GI hemorrhage is to
A) Obtain a CT scan of the abdomen
B) Perform a bleeding scan
C) Resuscitate the unstable patient
D) Perform a colonoscopy
E) Obtain a surgical consult

Answer and Discussion

The answer is C. The incidence of massive lower GI bleeding is 20% to 27% episodes per 100,000 persons annually, with a mortality rate of 4% to 10%. The clinical evaluation of GI bleeding depends on the hemodynamic status of the patient and the suspected source of the bleeding. Patients presenting with upper GI or massive lower GI bleeding, postural hypotension, or hemodynamic instability require inpatient stabilization and evaluation. The immediate response to significant bleeding is to resuscitate the patient if they are unstable. Hospitalization is also required in patients who are hemodynamically unstable or elderly and those who have comorbidities. GI bleeding suspected from a lower source may be secondary to diverticular disease, angiodysplasia, ulcerative colitis, ischemic colitis, neoplasm, colorectal polyps, proctitis, a/v malformations, anal and rectal neoplasia, and hemorrhoids. Acute massive rectal bleeding frequently arises form an upper GI source. Colonoscopy identifies definitive bleeding in more than 70% of patients. A technetium-99-tagged RBC scans may be helpful in identifying the site of bleeding if the volume is >0.1 to 0.4 mL/min. However, positive findings in this type of testing must be verified with an alternative test because of a relatively high number of false-positive results. Angiography may be useful in patients with active bleeding >0.5 mL/min and can identify highly vascular nonbleeding lesions such as angiodysplasia and neoplasms.

Additional Reading: Approach to acute lower gastrointestinal bleeding in adults. In: Basow DS, ed. *UpToDate*. Waltham, MA: UpToDate; 2013.

Category: Gastroenterology system

69. The primary indication for joint replacement surgery in patients with osteoarthritis is
A) Intractable pain
B) Joint laxity
C) Limited range of motion
D) Recurrent subluxation

Answer and Discussion

The answer is A. Knee osteoarthritis is a common disabling condition that affects 33.6% of persons older than 65 years. Osteoarthritis is a degenerative disease characterize by erosion of the articular cartilage, hyperthrophy of bone at the margins (osteophytes), and subcondral sclerosis. Twenty-five percent cannot perform major activities of daily living. Exercise, weight loss, physical therapy, intra-articular corticosteroid injections, and the use of NSAIDs and braces or heel wedges decrease pain and improve function.

Total joint arthroplasty of the knee should be considered when conservative symptomatic management is ineffective. According to the American Academy of Orthopedic Surgeons, the main indication for total knee arthroplasty is relief of pain, which is almost always relieved by the surgery. Joint replacement may also be appropriate for patients with significant limitations of joint function or with altered limb alignment. Range of motion, joint laxity, and recurrent subluxations relate to musculotendinous function and are not reliably improved by joint replacement. Arthroscopic surgery is not an appropriate treatment for knee osteoarthritis unless there is evidence of loose bodies or mechanical symptoms such as locking, giving way, or catching. The life expectancy of the replaced joint varies, but is usually between 15 and 20 years.

Additional Reading: Treatment of knee osteoarthritis. *Am Fam Physician*. 2011;83(11):1287–1292.

Category: Musculoskeletal system

70. Which of the following is *false* regarding latex allergies?
A) Approximately 10% of health care workers experience some form of allergic reaction to latex.
B) Latex is not found in catheters.
C) Persons allergic to latex also may be sensitive to fruits such as bananas, kiwis, pears, pineapples, grapes, and papayas.
D) Latex allergies became an important problem with the institution of universal precautions.
E) Many consumer products contain latex.

Answer and Discussion

The answer is B. Latex allergy has become a significant problem since the widespread adoption of universal precautions against infection. The incidence is 1% to 2% in the general population. As many as 17% of health care workers experience some form of allergic reaction to latex, although not all are anaphylaxis. Recognizing latex

allergy is crucial because physicians may inadvertently expose the patient to more latex during treatment. Latex is in gloves, catheters, and numerous other medical supplies (bandages, blood pressure cuffs, condoms, dental dams, diaphragms, tourniques, stethoscope tubing, pacifiers, gutta-percha and gutta-balata [to seal root canals]), as well as consumer products. Persons allergic to latex also may be sensitive to fruits such as bananas, kiwis, pears, pineapples, grapes, and papayas. Reactions to latex allergy can range from type IV delayed hypersensitivity (contact dermatitis) to type I immediate hypersensitivity (urticaria, bronchospasm, anaphylaxis). Main risk factors for latex allergy are occupational exposure and an atopic tendency. Occupations in which latex allergy are commonly used include health care workers, food handlers/restaurant workers, domestic workers, hairdressers, security personnel, construction workers, greenhouse workers, gardeners, painters, funeral home workers, and first-responders such as police officers, firefighters, and ambulance attendants. The most reliable indicator of allergy is a strong clinical history, associating exposure with the symptoms. Skin testing with extracts prepared from latex C-serum is a safe and effective diagnostic procedure when extracts are standardized in terms of their allergen content and stability.

Additional Reading: Latex allergy. *Am Fam Physician*. 2009; 80(12);1413–1418.

Category: Nonspecific system

71. Major risk factors for colon cancer include all of the following *except*
A) History of breast cancer
B) Asian descent
C) Inflammatory bowel disease
D) Peutz–Jeghers syndrome
E) Prior villous polyps

Answer and Discussion

The answer is B. CRC is the leading cause of death due to cancer in the United States. The major factors that increase the risk of colon cancer include

1. Age: More than 90% of people diagnosed with CRC are older than 50 years.
2. Having a personal history of colorectal polyps (risk increases with multiple polyps, villous polyps, and larger polyps).
3. Having a personal history of cancer: Rectal cancer has a higher incidence of local recurrence than proximal cancer (20% to 30% vs. 2% to 4%).
4. A history of inflammatory bowel disease: Those with ulcerative colitis and Crohn's disease have a prevalence of ~3%, with a cumulative risk of CRC of 2% at 10 years, 8% at 20 years, and 18% at 30 years.
5. A family history of CRC is present in 10% of adults and about 25% of cases. Individuals with one or more first-degree or two or more second-degree relatives with CRC are at higher lifetime risk of developing CRC, which ranges from two- to sixfold.
6. Certain genetic syndromes:
   - Individuals with Lynch syndrome (hereditary nonpolyposis colorectal cancer [HNPCC]) have a 2% to 3% risk of developing CRC. They are also at an increased risk for endometrial, stomach, ovarian, pancreas, ureter and kidney, biliary tract, and brain cancers. This syndrome should be considered in people with more than one family member with CRC or other Lynch syndrome–related cancers of small bowel, ovary, or endometrium which has occurred at a young age (30s and 40s).

- Familial adenomatous polyposis (FAPP): Tumors beginning in the 20s, and nearly all will develop CRC (usually before age 50).
- Individuals with Peutz–Jeghers syndrome (often have freckles [mouth, hands, feet] and large polyps in GI tract) are at an increased risk of CRC.

7. A personal history of childhood cancer requiring abdominal radiation therapy.
8. Race and ethnicity issues:
   - African Americans have highest CRC incidence and mortality rates in the United States.
   - Several different gene mutations have been identified among Ashkenazi Jews.

Additional Reading: Colorectal cancer. In: Domino F, ed. *The 5-Minute Clinical Consult.* Philadelphia, PA: Lippincott Williams and Wilkins; 2014.

Category: Gastroenterology system

72. A 56-year-old man presents to your office. He reports persistent, severe chest pain after repeated bouts of vomiting over the past 24 hours. The most appropriate management involves
A) Chest X-ray
B) Administration of H$_2$ antagonists
C) Treadmill exercise testing
D) Administration of proton pump inhibitor
E) Observation with antiemetics

Answer and Discussion

The answer is A. Effort rupture of the esophagus is a spontaneous perforation of the esophagus that most commonly results from a sudden increase in intraesophageal pressure combined with negative intrathoracic pressure by straining or vomiting. Esophageal rupture, also known as *Boerhaave's syndrome*, is a rare, life-threatening condition that can lead to mediastinitis and pleural effusions. A delay in the diagnosis can lead to a poor prognosis. Symptoms include midsternal chest pain after a severe episode of vomiting. Associated conditions include peptic ulcer disease, alcoholism, and other neurologic disorders. The differential diagnosis includes myocardial infarction, pulmonary embolism, pancreatitis, peptic ulcer disease with rupture, or a dissecting aortic aneurysm. Chest radiographs and CT scans of the chest usually show pneumomediastinum, and a barium swallow showing communication between the esophagus and pleural space can be used to confirm the diagnosis. Treatment involves immediate surgery and drainage of any associated fluid collection.

Additional Reading: Boerhaave's syndrome: effort rupture of the esophagus. In: Basow DS, ed. *UpToDate.* Waltham, MA: UpToDate; 2013.

Category: Gastroenterology system

73. Facial sutures should be removed at
A) 24 hours
B) 3 to 5 days
C) 7 to 10 days
D) 14 days
E) Only absorbable sutures should be used on the face.

Answer and Discussion

The answer is B. Postoperative care for lacerations does not include routine use of prophylactic antibiotics unless there is evidence of bacterial contamination or a risk factor is evident. Sutured or stapled lacerations should be covered with a protective, nonadherent dressing for at least 24 to 48 hours to avoid contamination. Patients should be instructed to observe the wound for the presence of warmth, redness, swelling, or drainage. Sutures or staples should be removed after approximately 7 days. Facial sutures should be removed within 3 to 5 days. Sutures in areas subject to high tension should be left in place for 10 to 14 days.

Additional Reading: Essentials of skin laceration repair. *Am Fam Physician.* 2008;78(8):945–951.

Category: Nonspecific system

74. The most appropriate treatment for cholesteatoma is
A) Oral antibiotics
B) Antibiotic otic drops
C) Oral steroids
D) Tympanostomy tube placement
E) Surgical removal

Answer and Discussion

The answer is E. Cholesteatoma refers to a keratinized, desquamated epithelial collection in the middle ear or mastoid. A cholesteatoma results from a chronic otitis media and perforation of the tympanic membrane or as a primary lesion. Prolonged dysfunction of the eustachian tube with the development of chronic negative pressure results in the formation of a squamous epithelial lined sac, which remains chronically infected. Cholesteatomas may be recognized during otoscopic examination by the white debris in the middle ear and the destruction of the ear canal bone adjacent to the perforation. Bone destruction due to an otherwise unsuspected cholesteatoma may be demonstrated on a CT scan. Aural polyps are usually associated with cholesteatomas. A cholesteatoma, particularly with an attic perforation, greatly increases the probability of a serious complication (e.g., purulent labyrinthitis, facial paralysis, intracranial suppuration). A cholesteatoma typically erodes the temporal bone and may destroy the small ossicle bones. With time, they can erode into the facial nerve or into the brain. Treatment involves surgical removal.

Additional Reading: Diagnosis of ear pain. *Am Fam Physician.* 2008;77(5):621–628.

Category: Special sensory

A cholesteatoma typically erodes the temporal bone and may destroy the small ossicle bones.

75. A 27-year-old woman presents to the emergency room complaining of periumbilical pain, anorexia, and vomiting. Physical findings show a fever of 101.5°F, rebound tenderness, and extreme pain with rectal examination. The patient is also found to have positive psoas and obturator signs. The most likely diagnosis is
A) Bowel infarction
B) Acute appendicitis
C) Acute cholecystitis
D) Torsion of the ovary
E) Ectopic pregnancy

Answer and Discussion

The answer is B. Appendicitis is the most common acute surgical condition of the abdomen. Approximately 7% of the population will have appendicitis in their lifetime, with the peak incidence occurring between the ages of 10 and 30 years. Despite technologic advances, the diagnosis of appendicitis is still based primarily on the patient's history and the physical examination. Prompt diagnosis and surgical referral may reduce the risk of perforation and prevent complications. The mortality rate in nonperforated appendicitis is less than 1%, but it may be as high as 5% or more in young and elderly patients in whom diagnosis may often be delayed, thus making perforation more likely. Appendicitis occurs when there is an obstruction in the appendiceal lumen. Although the symptoms are not always consistent, the typical presentation involves dull periumbilical pain that migrates to the right lower abdomen. Anorexia, nausea, and vomiting usually accompany the onset of the abdominal pain. It is more common in adolescents; diagnosis in infants, the elderly, and obese and pregnant patients is often more difficult. Physical findings often include a low-grade fever, right lower quadrant pain, rebound tenderness, and spasms of the overlying abdominal muscles with guarding. A positive psoas sign (i.e., pain with passive extension of the right hip) and obturator sign (i.e., pain with internal and external rotation of the flexed right hip) are strongly supportive of the diagnosis. Rectal examination may reveal localized tenderness. Laboratory results usually show a moderate leukocytosis (10,000 to 20,000 WBCs/mm^3) with a left shift; however, this finding neither confirms nor excludes the diagnosis. Hematuria, proteinuria, and pyuria may be present. Visualization of the appendiceal lumen with a barium enema rules out the diagnosis.

Standard abdominal CT scanning shows enlarged appendiceal diameter >6 mm with an occluded lumen, appendiceal wall thickening >2 mm, periappendiceal fat stranding, appendiceal wall enhancement, and appendicolith. The sensitivity and specificity of CT with intravenous (IV) and oral contrast for acute appendicitis is in the range of 91% to 98% and 75% to 93%, respectively.

Appendiceal CT consists of a focused, helical, appendiceal CT after a gastrografin saline enema (with or without oral contrast) and can be performed and interpreted within 1 hour. Positive findings include right lower abdominal quadrant fat stranding (100% sensitivity), focal cecal thickening (69% specificity), and adenopathy (63% sensitivity). Appendiceal CT had 98% accuracy and sensitivity with rectal contrast along a limited area (15 mm).

Unenhanced CT had a sensitivity of 88% to 96%, specificity of 91% to 98%, and diagnostic accuracy of 94% to 97% for appendicitis. Ultrasound in the diagnosis of appendicitis ranges from 25% to 98%, respectively.

Additional Reading: Appendicitis acute. In: Domino F, ed. *The 5-Minute Clinical Consult*. Philadelphia, PA: Lippincott Williams and Wilkins; 2014.

Category: Gastroenterology system

76. Application of tissue adhesives is useful in repairing lacerations. Which of the following statements regarding adhesives is not true?
A) They are resistant to bacterial growth.
B) They have lower tensile strength when compared with sutures.
C) They are not useful on the hand.
D) Exposure to water has little effect on adhesives.
E) Adhesives are not recommended over high-tension areas.

Answer and Discussion

The answer is D. Tissue adhesives are used to close lacerations and have some advantages and disadvantages when compared with traditional suturing. Adhesives are resistant to bacterial growth and they have lower tensile strength when compared with sutures. They are not useful on the hand, and exposure to water is contraindicated. Adhesives are not recommended over high-tension areas.

Additional Reading: Essentials of skin laceration repair. *Am Fam Physician*. 2008;78(8):945–951.

Category: Nonspecific system

77. Diagnosis of corneal abrasions can best be accomplished in a family physician's office with
A) Fluorescein dye examination
B) Slit-lamp examination
C) Handheld ophthalmoscope
D) Visual field testing
E) Schiøtz's tonometer

Answer and Discussion

The answer is A. Eye injuries are frequently encountered in the family physician's office. The following are some of the most common:

- *Corneal abrasions.* Corneal abrasions occur when there is localized loss of epithelium from the cornea typically caused by trauma. Symptoms include pain, foreign body sensation, tearing, and injection and history of trauma. A fluorescein dye examination is used to diagnose corneal abrasions. The goals of treatment include pain control, prevention of infection, and healing. Physicians should carefully examine for foreign bodies and remove them. Pain relief may be achieved with topical NSAIDs or oral analgesics. Evidence does not support the use of topical cycloplegics for uncomplicated corneal abrasions. Patching is not recommended because it does not reduce pain and has the potential to delay healing. Although evidence are lacking, topical antibiotics are commonly prescribed to prevent bacterial superinfection. Contact lens–related abrasions should be treated with antipseudomona topical antibiotics. After fluorescein dye, a Wood's light is then used to examine all four quadrants of the globe. If an abrasion is detected, antibiotic drops are applied and the eye is covered for 24 hours. The patient should be reexamined in 24 hours. Visual acuity should be tested at the time of presentation and again the day after. Antibiotic drops are usually continued for an additional 5 days. Follow-up may not be necessary for a patient with small (4 mm or less), uncomplicated abrasions; normal vision; and resolving symptoms. Referral is indicated for any patient with symptoms that do not improve or that worsen, a corneal infiltrate or ulcer, significant vision loss, or a penetrating eye injury.

- *Foreign bodies.* Inspection of the entire cornea is necessary to identify foreign bodies. The upper and lower eyelid should also be inspected. Foreign bodies should be removed by flushing with normal saline, cotton swab, eye spud, or 25-gauge needle. Fluorescein dye examination should be performed to rule out an abrasion. Rust rings should be examined for and removed as much as possible by an ophthalmologist; however, complete removal is unnecessary.

- *Blunt trauma.* Blunt trauma can cause orbital wall fractures. Signs and symptoms include diplopia, epistaxis, ecchymosis, crepitus, hypesthesia in the infraorbital nerve distribution, and restricted upward gaze secondary to inferior rectus entrapment. CT of the orbits is necessary for diagnosis. Surgical referral is indicated.

- *Subconjunctival hemorrhage.* This condition is present when there is a well-demarcated area of injection from the rupture of small subconjunctival vessels. Causes include trauma, coughing, vomiting, straining, or viral hemorrhagic conjunctivitis. Blood in the anterior chamber indicates a hyphema and requires immediate ophthalmologic referral. Referral is indicated for any patient with symptoms that do not improve or that worsen, a corneal infiltrate or ulcer, significant vision loss, or a penetrating eye injury.

Additional Reading: Evaluation and management of corneal abrasions. *Am Fam Physician.* 2013;87(2):114–120.

Category: Special sensory

78. Which of the following statements about epistaxis is true?
A) Unless there are previous symptoms of infection, the use of antibiotics while nasal packs are in place is unwarranted.
B) Nasal packs should be left in place for at least 72 hours.
C) In most cases, anterior bleeding originates from Kiesselbach's area.
D) The use of silver nitrate or electric cautery is contraindicated in the nose.
E) Patients with chronic obstructive pulmonary disease are not affected by nasal packing because the majority are mouth breathers.

Answer and Discussion

The answer is C. Epistaxis has been reported to occur in up to 60% of the general population. Nosebleeds can be caused by a number of different mechanisms including trauma, nose picking, infection, foreign bodies, excessive drying of the nasal mucosa, and bleeding disorders. Most bleeding originates from a plexus of vessels in the anteroinferior septum called *Kiesselbach's plexus.* In most cases, pinching the nasal ala together for 10 to 15 minutes stops the bleeding. If nasal bleeding continues, local and/or systemic source should be identified. Treatment to be considered include topical vasoconstriction, chemical cautery, electrocautery, nasal packing (nasal tampon or gauze impregnated with petroleum jelly), posterior gauze packing, use of a balloon system (including a modified Foley catheter), and arterial ligation or embolization. Common local causes of epistaxis include chronic sinusitis, epistaxis digitorum, foreign bodies, intranasal neoplasm or polyps, irritants, medications (topical steroids), rhinitis, septal deviation, septal perforation, trauma, vascular malformation, or telangiectasia. Systemic causes include hemophilia, hypertension, leukemia, liver disease, medications (aspirin, anticoagulants, NSAIDs), platelets dysfunction, and thrombocytopenia. Once the source is located, nasal packing or cauterization with silver nitrate or electric cautery may be necessary. If the nose is packed, antibiotics such as trimethoprim-sulfamethoxazole should be started while the packing is in place. Packs should not be left in place for more than 48 hours. If bleeding continues, a posterior source is most likely the cause, and a posterior pack should be placed by an otolaryngologist. Hospitalization for observation is indicated with serial blood counts in posterior bleeds. For severe nosebleeds, a bleeding time and von Willebrand's factor should be checked to rule out bleeding disorders.

Referral to an otolaryngologist is appropriate when bleeding is refractory, complications are present, or specialized treatment (balloon placement, arterial ligation, angiographic arterial embolization) is required.

Additional Reading: Epistaxis. In: Domino F, ed. *The 5-Minute Clinical Consult.* Philadelphia, PA: Lippincott Williams and Wilkins; 2014.

Category: Special sensory

79. A 60-year-old man presents with pain in the upper legs that is exacerbated with walking. Symptoms are relieved with sitting. Peripheral pulses are intact. The most likely diagnosis is
A) Spinal stenosis
B) Claudication
C) Dissecting aortic aneurysm
D) Incarcerated inguinal hernia
E) Myasthenia gravis

Answer and Discussion

The answer is A. Spinal stenosis is a condition characterized by narrowing of the spinal canal and foramen. Pain in the legs, calves, thighs, and buttocks occurs with walking, running, or climbing stairs. Symptoms are often relieved by flexing at the spine or sitting. Conversely, lying prone or in any position that extends the lumbar spine exacerbates the symptoms, presumably because of ventral infolding of the ligamentum flavum in a canal already significantly narrowed by degenerative osseus changes. Middle-age patients and the elderly are most commonly affected. Typically, the earliest complaint is back pain, which is relatively nonspecific and may result in delayed diagnosis. Patients then often experience leg fatigue, pain, numbness, and weakness, sometimes several months to years after the back pain was first noticed. Patients may undergo minor trauma that can exacerbate symptoms, which may lead to a more rapid diagnosis. Once the leg pain begins, it is most commonly bilateral, involving the buttocks and thighs and spreading distally toward the feet, typically with the onset and progression of leg exercise. In some patients, the pain, paresthesias, and/or weakness are limited to the lower legs and feet, remaining present until movement ceases. The lower extremity symptoms are almost always described as burning, cramping, numbness, tingling, or dull fatigue in the thighs and legs. Disease onset is usually insidious; early symptoms may be mild and progress to become extremely disabling. Symptom severity does not always correlate with the degree of lumbar canal narrowing. Causes include osteoarthritis, spondylosis, spondylolisthesis with associated edema in the area of the cauda equina, and Paget's disease affecting the lower spine. Spinal stenosis may be difficult to distinguish from claudication; however, with spinal stenosis, there are usually neurologic deficits present and peripheral pulses are normal. MRI scanning, with its multiplanar-imaging capability, is currently the preferred modality for establishing a diagnosis and excluding other conditions. The MRI depicts soft tissues, including the cauda equina, spinal cord, ligaments, epidural fat, subarachnoid space, and intervertebral discs, with exquisite detail in most instances. Loss of epidural fat on T_1-weighted images, loss of cerebrospinal fluid signal around the dural sac on T_2-weighted images, and degenerative disc disease are common features of lumbar stenosis on MRI. Treatment for symptomatic lumbar stenosis is usually surgical decompression. Medical treatment alternatives such as bed rest, pain management, and physical therapy should be reserved for use in debilitated patients or patients whose surgical risk is prohibitive as a result of concomitant medical conditions.

Additional Reading: Spinal stenosis. In: Domino F, ed. *The 5-Minute Clinical Consult.* Philadelphia, PA: Lippincott Williams and Wilkins; 2014.

Category: Neurologic

80. A 31-year-old man is brought to the emergency room after suffering severe injuries in a motorcycle accident. A dipstick urinalysis shows hemoglobin. However, microscopic examination fails to show RBCs. The most likely diagnosis is
A) Renal trauma
B) Urethral rupture
C) Laboratory error
D) Myoglobinuria
E) Underlying urinary tract infection

Answer and Discussion

The answer is D. Myoglobinuria is a condition that results when there is massive muscle destruction known as *rhabdomyolysis.* The condition occurs as a result of severe infection, toxic insult, inflammation, or metabolic or traumatic damage to the muscles. Laboratory findings include elevated creatinine kinase, lactate dehydrogenase, AST, alanine aminotransferase, and a positive urine test for blood with the absence of RBCs. Specific tests for the detection of myoglobinuria are done with immunoassay. Treatment involves correcting the underlying causative factor and administering fluids. Renal failure may require further treatment.

Additional Reading: Clinical manifestations and diagnosis of rhabdomyolysis. In: Basow DS, ed. *UpToDate*. Waltham, MA: UpToDate; 2013.

Category: Nephrologic system

81. Duodenal obstruction is associated with which of the following radiographic signs?
A) Bird's beak sign
B) Hampton's hump
C) Double bubble sign
D) Kerley B lines
E) Scalloping of the diaphragm

Answer and Discussion
The answer is C. Duodenal obstruction is a congenital abnormality that can be caused by several different abnormalities, including duodenal atresia, duodenal stenosis, and malrotation of the intestine. In neonates, malrotation can also present as duodenal obstruction. The obstruction may be caused by Ladd bands or associated duodenal atresia. Infants with Down syndrome are at increased risk. Symptoms include projectile vomiting after the first few feedings. Polyhydramnios may also be present during pregnancy and is caused by a failure of absorption of amniotic fluid in the distal intestine. Diagnosis is usually made radiographically. Plain radiographs show the characteristic "double bubble" sign—one large bubble in the stomach with a smaller adjacent bubble that represents the duodenum. Upper GI contrast series is the best examination to visualize the duodenum. If atresia is present, no abdominal gas is seen in the distal bowel; however, if stenosis is present, a small amount of gas may be present. A barium swallow helps localize the site of obstruction. Treatment involves nasogastric suction to decompress the stomach and surgery to correct the obstruction.

Additional Reading: Approach to the infant or child with nausea and vomiting. In: Basow DS, ed. *UpToDate*. Waltham, MA: UpToDate; 2013.

Category: Gastroenterology system

Duodenal obstruction is associated with a "double bubble" radiographic sign.

82. When repairing a facial laceration, it is important to test all aspects of the facial nerve. Which of the following tasks tests the zygomatic branch?
A) Contract the forehead and elevate the eyebrow
B) Open and shut the eyes
C) Smile
D) Frown
E) Contract the platysma muscle

Answer and Discussion
The answer is B. When repairing a facial laceration, the facial nerve function should be tested in all five branches as follows:

- *Temporal:* Contract the forehead and elevate the eyebrow
- *Zygomatic:* Open and shut eyes

- *Buccal:* Smile
- *Mandibular:* Frown
- *Cervical:* Contract the platysma muscle

Additional Reading: Townsend CM Jr, Beauchamp RD, Evers BM, et al., eds. *Sabiston Textbook of Surgery*, 19th ed. Philadelphia, PA: Saunders/Elsevier; 2012.

Category: Special sensory

83. A man has longstanding gynecomastia and asks about having a breast reduction. He reports that his has been a problem for a dozen years and denies an associated galactorrhea. A careful drug history and physical examination, along with an endocrine and malignancy workup, are negative. Which one of the following is the treatment of choice?
A) Clomiphene (Clomid, Serophene)
B) Danazol
C) Tamoxifen (Soltamox)
D) Topical testosterone (AndroGel)
E) Surgery

Answer and Discussion
The answer is E. Surgery is indicated to treat longstanding gynecomastia as the initial glandular hyperplasia transforms into a progressive fibrotic state. Medical management is most useful when the onset is recent or to prevent the initial development of the problem. The listed drugs have been tried with varying success in this context, but their clinical usefulness is not established.

Additional Reading: Gynecomastia. *Am Fam Physician*. 2012;85(7):716–722.

Category: Integumentary

84. Which of the following foreign bodies should not be removed with irrigation from the ear?
A) A plastic bead
B) A small pebble
C) A BB gun pellet
D) A dried pea
E) A metal part from a matchbox car

Answer and Discussion
The answer is D. Most ear and nose foreign bodies can be removed in the office utilizing a variety of methods, which include use of forceps, water irrigation, and suction catheter. Small, inorganic objects can be removed from the external auditory canal by irrigation. The irrigation solution should be at body temperature, and the stream of water should be directed along the superior margin of the external ear canal and should deliver an adequate volume of water with brisk flow. This volume can be achieved using a 20 to 50 mL syringe attached to a flexible catheter or plastic tubing from a butterfly needle. This technique is contraindicated if the tympanic membrane is perforated or the foreign body is vegetable matter or an alkaline button battery. Organic matter swells as it absorbs water, leading to further obstruction. Irrigation of the button battery enhances leakage and potential for liquefaction necrosis.

Additional Reading: Foreign bodies in the ear, nose, and throat. *Am Fam Physician*. 2007;76(8):1185–1189.

Category: Special sensory

85. Regular breast self-examinations (BSE) to screen for breast cancer

A) Are performed by most American women
B) Reduce mortality due to breast cancer
C) Reduce all-cause mortality in women
D) Are recommended by the USPSTF
E) Increase the number of breast biopsies performed

Answer and Discussion

The answer is E. Performance of regular BSE (even by trained women) does not reduce breast cancer–specific mortality or all-cause mortality. The 2009 update to the USPSTF breast cancer screening recommendations recommended against teaching BSE. The rationale for this "D" recommendation is that there is moderate certainty that the harms outweigh the benefits. Trials have demonstrated that more additional imaging procedures and biopsies are done on women who performed BSE than for controls, with no gains in breast cancer detection or reduction in breast cancer–related mortality. Most women do not regularly perform BSE.

> **Additional Reading:** Breast cancer screening update. *Am Fam Physician.* 2013;87(4):274–278.

> Category: Integumentary

86. Which of the following is associated with a positive Tinel's sign?

A) Carpal tunnel syndrome
B) Scaphoid fracture
C) de Quervain's tenosynovitis
D) Raynaud's phenomenon
E) Gamekeeper's thumb

Answer and Discussion

The answer is A. Carpal tunnel syndrome occurs when there is an entrapment of the median nerve at the level of the wrist. Symptoms include pain, numbness, and paresthesia in the distribution of the median nerve, including the palmar surface of the first three fingers. Symptoms characteristically occur at night and may awaken the patient. Symptoms may also involve the forearm or shoulder. Women are more frequently affected than men, and the condition can involve one or both hands. Percussion of the median nerve at the area of the carpal tunnel (Tinel's sign), sustained flexion of the wrist (Phalen's sign), or extension of the wrist (reverse Phalen's sign) reproduces symptoms. Other clinical findings include weakness of the thumb and thenar atrophy. Carpal tunnel syndrome is associated with continuous repetitive flexion of the wrist, pregnancy (most cases resolve after delivery), acromegaly, rheumatoid arthritis, and myxedema. Nerve conduction tests are used to help make the diagnosis but are not always necessary. Treatment includes anti-inflammatory agents, wrist braces, and steroid injections; surgery is indicated in severe cases that are unresponsive to conservative therapy.

> **Additional Reading:** Carpal tunnel syndrome. In: Domino F, ed. *The 5-Minute Clinical Consult.* Philadelphia, PA: Lippincott Williams and Wilkins; 2014.

> Category: Musculoskeletal system

87. Which of the following is indicated immediately after a minor burn?

A) Application of butter
B) Rapid cooling with ice
C) Extensive debridement of nonviable skin
D) Application of room temperature water
E) Firm washing to remove particulate matter

Answer and Discussion

The answer is D. Initial treatment of minor thermal injuries consist mainly of cooling (with room temperature water, not with ice), simple gentle cleansing with mild soap and water, and appropriate dressing. Pain management and tetanus prophylaxis are important. Extensive debridement is generally not immediately necessary and may be deferred until the initial follow-up visit.

> **Additional Reading:** Burns. In: Domino F, ed. *The 5-Minute Clinical Consult.* Philadelphia, PA: Lippincott Williams and Wilkins; 2014.

> Category: Integumentary

88. A 17-year-old high school football player is knocked unconscious for a brief period during a game for which you provide medical coverage. Now, he is doing well and the results of his examination are normal. The most appropriate action is

A) Transfer the athlete to a local emergency room.
B) Keep the athlete out of the game for a full quarter; if he remains normal, he may return to play.
C) Prohibit the athlete from returning to play.
D) Allow the athlete to return to competition after 10 additional minutes of normal observation.
E) Prohibit the athlete from returning to play for the rest of the season.

Answer and Discussion

The answer is C. Any athlete with a suspected concussion should not be allowed to return to play on the same day. Return-to-play decisions for athletes should be individually graded and not made without follow-up evaluation. These include

- Complete rest until symptoms free
- Then beginning gradual reintroduction of activity as long as symptom free
- Doing each step generally 24 hours apart: light aerobic exercise; sport-specific exercise; noncontact training drills; full-contact training; game play
- Stopping all activity until again asymptomatic for 24 hours, if any signs or symptoms recur (i.e., exertional headache, visual disturbance, or disequilibrium). Restarting return-to-play plan at last step when patient was asymptomatic

Athletes who are high risk for more prolonged recovery include pediatric athletes, athletes with mood disorders, athletes with learning disabilities, and athletes with migraine headaches. These athletes should have a slower return-to-play progression and may require more intensive evaluation (formal neuropsycologic, balance, symptoms testing). Athletes with multiples concussions should have slower return to play and may benefit from sports medicine consultation or neurologic referral.

> **Additional Reading:** Concussion. In: Domino F, ed. *The 5-Minute Clinical Consult.* Philadelphia, PA: Lippincott Williams and Wilkins; 2014.

> Category: Neurologic

89. A 21-year-old is brought to the emergency room by ambulance after developing sudden shortness of breath. A chest radiograph shows a 10% pneumothorax. The patient remains stable. Appropriate management includes

A) Immediate chest tube placement
B) Intubation and mechanical ventilation
C) Pulmonary function testing
D) Large-bore needle placed in the second intercostal space
E) Observation

Answer and Discussion

The answer is E. Pneumothorax is the accumulation of air within the pleural space. The usual cause of pneumothorax is a penetrating wound such as a stabbing wound, gunshot wound, or deceleration-type injury (e.g., as seen in motor vehicle accidents). Spontaneous pneumothorax can also occur and typically affects tall, thin men or smokers (as a result of a ruptured bleb). Clinical findings include decreased breath sounds on the side affected, shortness of breath, chest pain (most common symptom), cough, distended neck veins, and hypotension. A chest radiograph is usually diagnostic. Treatment may require immediate intervention but in many cases depends on the extent of pneumothorax. If pneumothorax involves up to 15% to 20% of lung volume, observation is the only treatment necessary. Supplemental oxygen is usually administered, and most cases resolve in 10 days. For larger pneumothoraces, chest tube placement is necessary. Tension pneumothoraces require emergent decompression with a large-bore needle placed in the second intercostal space of the midclavicular line, followed by chest tube placement. Providing 100% O_2 accelerates the rate of pleural air absorption.

> **Additional Reading:** Pneumothorax. In: Domino F, ed. *The 5-Minute Clinical Consult*. Philadelphia, PA: Lippincott Williams and Wilkins; 2014.

Category: Respiratory system

90. The American Academy of Dermatology recommends a sunscreen protector with a sun protection factor (SPF) of _____ on the exposed skin to prevent sunburn.
A) SPF 8
B) SPF 30
C) SPF 45
D) SPF 60

Answer and Discussion

The answer is B. SPF is a measure of the ability of a blocking agent (typically clothing or sunscreen) to prevent erythema in response to sun exposure. The SPF can be multiplied by the time of exposure necessary to produce minimal erythema in an unprotected individual to get the expected time until minimal erythema using that protection. As an example, if an unprotected individual develops minimal erythema after 20 minutes of sun exposure, after use of an SPF-8 sunscreen, minimal erythema would be expected after 160 minutes of exposure. However, the duration of protection with sunscreen may be shorter in many circumstances than the SPF would indicate.

The American Academy of Dermatology recommends using a broad-spectrum sunscreen that protects against both UVA and UVB radiation with an SPF of 30 or greater on exposed skin. Other recommendations include staying out of the sun in the middle of the day (10 a.m. to 4 p.m.), wearing a wide-brimmed hat, long-sleeve shirt, or long pants, and avoiding tanning beds.

Apply sunscreen generously to all exposed skin 15 to 30 minutes before exposure. Reapply sunscreen after sweating, rubbing the skin, drying off with a towel, or swimming. Reapply sunscreen every 2 or 3 hours.

> **Additional Reading:** Sunscreens revisited. *Med Lett Drugs Ther.* 2011;53(1359):17–18.

Category: Integumentary

91. The most appropriate test for the detection of a sub-dural hematoma (SDH) SDH is
A) Skull radiographs change
B) CT of the head with and without contrast
C) CT of the head without contrast
D) MRI of the head
E) Lumbar puncture

Answer and Discussion

The answer is C. Acute SDH is readily visualized on head CT as a high-density crescentic collection across the hemispheric convexity. Subacute and chronic SDH appear as isodense or hypodense crescent collection-shaped lesion that deform the surface of the brain. Epidural hematoma produces a convex pattern on CT because its collection is limited by firm dural attachments at the cranial sutures. Brain MRI is more sensitive than head CT for the detection of intracranial hemorrhage. MRI is also more sensitive for the detection of small SDH, and tentorial and interhemispheric SDH. Brain MRI is used for situations in which there is a suspicion for SDH or other intracranial hemorrhage, but no clear evidence of hematoma by CT.

> **Additional Reading:** Subdural hematoma in adults: etiology, clinical features, and diagnosis. In: Basow DS, ed. *UpToDate*. Waltham, MA: UpToDate; 2013.

Category: Neurologic

92. A 21-year-old is brought to your clinic in status epilepticus. What drug should be administered initially?
A) Lorazepam
B) Phenytoin
C) Phenobarbital
D) Pentobarbital
E) Fosphenytoin

Answer and Discussion

The answer is A. Lorazepam should be administered intravenously, and approximately 1 minute is allowed to assess its effect. Diazepam or midazolam may be substituted if lorazepam is not available. If seizures continue at this point, additional doses of lorazepam should be infused and a second intravenous catheter placed in order to begin a concomitant phenytoin (or fosphenytoin) loading infusion. Even if seizures terminate after the initial lorazepam dose, therapy with phenytoin or fosphenytoin is generally indicated to prevent the recurrence of seizures.

> **Additional Reading:** Status epilepticus in adults. In: Basow DS, ed. *UpToDate*. Waltham, MA: UpToDate; 2013.

Category: Neurologic

93. Which of the following statements is *false* regarding the treatment of high-voltage lightning injuries?
A) Cervical spine immobilization and clearance should be performed.
B) Airway burns should be excluded.
C) Tetanus immunization should be administered.
D) Serum CK-MB measurements should be measured to assess myocardial injury.
E) Cardiac monitoring should be maintained after the injury.

Answer and Discussion

The answer is D. A patient exposed to a serious electrical burn or lightning strike should be treated as a trauma patient. Resuscitation should begin with a rapid assessment of airway and cardiopulmonary status. Cervical spine immobilization and clearance should be maintained, and tetanus vaccination should be administered. Coexisting smoke inhalation or airway burns should be excluded. Patients can have spontaneous cardiac activity but paralysis of the respiratory muscles. Prompt restoration of a secure airway may prevent secondary cardiac and neurologic dysfunction or death. Coma or neurologic deficit should include brain and/or spine imaging. An extensive head-to-toe and neurologic examination should be performed. The survivor of high-energy injury should have cardiac and hemodynamic monitoring due to the high incidence of arrhythmia and autonomic dysfunction, especially if there have been arrhythmias in the field or emergency department, loss of consciousness, or if the initial ECG is abnormal. Serum CK-MB measurements and ECG changes are poor measures of myocardial injury. The diagnostic and prognostic value of cardiac troponin levels has not been evaluated in this setting.

Additional Reading: Townsend CM Jr, Beauchamp RD, Evers BM, et al., eds. *Sabiston Textbook of Surgery,* 19th ed. Philadelphia, PA: Saunders/Elsevier; 2012.

Category: Nonspecific system

94. An 18-year-old with a history of von Willebrand's deficiency (vWD) is involved in a motor vehicle accident and presents to the emergency room. There is concern about bleeding; however, the patient is stable. Which of the following would be indicated to help correct the coagulation disorder?

A) Platelets
B) Cryoprecipitate
C) DDAVP
D) Fresh frozen plasma (FFP)
E) Packed RBCs

Answer and Discussion

The answer is C. Approaches to treating vWD include increasing plasma concentration of von Willebrand factor (vWF) by releasing endogenous vWF stores through stimulation of endothelial cells with desmopressin (DDAVP); use of vWF concentrates; and promoting hemostasis using hemostatic agents with mechanisms other than increasing vWF.

For minor bleeding and minor surgery, the use of IV or intranasal DDAVP is the initial treatment of bleeding or at the time of surgery in patients who have shown a prior response to this agent. For major bleeding or major surgical procedures, it is recommended to use vWF concentrate over DDAVP in order to reach a target level of approximately 100 IU/dL or VWF ristocetin cofactor activity. The above levels should be maintained for 7 to 14 days or as needed. Packed RBCs can be stored in cooled storage for up to 35 days; however, refrigerated temperatures cause platelets to degenerate, so banked, packed RBCs contain essentially no functioning platelets. Also, factors V and VII decrease with refrigeration; however, other factors remain unchanged. Packed RBC transfusion should be used only when time or the clinical situation precludes other therapy. Each unit of packed RBCs usually raises the hematocrit by 2% to 3% in a 70-kg adult, although this varies depending on the donor, the recipient's fluid status, the method of storage, and its duration. Leukocyte-poor RBCs may be given to help reduce transfusion reactions in those who have experienced reactions with previous transfusions.

Platelet transfusions are indicated if patients have thrombocytopenia or platelet dysfunction, or both. Patients are usually administered 6 or 10 units at one time (*6-pack* or *10-pack*). Multiple-unit, single-donor platelets are harvested from one donor using apheresis. After platelet transfusion in the adult, the platelet count obtained at 1 hour should rise at least 5,000 platelets/mm^3 for each unit of platelets transfused. Patients may experience a smaller response after multiple transfusions. Platelets should not be routinely given for bleeding prophylaxis unless there is evidence of microvascular bleeding or planned surgery and the platelet count is <50,000/mm^3 or the platelet count is <10,000/mm^3 (for prophylaxis against bleeding). Previous guidelines of 20,000/mm^3 are no longer used. Patients receiving massive transfusion should not automatically receive platelets in the

absence of microvascular bleeding. Additionally, body temperature can affect platelets' ability to function, and, ideally, body temperature should be restored before consideration of platelet transfusion.

FFP is used to replace labile clotting factors. A unit of FFP contains near-normal levels of all clotting factors, including approximately 400 mg of fibrinogen. A unit of FFP increases clotting factors by approximately 3%. Adequate clotting is usually obtained with factor levels >30%. FFP is used to correct PT and activated PTT.

Additional Reading: Diagnosis and management of von Willebrand disease: guidelines for primary care. *Am Fam Physician.* 2009;80(11):1261–1268.

Category: Hematologic system

95. A 4-year-old girl is seen in the emergency room and is suspected of having meningitis. A positive Brudzinski's sign is noted. Which of the following describes a positive Brudzinski's sign?

A) The child dorsiflexes her feet when her head is flexed forward.
B) The child shows resistance when her legs are extended from a flexed position.
C) The child involuntarily flexes the hips with flexion of the neck.
D) The child involuntarily blinks with gentle tapping of the forehead.
E) The child shows extension-type posturing when her arms are flexed.

Answer and Discussion

The answer is C. Symptoms of bacterial meningitis include high-pitched cry, fever, anorexia, irritability, obtundation, lethargy, nausea, vomiting, neck stiffness, and a full fontanel (in infants).

In neonates, clinical clues to the presence of meningitis include temperature instability (hypothermia or hyperthermia), listlessness, high-pitched crying, fretfulness, lethargy, refusal to eat, a weak sucking response, irritability, vomiting, diarrhea, and respiratory distress. Because neonates usually do not have meningismus, a change in the child's affect or state of alertness is one of the most important signs. A bulging fontanel may occur late in the course of the disease in one-third of neonates. About 30% of neonates have seizures. Meningeal signs and fever are not always present in infants; however, meningeal signs are more reliable in older children and include the following:

- Brudzinski's sign: Flexion of neck with the patient supine causes involuntary flexion at the hips.
- Kernig's sign: Attempts to extend the knees from a flexed position are met with resistance.

The most common causes of bacterial meningitis include the following:

- *Neisseria meningitidis* (meningococcal meningitis): Usually seen in the first year of life.
- *H. influenzae:* The Hib vaccination has dramatically reduced the incidence.
- *Streptococcal pneumoniae:* The most common form of adult meningitis; immunization can help prevent this in children and adults.
- Group B or D streptococci and gram-negative organisms: Most common in neonates.

Among U.S. children, there has been a substantial decrease in deaths and hospitalization from *H. influenzae* meningitis but not *S. pneumoniae* or *N. meningitidis* meningitis in the years after Hib conjugate vaccine licensure. This observation suggests that the declines in *H. influenzae* meningitis are due primarily to the use of Hib conjugate vaccines. The most common sequelae after meningitis include hearing loss and seizure disorders.

Additional Reading: Meningitis. *The Merck Manual of Diagnosis and Therapy*. 19th ed. Merck Research Laboratories. 2011.

Category: Neurologic

96. Which of the following statements regarding acute pancreatitis is true?
A) All patients should receive nasogastric suction to maintain strict bowel rest.
B) Anticholinergics are useful in the treatment of acute pancreatitis.
C) Amylase is the most sensitive and specific test for the detection of acute pancreatitis.
D) Enteral feedings (distal to the ligament of Treitz) can be beneficial after 48 hours for severe cases.
E) Nausea and vomiting are rarely present.

Answer and Discussion

The answer is D. Acute pancreatitis usually results from alcohol abuse, bile duct obstruction, or severe hypertriglyceridemia. Patients with acute pancreatitis present with mild-to-severe epigastric pain with radiation to the flank, back, or both. Classically, the pain is characterized as constant, dull, and boring and is worse when the patient is supine. The discomfort may lessen when the patient assumes a sitting or fetal position. A heavy meal or drinking binge often triggers the pain. Nausea and nonfeculent vomiting are present in the vast majority of patients. Serum amylase and lipase (the most sensitive and specific laboratory indicator for pancreatitis) levels are used to confirm the diagnosis of acute pancreatitis. CT will confirm the diagnosis, assess severity, establish a baseline, and rule out other possibilities. CT scan with IV contrast at day 3 can assess the degree of necrosis when necrotizing pancreatitis is suspected (O_2 saturation <90%, systolic BP <90, worsening symptoms). Intravenous rehydration should usually be aggressive, with close attention to blood pressure and cardiac and pulmonary status. Withholding food by mouth does reduce pain; however, the use of a nasogastric tube with suction is indicated only for intractable emesis. In mild pancreatitis, oral intake should be withheld until the nausea and vomiting subside. Total enteral feeding beyond the ligament of Treitz is considered after 48 hours, if oral feeding will not be possible within 5 to 7 days. Systemic antibiotics remain controversial.

Additional Reading: Acute pancreatitis: diagnosis, prognosis and treatment. *Am Fam Physician*. 2007;75(10):1513–1520.

Category: Gastroenterology system

97. A 75-year-old presents to your office complaining of anorexia, nausea, abdominal pain, and muscle weakness. Laboratory tests show an elevated calcium level. The most likely diagnosis is
A) Osteoporosis
B) Paget's disease
C) Hyperparathyroidism
D) Myasthenia gravis
E) Chronic fatigue syndrome

Answer and Discussion

The answer is C. Hyperparathyroidism is a common cause of hypercalcemia. The incidence of hyperparathyroidism increases with age. Women are more commonly affected. The hypercalcemia usually is discovered during a routine serum chemistry profile. Primary hyperparathyroidism results from excessive secretion of parathyroid hormone (PTH) with a lack of response feedback inhibition by elevated calcium. Secondary hyperparathyroidism with excessive secretion of parathyroid hormone from the parathyroid gland occurs in response to hypocalcemia, which usually can be caused by vitamin D deficiency or renal failure. Tertiary hyperparathyroidism results from autonomous hyperfunction of the parathyroid gland in the setting of longstanding secondary parathyroid hormone. Most patients are asymptomatic. In the majority of cases, primary hyperparathyroidism is the result of an adenoma in a single parathyroid gland. Hypertrophy of all four parathyroid glands causes hyperparathyroidism in a smaller percentage of patients. The incidence of hyperparathyroidism is higher in patients with type I and type II multiple endocrine neoplasia syndromes, in patients with familial hyperparathyroidism, and in patients who received radiation therapy to the head and neck area for benign diseases during childhood. Chronic renal failure, rickets, and malabsorption syndromes are the most frequent conditions leading to secondary hyperparathyroidism. The symptoms of hyperparathyroidism are vague and often similar to symptoms of depression, irritable bowel syndrome, fibromyalgia, or stress reaction. Some combination of headaches, fatigue, anorexia, nausea, paresthesias, muscular weakness, pain in the extremities, pain in the abdomen, and other such nonspecific symptoms appears to be the most common presentation of primary hyperparathyroidism.

Complications of primary hyperparathyroidism include peptic ulcers, nephrolithiasis, pancreatitis, dehydration, and nephrocalcinosis. Intravenous hydration is the most critical treatment for a patient with an acute presentation of hyperparathyroidism and hypercalcemia. The addition of furosemide (Lasix) increases urinary calcium loss. Such patients can be treated with biphosphonates (alendronate) to reduce bone turnover and maintain bone density. When medical management is used, routine monitoring for clinical deterioration is recommended. Critical hypercalcemia requires IV fluid rehydration, IV biphosphonate therapy, and SC calcitonin (4 U/kg q 12 h) for severe symptoms. Surgical management is indicated in cases of hyperparathyroidism, associated with nephrolitiasis, nephrocalcinosis, and/or osteitis fibrosa.

Additional Reading: Hyperparathyroidism. In: Domino F, ed. *The 5-Minute Clinical Consult*. Philadelphia, PA: Lippincott Williams and Wilkins; 2014.

Category: Endocrine system

98. Patients who have been scuba diving should wait at least _____ before flying because of the risk of decompression illness.
A) 4 hours
B) 12 hours
C) 24 hours
D) 72 hours
E) 1 week

Answer and Discussion

The answer is B. Patients who travel by air soon after scuba diving are at increased risk for developing decompression sickness (DCS) in-flight. Such a passenger should be advised to wait 12 hours before flying, if he or she has been making only 1 dive/day. Individuals who have participated in multiple dives or those requiring decompression stops should consider waiting up to 48 hours before flying.

Additional Reading: Decompression sickness. In: Domino F, ed. *The 5-Minute Clinical Consult*. Philadelphia, PA: Lippincott Williams and Wilkins; 2014.

Category: Nonspecific system

99. Which of the following statements is true regarding breast implants?

A) There is a higher incidence of connective tissue disease in patients who received silicone breast implants.

B) There is a higher incidence of breast cancer in women who have had breast augmentation.

C) Mammography with Eklund views can be helpful in assessing breast lumps after augmentation.

D) MRI is not helpful in detecting rupture of breast implants.

E) According to the U.S. Food and Drug Administration, all women with silicone breast implants should have them removed.

Answer and Discussion

The answer is C. Women who have undergone augmentation mammoplasty with silicone gel or others implants may present for routine breast cancer screening with palpable breast lumps. Standard imaging technique in women with breast implant involves four views, rather than the usual two views per breast. Standard cranial-caudal (CC) and mediolateral oblique (MLO) projections of each breast are obtained with the implant included. The Eklund technique consists of postero-superior displacement of the implants simultaneously to an anterior traction of the breast, pushing the implants toward the chest wall up to flatten. These additional views permit evaluation of the implant as well as the deep breast tissues. MRI is the most accurate imaging examination for detecting rupture of breast implants.

Numerous meta-analysis have concluded that there is no evidence of an increased risk of any specific connective tissue diseases or other autoimmune conditions associated with the use of breast implants, including nonsilicone and silicone implants. There is no increased risk of breast cancer.

Additional Reading: Breast implant complications. From: http://www.fda.gov/MedicalDevices/ProductsandMedicalProcedures/ImplantsandProsthetics/BreastImplants/ucm259296.htm.

Category: Integumentary

100. Bariatric surgery can be considered in individuals who have a body mass index (BMI) that exceeds

A) 10 kg/mm^2

B) 20 kg/mm^2

C) 30 kg/mm^2

D) 40 kg/mm^2

E) 50 kg/mm^2

Answer and Discussion

The answer is D. A body mass index of greater than 40 kg/m^2 or a body mass index of 35 kg/m^2 with an obesity-related comorbidity (e.g., diabetes, hypertension) are indications of bariatric surgery and are able to adhere to postoperative care.

Exclusion criteria include cardiopulmonary disease that would make the risk prohibitive; current drug or alcohol abuse; lack of comprehension of risks, benefits, expected outcomes, alternatives, and required lifestyle changes; reversible endocrine or other disorders that can cause obesity; and uncontrolled severe phychiatric illness.

Bariatric surgery procedures, including laparoscopic adjustable gastric banding, laparoscopic sleeve gastrectomy, and Roux-e-Y bypass results in an average weight loss of 50% of excess body weight. Remission of diabetes mellitus occurs in approximately 80% of patient after Roux-en-Y bypass. Other obesity-related comorbidities are greatly reduced, and health-related quality of life improves. The Obesity Surgery Mortality Risk score identify patients with increased risk from bariatric surgery. The Roux-en-Y procedure carries an increased risk of malabsorption sequelae but lead to the greatest weight loss (up to 10 lb (4.5 Kg.) per month) during the first one to two postsurgical years, followed by laparoscopic sleeve gastrectomy (LSG) and laparoscopic adjustable gastric banding (LAGB). After bariatric surgery, many patients maintain a long-term (8 to 10 years) weight loss of greater than 50% of excess body weight. Hyperlipidemia, hypertension, diabetes, and most other obesity-related conditions are significantly improved after bariatric surgery. Overall, these procedures have a mortality risk of less than 0.5%.

Additional Reading: Treatment of adults obesity with bariatric surgery. *Am Fam Physician*. 2011;84(7):805–814.

Category: Endocrine system

101. The mother of a 12-year-old calls to report that her child was bitten by a pet hamster. Which of the following is the appropriate management?

A) Human diploid cell vaccine

B) Rabies immune globulin

C) Reassurance to the mother with no further treatment

D) Immediate sacrifice of the hamster for pathologic evaluation

E) Hospitalization and close observation of the child for abnormal behavior

Answer and Discussion

The answer is C. Rabies is an infectious viral infection that is often transmitted by the bite of an infected animal or, rarely, by exposure of mucous membranes and saliva with a skin abrasion. The rabies virus affects the central nervous system (CNS), and the presence of intracytoplasmic Negri bodies seen microscopically is pathognomonic for the infection. Symptoms affecting humans include depression, difficulty with concentration, malaise, fever, extreme restlessness with excessive salivation, painful laryngeal and pharyngeal muscle spasms, and convulsions. Although patients often experience extreme thirst, they are hydrophobic because drinking can often precipitate pharyngeal spasms. Death usually occurs secondary to exhaustion and asphyxia with generalized paralysis. The disease is usually found in wild animals such as skunks, foxes, coyotes, raccoons, bobcats, and bats, but is also seen in domestic dogs and cats. Other animals affected include livestock. Treatment of those bitten includes confining the animal that bit the patient for at least 10 days to look for abnormal behavior. If no changes are seen, the patient usually does not need treatment. Animals with abnormal behavior should be sacrificed and examined pathologically for rabies infection. If the animal cannot be caught or if the animal exhibits abnormal behavior and has evidence of rabies infection, the patient should be treated with human diploid cell vaccine or rabies vaccine, adsorbed: 1 mL administered intramuscularly at the time of presentation and then at days 3, 7, 14, and 28 for a total of five doses. Rabies vaccine (adsorbed) should not be given intradermally. Also, to bridge the gap of time it takes for the patient to develop antibodies to the rabies vaccine, 20 IU/kg of rabies immune globulin is given, with much of the dose administered at the site of the bite and the rest administered at a distant site from vaccine inoculation intramuscularly. In most cases, the wound should not be sutured. If rabies does develop, aggressive symptomatic treatment is required. The prognosis is not universally fatal, but there is significant mortality associated with rabies. Prophylaxis for rabies should be considered for high-risk populations such as veterinarians, animal handlers, technicians in laboratories in which rabies is present, and travelers spending a month or more in countries in which rabies is common. Bites of rodents such as squirrels, opossums, rats, mice, guinea pigs, gerbils, hamsters, rabbits, and hares rarely, if ever, require rabies prophylaxis.

Additional Reading: Rabies, 2011. From: http://www.cdc.gov/rabies/specific_groups/doctors/index.html.

Category: Nonspecific system

102. A 16-year-old girl presents to the office complaining of throat pain, difficulty swallowing, and trismus. Physical examination shows erythema and enlargement of the left tonsillar pillar. In addition, the patient holds her head to the left side and has muffled speech. The most likely diagnosis is
A) Peritonsillar abscess
B) Streptococcal pharyngitis
C) Tonsillar cancer
D) Epiglottitis
E) Retropharyngeal abscess

Answer and Discussion

The answer is A. Peritonsillar abscess (also known as *quinsy*) is the most common ear, nose, and throat abscess. It is seen most commonly in teenagers and young adults and is rare in children below the age of 5 years. The condition occurs when an abscess develops between the tonsil and the superior constrictor muscle. Symptoms include worsening throat pain, muffled speech (hot-potato voice), trismus, and difficulty swallowing. The patient often holds his or her head toward the side that the abscess affects. If the abscess is large, airway compromise may occur. Ultrasound or CT scanning can help distinguish between cellulitis and abscess formation. Treatment of peritonsillar abscess is accomplished by lancing a fluctuant area, if present, with an 18-gauge needle (making certain not to go deeper than 1 cm where the internal carotid artery passes) and prescribing penicillin-containing antibiotics. The fluid should be cultured before initiation of antibiotics. Common infecting organisms include group A *Streptococcus* and anaerobes. Recurrent episodes necessitate tonsillectomy.

Additional Reading: Peritonsillar abscess. *Am Fam Physician*. 2008;77(2):199–202.

Category: Nonspecific system

103. A boy who plays little league baseball presents with swelling over the medial elbow and pain with valgus and varus stress while flexing and extending the elbow. The patient reports locking of the elbow. In addition, radiographs show the presence of loose bodies. The most likely diagnosis is
A) Osteochondritis dissecans
B) Chondromalacia
C) Nursemaid's elbow
D) Lateral epicondylitis

Answer and Discussion

The answer is A. Little league elbow is an overuse injury caused by compressive forces at the radiocapitellar joint and opposite pulling forces at the medial aspect of the elbow. These injuries usually occur in adolescents who use motions such as overhand pitching in sports such as baseball. The repetitive forces may lead to damage of the articular surface of the capitellum, ligamentous injury of the medial elbow, and ulnar nerve dysfunction. In severe cases, osteochondritis dissecans of the capitellum with the formation of loose bodies can occur and result in locking of the elbow joint. Other symptoms include pain with valgus and varus stress while flexing and extending the elbow. For most cases, treatment involves rest (no throwing for

4 to 6 weeks), ice, elevation, and NSAIDs. However, if there are signs of osteochondritis dissecans, orthopedic referral for possible surgical intervention is necessary.

Additional Reading: Busconi BD, Stevenson JH. Approach to the athlete with little league elbow. *Sports Medicine Consult: A Problem-Based Approach to Sports Medicine for the Primary Care Physician*. Philadelphia, PA: Lippincott, Williams & Wilkins; 2009.

Category: Musculoskeletal system

104. A 23-year-old woman was bitten on the finger by her neighbor's cat 1 hour ago. There are small puncture bites with minimal inflammation at the site. She is allergic to penicillin. Appropriate management at this time includes
A) Observation only
B) Topical antibiotic ointment
C) Oral doxycycline (Vibramycin)
D) IV ceftriaxone (Rocephin)
E) Oral amoxicillin-clavulanate (Augmentin)

Answer and Discussion

The answer is C. The oral flora of humans and animals contains a mixture of potential pathogens: *Eikenella corrodens* is frequently isolated from human bites, and *Pasteurella multocida* from many animal bites, particularly those of cats. Amoxicillin-clavulanate potassium is the antibiotic of choice for both dog and cat bites when infection is present. For patients who are allergic to penicillin, doxycycline is an acceptable alternative, except for children younger than 8 years and pregnant women. Erythromycin can also be used, but the risk of treatment failure is greater because of antimicrobial resistance. Other acceptable combinations include clindamycin (Cleocin) and a fluoroquinolone in adults or clindamycin and trimethoprim-sulfamethoxazole (Bactrim, Septra) in children. When compliance is a concern, daily intramuscular injections of ceftriaxone are appropriate. All bite injuries are potentially dangerous and can cause significant infection. They should be debrided surgically, with the wounds left open. Currently there is insufficient evidence to support antibiotic prophylaxis in dog and cat bites, and minimal evidence supports its use for human bites. However, there is evidence that antibiotics reduce the risk of infection in hand bites.

Additional Reading: Pet-related infections. *Am Fam Physician*. 2007;76(9):1314–1322.

Category: Nonspecific system

105. A 56-year-old woman is found to have biliary colic. You explain to her that the risk of developing acute cholecystitis is
A) 10%
B) 25%
C) 50%
D) 75%
E) 90%

Answer and Discussion

The answer is A. Acute cholecystitis develops in up to 10% of patients with symptomatic gallstones and is caused by the complete obstruction of the cystic duct. Patients with incidental gallstones by Ultrasonogram, 20% will become symptomatic during up to 15 years of follow-up.

Additional Reading: Cholelithiasis. In: Domino F, ed. *The 5-Minute Clinical Consult*. Philadelphia, PA: Lippincott Williams and Wilkins; 2014.

Category: Gastroenterology system

106. Diverticulosis is a condition associated with
A) Increased risk of colon cancer
B) Herniations of the bowel mucosa and submucosa through the muscular layers of the bowel wall
C) Inflammatory bowel disease
D) A 90% risk of developing diverticulitis
E) Predominantly the proximal colon

Answer and Discussion

The answer is B. Diverticulosis, an outpouching of the bowel wall, increases in frequency after 40 years of age. Acquired diverticular disease affects approximately 5% to 10% of the Western population older than 45 years and approximately 80% of persons older than 85 years. It is more common in the sigmoid and distal colon. Colonic diverticula are related primarily to two factors: increased intraluminal pressure and a weakening of the bowel wall. Patients with known diverticula have been found to have elevated resting colonic pressures. The Western diet, which tends to be low in dietary fiber and high in refined carbohydrates, is also believed to be a contributing factor. The condition occurs when there is herniation of bowel mucosa and submucosa through muscular layers of the colon. Inflammation of the small herniations, referred to as *diverticulitis*, occurs in approximately 10% to 20% of patients with diverticulosis and more commonly in men. Most patients with diverticulosis remain asymptomatic. Symptoms of diverticulitis include lower abdominal pain usually located on the left that may be steady or cramping and is sometimes relieved with a bowel movement, anorexia, nausea, vomiting, and constipation. Physical examination usually shows abdominal tenderness and guarding and, occasionally, a palpable abdominal or rectal mass with abscess formation. Occult blood is present in approximately 20% of patients. Diverticular hemorrhage occurs in 3% to 5% of patients with diverticular disease. Fever and an increased WBC count may also be present. Previously, diverticular disease was diagnosed using a contrast barium enema. However, because of the possibility of an obstructing fecalith being dislodged by insufflation and causing bowel perforation, CT scanning is now the diagnostic procedure of choice. Treatment of diverticulitis can take place on an outpatient basis for a patient with a mild first attack who is able to tolerate oral hydration and an antibiotic. Treatment consists of a liquid diet and 7 to 10 days of therapy with broad-spectrum antimicrobials such as metronidazole and ciprofloxacin. Patients with severe illness, or those who cannot tolerate oral hydration or who have pain severe enough to require narcotic analgesia, should be hospitalized. Because feeding increases intracolonic pressure, patients should receive nothing by mouth and should be treated with intravenous triple therapy consisting of ampicillin, gentamicin, and metronidazole. Alternative monotherapy includes piperacillin or tazobactam. If narcotics are required for pain control, meperidine is recommended because morphine sulfate causes colonic spasm. If the pain, fever, and leukocytosis do not resolve within 3 days, further imaging studies are indicated. If an abscess is uncovered and is >5 cm in size, CT-guided drainage and adequate antibiotic coverage should be considered. Approximately 20% of patients with diverticulitis require surgery. Indications for emergent surgery include peritonitis, uncontrolled sepsis, visceral perforation, colonic obstruction, or acute deterioration. Bowel resection is usually recommended for recurrent episodes of diverticulitis or if fistulas are present.

Additional Reading: Diverticular disease. In: Domino F, ed. *The 5-Minute Clinical Consult*. Philadelphia, PA: Lippincott Williams and Wilkins; 2014.

Category: Gastroenterology system

107. The most common form of malignant melanoma is
A) Lentigo maligna melanoma
B) Superficial spreading melanoma
C) Nodular melanoma
D) Acrolentiginous melanoma

Answer and Discussion

The answer is B. Cutaneous malignant melanoma accounts for 3% to 5% of all skin cancers and is responsible for approximately 75% of all deaths from skin cancer. It is a serious and life-threatening condition because of the potential for distant metastasis. Studies have shown that the prevalence of melanoma increases with proximity to the equator. Persons with skin types that are sensitive to the effects of ultraviolet radiation—red or blond hair, freckles, and fair skin that burns easily and tans with difficulty—are at higher risk. Although cumulative sun exposure is linked to nonmelanoma skin cancer, intermittent intense sun exposure seems to be more related to melanoma risk. Persons with an increased number of moles, dysplastic nevi, or a family history of the disease and immunosupression are at increased risk compared with the general population. Melanomas are classified into the following:

- *Lentigo maligna melanoma.* This usually affects older patients in their 60s and 70s. These lesions usually show variegation of color including black, brown, reddish lesions and are rather large (measuring 2 to 6 cm).
- *Superficial spreading melanoma.* This is the most common type. These lesions are usually smaller (2 to 3 cm in diameter) and tend to affect patients in their 50s and 60s.
- *Nodular melanoma.* These patients are usually younger (average, 30 to 50 years of age). These lesions are usually smaller than the other two types and are slightly raised and uniform in color. Unfortunately, these lesions tend to spread deeply into the underlying tissue and have the worst prognosis.
- *Acrolentiginous melanoma.* This condition is rare and is associated with lesions affecting the palmar and plantar surface of the extremities as well as the subungual skin. It is similar to lentigo maligna melanoma.

The ABCDE mnemonic stands for: **A**symmetry, **B**orders irregularities, **C**olor variation, **D**iameter, and **E**volution/Elevation. Any suspicious pigmented lesion should be biopsied. Malignant melanoma may tend to bleed or ulcerate. Early metastasis occurs through the lymph nodes; late metastasis occurs through a hematogenous route and may affect the skin, liver, or lungs. A properly performed biopsy is essential for the diagnosis. If melanoma is diagnosed, the histologic interpretation of the biopsy determines the prognosis and treatment plan. General recommendations include performing an excisional biopsy whenever possible. Accepted techniques for biopsy include punch, saucerization, and elliptic excision. Shave biopsy will not miss a diagnosis of melanoma, but may interfere with the staging process of determining the depth of invasion, the Breslow depth. The Breslow depth is the most important prognostic parameter in evaluating the primary tumor. Because early detection and treatment can lead to identification of thinner lesions, which may increase survival, it is critical that physicians be comfortable with evaluating suspicious pigmented lesions and providing treatment or referral as necessary.

Additional Reading: Cutaneous malignant melanoma: a primary care perspective. *Am Fam Physician.* 2012;85(2):161–168.

Category: Integumentary

108. A 72-year-old man complains that he cannot void the day after his knee-replacement surgery. He has not voided in the past

12 hours. A urethral catheter is placed and 500 mL of urine is removed from his bladder. Which one of the following is most likely to improve the success rate of a voiding trial?

A) Using a specialized catheter could instead of a standard catheter
B) Leaving the catheter in place for at least 2 weeks
C) Immediately removing the catheter
D) Starting tamsulosin (Flomax), 0.4 mg daily, at the time of catheter insertion
E) Starting antibiotic prophylaxis at the time of catheter insertion

Answer and Discussion

The answer is D. Urinary retention is a common problem in hospitalized patients, especially following certain types of surgery. Starting an alpha-blocker (like tamsulosin) at the time of insertion of the urethral catheter has been shown to increase the success of a voiding trial. Voiding trial success rates have not been shown to be improved by immediate removal of the catheter or by leaving the catheter in for 2 weeks. Specialized catheters, such as a coudé catheter, which is designed with a curved tip that makes it easier to pass through the curvature of the prostatic urethra, has not been shown to make a difference. Antibiotic prophylaxis has no impact on urinary retention.

Additional Reading: Urinary retention in adults: diagnosis and initial management. *Am Fam Physician.* 2008;77(5):643–650.

Category: Nephrologic system

109. An 18-month-old is brought into your emergency room after being involved in a motor vehicle accident. The child's blood pressure is low, and he is tachycardic and lethargic. His capillary refill is delayed and his mucous membranes are dry. Appropriate management consists of

A) Oral rehydration
B) Intravenous lactated Ringer's, 20 mL/kg bolus
C) Intravenous 0.45 normal saline, 20 mL/kg given over 30 to 60 minutes
D) Intravenous D5 with normal saline, 20 mL/kg given over 30 to 60 minutes
E) Intravenous D5 W, 20 mL/kg given over 30 to 60 minutes

Answer and Discussion

The answer is B. Emergent resuscitation of infants and children typically involves fluid replacement. Fluid deficits can result from a host of conditions including infection, trauma, or dehydration. A short-term weight loss >1% body weight/day is presumed to represent a fluid deficit. The rate at which the deficit is replaced depends on the severity of dehydration and the rate of fluid loss. In general, when signs of circulatory compromise exist, 20 mL/kg of lactated Ringer's solution or 0.9% sodium chloride solution is rapidly infused intravenously to restore adequate perfusion. If circulation does not improve satisfactorily, more fluid is infused. Children in severe hypovolemic shock may require and tolerate fluid boluses totaling 60 to 80 mL/kg within the first 1 to 2 hours of presentation. The need for additional fluid should alert the physician to anticipate complications of acute shock. The remainder of the deficit can be replaced over 8 to 48 hours, depending on clinical need.

Additional Reading: Deficit therapy. In: Basow DS, ed. *UpToDate.* Waltham, MA: UpToDate; 2013.

Category: Nonspecific system

Care of the Elderly Patient

QUESTIONS

Each of the following questions or incomplete statements is followed by suggested answers or completions. Select the ONE BEST ANSWER in each case.

1. Which of the following symptoms is more likely to represent myocardial ischemia in older patients?
A) Chest pain
B) Dyspnea
C) Diaphoresis
D) Back pain
E) Jaw pain

Answer and Discussion

The answer is B. Exertional angina (chest pain) is the most common manifestation of myocardial ischemia in young and middle-age persons. Because of their more sedentary lifestyle or possibly a difference in pathophysiology, this may not be true in elderly patients. Instead of exertional chest pain, ischemia may be more commonly manifested as dyspnea in elderly patients. Other elderly patients with coronary artery disease (CAD) may be completely asymptomatic, although silent ischemia may be demonstrated by stress testing or Holter monitoring.

> **Additional Reading:** Evaluation of the adult with dyspnea in the emergency department. In: Basow DS, ed. *UpToDate*. Waltham, MA: UpToDate; 2013.
>
> Category: Cardiovascular system

> 🌀 Instead of exertional chest pain, ischemia may be more commonly manifested as dyspnea in elderly patients.

2. Which of the following statements is true regarding thrombolytic therapy when treating elderly patients with myocardial infarction (MI)?
A) Elderly patients are frequently overtreated with thrombolytics.
B) Elderly patients with non-Q-wave MIs should receive thrombolytics.

C) Streptokinase is more expensive to use than tPA.
D) tPA is associated with a higher risk of hemorrhagic stroke when compared with streptokinase in elderly patients.
E) Up to 75% of elderly patients have absolute contraindications to thrombolytics.

Answer and Discussion

The answer is D. Despite a wealth of evidence in favor of thrombolytic treatment for elderly MI patients, the therapy is commonly not used in this age group. The reasons for this are numerous and include delay in seeking medical assistance, misdiagnoses due to atypical presentation, increased contraindications, and higher prevalence of non-Q-wave MIs. Additionally, physicians are reluctant to use thrombolytics in the elderly population for fear of hemorrhage, although most studies show that intracerebral hemorrhage is not significantly increased in elderly MI patients who receive thrombolytics. Only approximately one-third of elderly patients presenting with acute MI have any contraindications to thrombolytic therapy, and less than 5% have absolute contraindications. In regard to patients with non-Q-wave infarction or unstable angina, repeated studies have demonstrated that thrombolytic therapy has no benefits in these patients regardless of age. In regard to choice of specific thrombolytic agent, initial studies comparing streptokinase to the much more expensive tissue-type plasminogen activator found that both drugs increased the survival rate equally. The Global Utilization of Streptokinase and Tissue Plasminogen Activator (tPA) for Occluded Coronary Arteries (GUSTO) trial, which was designed specifically to compare thrombolytic agents, reported a significant advantage with tPA for the overall study population. Patients above age 75, however, had a significantly higher risk of hemorrhagic stroke when treated with tPA than with streptokinase, and the incidence of death or nonfatal disabling stroke was not significantly different between the two therapies in this age group. Therefore, streptokinase may be appropriate in patients above the age of 75 years.

> **Additional Reading:** Coronary reperfusion for acute myocardial infarction in older adults. In: Basow DS, ed. *UpToDate*. Waltham, MA: UpToDate; 2013.
>
> Category: Cardiovascular system

3. A 75-year-old man presents with exertional dyspnea and generalized weakness. On examination, you discover a high-pitched, blowing diastolic murmur and a wide pulse pressure with bounding pulses. The most likely diagnosis is
A) Aortic stenosis
B) Aortic insufficiency
C) Mitral stenosis
D) Mitral insufficiency
E) Coarctation of the aorta

Answer and Discussion
The answer is B. The prevalence of aortic regurgitation increases with age. Unlike aortic valve stenosis, aortic valvular insufficiency is rarely caused by degenerative aortic valve disease. Acute aortic valvular insufficiency may be due to infective endocarditis, aortic dissection, trauma, or rupture of the sinus of Valsalva. Chronic aortic insufficiency may be caused by aortic root disease secondary to systemic hypertension, syphilitic aortitis, cystic medial necrosis, ankylosing spondylitis, rheumatoid arthritis, Reiter's disease, systemic lupus erythematosus, Ehlers–Danlos syndrome, and pseudoxanthoma elasticum. Chronic aortic insufficiency can be caused by valve leaflet disease, including rheumatic heart disease, congenital heart disease, rheumatoid arthritis, ankylosing spondylitis, or myxomatous degeneration. Symptoms of aortic valvular insufficiency are the same in older persons as they are in younger ones. Usually, the main symptoms are related to heart failure, with exertional dyspnea and weakness being common symptoms. In some elderly patients, symptoms of dyspnea and palpitations may be more common at rest than with exertion. Nocturnal angina pectoris, often accompanied by flushing, diaphoresis, and palpitations, may occur; this is thought to be related to the slowing of the heart rate and the drop of arterial diastolic pressure. The classic findings of a high-pitched, blowing diastolic murmur and a wide pulse pressure with an abruptly rising and collapsing pulse should make the diagnosis of aortic valvular insufficiency easily recognized in elderly patients.

Additional Reading: Adult aortic regurgitation. In: Domino F, ed. *The 5-Minute Clinical Consult.* Philadelphia, PA: Lippincott Williams and Wilkins; 2014.

Category: Cardiovascular system

4. Once symptoms develop in elderly patients with aortic stenosis (without intervention), the survival is approximately
A) 6 months or less
B) 1 to 3 years
C) 3 to 5 years
D) 5 to 7 years
E) Survival is unaffected with symptomatic aortic stenosis

Answer and Discussion
The answer is B. Once symptoms develop in patients with critical aortic valve stenosis, the clinical course is rapidly downhill. Symptoms and left ventricular dysfunction are progressive, and the average survival is approximately 1 to 3 years. Aggressive treatment should be considered.

Additional Reading: Aortic stenosis. In: Domino F, ed. *The 5-Minute Clinical Consult.* Philadelphia, PA: Lippincott Williams and Wilkins; 2014.

Category: Cardiovascular system

5. A 69-year-old woman presents with peripheral edema, orthopnea, and dypsnea on exertion. She has gained 10 pounds in the last 3 days. She is otherwise healthy. You suspect congestive heart failure. Appropriate first-line medication includes which of the following?
A) Diltiazem
B) Lisinopril
C) Nitroglyercin
D) Verapamil
E) Hydralazine

Answer and Discussion
The answer is B. Due to the results of numerous studies showing that angiotensin-converting-enzyme (ACE) inhibitors are beneficial in relieving symptoms and preventing progressive ventricular deterioration, it is recommended that they should be the initial therapy utilized in patients with heart failure. In patients with moderate to severe heart failure due to systolic left ventricular dysfunction, the use of ACE inhibitors alone has not been found to be successful in relieving the signs and symptoms of volume overload. There is no question, however, that ACE inhibitors, digitalis, and diuretics are beneficial in improving the symptoms and prolonging survival in symptomatic patients with left ventricular systolic dysfunction. In the CONSENSUS trial, which demonstrated significant benefits in the use of ACE inhibitors in symptomatic patients, the mean age of the patients was above 70 years, and, at this age, ACE inhibitors were well tolerated. In asymptomatic elderly patients with depressed left ventricular systolic dysfunction, the use of ACE inhibitors is more controversial. The SOLVD trial demonstrated that asymptomatic patients with a depressed left ventricular ejection fraction of less than 35% demonstrated no benefit in survival, although a significant reduction in progression to clinical heart failure with a decrease in hospitalizations was noted. In the SAVE trial, ACE inhibitors were found to be beneficial in improving long-term survival and reducing the development of heart failure and recurrent MI in patients with reduced left ventricular systolic function following acute MI, regardless of the patient's age.

Additional Reading: Ace inhibitors in heart failure due to systolic dysfunction: therapeutic use. In: Basow DS, ed. *UpToDate.* Waltham, MA: UpToDate; 2013.

Category: Cardiovascular system

6. A 75-year-old man is brought in to your office by his wife. She complains that he is not the same over the last 6 months. His memory is failing him, he has difficulty walking (especially when he initiates walking), and he is incontinent of urine. Which of the following is the most likely diagnosis based on his history?
A) Alzheimer's disease (AD)
B) Parkinson's disease
C) Normal-pressure hydrocephalus (NPH)
D) Pick's disease
E) Progressive supranuclear palsy

Answer and Discussion
The answer is C. NPH is a cause of dementia in the elderly. It may be caused by previous insult to the brain, usually as a result of a subarachnoid hemorrhage or diffuse meningitis that presumably results in scarring of the arachnoid villi over the brain convexities where cerebrospinal fluid (CSF) absorption usually occurs. However, elderly NPH patients seldom have a history of predisposing disease. NPH classically consists of dementia, apraxia of gait, and incontinence ("Wacky, wobbly, wet"), but many patients with these symptoms do not have NPH. Typically, motor weakness and staggering are absent, but initiation of

gait is hesitant—described as a "slipping clutch" or "feet stuck to the floor" gait—and walking eventually occurs. NPH has also been associated with various psychiatric manifestations that are not categorical. NPH should be considered in the differential diagnosis of any new mental status changes in the elderly. Computed tomography (CT) or magnetic resonance imaging (MRI) and a lumbar puncture are necessary for diagnosis. On CT or MRI, the ventricles are dilated. CSF pressure measured by a lumbar puncture is normal. A limited improvement after removing about 50 mL of CSF indicates a better prognosis with shunting. Radiographic or pressure measurements alone do not seem to predict response to shunting. Shunting CSF from the dilated ventricles sometimes results in clinical improvement, but the longer the disease has been present, the less likely shunting will be curative.

> **Additional Reading:** Normal pressure hydrocephalus. In: Basow DS, ed. *UpToDate*. Waltham, MA: UpToDate; 2013.

> **Category:** Neurologic

7. Which of the following is more commonly seen in patients with Lewy body dementia when compared with AD?
A) Hallucinations
B) Lip smacking
C) Tremor
D) Emotional lability
E) Repetitive behavior

Answer and Discussion

The answer is A. Although difficult to know for sure, Lewy body dementia may be the second most common dementia after AD. Lewy bodies are hallmark lesions of degenerating neurons in Parkinson's disease and occur in dementia with or without features of Parkinson's disease. In Lewy body dementia, Lewy bodies may predominate markedly or be intermixed with classic pathologic changes of AD. Symptoms, signs, and course of Lewy body dementia resemble those of AD, except that hallucinations (mainly visual) are more common and patients appear to have an exquisite sensitivity to antipsychotic-induced extrapyramidal adverse effects.

> **Additional Reading:** Clinical features and diagnosis of dementia with Lewy bodies. In: Basow DS, ed. *UpToDate*. Waltham, MA: UpToDate; 2013.

> **Category:** Neurologic

8. A patient with Pick's disease is brought in by his caregiver. She complains that he has become increasingly more apathetic and, at times, sexually inappropriate, and is smacking his lips more frequently. You suspect
A) Elder abuse
B) Medication side effects
C) Development of Klüver–Bucy syndrome
D) Toxin exposure
E) Chronic hypoxia

Answer and Discussion

The answer is C. Pick's disease is a less common form of dementia affecting predominantly the frontal and temporal lobes of the cortex. Patients have prominent apathy and memory disturbances. They may show increased carelessness, poor personal hygiene, and decreased attention span. Although the clinical presentation and CT findings in Pick's disease can be quite distinctive, definitive diagnosis is possible only at autopsy. The Klüver–Bucy syndrome can occur early in the course of Pick's disease, with emotional blunting, hypersexual activity, hyperorality (bulimia and sucking and smacking of

lips), and visual agnosias. A variety of terms are also used to describe the clinical syndrome associated with Pick's disease, including frontal lobe dementia, frontotemporal lobar degeneration, but the preferred terminology is frontotemporal dementia.

> **Additional Reading:** Frontotemporal dementia: clinical features and diagnosis. In: Basow DS, ed. *UpToDate*. Waltham, MA: UpToDate; 2013.

> **Category:** Neurologic

9. A 75-year-old woman presents with rather severe shoulder and hip pain that has been progressively worse over the last 3 months. She complains of morning stiffness and low-grade fevers, malaise, and weight loss. She has no headache or visual disturbance, and electromyogram (EMG) study of her lower extremities was normal. Her labs reveal a normocytic–normochromic anemia and her erythrocyte sedimentation rate (ESR) was found to be 60 mm/h. Appropriate management at this time includes
A) Referral for a temporal artery biopsy
B) Initiation of prednisone
C) Initiation of an NSAID
D) Referral to physical therapy
E) Referral to orthopaedics for consideration of joint replacement

Answer and Discussion

The answer is B. The true prevalence, etiology, and pathogenesis of polymyalgia rheumatica (PMR) are not entirely known. In some, the condition is a manifestation of underlying temporal arteritis. Although most patients are not at significant risk for the complications of temporal arteritis, they should be warned of the possibility and should immediately report such symptoms as headache, visual disturbance, and jaw muscle pain on chewing. PMR usually occurs in patients older than 60 years, and the female:male ratio is 2:1. Onset may be acute or subacute. PMR is characterized by severe pain and stiffness of the neck and shoulders and hips; morning stiffness; stiffness after inactivity; and systemic complaints, such as malaise, fever, depression, and weight loss. There is no selective muscle weakness or evidence of muscle disease on EMG or biopsy. Normochromic–normocytic anemia may be present. In most patients, the ESR is dramatically elevated, often >100 mm/h, usually >50 mm/h. C-reactive protein levels are usually elevated (>0.7 mg/dL) and may be a more sensitive marker of disease activity in certain patients than is ESR. PMR is distinguished from rheumatoid arthritis (RA) by the usual absence of small joint synovitis (although some joint swelling may be present), erosive or destructive disease, rheumatoid factor, or rheumatoid nodules. PMR is differentiated from polymyositis by usually normal muscle enzymes, EMG, and muscle biopsy, as well as by the prominence of pain over weakness. Hypothyroidism can present as myalgia, with abnormal thyroid function tests and elevated creatine kinase (CK). PMR is differentiated from myeloma by the absence of monoclonal gammopathy and from fibromyalgia by the systemic features and elevated ESR. PMR usually responds dramatically to prednisone initiated at doses of at least 15 mg/day. If temporal arteritis is suspected, treatment should be started immediately, with 60 mg/day to prevent blindness. As symptoms subside, corticosteroids are tapered to the lowest effective dose, regardless of ESR. Some patients are able to discontinue corticosteroids in less than 2 years, whereas others require small amounts for years. Rarely do patients respond adequately to salicylates or other NSAIDs.

> **Additional Reading:** Polymyalgia rheumatica. In: Domino F, ed. *The 5-Minute Clinical Consult*. Philadelphia, PA: Lippincott Williams and Wilkins; 2014.

> **Category:** Musculoskeletal system

10. When dealing with a dying patient, the patient's family should
A) Be contacted only when they request it
B) Be thoroughly informed of the physical findings that occur during the dying process
C) Be kept away from the patient to prevent bad associations and memories
D) Be contacted about an autopsy only after death has occurred
E) Never be approached about organ donation until after death has occurred

Answer and Discussion

The answer is B. The family should be thoroughly informed of the changes that the patient's body may exhibit directly before and after death. They should not be surprised by irregular breathing, cool extremities, confusion, a purplish skin color, or somnolence in the last hours. A discussion about autopsy can occur either before or just after death. Families may have strong feelings, either in favor of or against it. The discussion of autopsy should not be left to a covering physician or house officer who has not had previous contact with the family. Discussions about organ donation, if appropriate, should take place before death or immediately after death.

Additional Reading: Palliative care. In: Domino F, ed. *The 5-Minute Clinical Consult*. Philadelphia, PA: Lippincott Williams and Wilkins; 2014.

Category: Patient/population-based care

> The family should be thoroughly informed of the changes that the patient's body may exhibit directly before and after death.

11. In the elderly, a rise in the systolic blood pressure with no change in the diastolic blood pressure most likely suggests
A) Anemia
B) Thyrotoxicosis
C) Aortic insufficiency
D) Stiffening of the arteries
E) None of the above

Answer and Discussion

The answer is D. Stiffened blood vessels also have an impact for blood pressure determination in later life. Systolic blood pressure rises throughout life in Western populations, whereas diastolic pressure peaks and plateaus in middle age and later life. "Normal" blood pressure has been defined by determining the cardiovascular risk associated with a given blood pressure. The presence of an isolated rise in the systolic pressure without a diastolic rise (isolated systolic hypertension) is fairly unique to older patients and, unlike younger patients, does not necessarily imply anemia, thyrotoxicosis, or aortic insufficiency, which can cause a bounding pulse and wide pulse pressure in the young.

Additional Reading: Treatment of hypertension in the elderly patient, particularly isolated systolic hypertension. In: Basow DS, ed. *UpToDate*. Waltham, MA: UpToDate; 2013.

Category: Cardiovascular system

12. Causes for orthostatic hypotension in the elderly include all of the following *except*
A) Declining baroreceptor sensitivity
B) Decreased arterial compliance
C) Increased venous tortuosity
D) Decreased renal sodium conservation
E) Increased plasma volume

Answer and Discussion

The answer is E. Determination of orthostatic hypotension should be routinely performed in geriatric patients. Although a number of factors, such as declining baroreceptor sensitivity, diminished arterial compliance, increased venous tortuosity, decreased renal sodium conservation, and diminished plasma volume, could combine to cause a drop in orthostatic blood pressure among older patients, there is no clear evidence that the pressure drops solely as a function of age. However, a blood pressure drop when changing from the supine to the upright position is common among geriatric patients (possibly as many as 30% of unselected patients may experience a 20 mm Hg or more drop in systolic pressure). Diseases and medications that cause the problem are common offenders.

Additional Reading: Orthostatic hypotension. In: Domino F, ed. *The 5-Minute Clinical Consult*. Philadelphia, PA: Lippincott Williams and Wilkins; 2014. Category: Cardiovascular system.

13. When caring for the elderly, it is important to remember which of the following about measurement of body temperature?
A) Serious infections often adversely affect the patient's temperature.
B) Norms for fever are adjusted on the basis of the patient's age.
C) Temperature in the elderly may not accurately reflect their health status.
D) Temperature variations do not occur in the elderly population on the basis of comparisons with younger patients.
E) Temperatures should not be recorded in the elderly because of their notorious inaccuracy.

Answer and Discussion

The answer is C. Temperature determination in the elderly is the same as it is in other patients. Norms for fever or hypothermia have not been adjusted for age. Elderly people do have a tendency toward disturbances of temperature regulation (hypothermia or hyperthermia). It is possible that some elderly patients, like others, may present with serious infections that do not produce much temperature rise.

Additional Reading: Evaluation of infection in the older adult. In: Basow DS, ed. *UpToDate*. Waltham, MA: UpToDate; 2013.

Category: Nonspecific system

14. Which one of the following is true regarding respiratory rate in the elderly?
A) Subtle differences in age-adjusted respiratory rate are present and should be adjusted for in the evaluation of the elderly patient.
B) Respiratory rates in the elderly are 5% higher than age-adjusted controls.
C) Respiratory rates and patterns do not change as the patient ages.
D) Elevated respiratory rates do not represent concern in elderly patients.
E) Respiratory rates do not correlate with disease in elderly patients.

Answer and Discussion

The answer is C. Respiratory rate and patterns do not change significantly with age. An elevated respiratory rate may be a subtle clue to a serious medical illness (e.g., acidosis, hypoxia, central nervous system [CNS] disturbance) and should be detected and evaluated as in any other patient.

Additional Reading: The geriatric assessment. *Am Fam Physician*. 2011;83(1):48–56.

Category: Respiratory system

15. While examining a relatively healthy 65-year-old woman for her yearly well-woman exam, you note a palpable right ovary on pelvic exam. The remainder of her examination is entirely normal. The most likely diagnosis is
A) Cecal fecalith
B) Polycystic ovary syndrome
C) Normal variant
D) Ovarian carcinoma
E) Fibroid tumor

Answer and Discussion

The answer is D. The presence of a palpable ovary in an elderly woman should raise a suspicion of some pathology, especially malignancy. Given the enlarged ovary, it is likely that she has an ovarian carcinoma, which often starts silently, not showing signs until later stages. The average age of diagnosis is about 63 years. Polycystic ovary syndrome would include other findings (e.g., acne, hirsutism, menstrual irregularities, and infertility) and is typically diagnosed at a much younger age. Fecaliths are often associated with acute illnesses such as appendicitis, intussusception, and diverticulitis.

> **Additional Reading:** Ovarian cancer. In: Domino F, ed. *The 5-Minute Clinical Consult.* Philadelphia, PA: Lippincott Williams and Wilkins; 2014.

> **Category:** Reproductive system

16. From admission to discharge, what percentage of elderly patients lose independence in one or more of the basic activities of daily living?
A) Approximately 1% to 3%
B) 10%
C) 25% to 35%
D) 50%
E) More than 75%

Answer and Discussion

The answer is C. From hospital admission to discharge, 25% to 35% of elderly patients lose independence in one or more of the basic activities of daily living. The loss of independent functioning during hospitalization is associated with important complications including prolonged length of hospital stay, greater risk of institutionalization, and higher mortality rates.

> **Additional Reading:** The geriatric assessment. *Am Fam Physician.* 2011;83(1):48–56.

> **Category:** Nonspecific system

17. Factors known to precipitate delirium in elderly hospitalized patients include use of restraints, presence of a bladder catheter, malnutrition, and which of the following?
A) Recent X-ray or computed axial tomography (CAT) scan
B) Taking three or more medications
C) Family history of dementia
D) Loud noise
E) Visit from close family members

Answer and Discussion

The answer is B. Dementia is the single most important risk factor for the development of delirium or acute confused state. Delirium is found at admission or during hospitalization in about 25% of elderly patients admitted for acute medical illnesses. Patients with baseline dementia and severe systemic illness are predisposed to delirium. Factors known to precipitate delirium include the use of physical restraints, the addition of more than three medications to the regimen, the use of a bladder catheter, malnutrition, and any iatrogenic event.

> **Additional Reading:** Delirium. In: Domino F, ed. *The 5-Minute Clinical Consult.* Philadelphia, PA: Lippincott Williams and Wilkins; 2014.

> **Category:** Neurologic

18. A 65-year-old man presents to your office complaining of a right-hand tremor. The patient reports the tremor is worse with sustained positions and stressful situations. Surprisingly, a shot of scotch makes the tremor better. He also reports a positive family history for tremors. There are no signs of bradykinesia or rigidity. The most likely diagnosis is
A) Parkinson's disease
B) Essential tremor
C) Huntington's disease
D) Caffeine withdrawal
E) Alcohol withdrawal

Answer and Discussion

The answer is B. Essential tremor is the most common movement disorder. This postural tremor may have its onset anywhere between the second and sixth decades of life, and its prevalence increases with age. It is slowly progressive over a period of years. An essential tremor is characterized by a rapid, fine tremor that is made worse with sustained positions. The frequency of essential tremor is 4 to 11 Hz, depending on which body segment is affected. Proximal segments are affected at lower frequencies, and distal segments are affected at higher frequencies. Although typically a postural tremor, essential tremor may occur at rest in severe and very advanced cases. It most commonly affects the hands but can also affect the head, voice, tongue, and legs. It usually affects patients older than 50 years. The tremor may be intensified by stress, anxiety, excessive fatigue, drugs (e.g., caffeine, alcohol withdrawal, steroids), or thyroid disorders. In many cases, the patient may report relief with alcohol use and a positive family history for tremors. Senile tremors tend to increase with age. Parkinson's disease is differentiated by the presence of a pill-rolling tremor at rest, masked face, bradykinesias, and rigidity. Parkinson's also shows a favorable response to the administration of L-dopamine and does not improve with the use of alcohol. Treatment of essential tremors involves the treatment of the underlying disorder and the use of propranolol (Inderal), or primidone (Mysoline). Primidone may be preferred because of the exercise intolerance associated with the high-dose β-blockers. Some data suggest newer antiseizure agents (topirimate, gabapentin) have efficacy. Patients who have a very-low-amplitude rapid tremor are generally more responsive to these agents than those who have a slower tremor with greater amplitude. Patients who have a tremor of the head and voice may also be more resistant to treatment than do patients with an essential tremor of the hands. In severe cases, surgery may be considered.

> **Additional Reading:** Differentiation and Diagnosis of Tremor. *Am Fam Physician.* 2011 Mar 15;83(6):697–702

> **Category:** Neurologic

19. Which of the following is indicated in the initial workup of urinary incontinence in the elderly?
A) Voiding and bowel diary
B) Urodynamic studies
C) Renal ultrasound
D) Urine cytology
E) Intravenous pyelogram

Answer and Discussion

The answer is A. Urinary incontinence is often seen in the elderly. In most cases, the evaluation of urinary incontinence requires only a history (including frequency of urination and bowel movements, fluid and caffeine intake, and medication review), physical examination, urinalysis and culture, and, if no cause is easily identified, the measurement of postvoid residual urine volume. The initial purposes of the evaluation are to identify conditions requiring referral or specialized workup and to detect and treat reversible causes that may be present. Causes may include infection, atrophic urethritis, pelvic floor weakness (usually related to previous childbirth), medications (e.g., diuretics), altered mental status, or overflow incontinence related to obstruction (e.g., fecal impaction, prostatic hypertrophy). If the patient does not require referral and a reversible cause is not identified, the next step is to categorize the patient's symptoms as typical of urge or stress incontinence and treat the patient accordingly. *Urge incontinence* results from bladder contractions that overwhelm the ability of the cerebral centers to inhibit them. These uncontrollable contractions can occur because of inflammation or irritation within the bladder resulting from calculi, malignancy, infection, or atrophic vaginitis–urethritis. They can also occur when the brain centers that inhibit bladder contractions are impaired by neurologic conditions such as stroke, Parkinson's disease, or dementia; drugs such as hypnotics or narcotics; or metabolic disorders such as hypoxemia and encephalopathy. *Stress incontinence* is caused by a malfunction of the urethral sphincter that causes urine to leak from the bladder when intra-abdominal pressure increases, such as during coughing or sneezing. Classic or genuine stress incontinence is caused by pelvic prolapse, urethral hypermobility, or displacement of the urethra and bladder neck from their normal anatomic alignment. Stress incontinence can also occur as a result of intrinsic sphincter deficiency in which the sphincter is weak because of a congenital condition or denervation resulting from α-adrenergic-blocking drugs, surgical trauma, or radiation damage. Treatment involves the strengthening of pelvic floor muscles with Kegel exercises, voiding schedules, and biofeedback. Tolterodine (Detrol) and extended-release oxybutynin chloride (Ditropan XL) are used as a first-line treatment option for overactive bladder, which contributes to incontinence because of favorable side-effect profiles. A trial of therapy may be attempted before formal urodynamic studies are ordered. If treatment fails or a presumptive diagnosis of urge or stress incontinence cannot be reached, the final step would be to perform more sophisticated tests or refer the patient for testing to define the cause and determine the best treatment.

Additional Reading: Incontinence, urinary adult female. In: Domino F, ed. *The 5-Minute Clinical Consult.* Philadelphia, PA: Lippincott Williams and Wilkins; 2014.

Category: Nephrologic system

20. Increasing age is associated with many effects on the kidney. These effects include which of the following?
A) Increase in renal size
B) Increase in serum creatinine
C) Decreased glomerular filtration rate
D) Increase in renal blood flow
E) Decreased threshold for glucose

Answer and Discussion

The answer is C. Many changes occur within the kidney as a result of increasing age. There is a gradual decrease in renal size; a decrease in renal blood flow; and, most importantly, a decrease in glomerular filtration rate, which can have a significant effect on drug metabolism. In most cases, serum creatinine remains essentially unchanged.

In many cases, the doses of renal-metabolized medications need to be reduced in patients with decreased creatinine clearance. Additionally, the renal threshold for glucose increases with increasing age, and there is a decrease in maximal urinary concentration.

Additional Reading: Reducing the risk of adverse drug events in older adults. *Am Fam Physician.* 2013;87(5):331–336.

Category: Nephrologic system

Many changes occur within the kidney as a result of increasing age. There is a gradual decrease in renal size; a decrease in renal blood flow; and, most importantly, a decrease in glomerular filtration rate, which can have a significant effect on drug metabolism. In most cases, serum creatinine remains essentially unchanged.

21. When comparing middle-aged patients with hyperthyroidism to elderly patients with hyperthyroidism, elderly patients are more likely to have
A) Restlessness
B) Hyperactive appearance
C) Atrial fibrillation
D) Weight gain
E) Goiter

Answer and Discussion

The answer is C. The most common cause of hyperthyroidism in the elderly is Graves' disease or toxic diffuse goiter. Graves' disease is an autoimmune disorder resulting from the action of a thyroid-stimulating antibody on thyroid-stimulating hormone receptors. Thyroid-stimulating hormone receptor antibodies are detectable in the serum of approximately 80% to 100% of untreated patients with Graves' disease. Hyperthyroidism in the elderly is often more difficult to diagnose than in younger patients. Only 25% of those affected present with symptoms typical in younger patients, such as restlessness and hyperactive appearance. Elderly patients are more likely to show weight loss, new-onset atrial fibrillation, and withdrawal or depression. Other complications include cardiac failure, angina, MI, and osteoporosis with an increased risk of bone fractures. Older patients have a lower incidence of goiter. Behavioral changes in younger patients include anxiety, emotional lability, insomnia, lack of concentration, restlessness, and tremulousness. In contrast, elderly patients show apathy, lethargy, pseudodementia, and depressed moods.

Additional Reading: Atrial fibrillation and atrial flutter. In: Domino F, ed. *The 5-Minute Clinical Consult.* Philadelphia, PA: Lippincott Williams and Wilkins; 2014.

Category: Endocrine system

22. Which of the following is a risk factor for the development of pressure ulcers in hospitalized patients?
A) Blanchable erythema
B) Lymphocytosis
C) Increased body weight
D) Moist skin
E) None of the above

Answer and Discussion

The answer is E. Pressure ulcers occur more often in patients who have nonblanchable erythema, lymphopenia, immobility, dry skin, and decreased body weight. Patients with these risk factors need aggressive mobilization to avoid developing pressure sores.

> **Additional Reading:** Pressure ulcers. In: Domino F, ed. *The 5-Minute Clinical Consult.* Philadelphia, PA: Lippincott Williams and Wilkins; 2014.

> Category: Integumentary

23. When assessing for urinary retention, which of the following postvoid residuals (PVR) represents the *threshold* for an abnormal finding?
A) 25 mL
B) 50 mL
C) 100 mL
D) 200 mL
E) 500 mL

Answer and Discussion

The answer is B. In general, a patient should be able to void 80% of the total bladder volume and have a PVR of less than 50 mL immediately after emptying the bladder. High PVR volumes are suggestive of either detrusor weakness or obstruction.

> **Additional Reading:** Urodynamic evaluation of women with incontinence. In: Basow DS, ed. *UpToDate.* Waltham, MA: UpToDate; 2013.

> Category: Nephrologic system

24. An 80-year-old man is brought in by his wife. She complains her husband has had a noticeable change in his personality. He is impulsive and at times inappropriate with his behavior. Although he has difficulty naming objects, his memory, ability to calculate, and his visuospatial skills appear to be intact. The most likely diagnosis is
A) AD
B) Pick's disease
C) Parkinson's disease
D) Wilson's disease
E) Lewy body dementia

Answer and Discussion

The answer is B. Pick's disease and other frontotemporal dementias (FTD) are a heterogeneous group of disorders that share several clinical features with AD such as rate of progression and duration. Many frontotemporal dementias patients are also aphasic and manifest preserved motor integrity. The language disturbance characteristic of Pick's disease initially includes anomia, but there is a more stereotyped and perseverative verbal output than that found in AD. Unlike AD, in the early stages of frontotemporal dementias, memory, calculation, and visuospatial function are relatively well preserved. The most striking feature of this disorder is an extravagant change in the patient's personality, including disinhibition, impulsivity, inappropriate jocularity, and intrusiveness. Patients with Parkinson's disease with dementia typically show deficits on tests of executive function, visuospatial abilities, and verbal fluency. Symptoms in Wilson's disease usually appear between 6 and 20 years of age, and although cases in older people have been described, psychiatric symptoms are accompanied by neurological symptoms. Lewy body dementia is often accompanied by delirium.

> **Additional Reading:** Frontotemporal dementia: clinical features and diagnosis. In: Basow DS, ed. *UpToDate.* Waltham, MA: UpToDate; 2013.

> Category: Neurologic

25. Which of the following medications used in the treatment of benign prostatic hypertrophy (BPH) works by inhibiting the transformation of testosterone to dihydrotestosterone?
A) Finasteride (Proscar)
B) Doxazosin (Cardura)
C) Terazosin (Hytrin)
D) Tamsulosin (Flomax)
E) Prazosin (Minipress)

Answer and Discussion

The answer is A. BPH is a condition associated with enlargement of the prostate gland that gives rise to obstructive urinary symptoms. The condition affects men older than 50 years and is characterized as adenomatous hyperplasia. Enlargement of the gland is usually asymptomatic until bladder outlet obstruction occurs. Symptoms reported by patients include decreased force and caliber of the urinary stream, incomplete voiding, hesitancy, frequency, overflow incontinence, retention, nocturia, and dribbling after urination. Acute urinary retention may be precipitated by prolonged attempts to retain urine, immobilization, exposure to cold, anesthetics, anticholinergic and sympathomimetic drugs, or ingestion of alcohol. Physical examination consistent with BPH shows an enlarged bladder and an enlarged prostate, which is usually firm and symmetrical. The median furrow may be absent. Hard nodules found within the gland are more worrisome for cancer. Laboratory findings with BPH may show an elevated prostate-specific antigen (PSA), usually <10 ng/dL, and elevated creatine when there is obstruction severe enough to lead to renal impairment. Postvoid residuals are usually large and may predispose to infection. The most common cause of hematuria in older men is BPH. Medical treatment involves the use of 5-alpha reductase inhibitors finasteride or dutasteride, which may help to shrink the prostate by blocking the transformation of testosterone to dihydrotestosterone. The drawbacks of the 5-alpha reductase inhibitors are that they require 6 to 12 months to work and regrowth of the prostate occurs after the discontinuation of the medication. Other medications that help with voiding dysfunction are the α-adrenergic blockers prazosin, doxazosin, and terazosin, which are also used in the treatment of hypertension. Tamsulosin is a newer α-adrenergic blocker that does not significantly affect blood pressure. Definitive therapy is surgical. Although sexual potency and continence are usually retained, approximately 5% to 10% of patients experience some postsurgical problems. Transurethral resection of the prostate is preferred. Larger prostates (usually >75 g) may require open surgery using the suprapubic or retropubic approach, permitting enucleation of the adenomatous tissue from within the surgical capsule. The incidence of impotence and incontinence is much higher than after transurethral resection of the prostate. Alternative surgical approaches include intraurethral stents, microwave thermotherapy, high-intensity focused ultrasound thermotherapy, laser ablation, electrovaporization, and radiofrequency vaporization.

> **Additional Reading:** Dutasteride (Avodart) with Tamsulosin (Flomax) for benign prostatic hyperplasia. *Med Lett Drugs Ther.* 2008;50(1296):79–80.

> Category: Reproductive system

26. Which of the following statements regarding osteoporosis is true?
A) Routine screening of women older than 65 years is not recommended.
B) Dual-energy X-ray absorptiometry (DEXA) scans result in more radiation exposure than qualitative CT.
C) T scores are used to diagnose osteoporosis.
D) Plain X-rays are a good diagnostic test for assessment of osteoporosis.
E) Medicare will not pay for bone-density examination.

Answer and Discussion

The answer is C. Osteoporosis afflicts 75 million persons in the United States, Europe, and Japan and results in more than 1.3 million fractures annually in the United States. Osteoporosis is defined as the loss of bone below the density for mechanical support. It occurs when there is a loss of bony matrix and mineral composition of the bone, which is defined as osteopenia. Those most commonly affected are white and Asian postmenopausal women. Bones typically affected include vertebrae, wrist, humerus, hip, and tibia. Risk factors include menopausal state, positive family history, small bone structure, decreased calcium intake, lack of exercise, smoking, excessive alcohol use, and chronic steroid use. Physicians should recommend bone mineral density testing to all women at age 65, postmenopausal women who present with fractures, and women 60 and older who have multiple risk factors. The most widely used techniques of assessing bone mineral density are DEXA and quantitative CT. Of these methods, DEXA is the most precise and the diagnostic measure of choice. Quantitative CT is the most sensitive method but results in substantially greater radiation exposure than DEXA. Bone densitometry reports provide a T score (the number of standard deviations above or below the mean bone mineral density for gender and race matched to young controls) or a Z score (comparing the patient with a population adjusted for age, gender, and race). Osteoporosis is the classification for a T score of more than 2.5 standard deviations below the gender-adjusted mean for normal young adults at peak bone mass. A T score of −1.0 to −2.5 represents osteopenia. Z scores are not used for the diagnosis. Medicare pays for bone-density examination at age 65 for initial diagnosis and for follow-up after 24 months. Other indications for screening at an earlier age include when estrogen deficiency is present in a woman at clinical risk for osteoporosis, vertebral abnormalities are present (e.g., osteopenia, vertebral fractures, osteoporosis), the patient has been exposed to long-term (more than 3 months' duration) glucocorticoid therapy, the patient has primary hyperparathyroidism, or the patient requires monitoring to assess response to osteoporosis drug therapy. Plain X-rays are not adequate for the detection of osteoporosis because as much as 30% of bone mass can be lost before it becomes apparent on X-ray. More advanced cases may reveal decreased radiodensity of vertebrae, anterior wedging of vertebrae, and compression fractures. Prevention involves the use of vitamin D supplementation, exercise, and avoidance of smoking and heavy alcohol use. Thiazide diuretics may also help to decrease urinary excretion of calcium in patients with secondary hyperparathyroidism. In established cases, the bisphosphonates (alendronate [Fosamax] and risedronate [Actonel]) and a selective estrogen receptor modulator (SERM) (raloxifene [Evista]) are used for treatment. Monoclonal antibodies that inhibit osteoclast formation (Denosumab) are new to the market, effective, but very costly. Additionally, calcitonin (Calcimar) may also be used to prevent vertebral fractures; it does not appear to prevent nonvertebral fractures.

> Additional Reading: Osteoporosis. In: Domino F, ed. *The 5-Minute Clinical Consult*. Philadelphia, PA: Lippincott Williams and Wilkins; 2014.

Category: Endocrine system

27. Which of the following is associated with reducing the risk of falls in elderly patients?
A) Vitamin C
B) Vitamin D
C) Folate
D) Vitamin B_{12}
E) Calcium

Answer and Discussion

The answer is B. Falls are a major cause of injury-related visits to emergency departments in the United States and the primary cause of accidental deaths in persons older than 65 years. The mortality rate for falls increases dramatically with age in both sexes and in all racial and ethnic groups. Falls can be an indication of poor health and declining function, and they are often associated with significant morbidity. More than 90% of hip fractures occur as a result of falls, with most of these fractures occurring in persons older than 70 years of age. Risk factors for falls in the elderly include increasing age, arthritis, medication use (more than four medications, including tricyclic antidepressants, neuroleptics, benzodiazepines, and type IA antiarrythmics), cognitive impairment (dementia and depression), and sensory deficits. Outpatient evaluation of a patient who has fallen includes a focused history with an emphasis on medications, a directed physical examination, and tests of postural control and overall physical function. Treatment is directed at the underlying cause of the fall, with the goal to return the patient to baseline function. Vitamin D deficiency has been associated with an increased risk of falls, and empiric supplementation can reduce the risk.

> Additional Reading: Management of falls in older persons: a prescription for prevention. *Am Fam Physician*. 2011;84(11): 1267–1276.

Category: Nonspecific system

28. Which one of the following statements about presbycusis is true?
A) Women are more commonly affected than men.
B) Low-frequency tones are affected first.
C) The condition cannot be treated with amplification.
D) The condition can lead to depression.
E) The condition does not affect the ability to interpret speech.

Answer and Discussion

The answer is D. Presbycusis, a progressive, high-frequency hearing loss, is the most common cause of hearing impairment in geriatric patients. Exposure to loud noises and genetic factors play a role in the etiology. Men are more commonly affected with sensory neural hearing loss. It usually begins after 20 years of age and affects the high-frequency tones first (18 to 20 kHz). Patients often report trouble hearing normal conversations in crowds. This type of hearing loss decreases the ability to interpret speech, which can lead to a decreased ability to communicate and a subsequent increased risk for social isolation and depression. Hearing loss in the elderly can also adversely affect physical, emotional, and cognitive well-being. Questionnaires such as the Hearing Handicap Inventory for the Elderly–Screening Version have been shown to accurately identify persons with hearing impairment. The reference standard for establishing hearing impairment, however, remains pure tone audiometry, which can be performed in the physician's office. Combining the Hearing Handicap Inventory for the Elderly–Screening Version questionnaire with pure tone audiometry has been shown to improve screening effectiveness. Appropriate interventions include periodic screening to provide early detection of hearing impairment, cautious use or avoidance of ototoxic drugs, and support for obtaining and continued use of the hearing aids.

> Additional Reading: Presbycusis. In: Domino F, ed. *The 5-Minute Clinical Consult*. Philadelphia, PA: Lippincott Williams and Wilkins; 2014.

Category: Special sensory

🔵 Presbycusis, a progressive, high-frequency hearing loss, is the most common cause of hearing impairment in geriatric patients.

29. Which of the following statements is true regarding the abdominal aortic aneurysms (AAAs)?
A) Screening has not been shown to be cost effective.
B) CT is the test recommended for screening of AAA.
C) All women and men who are 65 years or older should be screened once for AAA.
D) One-time screening with ultrasound for AAA in men 65 to 75 years of age who have ever smoked is recommended.
E) Ultrasound is specific but not sensitive for the screening of AAA.

Answer and Discussion

The answer is D. Ultrasound is the standard imaging tool for the detection of an AAA. In experienced hands, it has a sensitivity and specificity approaching 100% and 96%, respectively, for the detection of infrarenal AAA. The U.S. Preventive Services Task Force (USPSTF) recommends screening for AAA in patients who have a relatively high risk of dying from an aneurysm. Major risk factors include age 65 years or older, male sex, and smoking at least 100 cigarettes in a lifetime. The guideline recommends one-time screening with ultrasound for AAA in men 65 to 75 years of age who have ever smoked. No recommendation was made for or against screening in men 65 to 75 years of age who have never smoked, and it recommended against screening women. Men with a strong family history of AAA should be counseled about the risks and benefits of screening as they approach 65 years of age.

> Additional Reading: Screening for abdominal aortic aneurysm. *US Preventive Service Task Force*, 2005 update. From: http://www.uspreventiveservicestaskforce.org/uspstf/uspsasco.htm.

> Category: Cardiovascular system

30. The threshold for considering elective repair of an AAA is
A) 4.5 cm
B) 5.5 cm
C) 6.5 cm
D) 7.5 cm
E) 8.5 cm

Answer and Discussion

The answer is B. Patients with aneurysms >5.5 cm should be considered for elective AAA repair. Because most clinically diagnosed AAAs are repaired, their long-term natural history is difficult to predict. The 1-year incidence of rupture is 9% for aneurysms 5.5 to 6.0 cm in diameter, 10% for 6.0 to 6.9 cm, and 33% for AAAs of 7.0 cm or more. Patients with an aneurysm <5.5 cm in diameter should have follow-up serial ultrasounds. Smoking is the biggest risk factor for the development of aneurysms.

> Additional Reading: Abdominal aortic aneurysm. *Am Fam Physician*. 2006;73:1198–1206.

> Category: Cardiovascular system

31. Which of the following classes of drugs has shown modest improvement in cognitive symptoms associated with AD?
A) Cholinesterase inhibitors
B) Dopamine agonists
C) Norepinephrine antagonist
D) Serotonin reuptake inhibitors
E) None of the above

Answer and Discussion

The answer is A. Treatment with cholinesterase inhibitors can provide mild improvement of symptoms, temporary stabilization of cognition, or reduction in the rate of cognitive decline in some patients with mild to moderate AD. Approximately 20% to 35% of patients treated with these agents exhibit a 7-point improvement on neuropsychologic tests (equivalent to 1 year's decline and representing a 5% to 15% benefit over placebo). Before treatment is started, it is important to inform the family of the expected (modest) benefits of cholinesterase inhibitors. Some cholinesterase inhibitors include donepezil (Aricept), rivastigmine (Exelon), galantamine (Reminyl), and tacrine (Cognex). These agents raise acetylcholine levels in the brain by inhibiting acetylcholinesterase.

> Additional Reading: Drugs for cognitive loss and dementia. *Treat Guidel Med Lett*. 2010;8(91):19–24.

> Category: Neurologic

32. Which of the following is most consistent with signs and symptoms of retinal detachment?
A) Pain associated with the eye
B) Seeing flashes of light
C) Photophobia
D) Excessive tearing
E) Conjunctival injection

Answer and Discussion

The answer is B. Retinal detachment usually affects individuals older than 50 years. It does not cause pain or erythema of the eye. Bilateral spontaneous detachments are present in as much as 25% of those affected. Retinal detachment can be caused by retinal tears, retinal holes, or by other causes, including ocular melanoma and metastatic tumors. Warning symptoms include floaters, flashes of light (photopsia), or blurred vision. As detachment progresses, the patient may report a "curtain or shade coming down" phenomenon. Macular involvement leads to central visual loss and a worse prognosis. Patients suspected of retinal detachment should undergo emergent ophthalmologic evaluation. Prognosis is best if there is no macular involvement. Without treatment, total detachment usually occurs within 6 months. Treatment of retinal tears or holes is accomplished with laser photocoagulation, cryotherapy, or a scleral buckle. Uncomplicated retinal detachment can be repaired in up to 90% of cases.

> Additional Reading: Retinal detachment. In: Domino F, ed. *The 5-Minute Clinical Consult*. Philadelphia, PA: Lippincott Williams and Wilkins; 2014.

> Category: Special sensory

33. Which of the following statements about pharmacokinetics in the elderly is true?
A) Body fat stores decrease, and, thus, fat-soluble medications have decreased distribution, and there is less risk for toxicity.
B) The glomerular filtration rate is reduced in the elderly, which can lead to a decreased clearance of medication and an increased risk for toxicity.
C) The volume of body water is increased in the elderly, which may require increased dosages of water-soluble medications.
D) Accumulation of active metabolites does not occur in the elderly secondary to rapid clearance.
E) Hepatic metabolism of drugs increases as patients age.

Answer and Discussion

The answer is B. In the United States, approximately two-thirds of persons 65 years or older take prescription and nonprescription (over-the-counter) medications. Women take more drugs than men because they are, on average, older, and they use more psychoactive and anti-arthritic drugs. At any given time, an average older person uses four to five prescription drugs, two over-the-counter drugs, and fills 12 to 17 prescriptions a year. The frail elderly use the most drugs. Drug use is greater in hospitals and nursing homes than in the community; typically, a nursing home resident receives seven or eight drugs. Changes that occur in the elderly often affect the medications that are administered to them. As patients age, they increase their body stores of fat. Because of this, fat-soluble medications have increased distribution and a longer half-life in the body. Although expression of drug-metabolizing enzymes in the cytochrome P450 systems does not appear to decline with age, the overall hepatic metabolism of many drugs by these enzymes is reduced. The glomerular filtration rate in the elderly is also reduced, which can lead to a decreased clearance of medications and an increased risk for toxicity. The volume of body water is also reduced in the elderly, and the administration of water-soluble medications can lead to toxicity with some medications. All these changes must be considered when administering medication to the elderly. Increased sensitivity with aging must be considered when drugs that can have serious adverse effects are used. These drugs include morphine, pentazocine, warfarin, ACE inhibitors, diazepam (especially given parenterally), and levodopa. Some drugs' effects are reduced with aging (e.g., glyburide, β-blockers) and should also be used with caution because serious dose-related toxicity can still occur and signs of toxicity may be delayed. Many drugs produce active metabolites in clinically relevant concentrations. Examples are some benzodiazepines (e.g., diazepam, chlordiazepoxide), tertiary amine antidepressants (e.g., amitriptyline, imipramine), antipsychotics (e.g., chlorpromazine, thioridazine; not haloperidol), and opioid analgesics (e.g., morphine, meperidine, propoxyphene). The accumulation of active metabolites (e.g., N-acetylprocainamide, morphine-6-glucuronide) can cause toxicity in the elderly as a result of age-related decreases in renal clearance; toxicity is likely to be severe in those with renal disease.

> **Additional Reading:** Reducing the risk of adverse drug events in older adults. *Am Fam Physician.* 2013;87(5):331–336.

> **Category:** Nonspecific system

34. Which one of the following features can usually distinguish delirium from dementia?
A) There is a lack of long-term memory loss with delirium.
B) The time span over which symptoms develop differs.
C) There is an absence of long-term memory loss with dementia.
D) There is a loss of orientation with delirium.
E) None of the above.

Answer and Discussion

The answer is B. Delirium is a condition that usually develops in an acute situation (over a period of hours to days) and is characterized by confusion, agitation, loss of orientation, lack of attention, hallucinations, paranoia, disturbed sleep–wake cycles, and loss of perception. The condition is a transient global disorder of cognition and consciousness. The delirious patient may also have psychomotor and emotional disturbances. In most patients, delirium due to a medical disease is reversible with treatment of the underlying condition. The symptoms of delirium tend to fluctuate in their course. The etiology may be related to toxin exposure, withdrawal from narcotics or alcohol, medications, vitamin deficiencies, infection, trauma, or structural

abnormalities affecting the brain (e.g., tumor, abscess). The best treatment is to correct the underlying cause. Dementia, however, is a slow, progressive condition that may take months to years to develop.

> **Additional Reading:** Delirium. In: Domino F, ed. *The 5-Minute Clinical Consult.* Philadelphia, PA: Lippincott Williams and Wilkins; 2014.

> **Category:** Neurologic

35. Which of the following is the predominant component of dementia?
A) Confusion
B) Anxiety
C) Depression
D) Memory loss
E) Paranoia

Answer and Discussion

The answer is D. Dementia is a condition characterized by the loss of intellectual abilities and the impairment of usually short-term memory. Most patients are older than 65 years. Dementia usually has a slow, progressive, and remitting course. The condition is characterized by a decline in intellectual functioning to the extent that the patient is unable to perform the usual activities of daily living. Memory deficit is a predominant component of dementia, and the deterioration of intellectual functioning may occur over months to years. Dementing diseases in the elderly include AD (now known as *dementia of the Alzheimer's type*), vascular dementia (previously called *multiinfarct dementia*), and other disorders. The precise mechanisms of the dementias are generally unclear, and no effective cures are available. There is usually no history of prior psychiatric illness, and patients affected typically perform poorly on cognitive tests. *Sundowning* (confusion, loss of orientation) at night in unfamiliar surroundings is common. As many as 15% of dementias are reversible, and, thus, physiologic causes must be ruled out. Treatable causes include medication side effects, depression, hypothyroidism, dehydration, infection, schizophrenia, Wernicke–Korsakoff syndrome, liver or kidney failure, electrolyte abnormalities, hypoglycemia, vitamin deficiency (e.g., vitamin B_{12}), subdural hematoma, NPH, neoplasm, and stroke. The workup should be individualized but in many cases consists of electrolytes, complete blood count, thyroid-stimulating hormone, vitamin B_{12}, Venereal Disease Research Laboratory (VDRL), liver function tests, ESR, urine and plasma heavy metal screens, electrocardiogram, CT or MRI of the head, chest X-ray, electroencephalogram, O_2 saturation, and lumbar puncture.

> **Additional Reading:** Evaluation of cognitive impairment and dementia. In: Basow DS, ed. *UpToDate.* Waltham, MA: UpToDate; 2013.

> **Category:** Neurologic

36. Which of the following is true regarding the use of tacrine (Cognex)?
A) The drug has been shown to cause renal failure and thus serum creatinine must be monitored.
B) The drug is associated with hepatotoxicity and requires the monitoring of liver function tests.
C) The drug is favored over others in its class due to its once-daily dosing.
D) The drug has an exceptionally long half-life.
E) Tacrine is considered a first-line agent in the treatment of AD.

Answer and Discussion

The answer is B. The pharmacologic characteristics and side effects of tacrine make it a second-line agent. Unlike the newer cholinesterase inhibitors, tacrine causes elevation of liver enzyme levels in 40%

of treated patients; thus, biweekly liver tests are necessary during the period of dosage escalations and every 3 months thereafter. Because tacrine has a short half-life, it must be administered four times daily.

> **Additional Reading:** Drugs for cognitive loss and dementia. *Treat Guidel Med Lett.* 2010;8(91):19–24.

> Category: Neurologic

37. Which of the following is the most common cause of cognitive impairment in elderly patients?
A) Alcohol-induced encephalopathy
B) Multi-infarct dementia
C) Alzheimer's Disease
D) Parkinson's associated dementia
E) Pick's disease

Answer and Discussion

The answer is C. Alzheimer's Disease is the most common cause of cognitive impairment in elderly persons, with an incidence that doubles every 5 years after the age of 60 years. This disease afflicts approximately 4 million Americans and is estimated to cost the U.S. economy $60 billion annually.

> **Additional Reading:** Evaluation of cognitive impairment and dementia. In: Basow DS, ed. *UpToDate.* Waltham, MA: UpToDate; 2013.

> Category: Neurologic

38. Which of the following is not commonly seen in Lewy body dementia?
A) Dementia
B) Delirium
C) Visual hallucinations
D) Bradykinesia
E) Tremor

Answer and Discussion

The answer is E. A useful mnemonic to remember the cardinal features of dementia with Lewy bodies is DDaVP (Dementia, Delirium and Visual hallucinations with Parkinsonism). Although bradykinesia, rigidity, and falls are common to those affected, tremor often is absent in dementia with Lewy bodies.

> **Additional Reading:** Dementia with Lewy bodies: an emerging disease. *Am Fam Physician.* 2006;73:1223–1230.

> Category: Neurologic

> A useful mnemonic to remember the cardinal features of dementia with Lewy bodies is DDaVP: Dementia, Delirium and Visual hallucinations with Parkinsonism.

39. The leading cause of injury-related visits (in patients older than 65 years) to the emergency room in the United States is which of the following?
A) Motor vehicle accidents
B) Falls
C) Elder abuse
D) Exposure to extremes of temperature
E) Self-induced injury related to depression

Answer and Discussion

The answer is B. Falls affecting the elderly are a major cause of morbidity. Falls are the leading cause of injury-related visits to emergency

departments in the United States and the primary etiology of accidental deaths in persons older than 65 years. They may result in severe injury, including hip or other bone fractures; bruises; and subdural hematomas as well as dehydration and hypothermia if the patient is not found. Many factors play a role in the cause of falls, including muscle weakness, lack of coordination, poor vision, joint stiffness, autonomic dysfunction, increased reaction time, dementia or delirium, and medications. The physician should always search for precipitating causes such as stroke, cardiac arrhythmias, hypoglycemia, orthostasis, or environmental causes. Precautions should include supplementation of vitamin D 800 IU/day, proper lighting, short-pile carpet, railings, and walkers or canes for those with gait disorders. A visit to the patient's home or living environment may be helpful in determining dangerous conditions. All reversible problems should be corrected. When the cause of a fall is not determined or a patient remains at high risk for falls, referral to a falls-prevention program may be warranted.

> **Additional Reading:** The U.S. Preventive Services Task Force (USPSTF) recommendations on prevention of falls in community-dwelling older adults. May 2012. From; http://www.uspreventiveservicestaskforce.org/uspstf/uspsfalls.htm.

> Category: Patient/population-based care

40. Which one of the following laboratory findings is seen with aging?
A) Increase in creatinine clearance
B) Increased aspartate aminotransferase
C) Decreased serum creatinine
D) Decreased incidence of false-positive rapid plasma reagin tests
E) Increase in fasting glucose levels

Answer and Discussion

The answer is E. For the most part, many laboratory normal values remain the same for elderly patients. However, there are some exceptions. With increasing age, there is usually

1. decline in renal function, as is evident by a 10% decrease in creatinine clearance per 10 years after 40 years of age;
2. increase in fasting blood glucose (1 mg/dL for every 10 years), although most patients remain within the normal limit values;
3. increased alkaline phosphatase;
4. increased incidence of false-positive rapid plasma reagin tests for syphilis;
5. other tests, including electrolytes, serum creatinine, and liver function tests, usually remaining the same.

> **Additional Reading:** *Wallach's Interpretation of Laboratory Tests,* 9th ed. Philadelphia, PA: Lippincott Williams and Wilkins; 2012.

> Category: Nonspecific system

41. Which one of the following defines a stage II pressure ulcer?
A) A break in the skin with surrounding erythema and induration
B) An ulcer with penetration of the deep fascia, exposing bone or underlying muscle
C) A localized area of nonblanchable, erythematous skin
D) A full-thickness ulcer that extends to the subcutaneous layer but not through the underlying fascia

Answer and Discussion

The answer is A. Pressure ulcers are quite common in elderly debilitated patients if they are not adequately cared for. Between 3% and 11% of nursing home and hospital patients suffer from pressure ulcers. Precipitating factors include constant pressure, moisture (incontinence), shearing forces, and friction. The ulcers may form as quickly as in 2 to 3 hours if the patient is not repositioned. If patients are placed on their sides, they should be positioned at a 30-degree angle to avoid excessive pressure over the greater trochanter and lateral malleolus. Soft pillows, padded chairs, and egg-crate mattresses can help decrease the risk of ulcer formation but are not a substitute for repositioning. Doughnut-type cushions are not helpful and can cause decreased circulation to the tissue in the center of the doughnut and worsening of any existing ulcers. Alternating air mattresses and waterbeds have been shown to help reduce the incidence of pressure ulcers.

Pressure ulcers are classified as follows:

Stage 1: a localized area of nonblanchable, erythematous skin.
Stage 2: a break in the skin with surrounding erythema and induration.
Stage 3: a full-thickness ulcer that extends to the subcutaneous layer but not through the underlying fascia. Risk for infection is high, and the use of antibiotics may be required.
Stage 4: ulcer penetrates the deep fascia exposing bone or underlying muscle.

Mild pressure sores (stages I and II) require all the prophylactic measures mentioned previously to prevent necrosis. The area should be kept exposed, free from pressure, and dry. Stimulating the circulation by gentle massage can accelerate healing. Ulcers that have not advanced beyond stage III may heal spontaneously if the pressure is removed and the area is small. New hydrophilic gels and hydrocolloid dressings speed healing. Stage IV ulcers require debridement or more extensive surgery. When the ulcers are filled with pus or necrotic debris, dextranomer beads or newer hydrophilic polymers may hasten debridement without surgery. Conservative debridement of necrotic tissue with forceps and scissors should be instituted. Some ulcers may be debrided by cleansing with 1.5% hydrogen peroxide. Whirlpool baths may assist debridement. More advanced ulcers with fat and muscle involvement require surgical debridement and closure. For cellulitis, a penicillinase-resistant penicillin or a cephalosporin is necessary. A culture is generally not helpful in choosing an antibiotic because surface growth is often polymicrobial.

Additional Reading: Pressure ulcers: prevention, evaluation, and management. *Am Fam Physician.* 2008;78(10):1186–1194.

Category: Integumentary

42. An 85-year-old nursing home patient was seen in a local physician's office during the day for a corneal abrasion. The patient had antibiotic drops instilled, and the eye was patched. At 10:00 p.m., the nursing staff calls reporting the patient is very confused. The most appropriate action is to
A) Remove the eye patch
B) Prescribe haloperidol
C) Have the patient taken to the emergency room
D) Reassure the nursing staff and see the patient the next day
E) Restrain the patient to protect him from injury

Answer and Discussion

The answer is A. Sensory deprivation, such as patching an elderly patient's eyes, may lead to an acute case of delirium. Even small alterations in the elderly patient's environment can lead to confusion. In cases of corneal abrasions, an elderly patient should receive topical ophthalmic antibiotics. Although eye patching traditionally has been recommended in the treatment of corneal abrasions,

multiple well-designed studies show that patching does not help and may hinder healing. Topical anesthetics should not be used for corneal abrasions because they interfere with the healing process; however, they may be useful in the initial evaluation to help relieve discomfort.

Additional Reading: Management of corneal abrasions. *Am Fam Physician.* 2004;70:123–130.

Category: Special sensory

43. Which of the following defines a *durable power of attorney*?
A) A written advance directive that assigns one person as a decision-making proxy should the user become incapacitated
B) A written advance directive in which a competent person indicates health care preferences while cognitively and physically intact
C) A detailed written directive that describes in questionnaire format what type of treatment a person would or would not want in various medical situations
D) The ability of attorneys to sue physicians for negligence
E) None of the above

Answer and Discussion

The answer is A. A *durable power of attorney* is defined as a written advance directive that assigns one person as a decision-making proxy should the user becomes incapacitated. A *living will* is a written advance directive in which a competent person indicates health care preferences while cognitively and physically intact. A *medical directive* is a detailed written directive that describes in questionnaire format what type of treatment a person would or would not want in various medical situations.

Additional Reading: Respecting end-of-life treatment preferences. *Am Fam Physician.* 2005;72:1263–1268, 1270.

Category: Patient/population-based care

44. You are called by the nursing supervisor at the local nursing home where you manage patients. She reports the outbreak of influenza A in three of the patients. What is your most appropriate response?
A) You place patients in isolation and call if any further episodes occur.
B) You order amantadine (Symmetrel) for all contacts.
C) You order rimantadine (Flumadine) for all contacts.
D) You order zanamivir (Relenza) for all contacts.
E) You order treatment with oseltamivir (Tamiflu) for any patient who develops symptoms of influenza.

Answer and Discussion

The answer is D. Chronically ill and elderly persons have a higher incidence of side effects while taking amantadine and rimantadine. Both medications can cause gastrointestinal effects such as anorexia and nausea. However, amantadine has significantly more side effects relating to the CNS than rimantadine, including confusion, anxiety, insomnia, hallucinations, and falls in nursing home residents. Amantadine also has significantly higher discontinuation rates (up to 17%). Rimantadine resistance is increasing, so the Center for Disease Control and Prevention (CDC) currently recommends rimantadine or oseltamivir to all contacts (do not wait till there are symptoms, especially if unvaccinated).

Additional Reading: Influenza antiviral medications. *Centers for Disease Control and Prevention;* 2013. From: http://www.cdc.gov/flu/professionals/antivirals/summary-clinicians.htm.

Category: Respiratory system

45. Patients with gallbladder carcinoma
A) Typically have a life expectancy of more than 5 years
B) May have a history of chronic cholecystitis
C) Rarely develop jaundice
D) Rarely have metastasis at the time of diagnosis
E) Are typically of middle age (35 to 65 years of age)

Answer and Discussion

The answer is B. Cancer of the gallbladder is rare, affects predominantly the elderly, and is very difficult to detect clinically. In most cases, it is found during surgery (1% of cases undergoing exploration for cholelithiasis) and has metastasized at the time of diagnosis. Ninety percent are adenocarcinomas. Symptoms, when they are present, include right-upper-quadrant pain that radiates to the back, jaundice, weight loss, and anorexia. A palpable gallbladder with obstructive jaundice usually signifies cancer of the gallbladder. Treatment is limited, and surgery is used only in certain situations to relieve biliary obstruction. The prognosis is poor; few patients survive longer than 6 months. Chronic calculus cholecystitis increases the risk for cancer of the gallbladder, and cholecystectomy is recommended.

> **Additional Reading:** Gallbladder cancer: epidemiology, risk factors, clinical features, and diagnosis. In: Basow DS, ed. *UpToDate*. Waltham, MA: UpToDate; 2013.

> **Category:** Gastroenterology system

46. Which of the following is necessary to diagnose menopause?
A) Estrogen levels <30 mg/dL
B) FSH level >35 mg/dL
C) An abnormal progesterone challenge test
D) The absence of menses for 6 months

Answer and Discussion

The answer is D. *Menopause* is defined as the absence of menses for 6 months. The average age of onset is 51 years. Symptoms of menopause are common and include hot flashes, night sweats, mood swings with emotional lability and irritability, depression, insomnia, vaginal dryness, dyspareunia, dysuria, and urinary incontinence. Hormone-replacement therapy (estrogen with or without progestin) was the primary treatment for the symptoms and long-term risks associated with menopause. However, recent evidence fails to confirm the protective effect of estrogen on cardiovascular disease risk. Menopause can be confirmed by measuring follicle-stimulating hormone levels; however, this is not necessary for the diagnosis. Follicle-stimulating hormone levels higher than 35 support a menopausal state. Also, a progesterone challenge test (13 days of progestin) resulting in no withdrawal bleeding indicates a lack of estrogen and the menopausal state.

> **Additional Reading:** Clinical manifestations and diagnosis of menopause. In: Basow DS, ed. *UpToDate*. Waltham, MA: UpToDate; 2013.

> **Category:** Endocrine system

> 🌀 *Menopause* is defined as the absence of menses for 6 months.

47. Which one of the following statements concerning cataracts is true?
A) They are usually unilateral.
B) Asymptomatic lens opacities should be removed because of risk to the retina.
C) Ultraviolet light exposure may contribute to the progression of cataract formation.
D) The cataracts require a slit-lamp examination to be seen.
E) Surgery is rarely helpful for advanced cataract formation.

Answer and Discussion

The answer is C. Cataracts are lens opacities that result in a painless loss of vision in patients usually older than 60 years. The prevalence of cataract increases with age from <5% in persons younger than 65 years to approximately 50% in those 75 years of age and older. They are usually bilateral and develop gradually over many years. Exposure to ultraviolet light may contribute to the progression of cataract formation. Typical symptoms related to cataracts include decreased visual acuity, particularly at night, with excessive glare in bright light or sunlight. Most cataracts can be visualized with a handheld ophthalmoscope; however, slit-lamp examination may be more revealing. Cataract surgery is the most common surgical procedure covered by Medicare, with more than 1 million procedures performed annually. This surgery should be considered when the cataract reduces vision function to a level that interferes with everyday activities. The mere presence of lens opacities—that is, lens opacities not associated with decreased visual function—is not an indication for surgery in most instances. Cataract surgery is an outpatient procedure performed under local or topical anesthesia. More than 90% of patients undergoing cataract surgery experience visual improvement and improved quality of life if there is no ocular comorbidity. Complications of cataract surgery are unusual and occur in less than 1% of surgeries. Potentially serious complications include glaucoma, bleeding, infection, vitreous loss, retinal detachment, and loss of vision.

> **Additional Reading:** Cataract in adults. In: Basow DS, ed. *UpToDate*. Waltham, MA: UpToDate; 2013.

> **Category:** Special sensory

48. A nurse calls to report that a hospitalized patient fell and is now complaining of severe left-hip pain. On arriving at the patient's room, you noticed the woman's left leg is shorter than the right and is externally rotated. The most likely diagnosis is
A) Left-fibular fracture
B) Stable left-hip fracture
C) Left-anterior cruciate ligament injury
D) Unstable left-hip fracture
E) Unstable right-hip fracture

Answer and Discussion

The answer is D. Hip fractures represent significant morbidity and mortality as well as health care costs to the elderly. Fractures of the femoral neck are classified as being stable or unstable. Stable fractures include stress or impacted fractures. Patients usually report minimal pain and may be able to walk with only mild groin pain and perhaps a limp. The physical exam is unremarkable. Both stress and impacted fractures may be treated nonoperatively; however, impacted fractures are at an increased risk to become displaced and are, therefore, usually corrected with internal fixation to stabilize a reduction and allow earlier weight bearing. Patients who are demented, nonambulatory, or poor surgical candidates should be treated by nonsurgical means. Conservative measures to protect the injured extremity, prevent decubitus ulcers, and avoid pneumonia should be instituted. Unstable fractures include displaced and comminuted fractures that can be life threatening for the elderly. Most patients report considerable pain with any movement of the hip. The physical exam usually shows the affected extremity is externally rotated and shorter in length than the unaffected side. Treatment consists of surgical reduction and internal fixation followed by traction.

> **Additional Reading:** Hip fracture. In: Domino F, ed. *The 5-Minute Clinical Consult*. Philadelphia, PA: Lippincott Williams and Wilkins; 2014.

> **Category:** Musculoskeletal system

49. A 65-year-old woman presents to your office complaining of leakage of urine when she coughs or sneezes. The most likely diagnosis is
A) Urinary tract infection
B) Urge incontinence
C) Neurogenic bladder
D) Stress incontinence
E) Interstitial cystitis

Answer and Discussion

The answer is D. *Stress urinary incontinence* is defined as bladder outlet incompetence and the loss of urine with coughing, sneezing, straining, lifting, or any activity that requires a Valsalva maneuver and associated increased abdominal pressure. In women, the usual cause is a loss in the normal posterior ureterovesical angle as a result of pelvic floor muscle laxity. Pelvic floor weakness is a common result of aging and multiparity. Treatment may involve the use of Kegel exercises (multiple contractions of the pelvic floor muscles as if the patient were shutting off the flow of urine) and α-adrenergic medications (e.g., pseudoephedrine). Estrogens may also be effective in treating women with stress incontinence. The presence of estrogen receptors in high concentrations throughout the lower urinary tract makes it possible to treat women with stress incontinence by localized estrogen-replacement therapy. Estrogen-replacement therapy causes engorgement of the periurethral blood supply and subsequent thickening of the urethral mucosa. Localized estrogen-replacement therapy can be given in the form of estrogen cream or an estradiol-impregnated vaginal ring (Estring). Surgery (Marshall–Marchetti procedure) may be considered if the condition is severe and refractive to medication. In some cases, the use of a pessary may be beneficial. The U.S. Food and Drug Administration recently approved extracorporeal magnetic innervation, a noninvasive procedure for the treatment of incontinence caused by pelvic floor weakness. The patient sits fully clothed in a pulsating magnetic chair that stimulates the pelvic floor. A typical treatment session lasts approximately 20 minutes and includes high- and low-frequency stimulation. Preliminary results from one uncontrolled trial suggest that extracorporeal magnetic innervation may have a place in the treatment of women with stress and urge incontinence. Another minimally invasive procedure for the treatment of stress incontinence is periurethral injection. This procedure involves injection of material at the bladder neck just under the urothelium and is performed in an office setting under local anesthesia. Pharmacologic agents may be given empirically to women with symptoms of overactive bladder. Two new medications, tolterodine and extended-release oxybutynin chloride, have largely replaced generic oxybutynin as a first-line treatment option for overactive bladder because of favorable side-effect profiles.

> Additional Reading: Urinary incontinence. In: Domino F, ed. *The 5-Minute Clinical Consult*. Philadelphia, PA: Lippincott Williams and Wilkins; 2014.

Category: Nephrologic system

50. An 85-year-old man complains of chronic insomnia. On the basis of study results, you know that
A) Insomnia is relatively rare in the elderly
B) Insomnia is a natural progression of aging and has little effect on the well-being of elderly patients
C) Chronic insomnia is an independent risk factor for cognitive decline in elderly men
D) Insomnia has no impact on the risk of falls
E) Insomnia does not lead to nursing home placement

Answer and Discussion

The answer is C. Chronic insomnia is an independent risk factor for cognitive decline in patients 65 years and older, especially in men. Insomnia is often associated with dependence on sleep medications, chronic fatigue, and increased risk of falls. Chronic sleep disturbances may lead to nursing home placement.

> Additional Reading: The impact of insomnia on cognitive functioning in older adults. *J Am Geriatr Soc.* 2001;49:1185–1189.

Category: Neurologic

51. Which of the following tests may help identify elders who are at increased risk for falling?
A) Straight line test
B) One foot hop test
C) Two hand one foot test
D) Sit down and stop test
E) Get up and go test

Answer and Discussion

The answer is E. Approximately one-third of noninstitutionalized elders fall each year. The annual incidence of falls approaches 50% in patients above 80 years of age. Factors contributing to falls include age-related postural changes, decreased vision, certain medications (particularly anticholinergic, sedative, and diuretic medications), and diseases affecting muscle strength and coordination. A straightforward physical examination maneuver called the "get up and go" test can help identify those at risk for falls. In this test, the patient is instructed to arise from a sitting position, walk 10 feet, turn, and return to the chair to sit. A requirement of >16 seconds to complete the process or observation of postural instability or gait impairment suggests an increased risk of falling. A number of effective interventions are available for people with a history of falls or who are at risk for falling.

> Additional Reading: Falls in older persons: risk factors and patient evaluation. In: Basow DS, ed. *UpToDate*. Waltham, MA: UpToDate; 2013.

Category: Patient/population-based care

52. A 70-year-old man is recently diagnosed with early Alzheimer's Disease (AD). His family is very concerned with his ability to drive. You explain to them:
A) In the first year after the diagnosis is made, patients with AD have a similar rate of accidents as registered drivers of all ages.
B) The risk of accidents rarely changes as AD patients grow older.
C) The department of transportation is the only group that has a role in the determination of driving skills.
D) Roadside testing should not be used to determine the ability to drive.
E) Accident rates may be overestimated because of the number of miles elderly people drive.

Answer and Discussion

The answer is A. In many situations, one of the first safety issues to be confronted with elderly patients affected with dementia is their driving. In the first year after diagnosis, patients affected with AD have a similar rate of accidents as registered drivers of all ages, although higher than age-matched controls. The risk of motor vehicle accidents increases dramatically in the following years. This increase is likely underrepresented in that the risk per mile driven is much greater because patients substantially reduce their driving. Discussions of driving cessation are often difficult. Patients are generally unaware of their deficits (particularly their deficits in judgment), and surrendering a license often represents a severe loss of independence. With early diagnosis, many patients will still be able to drive safely for a period of time, but all will eventually progress to the point where it is no longer safe to drive. Discussions with patients in the intermediate stages of dementia pose the greatest difficulty. Only the state of California currently has a requirement that physicians notify authorities when a patient is diagnosed with dementia. Although a number of driving safety tests have been suggested, no general guidelines have been broadly instituted. Local programs may exist to evaluate these patients with neuropsychological and roadside tests. In the absence of these programs, the department of motor vehicles often performs roadside testing, but patients must be informed that even if they pass they must be retested at regular intervals as their disease progresses. Families must be warned about potential liability for accidents. They may need to take possession of car keys, or even the cars, and restrict all driving. The American Academy of Neurology has issued guidelines for driving in patients with AD based on the clinical dementia rating scale.

> **Additional Reading:** Dubinsky RM, Stein AC, Lyons K. Practice parameter: risk of driving and Alzheimer's disease (an evidence-based review): report of the quality standards subcommittee of the American Academy of Neurology. *Neurology.* 2000;54:2205.

> Category: Patient/population-based care

53. Which of the following statements about rehabilitation after a stroke is true?
A) Physical therapy should be instituted for stretching and strengthening once supporting muscles are strong enough to support appropriate loads.
B) Tennis ball exercises can be used to strengthen the hand muscles.
C) Most motor function improvement occurs more than 6 months after a cerebral vascular accident.
D) A walking cane used on the affected side can help with ambulation and balance.
E) Bladder or bowel incontinence has no effect on prognosis after stroke.

Answer and Discussion

The answer is A. Rehabilitation after a stroke is often a difficult and lengthy process. Most improvement in motor function occurs in the first 6 to 12 weeks after a stroke; speech may continue to improve significantly after this period. Stretching and strengthening exercises should be instituted when the supporting muscles are capable of supporting the appropriate loads. Gait training should take place as soon as the hip musculature is capable of supporting the patient's weight. In many cases, the patient can use a cane in the hand opposite to the side the stroke affected to help support the weaker side. Squeezing a tennis ball as a hand exercise should be discouraged because it favors finger flexors over extensors and can lead to contractures. Using a team approach with a physical therapist, occupational therapist, speech therapist, and social workers is often beneficial. The outcome after a stroke is most likely to be positive when patients have bladder and bowel continence, are able to feed themselves, and have a healthy and caring spouse. Stroke rehabilitation must include the prevention or early diagnosis of medical complications, as well as patient and family education concerning the prevention of recurrent stroke.

> **Additional Reading:** Stroke rehabilitation. In: Domino F, ed. *The 5-Minute Clinical Consult.* Philadelphia, PA: Lippincott Williams and Wilkins; 2014.

> Category: Neurologic

> **Most improvement in motor function occurs in the first 6 to 12 weeks after a stroke; speech may continue to improve significantly after this period.**

54. Pernicious anemia is associated with
A) Vitamin B_{12} malabsorption
B) Chronic blood loss
C) Myelofibrosis
D) Iron deficiency
E) Malignancy

Answer and Discussion

The answer is A. Anemia should not be accepted as an unavoidable consequence of aging. A cause is found in approximately 80% of elderly patients. The most common causes of anemia in the elderly are chronic disease and iron deficiency. Vitamin B_{12} deficiency, folate deficiency, gastrointestinal bleeding, and myelodysplastic syndrome are among other causes of anemia in the elderly. Serum ferritin is the most useful test to differentiate iron-deficiency anemia from anemia of chronic disease. The condition of pernicious anemia is the result of malabsorption or lack of ingestion of vitamin B_{12}. The lack of absorption is usually the result of atrophic gastric mucosa, which fails to produce the intrinsic factor that is required for the absorption of vitamin B_{12}. With pernicious anemia, the lack of intrinsic factor results from destruction of the gastric parietal cells by autoimmune antibodies. Previous gastrectomy, blind-loop syndrome, fish tapeworm infections, or thyroid abnormalities may also decrease intrinsic factor secretion. The anemia usually develops over time and is associated with macrocytic features, basophilic stippling of red blood cells, and an increased red blood cell distribution width index. *Achlorhydria* (lack of acid production) is usually associated with pernicious anemia. Symptoms of pernicious anemia include anorexia, constipation, diarrhea, and abdominal pain; glossitis; loss of sensation involving the distal extremities; weight loss; and generalized fatigue. Previously, the Schilling test would have been used to identify the cause of inadequate vitamin B_{12} absorption. Recent studies, however, show that high-dose oral vitamin B_{12} effectively treats the deficiency regardless of the cause. Vitamin B_{12} deficiency is effectively treated with high-dose oral or parenteral vitamin B_{12} supplementation.

> **Additional Reading:** Update on Vitamin B12 Deficiency. *Am Fam Physician.* 2011;83(12):1425–1430.

> Category: Hematologic system

55. Which one of the following statements about Alzheimer's Disease (AD) is true?
A) It is associated with microscopic senile plaques and neurofibrillary tangles, in the brain.
B) It is associated with birth trauma.
C) It is usually reversible.
D) It is associated with tremor, ataxia, and muscle rigidity.
E) It is not familial.

Answer and Discussion

The answer is A. AD is a progressive, irreversible cause of dementia. It is the most common type of dementia. Symptoms include memory difficulties, disorientation, impaired judgment, aphasia, and apraxia. Histopathologic changes seen in the brain with AD include microscopic senile plaques, neurofibrillary tangles, and granulovacuolar degeneration of neurons. A CT scan usually shows cerebral cortical atrophy and ventricular dilation. There is no identifiable cause, and other causes for dementia must be ruled out before a diagnosis of AD is made. It is important to remember that 5% to 15% of dementias are reversible and may be caused by factors such as meningiomas, subdural hematomas, systemic illnesses, deficiency states and endocrinopathies, heavy metal and drug poisonings, and infections. AD is familial, and no specific cause has been identified. Treatment is supportive. Efforts should be made to provide regular routines that the patient becomes accustomed to. The mainstay of treatment options is acetylcholinesterase inhibitors, which increase the duration of acetylcholine action in synapses. Tacrine, the earliest drug in this group, has only limited benefit and a poor side-effect profile, including hepatotoxicity. Donepezil is a highly selective acetylcholinesterase inhibitor that significantly improved cognitive scores (during phases 2 and 3 clinical trials) with a better side-effect profile. A newer acetylcholinesterase inhibitor, rivastigmine, has a good side-effect profile but requires more time for dosage titration than donepezil. Estrogen therapy increases acetylcholine concentrations and has antioxidant activity, but proof of its ability to reduce the risk of AD has not been shown. Anti-inflammatory drugs are under investigation. Antioxidants, including selegiline and Ginkgo biloba, have demonstrated some benefits in improving cognition and delaying progression of the disease, but the outcome measures used have been variable, making treatment recommendations difficult.

Additional Reading: Evaluation of cognitive impairment and dementia. In: Basow DS, ed. *UpToDate*. Waltham, MA: UpToDate; 2013.

Category: Neurologic

56. Which one of the following is most likely to cause hypoglycemia in the elderly treated for diabetes mellitus?
A) Metformin (Glucophage)
B) Glyburide (Micronase, DiaBeta)
C) Glipizide (Glucotrol)
D) None of the above

Answer and Discussion
The answer is B. Diabetes in the elderly poses some additional concern. The elderly develop microvascular complications such as diabetic retinopathy and peripheral neuropathy more quickly than do younger patients. Diabetes also represents a major risk factor for the development of atherosclerosis. The renal threshold for glucose is also increased in the elderly, allowing higher levels of blood glucose before glycosuria is seen. The use of glyburide has shown a twofold relative risk of hypoglycemia when compared with glipizide. Metformin does not cause hypoglycemia with monotherapy.

Additional Reading: Management of hypoglycemia during treatment of diabetes mellitus. In: Basow DS, ed. *UpToDate*. Waltham, MA: UpToDate; 2013.

Category: Endocrine system

57. An 85-year-old Alzheimer's Disease patient is reported missing from a local nursing home. You are contacted about directions for a search. You make all of following statements *except*
A) Most people found alive are found within 24 hours.
B) Of those who die, >90% are found in natural areas.
C) Night searches should be avoided because individuals are unlikely to wander when it is dark.
D) The first areas searched should be concentrated on open, populated areas.
E) The hottest and coldest times of the year are associated with the highest risk of death.

Answer and Discussion
The answer is C. The issue of wandering and becoming lost, with the possibility of physical harm or death, is one of the concerns that often leads families and caregivers to place demented patients in nursing homes. A review of this issue that analyzed data from several available studies produced the following observations. All persons with dementia are at risk of becoming lost. The risk may be higher for demented men than for women. Individuals residing in professional care settings are at risk as well as those at home. Wandering is only a risk factor; individuals who had never wandered have become lost. The risk of becoming lost is increased when demented persons are unattended, even in their own residences. However, about 65% of people with dementia are in the presence of a caregiver at the time they become lost. Becoming lost appears to be a highly unpredictable event and can occur even when individuals with dementia are in their own homes or are participating in activities they had routinely performed many times in the past without incident. Most individuals who are found alive remain out in the open in populated areas of the community. The risk of death is increased if the demented person ends up secluded in natural or sparsely populated areas. About 91% of persons with dementia who died were found in natural areas such as woods, fields, ditches, bodies of water (approximately 20% drowned), or abandoned vehicles. The risk of death also appears to be associated with the hottest and coldest times of the year. The time it took to search for and locate a missing person with dementia also correlated with the risk of death, as most individuals found alive were located within 24 hours, and all were found within 4 days. Locating a person with dementia who becomes lost can be difficult, and this problem is complicated by several factors related to the increased likelihood of abnormal behavior. People with dementia are often unpredictable when lost. The accuracy of the search is usually not enhanced by predictions from families and caregivers. The lost persons rarely call for help or respond to searcher's calls. Search strategies should not be based on the individual characteristics of the missing person because the unpredictable and abnormal behavior is likely to negate any prior individual patterns. Caregivers should report the person missing immediately to local authorities. An exhaustive search should begin immediately so that the individual has less time to find a secluded hiding place and has reduced exposure to the environment. Searches should continue through the night as individuals often continue to wander. The initial 6 to 12 hours of the search should cover a 5-mile radius around the location where the lost person was last seen, concentrating on open, populated areas, including the inside of easily accessible buildings. If initial search efforts fail, the subsequent efforts should be devoted to an intensive foot search of natural and sparsely populated areas beginning within a 1-mile radius of the last known location and extending from there. If the person with dementia traveled by car, initial search efforts should focus on locating the vehicle. Caregivers, both formal and informal, must be informed that all persons with dementia are at risk of becoming lost, even if the individual has never wandered or exhibited "risky" behavior in the past. Because the risk is highest when persons with dementia are left unattended, every effort should be made to ensure continuous supervision. Community resources, adult day care and respite care facilities, and caregiver support groups may be utilized, if available, to reduce the burden on families and caregivers.

Additional Reading: Persons with dementia who become lost in the community: a case study, current research, and recommendations. *Mayo Clin Proc.* 2004;79:1417.

Category: Patient/population-based care

58. Which of the following supplements has been shown to decrease the risk of falls?
A) Glucosamine/chondroitin
B) Vitamin C
C) Ginkgo biloba
D) Vitamin D
E) Vitamin B_{12}

Answer and Discussion

The answer is D. Vitamin D supplementation, with or without calcium, has been shown to decrease the risk of falls in elderly patients. A subsequent meta-analysis focused specifically on vitamin D supplementation and concluded that such supplementation reduces the risk of falls (odds ratio 0.78, 95% CI 0.64–0.92); the proposed mechanism is through improvements in muscle strength with supplementation.

> **Additional Reading:** Effect of vitamin D on falls: a meta-analysis. *JAMA.* 2004;291:1999.

> **Category:** Nonspecific system

59. When performing an initial evaluation of urinary incontinence in elderly patients, which of the following tests is *not* indicated?
A) Urinalysis
B) Urine culture
C) Serum glucose
D) Vitamin B_{12} levels
E) Urodynamic testing

Answer and Discussion

The answer is D. Physicians must initiate a discussion of voiding symptoms because at least one-half of incontinent individuals do not report the problem to their providers. A physical examination for incontinence should be comprehensive and extend "above the waistline." In persons with symptoms of stress incontinence, a clinical stress test may be performed by having the patient (who should not have recently voided) give a single vigorous cough while standing and maintaining a relaxed perineum. Instantaneous leakage suggests stress incontinence, whereas a delay of several seconds before leakage suggests stress-induced detrusor overactivity. If urinary retention is suspected, it is important to consider postvoid residual testing, either by catheterization or ultrasound. A postvoid residual >200 mL suggests detrusor weakness or obstruction and in men should prompt a renal ultrasound examination to exclude hydronephrosis. If not recorded recently, it is necessary to measure renal function, glucose, and, in older people, vitamin B_{12} levels. A urinalysis should be obtained in all patients and a urine culture if infection is suspected. Routine urodynamic testing is not recommended as part of the initial evaluation.

> **Additional Reading:** Clinical presentation and diagnosis of urinary incontinence. In: Basow DS, ed. *UpToDate.* Waltham, MA: UpToDate; 2013.

> **Category:** Nephrologic system

60. A 79-year-old woman with a history of atherosclerosis and hypertension is seen in the emergency room. The patient reports she suddenly lost her vision in her left eye on awakening this morning. She reports no pain associated with the eye and has no other symptoms. Funduscopic examination shows disk swelling, extensive retinal hemorrhages, and cotton-wool spots. The most likely diagnosis is
A) Cerebrovascular accident
B) Central retinal vein occlusion
C) Closed-angle glaucoma
D) Macular degeneration
E) Transient ischemic attack

Answer and Discussion

The answer is B. Central vein occlusion usually affects elderly patients with atherosclerosis. The severity is variable; older individuals are usually affected more severely. Predisposing factors include hypertension, diabetes mellitus, glaucoma, increased blood viscosity, and elevated hematocrit. Symptoms include a sudden, dramatic, painless loss of vision usually first noticed on awakening in the morning. Physical findings include disk swelling, venous dilation, retinal hemorrhages, and cotton-wool spots. Those with poor visual acuity at the onset have the worst prognosis. These patients usually have extensive hemorrhages and cotton-wool spots, indicating retinal ischemia, and they may develop neovascular (rubeotic) glaucoma within 3 months after the initial occlusion. Should this occur, laser photocoagulation should be performed; otherwise, there is no medical therapy available. Underlying predisposing factors should be ruled out and treated appropriately if present. Branch vein occlusions may show varying degrees of visual loss and have a better prognosis than central vein occlusion.

> **Additional Reading:** Retinal vein occlusion: epidemiology, clinical manifestations, and diagnosis. In: Basow DS, ed. *UpToDate.* Waltham, MA: UpToDate; 2013.

> **Category:** Special sensory

> Symptoms of central vein occlusion include a sudden, dramatic, painless loss of vision usually first noticed on awakening in the morning.

61. Which of the following statements about hip fractures associated with osteoporosis is true?
A) African Americans have a higher incidence of osteoporosis and associated fractures.
B) The affected leg is usually shortened, abducted, and externally rotated.
C) Most fractures result from compression-type injuries rather than from falls laterally.
D) Bisphosphonates have not been found to be beneficial in preventing hip fractures.
E) The risk is highest for elderly men who have vision problems.

Answer and Discussion

The answer is B. Hip fractures as a result of osteoporosis represent a major morbidity for the elderly. The cost for treatment is excessive. Elderly persons are rightfully concerned about the loss of independence associated with fractures. Six months after a hip fracture, many older persons still require assistance with the activities of daily living. Furthermore, >10% of persons with hip fractures die. In the United States alone, hip fractures are responsible for 31,000 deaths each year. The risk is greatest for postmenopausal women who suffer from osteoporosis. Whites have a higher incidence of osteoporosis and associated fractures than African Americans. Most hip fractures occur as a result of falling sideways and not from compression. This mechanism of injury has a direct impact on the greater trochanter at the proximal femur. Most hip fractures present with the affected leg shortened, abducted, and externally rotated. Other fracture sites, including the spine (compression type), wrist, humerus, and tibia, are also affected. The use of estrogen-replacement therapy and calcium supplementation with vitamin D in postmenopausal women has a protective effect; however, because of controversy over estrogen risk, many avoid this treatment. The use of bisphosphonates, such as alendronate (Fosamax), risedronate (Actonel), etidronate (Didronel), once-monthly ibandronate (Boniva), calcitonin (Miacalcin), or raloxifene (Evista), a selective estrogen receptor modulator, can be beneficial in preventing further bone loss. Hip protectors may also help prevent hip fractures, although recent evidence is controversial.

Additional Reading: Hip fractures. In: Domino F, ed. *The 5-Minute Clinical Consult.* Philadelphia, PA: Lippincott Williams and Wilkins; 2014.

Category: Musculoskeletal system

62. The solid tumor malignancy most frequently diagnosed in elderly men is
A) Lung cancer
B) Colon cancer
C) Prostate cancer
D) Lymphoma
E) Esophageal cancer

Answer and Discussion

The **answer is C.** In the United States, prostate cancer is the most common solid tumor malignancy in men and is the second leading cause of cancer deaths (lung cancer is the first) in this group. African Americans are at higher risk than whites. The risk increases with age, and 70% of men older than 80 years are affected. Diagnosis is usually made by the detection of a palpable prostate nodule on physical examination followed by a PSA determination, which is elevated. The combination of a digital rectal examination and PSA test is more accurate in diagnosing early prostate cancer than either alone. The main problem with prostate cancer screening is that although this malignancy is extremely common, it is the actual cause of death in only a small proportion of patients who have histologic evidence of prostate cancer. Prostate cancer screening programs may result in the detection and treatment of many asymptomatic cancers that have no impact on length of life. The decision to offer prostate cancer screening must be made on an individual basis, depending on the patient's age, health status, family history, risk of prostate cancer, and personal beliefs. The patient must be informed about the risks and potential benefits of screening. The patient also must be helped to realize that although prostate cancer can grow quickly, it generally grows quite slowly.

Ultrasound examination with possible biopsy should be performed if the physical exam or PSA determination is abnormal. Disease progression is usually local extension or metastasis to bone; and may manifest itself in low-back pain as the presenting complaint in an elderly man. Treatment consists of surgery, radiation, and hormonal manipulation, depending on the stage and type of tumor identified. In radical prostatectomy, the entire prostate is excised from the urethra and bladder, which are then reconnected. Severe complications from radical prostatectomy are relatively uncommon. However, damage to the urinary sphincter and penile nerves during surgery can result in postoperative urinary incontinence and impotence. External-beam radiotherapy appears to be as effective as surgery in curing prostate cancer, at least for the first 10 years after treatment. Radiotherapy is well tolerated, and it is associated with no hemorrhagic or anesthetic risks. Furthermore, this treatment option does not require hospitalization or a significant recovery period. Normal activity can usually be maintained during radiotherapy. However, treatment is administered daily for 4 to 6 weeks, and many patients report feeling fatigued at the end of this period. It is associated with severe bladder irritation (urgency, pain, and frequency) in as much as 5% of patients. Rectal irritations (diarrhea, urgency, tenesmus, and bleeding) occur in 3% to 10% of patients who receive radiotherapy

for prostate cancer, and impotence is a problem in 40% to 50% of patients receiving this treatment. The two types of radiotherapy are external-beam irradiation and implantation of radioactive pellets (seeds). Although neither approach has been shown to be superior in terms of long-term outcome, seed implant therapy has been gaining in popularity since its introduction. Because of controversy surrounding outcomes and the potential for complications, the patient should be informed of the risks and benefits and participate in the decision-making process.

Additional Reading: Treatment options for localized prostate cancer. *Am Fam Physician.* 2011;84(4):413–420.

Category: Reproductive system

63. Which one of the following statements about herpes zoster is true?
A) The virus remains dormant in the muscle fibers and can be reactivated by stress.
B) The rash is usually maculopapular, bilateral, and typically affects the lower abdomen.
C) The virus can lead to chronic, debilitating pain for an extended period after resolution of the rash.
D) Steroids should always be used for treatment.
E) Exposure to patients with varicella (chickenpox) can cause herpes zoster.

Answer and Discussion

The **answer is C.** Herpes zoster, also known as *shingles*, is caused by a reactivation of the virus that causes varicella (chickenpox). The virus remains dormant in the nerve endings and reactivates itself, in some cases, as a result of stress or infection. In most cases, a vesicular, painful rash develops in a single, unilateral, dermatomal pattern. Herpes zoster typically presents with a prodrome consisting of hyperesthesia, paresthesias, burning dysesthesias, or pruritus along the affected dermatome(s). The prodrome generally lasts 1 to 2 days but may precede the appearance of skin lesions by up to 3 weeks.

The elderly are most frequently affected. Areas of involvement usually include the trunk; however, it may occur on the face (in the distribution of the trigeminal nerve). Other symptoms include fatigue, fever, and headache. After the resolution of the rash, many patients develop postherpetic neuralgia, which can be chronic and debilitating. For acute herpes zoster, the antivirals acyclovir (Zovirax), valacyclovir (Valtrex), and famciclovir (Famvir) are useful for treatment, particularly if administered early in the course of the disease. If the use of orally administered prednisone is not contraindicated, adjunctive treatment with this agent is justified on the basis of its effects in reducing pain, despite questionable evidence for its benefits in decreasing the incidence of postherpetic neuralgia. Given the theoretic risk of immunosuppression with corticosteroids, some investigators believe that these agents should be used only in patients older than 50 years because they are at greater risk of developing postherpetic neuralgia and prednisone may be beneficial. Treatment of postherpetic neuralgia consists of topical capsaicin (Zostrix) and amitriptyline. Pregabalin (Lyrica) is a relatively new medication approved for the treatment of postherpetic neuralgia. Additionally, the immunization (Zostavax) has been approved for the prevention of herpes zoster in patients above the age of 60. Those not immune to varicella can develop varicella after exposure to herpes zoster.

Additional Reading: Herpes zoster. In: Domino F, ed. *The 5-Minute Clinical Consult.* Philadelphia, PA: Lippincott Williams and Wilkins; 2014.

Category: Nonspecific system

64. The misuse and overprescribing of psychotropics lead to adverse effects and deteriorating medical and cognitive status. To combat the problem in the United States, nursing home reform legislation, the Omnibus Budget Reconciliation Act of 1987 (OBRA-87), mandated freedom for every resident from medically unnecessary "physical or chemical restraints imposed for purposes of discipline or convenience." After institution of this legislated action, which of the following occurred?

A) The use of selective serotonin reuptake inhibitors (SSRIs) increased.
B) The use of long-acting benzodiazepines (e.g., diazepam) increased.
C) The use of neuroleptics increased.
D) Antipsychotic medication use increased.
E) There was no effect noted on physician's prescribing practices.

Answer and Discussion

The answer is A. Several multiyear, multifacility reviews have examined the impact of OBRA regulations on psychotropic prescribing in nursing homes. These confirm an encouraging trend, including increased awareness of neuroleptic indications and side effects. After OBRA, overall antipsychotic use declined by nearly one-third. Prescribing antidepressant increased (by almost 85% in one study), with significant increases in the use of selective serotonin reuptake inhibitors, nortriptyline, and trazodone, and decreases in amitriptyline and doxepin. Anxiolytic/hypnotic prescribing patterns are less consistent. A large study documented a 12% increase in anxiolytics but decreases in particular agents (e.g., diazepam, diphenhydramine). Two studies identified the implementation of OBRA regulations alone as responsible for decreased neuroleptic dosing.

> **Additional Reading:** Medical care of the nursing home patient. In: Basow DS, ed. *UpToDate*. Waltham, MA: UpToDate; 2013.

> **Category:** Patient/population-based care

65. When considering treatment of hyperlipidemia in elderly patients, which of the following is true?

A) Elderly patients should not receive lipid-lowering medication above age 85 because of the risk involved with the use of the medications.
B) In the presence of a terminal illness, the use of lipid-lowering medication should not be withheld.
C) The decision to use lipid-lowering medications should be individualized to the patient.
D) All patients with a history of coronary artery disease should be treated with lipid-lowering medications regardless of their comorbid conditions.
E) None of the above.

Answer and Discussion

The answer is C. The decision whether to treat high or high-normal serum cholesterol in an elderly individual must be individualized, being based on both chronologic and physiologic age. As an example, a patient with a limited life span from a concomitant illness is probably not a candidate for drug therapy. However, an otherwise healthy elderly individual should not be denied drug therapy simply on the basis of age alone.

> **Additional Reading:** Treatment of dyslipidemia in the elderly. In: Basow DS, ed. *UpToDate*. Waltham, MA: UpToDate; 2013.

> **Category:** Patient/population-based care

66. Which of the following *increases* as men age?

A) Sex hormone–binding globulin (SHBG)
B) Serum-free testosterone
C) Bone mineral density
D) Muscle mass
E) Muscle strength

Answer and Discussion

The answer is A. Serum sex hormone–binding globulin (SHBG) concentrations increase gradually as a function of age. The clinical implication, because SHBG binds testosterone with high affinity, is that with increasing age, less of the total testosterone is free (i.e., biologically active). Because of the increase in SHBG with age, it is not surprising that the serum-free testosterone concentration decreases with increasing age to a greater degree than the total testosterone. No consequences of the decline in serum testosterone with age are known with certainty, but several parallels between the effects of aging and those of hypogonadism suggest that the decline in serum testosterone might be related to decreased frequency of orgasm or intercourse. Men with hypogonadism due to known disease also have a decline in sexual function, as illustrated by an improvement after testosterone treatment. As men age, their bone mineral density also declines. In a study of healthy men who had never had any fractures, the bone mineral density of the femur and, to a lesser extent, the spine declined from age 20 to age 90. Men who are hypogonadal due to disease or whose testosterone has been lowered surgically or medically also have a decline in bone mineral density. As men age, their muscle mass declines and fat mass increases. Hypogonadal men also have less muscle mass and more fat mass than normal men; testosterone treatment in men with hypogonadism tends to reverse these changes. Men ages 60 to 79 years have less muscle strength than those ages 20 to 39 years. The decrease in serum testosterone concentrations that occurs with aging in men may be associated with a decline in neuropsychological function.

> **Additional Reading:** Decline in testicular function with aging. In: Basow DS, ed. *UpToDate*. Waltham, MA: UpToDate; 2013.

> **Category:** Reproductive system

67. Which one of the following is typically associated with NPH?

A) Tremor
B) Small ventricles
C) Short stature
D) Urinary incontinence
E) Macrocephaly

Answer and Discussion

The answer is D. NPH is a relatively rare disorder characterized by the following triad: dementia, gait ataxia, and urinary incontinence. Lumbar CSF pressure must be normal, and there is usually ventricular dilation noted on the CT or MRI examination that is disproportionate to cortical atrophy. The etiology is unknown, but there appears to be inadequate absorption of CSF, which leads to hydrocephalus. It may follow head injury, subarachnoid hemorrhage, or meningoencephalitis; however, in many cases there are no preceding conditions. The patient shows no weakness, but has a stuttering gait in which the initiation of gait is hesitant but gives way to walking. In addition, the patient may show lower-extremity spasticity and upgoing toes. Treatment has included shunting of CSF fluid from the dilated ventricles, which has shown some clinical benefit but little effect with long-standing hydrocephalus. Brief improvement after removing approximately 50 mL of CSF indicates a better prognosis with shunting.

Radiographic or pressure measurements alone do not seem to predict the response to shunting. Shunting CSF from the dilated ventricles sometimes results in clinical improvement, but the longer the disease has been present, the less likely shunting will be curative.

Additional Reading: Normal pressure hydrocephalus. In: Domino F, ed. *The 5-Minute Clinical Consult*. Philadelphia, PA: Lippincott Williams and Wilkins; 2014.

Category: Neurologic

> ⟳ NPH is a relatively rare disorder characterized by the following triad: dementia, gait ataxia, and urinary incontinence.

68. A 65-year-old otherwise healthy woman presents to your office complaining of dyspareunia. The examination shows a pale-pink vaginal mucosa, loss of rugae, and a friable cervix. The most appropriate treatment is
A) Trichloroacetic acid application
B) Cryotherapy
C) Estrogen vaginal cream
D) Psychotherapy
E) Vaginal dilation

Answer and Discussion

The answer is C. Atrophic vaginitis is the result of a lack of estrogen on the vaginal tissue. Up to 40% of postmenopausal women have symptoms of atrophic vaginitis. Related to estrogen deficiency, the condition may occur in premenopausal women who take anti-estrogenic medications (medroxyprogesterone [Provera], tamoxifen [Nolvadex], danazol [Danocrine], leuprolide [Lupron], and nafarelin [Synarel]) or who have medical or surgical conditions that result in decreased levels of estrogen. The thinned endometrium and increased vaginal pH level induced by estrogen deficiency predispose the vagina and urinary tract to infection and mechanical weakness. The earliest symptoms are decreased vaginal lubrication, followed by other vaginal and urinary symptoms that may be exacerbated by superimposed infection. Patients often report vaginal pruritus, burning, discharge, and excessive dryness with dyspareunia. Urethritis with urinary incontinence, dysuria, and frequency may also occur. Physical findings include a pale-pink vaginal mucosa with friable or atrophic cervix. Once other causes of symptoms have been eliminated, treatment usually depends on estrogen administration. Estrogen-replacement therapy may be provided systemically or locally (preferred), but the dosage and delivery method must be individualized. Vaginal moisturizers and lubricants and participation in coitus may also be beneficial in the treatment of women with atrophic vaginitis.

Additional Reading: Atrophic vaginitis. In: Domino F, ed. *The 5-Minute Clinical Consult*. Philadelphia, PA: Lippincott Williams and Wilkins; 2014.

Category: Reproductive system

69. Which of the following statements is true regarding insomnia in the elderly?
A) Women are more commonly affected.
B) The condition is associated with inadequate tryptophan ingestion.
C) Exercise before bedtime can help relieve symptoms of insomnia.
D) Low-dose trazodone (Desyrel) is recommended for treating insomnia.
E) Small doses of alcohol given at bedtime can be used to treat insomnia.

Answer and Discussion

The answer is A. Elderly patients often sleep more than younger patients; however, some elderly patients suffer great difficulty with sleep patterns. The number of those patients receiving <5 hours of sleep per night dramatically increases as patients grow older. Women are more commonly affected. Patients with insomnia may experience one or more of the following problems: difficulty falling asleep, difficulty maintaining sleep, waking up too early in the morning, and nonrefreshing sleep. In addition, daytime consequences such as fatigue, lack of energy, difficulty concentrating, and irritability are often present. Behavior and pharmacologic therapies are used in treating insomnia. Behavior approaches take a few weeks to improve sleep but continue to provide relief even after training sessions have ended. Patients should be encouraged to keep a sleep diary for several weeks. Sleep diaries usually record bedtime, total sleep time, time until sleep onset, number of awakenings, use of sleep medications, time out of bed in the morning, and a rating of quality of sleep and daytime symptoms. The sleep diary provides a nightly record of the patient's sleep schedule and perception of sleep. Moreover, it may serve as a baseline for assessment of treatment effects. Treatment involves attention to contributing factors for insomnia, including depression, caffeine use, tobacco or alcohol use, and lack of exercise or exercise before bedtime. Medications include tricyclic antidepressants or trazodone given in low doses 1 hour before bed. Zolpidem (Ambien) has less tendency for rebound and habituation and may be a suitable alternative to other medications. Other medications that are used include eszopiclone (Lunesta) and zaleplon (Sonata) and the melatonin receptor agonist ramelteon (Rozerem).

Additional Reading: Treatment of insomnia. In: Basow DS, ed. *UpToDate*. Waltham, MA: UpToDate; 2013.

Category: Neurologic

70. Which of the following is a risk factor for fecal incontinence?
A) Running
B) Prolonged sitting
C) Childbirth
D) High-fiber diet

Answer and Discussion

The answer is C. Fecal incontinence is a serious and embarrassing problem that affects up to 5% of the general population and up to 39% of nursing home residents. Providing effective treatment is challenging because of the difficulties in identifying the underlying etiology. Risk factors include female gender, older age, physical limitations, and poor health. Previous studies in women have shown that obstetric or iatrogenic surgical injuries damage the internal or external sphincters, and straining or childbirth can injure the pudendal nerves. Anal ultrasound detects defects in the sphincter complex in up to 87% of incontinent women. Anorectal physiologic studies can identify pudendal nerve injuries in many of the remaining patients. Fecal incontinence may be associated with other causes, including spinal cord injuries, diabetes, dementia, fecal impaction, tumors, trauma, chronic constipation, or previous rectal surgery. All of these conditions result in a low anal sphincter resting tone. Physical examination should include a rectal examination to check for adequate anal sphincter tone and sensation. Further tests include EMG studies of the pelvic floor and anal manometry. Treatment involves a strict bowel program to develop predictable bowel movements. Adequate diet with fiber and bulk, proper positioning when defecating, and occasional bowel stimulants can be used to help regulate bowel movements into a regular pattern. For resistant cases, loperamide (Imodium) or diphenoxylate with atropine (Lomotil) may be used to control bowel movements. Other methods to help with rectal incontinence include Kegel exercises to strengthen the pelvic floor muscles and biofeedback; surgery can be considered for resistant cases.

Additional Reading: Fecal incontinence in adults. In: Basow DS, ed. *UpToDate*. Waltham, MA: UpToDate; 2013.

Category: Gastroenterology system

71. A 66-year-old otherwise healthy man presents to your office for a general examination. He had a pneumococcal vaccine 7 years ago and inquires whether he needs another one. You correctly answer
A) Further immunizations are not needed.
B) He should receive only one booster at 10 years.
C) He should receive one more booster and no further immunizations are needed.
D) He should receive boosters every 7 years indefinitely.
E) He should receive boosters every 10 years indefinitely.

Answer and Discussion
The answer is C. The 23-valent pneumococcal vaccine provides protection from 85% to 90% of the serotypes that cause invasive disease in the United States. The vaccine is 56% to 81% effective in preventing invasive bacteremia. Current guidelines from the Advisory Committee on Immunization Practices (ACIP) recommend that persons ages 65 or older who were vaccinated before age 65 should receive one revaccination 5 years after the initial vaccination, and previously unvaccinated individuals should receive one dose at age 65.

Additional Reading: Vaccines and preventable diseases: pneumococcal vaccination. *Centers for Disease Control and Prevention.* From: http://www.cdc.gov/vaccines/vpd-vac/pneumo/.

Category: Patient/population-based care

72. Based on the results of the Women's Health Initiative Study, which of the following is a correct statement?
A) Those taking conjugated estrogen combined with medroxyprogesterone had an increased risk of breast cancer, coronary artery disease, stroke, and pulmonary embolism than did the control group.
B) Those taking conjugated estrogen combined with medroxyprogesterone had an increased risk of breast cancer alone.
C) Those taking conjugated estrogen combined with medroxyprogesterone had an increased risk of coronary artery disease alone.
D) Those taking conjugated estrogen combined with medroxyprogesterone had an increased risk only of stroke and pulmonary embolism than did controls.
E) Those taking conjugated estrogen alone had an increased risk of breast cancer, coronary artery disease, stroke, and pulmonary embolism than did the control group.

Answer and Discussion
The answer is A. The conjugated estrogen/medroxyprogesterone acetate arm of the Women's Health Initiative Study was terminated early because of excess risk of breast cancer, and overall risks exceeded benefits (rates of coronary artery disease, stroke, and pulmonary embolism were also higher than the control group).

Additional Reading: Long-term follow-up after the women's health initiative study. *Am Fam Physician.* 2012;85(7):727–728.

Category: Reproductive system

73. Which of the following is true regarding hospice services?
A) Patients that use hospice must be eligible for Medicare Part A.
B) Patients enrolled in hospice must be terminally ill.
C) Patients enrolled are expected to die within 6 months.
D) Patients must sign a statement choosing hospice care instead of routine Medicare benefits for the specified illness.
E) All of the above.

Answer and Discussion
The answer is E. Medicare patients may choose to use the Medicare Hospice Benefit in situations of terminal illness. Terminal illness is defined as a life expectancy of 6 months or less if the condition progresses as expected. Patients who decide to use the hospice benefit must be eligible for Medicare Part A, be certified by their physician and hospice medical director as terminally ill, sign a statement choosing hospice care instead of routine Medicare benefits for the specified illness, and receive care of their terminal illness through a Medicare-approved hospice program.

Additional Reading: Hospice: what you should know. *Am Fam Physician.* 2008;77(6):817–818.

Category: Patient/population-based care

74. A 60-year-old multiparous woman presents to your office complaining of the sudden need to urinate followed by the loss of urine. The most likely diagnosis is
A) Urge incontinence
B) Stress incontinence
C) Overflow incontinence
D) Interstitial cystitis
E) Multiple sclerosis

Answer and Discussion
The answer is A. There are three basic types of urinary incontinence:

1. *Urge incontinence.* Also known as *detrusor hyperactivity,* the patient suddenly feels the urge to urinate, and involuntary loss of urine follows. It is the most common form of incontinence in elderly patients. Causes include multiple sclerosis, neurogenic bladder dysfunction, interstitial cystitis, urinary obstruction, urinary stones, urinary neoplasm, and urinary infections. In most cases, the cause is idiopathic with no clear etiologic reason. Urge incontinence may occur alone or together with stress incontinence. Treatment involves determining and correcting the underlying cause. If the cause is idiopathic, a trial of anticholinergic medication such as oxybutynin (Ditropan), imipramine (Tofranil), or propantheline (Pro-Banthine) can be used. Routine voiding schedules may also be helpful. Tolterodine and extended-release oxybutynin chloride have largely replaced generic oxybutynin as a first-line treatment option for overactive bladder that contributes to incontinence because of favorable side-effect profiles.

2. *Stress incontinence* occurs when there is incompetence in the urinary sphincter. The symptoms include an involuntary loss of urine with sudden and forceful Valsalva-type maneuvers such as sneezing, coughing, laughing, or lifting heavy objects. In women, pelvic floor muscle relaxation (seen with the development of cystoceles as a result of increasing age or multiparity) contributes to the symptoms. In men, who are less commonly affected, the symptoms are usually the result of previous prostate surgery that may have damaged the nerves responsible for urinary continence. Diagnosis is usually made by the observation of involuntary urinary loss with coughing

while performing a pelvic examination or the loss of urine when a patient is standing and performs a Valsalva maneuver with a full bladder. Treatment involves the use of Kegel exercises (repeated tightening of the pelvic floor muscles as if one were shutting off the flow of urine), estrogen replacement, and α-adrenergic agonists (pseudoephedrine), which help improve the urinary sphincter tone. In some cases, the use of a pessary or surgical correction may be needed.

3. *Overflow incontinence* results when the bladder becomes overdistended and the pressure within the bladder increases and exceeds the pressure of the urinary sphincter, leading to involuntary incontinence. Causes include outlet obstruction as a result of severe constipation with fecal impaction, urethral strictures, or prostatic hypertrophy or carcinoma; in children, causes include urethral meatal stenosis, urethral valves, or urethral strictures. Patients often report hesitancy and incomplete voiding. Postvoid residuals usually exceed 100 mL. Treatment includes the use of α-blockers such as terazosin, doxazosin, and tamsulosin. Other treatments include relieving outlet obstruction with medication such as finasteride and dutasteride or surgery.

Additional Reading: Clinical management of urinary incontinence in women. *Am Fam Physician.* 2013;87(9):634–640.

Category: Nephrologic system

75. Which one of the following statements associated with Parkinson's disease is true?
A) The condition is associated with neurofibrillary tangles found in the substantia nigra.
B) The carbidopa component of Sinemet blocks peripheral dopa decarboxylase.
C) Amantadine is an antagonist of levodopa.
D) Benztropine (Cogentin) is helpful for the bradykinesia late in the course of Parkinson's disease.
E) Surgery for Parkinson's disease has not been shown to be beneficial.

Answer and Discussion

The answer is B. Parkinson's disease is a progressive neurologic disorder that is associated with the loss of dopamine-containing neurons in the substantia nigra. It usually affects older patients, and there is usually no family history. The diagnosis is usually made clinically. Symptoms include a resting, pill-rolling tremor, bradykinesia (the most common complaint), and cogwheel or lead-pipe rigidity. Other manifestations include infrequent blinking, a distinguishing blank stare, festinating gait (shuffling gait with a rapid initiation and the inability to stop once started), and increased salivation. The patient may also show signs of depression or dementia. Dopamine replacement is still considered the most efficacious treatment for Parkinson's disease. Because dopamine itself does not cross the blood–brain barrier, it is administered as the precursor levodopa in combination with carbidopa (Sinemet). Carbidopa blocks peripheral dopa decarboxylase, the enzyme that converts levodopa to dopamine within the blood–brain barrier. With the levodopa–carbidopa combination, more levodopa reaches the brain and is converted to dopamine. Amantadine, which has a longer half-life than levodopa, appears to act synergistically with levodopa and thus has been considered useful in the treatment of early Parkinson's disease. Dopamine receptor agonists were introduced as adjuncts to levodopa therapy to help control the motor fluctuations that occur in patients with Parkinson's disease. The dopamine agonists available

for the treatment of Parkinson's disease in the United States are bromocriptine (Parlodel), pergolide (Permax), pramipexole (Mirapex), and ropinirole (Requip). Dopamine enhancement through the inhibition of dopamine breakdown in the CNS was the mechanism behind the development of selegiline (Eldepryl), a monoamine oxidase B inhibitor. This agent is used as an adjunct to levodopa therapy. Theoretically, it allows levodopa to be administered less often, but this has not been observed in practice. Although selegiline has antioxidant properties, no evidence supports the earlier notion that the drug is neuroprotective and delays the natural progression of Parkinson's disease. Dopamine and its precursor, levodopa, are metabolized by the enzyme catechol *O*-methyltransferase in the liver, gastrointestinal tract, and other organs. By preventing this breakdown, catechol *O*-methyltransferase inhibitors (e.g., entacapone; tolcapone (Tasmar) has been associated with liver failure) enhance the amount of levodopa that reaches the CNS, thereby allowing more of the drug to be converted to dopamine. Although this mechanism parallels that of carbidopa, catechol *O*-methyltransferase inhibitors can be taken concurrently with the levodopa–carbidopa combination because a different enzyme is involved. Trihexyphenidyl (Artane) or benztropine may be prescribed as adjunctive therapy to levodopa. Either of these anticholinergic drugs may be helpful in managing significant tremor early in the course of Parkinson's disease. Anticholinergic agents have been used with mixed results in patients with essential tremor, dystonias, and certain dyskinesias. Elderly patients are often unable to tolerate the side effects of these drugs, which include cognitive impairment, dry mouth, and urinary retention. Levodopa–carbidopa (Sinemet) should be taken with a low-protein meal. Surgery is considered an option even in elderly patients as long as they meet medical screening criteria, including failure to respond to available medications and absence of cardiopulmonary risk factors for surgery. Thalamotomy effectively reduces tremor and sometimes rigidity on the contralateral side. Bilateral thalamotomy may result in speech, swallowing, and visual deficits. Thalamic stimulation can reproduce the benefits of thalamotomy without the risk of irreversible tissue loss because no physical lesion is created. Pallidotomy is a procedure in which a portion of the globus pallidus is treated permanently. The procedure has significant associated risks, including visual field deficits and hemiparesis (because of the proximity of the medial pallidum to the optic tracts and internal capsule). Bilateral procedures have a >15% complication rate and are associated with postoperative neuropsychiatric deficits in some patients. Compared with thalamic procedures, pallidotomy is less beneficial for tremors and more beneficial for dyskinesias. Pallidal and subthalamic nucleus stimulation procedures are being accepted as less invasive, more reversible alternatives to pallidotomy. Tissue transplantation procedures are also being evaluated for the treatment of Parkinson's disease. Additional adjunctive therapies include physical therapy, nutritional counseling, and techniques to help patients manage emotional and cognitive changes related to the disease.

Additional Reading: Parkinson's disease. In: Domino F, ed. *The 5-Minute Clinical Consult.* Philadelphia, PA: Lippincott Williams and Wilkins; 2014.

Category: Neurologic

Parkinson's disease is a progressive neurologic disorder associated with the loss of dopamine-containing neurons in the substantia nigra.

76. Which of the following statements concerning macular degeneration is true?
A) Peripheral vision is spared.
B) Drusen is a sign of late disease.
C) The exudative form is the most commonly seen.
D) Vision loss is usually sudden and irreversible.
E) Vision rehabilitation is not beneficial.

Answer and Discussion

The answer is A. Age-related macular degeneration is the leading cause of severe vision loss among the elderly. In this condition, central vision is lost, but peripheral vision almost always remains intact. Affected persons rarely require canes or guide dogs. However, the loss of central visual acuity can lead to a reduction of daily activities and mobility in the elderly and increases the risks of falls, fractures, and depression in this population. Patients with age-related macular degeneration may complain of acute loss of vision, blurred vision, scotomas (areas of lost vision), or chronic distortion of vision. All patients with vision loss should be referred to an ophthalmologist; those with acute loss of vision should be referred immediately. The diagnosis of age-related macular degeneration is based on symptoms and ophthalmoscopic findings. The disease is usually classified as early or late. Late disease can be divided into atrophic (dry) and exudative (wet) forms. In early disease, the macula shows yellowish-colored subretinal deposits called *drusen* and/or increased pigment. Drusen are thought to be byproducts of retinal pigment epithelium dysfunction. In most eyes with early disease, visual acuity remains stable for many years, and loss of vision is usually gradual. Late disease (atrophic and exudative) can lead to significant loss of vision. Exudative disease occurs in only 10% of patients with age-related macular degeneration, but it is responsible for the majority of cases of severe vision loss related to the disease. In atrophic disease, the macula usually shows areas of depigmentation. In the exudative form, fluid can accumulate underneath the retina, as in pigment epithelial detachments or subretinal neovascularization, and loss of vision is usually sudden. Fluorescein angiography can be used to help determine whether a patient has the atrophic or exudative form of the disease. The two currently proven treatments are laser photocoagulation and photodynamic therapy, but these measures are effective in only a small fraction of eyes with the exudative form of macular degeneration. Diet therapy and vitamin supplementation is still being investigated. Vision rehabilitation can help patients maximize their remaining vision and adapt so that they can perform activities of daily living. Families need encouragement in providing support and helping patients adjust to being partially sighted.

Additional Reading: Age related macular degeneration. In: Domino F, ed. *The 5-Minute Clinical Consult.* Philadelphia, PA: Lippincott Williams and Wilkins; 2014.

Category: Special sensory

77. Amyotrophic lateral sclerosis (ALS) is associated with
A) Sensory dysfunction
B) Cerebellar dysfunction
C) Atrophy of the muscles and fasciculations
D) Extraocular muscle dysfunction
E) Improved prognosis in elderly patients (older than 70 years)

Answer and Discussion

The answer is C. Amyotrophic lateral sclerosis (or Lou Gehrig's disease) affects upper and lower motor neurons. Two-thirds of patients present with symptoms associated with the limbs, and 25% have bulbar symptoms (usually in patients older than 70 years). Amyotrophic lateral sclerosis does not affect sensory, cerebellar, or extraocular muscle function. Men are more commonly affected. Most cases occur between the ages of 40 and 70 years. Rapidly fatal disease is associated with increasing age and bulbar symptoms. EMG studies show muscle denervation with preserved nerve conduction velocities. Treatment is primarily symptomatic. Attention should be focused on emotional support and "end-of-life" issues.

Additional Reading: Amyotrophic lateral sclerosis. In: Domino F, ed. *The 5-Minute Clinical Consult.* Philadelphia, PA: Lippincott Williams and Wilkins; 2014.

Category: Neurologic

78. The Minimum Data Set (MDS) is
A) A document that provides a comprehensive assessment of a nursing home resident and develops a plan of care
B) A list of vital signs for the nursing home resident
C) A document that describes the activities available to a nursing home resident
D) A set of minimum requirements that a nursing home has to abide by to receive state certification
E) A group of indicators that rank nursing homes based on safety and quality

Answer and Discussion

The answer is A. An MDS is a federally mandated document that is based on a comprehensive resident assessment. Information from the physician's history and physical and progress notes is used to complete an MDS. The MDS is then used to develop a plan of care and also is used to determine Medicare reimbursement for the patient.

Additional Reading: Medical care of nursing home patient. In: Basow DS, ed. *UpToDate.* Waltham, MA: UpToDate; 2013.

Category: Patient/population-based care

79. Physicians are required to see nursing home patients
A) Daily
B) Weekly
C) Monthly as long as they reside there
D) Monthly for 3 months and then every 2 months thereafter
E) Every 3 months

Answer and Discussion

The answer is D. Medicare regulations require that a physician make monthly visits for the first 3 months of a resident's nursing home stay and then every 2 months thereafter.

Additional Reading: Medical care of nursing home patient. In: Basow DS, ed. *UpToDate.* Waltham, MA: UpToDate; 2013.

Category: Patient/population-based care

80. Most of the gait disturbances identified in geriatric patients in the outpatient primary care setting are related to which one of the following?
A) Sensory ataxia
B) Parkinson's disease
C) Osteoarthritis
D) Multiple strokes
E) Myelopathy

Answer and Discussion

The answer is C. Problems with gait and balance increase in frequency with advancing age and are the result of a variety of individual or combined disease processes. Findings may be subtle initially, making it difficult to make an accurate diagnosis, and knowing the relative frequencies of primary causes may be useful for management. A cautious gait (broadened base, slight forward leaning of the trunk, and reduced arm swing) may be the first manifestation of many diseases, or it may just be somewhat physiologic if not excessive. In the past, a problematic gait abnormality in an elderly person was generally termed a senile gait if there was no clear diagnosis; it is more accurate, however, to describe this as an undifferentiated gait problem secondary to subclinical disease. From the long list of potential causes, arthritic joint disease is by far the most likely to be seen in the family physician's office, accounting for more than 40% of total cases. It most frequently causes an antalgic gait characterized by a reduced range of motion. The patient favors affected joints by limping or taking short, slow steps.

Additional Reading: Gait and balance disorders in older adults. *Am Fam Physician.* 2010;82(1):61–68.

Category: Neurologic

81. Which of the following statements is true regarding USPSTF screening guidelines for AAAs?
A) Screening is not beneficial for any subgroups of the populations.
B) Both women and men above the age of 50 should be screened.
C) Only men older than 75 should be screened.
D) Only men ages 65 to 75 with prior history of smoking should be screened.
E) Abdominal CT scanning is recommended for screening.

Answer and Discussion
The answer is D. The USPSTF recommends a single screening for AAA by ultrasonography in men ages 65 to 75 years who have previously smoked. The USPSTF found that there is a little benefit to repeat screening in men who had a negative ultrasound and that men above age 75 are unlikely to benefit from screening. The prevalence of AAA in men ages 65 to 75 who have never smoked is very low. Screening is not indicated. AAA screening is not recommended for women.

Additional Reading: Screening for abdominal aortic aneurysm. *US Preventive Service Task Force,* 2005 update. From: http://www.uspreventiveservicestaskforce.org/uspstf/uspsasco.htm.

Category: Cardiovascular system

82. Which of the following statements concerning advanced directives is true?
A) Once recorded, they cannot be changed.
B) Living wills are often easier for patients to complete than designating a health care power of attorney.
C) Advanced directives should be discussed only when life-threatening illnesses are present.
D) Physicians are not required to comply with patients' requests for treatment when they believe such requests are ill advised, harmful, or futile.
E) There is no need to update advance directives.

Answer and Discussion
The answer is D. An advance directive consists of a person's oral and written instructions about his or her future medical care in the event that he or she becomes unable to communicate, becomes incompetent to make health care decisions (during a terminal illness), or is in a persistent vegetative state. There are two types of advance

directives: a health care power of attorney and a living will. The health care ("durable") power of attorney, or *health care proxy,* is a document by which the patient appoints a trusted person to make decisions about his or her medical care if he or she cannot make those decisions. A *living will* is a written form of advance directive in which the patient's wishes regarding the administration of medical treatment are delineated in case the patient becomes unable to communicate his or her wishes.

Discussion of advanced directives should take place early on in the care of patients to discuss the patient's wishes should they become debilitated and cannot answer for themselves. The durable power of attorney allows the patient to designate a surrogate to make medical decisions if the patient loses decision-making capacity. The durable power of attorney is often less emotionally laden than outlining specific treatments to give or withhold. The five steps identified in the ideal process of advanced care planning are as follows: (1) Raise the topic and give information regarding the advance directive and health care proxy; (2) facilitate a structured discussion; (3) complete a statement, date and record it, and have the patient supply copies to the proxy and anyone else deemed appropriate (e.g., clergy); (4) periodically review and update the directive, and initial and date all changes; and (5) implement the plan by following the patient's wishes when the appropriate time comes. Finally, physicians are not automatically obliged to comply with patients' requests for treatment when they believe such requests are ill advised, harmful, or futile. Strict adherence to such requests may interfere with the physician's autonomy and ability to provide sound medical care.

Additional Reading: Implementing advance directives in office practice. *Am Fam Physician.* 2012;85(5):461–466.

Category: Patient/population-based care

83. A 70-year-old man with a history of atrial fibrillation now on warfarin therapy presents with a left-sided hemiparesis and a change in personality noted by his family. The nursing home reports a fall 2 weeks ago. A CT scan from the emergency room shows a small illuminated crescentic collection of fluid that is located adjacent to the convexity of the hemisphere. The most likely diagnosis is
A) Subdural hematoma
B) Epidural hematoma
C) Subarachnoid hemorrhage
D) Subdural abscess
E) Brain tumor

Answer and Discussion
The answer is A. Subdural hematomas are associated with rupturing of the bridging veins beneath the dura. The elderly and those taking anticoagulants are at increased risk. Acute subdural hematomas become symptomatic within minutes to hours after the injury. Patients may report a unilateral headache, and the examination shows a slightly enlarged pupil on the side affected. Stupor, coma, hemiparesis, and unilateral papillary enlargement are typical signs of larger hematomas. Pupillary dilation is contralateral in 5% to 10%. For the patient with a rapidly declining course, burr holes or emergency craniotomy is indicated to reduce intracerebral pressure from an expanding lesion. Most subdural hematomas appear as crescentic collections over the convexity of the hemisphere and are located in the frontotemporal region. Chronic subdural hematomas may develop as a result of mild trauma and manifest as chronic headaches, slowed thinking, change in personality, seizures, or a mild hemiparesis that develops weeks to months after the injury. Many are bilateral. Symptoms may resemble a cerebrovascular accident or transient ischemic attack. Epidural

hematomas develop more quickly than subdural hematomas and are more dangerous. They occur as a result of arterial bleeding between the dura mater and skull and are less common in the elderly. Most patients are comatose when first seen. The epidural hematoma forms a lenticular-shaped clot on CT. Treatment is surgical evacuation.

Additional Reading: Subdural hematoma in adults. In: Basow DS, ed. *UpToDate*. Waltham, MA: UpToDate; 2013.

Category: Neurologic

84. Which of the following statements regarding home visits is true?
A) They are increasing in frequency.
B) Reimbursement has increased their use.
C) Physicians who perform home visits have increased job satisfaction.
D) Home visits are not effective at managing patients because of a lack of resources.
E) Home visits rarely identify new medical problems, but are better suited to manage chronic medical problems.

Answer and Discussion

The answer is C. Years ago, the home visit was an essential part of primary care practice. More recently, the home visit has been used less frequently. The low frequency of home visits by physicians is the result of many coincident factors, including deficits in physician compensation for these visits, time constraints, perceived limitations of technologic support, concerns about the risk of litigation, lack of physician training and exposure, and corporate and individual attitudinal biases. Physicians most likely to perform home visits are older generalists in solo practices. Health care providers who have long-established relationships with their patients are also more likely to use house calls. Rural practice setting, older patient age, and need for terminal care correlate with an increased frequency of home visits. Studies suggest that home visits can lead to improved medical care through the discovery of undetected health care needs. Home assessment of elderly patients with relatively good health status and function can increase the detection of new medical problems and new intervention recommendations. There is also improved effectiveness of home visits in assessing unexpected problems in patient compliance with therapeutic regimens. Additionally, specific home-based interventions such as adjusting the elderly patient's home environment to prevent falls have also yielded health benefits. Beyond the potential benefit of improved patient care, family physicians who conduct home visits report a higher level of practice satisfaction than those who do not offer this service.

Additional Reading: A home visit. *Am Fam Physician.* 2011; 83(3):254.

Category: Patient/population-based care

85. Which of the following should be adjusted for when performing a Mini-Mental State Examination (MMSE)?
A) Location and sex of individual
B) Age and level of education
C) Support and living arrangement
D) Height and weight
E) Eyesight and hearing

Answer and Discussion

The answer is B. The Mini-Mental State Examination is a 30-point tool that tests orientation, immediate recall, delayed recall, concentration/calculation, and language and visuospatial domains. Adjustments should be made for age and level of education. As a general guideline

scores >26 are normal, scores of 24 to 26 may indicate mild cognitive impairment, and a score of <24 is consistent with dementia.

Additional Reading: Neurological exam. *Massachusetts General Hospital Handbook of Neurology.* Philadelphia, PA: Lippincott Williams and Wilkins; 2007

Category: Neurologic

> The Mini-Mental State Examination is a 30-point tool that tests orientation, immediate recall, delayed recall, concentration/calculation, and language and visuospatial domains. Adjustments should be made for age and level of education.

86. Which of the following blood test has been correlated with an increased risk of late onset Alzheimer's Disease (AD) ?
A) Apolipoprotein E—E4
B) Apolipoprotein E—E2
C) Homocystine
D) Sedimentation rate
E) C-reactive protein

Answer and Discussion

The answer is A. The association between apolipoprotein E (APOE) and AD is well established. The presence of one E4 allele increases the risk of AD about two to three times, whereas the E2 allele may be protective. The absence of an E4 allele does not rule out the diagnosis, nor does the presence of homozygous E4/E4 rule it in. The test is considered experimental.

Additional Reading: Alzheimer disease. In: Domino F, ed. *The 5-Minute Clinical Consult.* Philadelphia, PA: Lippincott Williams and Wilkins; 2014.

Category: Neurologic

87. When treating nursing home patients, it is important to remember that any antipsychotic medications must be reviewed and an attempt to withdraw or taper them made every
A) 30 days
B) 3 months
C) 6 months
D) Year
E) There is no need to withdraw or taper antipsychotic medications because of the risk to patient's safety.

Answer and Discussion

The answer is C. Federal regulations require an attempt to withdraw (or decrease) the dose of medications to manage agitation or psychosis in nursing homes every 6 months.

Additional Reading: Medical care of the nursing home patient in the United States. In: Basow DS, ed. *UpToDate*. Waltham, MA: UpToDate; 2013.

Category: Patient/population-based care

88. Which of the following is less likely to occur in elderly patients with influenza?
A) Headache
B) Muscle aches
C) Fatigue
D) Sore throat
E) Fever

Answer and Discussion

The answer is E. Influenza is a common respiratory infection that causes significant morbidity and mortality in older adults. Influenza is responsible for more than $1 billion in annual Medicare expenditures. Of deaths resulting from influenza, the vast majority occur in adults 65 years and older. Older adults are susceptible to severe and potentially fatal complications from this common illness because of coexisting chronic disease and weakened immunity. Older adults can benefit most from vaccination, early detection, and aggressive therapy. The signs and symptoms of influenza infection in older adults are similar to those occurring in younger patients, although a febrile response may be absent. Influenza is typically associated with rapid onset of headache, fever, chills, muscle aches, malaise, cough, and sore throat. Most people recover fully within 1 week, but older adults may develop a persistent weakness that can last for many weeks, and are also at higher risk for developing complications such as pneumonia. Diagnosis is usually made clinically. Several commercially produced rapid diagnostic tests intended for use in outpatient settings can detect influenza viruses within 30 minutes. In selected patients, obtaining a viral culture may be warranted to acquire specific information on influenza subtypes and strains. Four antiviral agents—amantadine, rimantadine, zanamivir, and oseltamivir—are approved for prevention or treatment of influenza. Zanamivir and oseltamivir are not approved for prophylactic use. It is unknown whether therapy with amantadine or rimantadine can prevent complications of influenza A among persons at high risk, including older adults. Rimantadine costs more than amantadine, but has fewer adverse effects on the CNS (e.g., confusion, nervousness, anxiety) and is less dependent on renal excretion. Zanamivir and oseltamivir are equally effective neuroaminidase inhibitors, but their place in therapy is yet to be determined. It has not yet been determined whether early initiation of treatment reduces hospital admission and mortality, particularly in elderly and high-risk patients.

> **Additional Reading:** Common infections in older adults. *Am Fam Physician.* 2001;63:257–268.

> **Category:** Patient/population-based care

89. Which of the following statements regarding the treatment of prostate cancer is true?
A) Radical prostatectomy appears to have a better cure rate than radiation therapy.
B) Radiation therapy has a better cure rate than surgery.
C) Surgery is better suited for younger patients.
D) Younger patients are typically observed to prevent risks associated with surgery or radiation.
E) Metastatic disease is not treatable.

Answer and Discussion

The answer is C. Young, healthy patients are most often encouraged to undergo radical prostatectomy, and older patients are steered toward observation or radiotherapy. However, the treatment choice must be based on the patient's preference, given his understanding of the benefits and side effects of each option. Overall, cure rates for radical prostatectomy generally fall between 60% and 70%. External-beam radiotherapy appears to be as effective as surgery in curing prostate cancer, at least for the first 10 years after treatment. Radiotherapy is well tolerated, and it is associated with no hemorrhagic or anesthetic risks. Furthermore, this treatment option does not require hospitalization or a significant recovery period. Normal activity can usually be maintained during radiotherapy. However, treatment is administered daily for 4 to 6 weeks, and many patients report fatigue at the end of this period. Compared with surgery, radiotherapy has several potential disadvantages. Radical prostatectomy provides more definitive information about long-term prognosis because the size of the tumor, the presence of cancer spread, and the presence of cancer in the lymph nodes can be determined from the surgical specimen. With radiotherapy, the posttreatment status of the tumor is unknown; serial PSA levels serve as surrogate markers to determine whether the treatment was curative. Radiotherapy can also have significant side effects. It is associated with severe bladder irritation (urgency, pain, and frequency) in as many as 5% of patients. Rectal irritations (diarrhea, urgency, tenesmus, and bleeding) occur in up to 10% of patients who receive radiotherapy for prostate cancer, and impotence is a problem in almost one-half of patients receiving this treatment. Thus, surgery is generally preferred for younger patients, whereas radiation treatment may be better suited for older patients who may not be good surgical candidates. Metastatic disease can be treated with hormonal manipulation, including surgical castration or medical castration using a luteinizing hormone–releasing agonist.

> **Additional Reading:** Prostate cancer. In: Domino F, ed. *The 5-Minute Clinical Consult.* Philadelphia, PA: Lippincott Williams and Wilkins; 2014.

> **Category:** Reproductive system

90. The Medicare Hospice Benefit covers all of the following expenses for patients in nursing homes *except*
A) All visits by hospice team members
B) The rental or purchase of durable medical equipment
C) Cost of supplies that are ordered by the hospice team
D) The costs of medication (except for a small copay)
E) Payment of room and board

Answer and Discussion

The answer is E. When a nursing home patient is identified as having a life-threatening illness or condition, it is appropriate to plan for end-of-life care. The Medicare Hospice Benefit can help greatly with the many tasks involved in providing palliative management of the dying patient's symptoms, attending to increased hygienic needs, and supplying bereavement services. For eligible terminally ill patients, the Medicare Hospice Benefit supplies an interdisciplinary team with skills in pain management, symptom control, and bereavement assistance. The services of the hospice team supplement the usual nursing home care at a time when staff, family members, and the patient are facing the increased and urgent needs associated with the dying process. The Medicare Hospice Benefit can make it much easier for physicians and nursing home staff to provide comprehensive palliative care for terminally ill patients. When a nursing home resident is referred for care under the Medicare Hospice Benefit, the hospice assumes responsibility for the professional management of many interdisciplinary services that supplement the usual care provided by nursing home staff. All medical treatments should have the goal of symptom control and they should be consistent with the hospice plan of treatment. The Medicare Hospice Benefit covers all visits by hospice team members, the rental or purchase of durable medical equipment, and the cost of supplies that are ordered by the hospice team. The hospice also supplies drugs for the palliation and management of the terminal illness, a benefit that normally is not available under the regular Medicare program. For each of these drugs, the beneficiary is only responsible for a small co-payment. Thus, hospice care is not an additional expense for many nursing home residents. Payment of room and board remains the responsibility of the patient and/or the family, or government assistance programs cover it for eligible residents (e.g., under Medicaid). The Medicare Hospice Benefit cannot be provided for nursing home residents who are receiving skilled Medicare coverage if their diagnoses for hospice and nursing home skilled care are the same. Before the Medicare Hospice Benefit can be initiated, these patients may choose to use all their skilled care days, or they may elect to waive their skilled coverage.

> **Additional Reading:** Hospice: what you should know. *Am Fam Physician.* 2008;77(6):817–818.

Category: Patient/population-based care

91. The drug of choice for the treatment of a serious methicillin-resistant *Staphylococcus aureus* (MRSA) infection is
A) Penicillin
B) Ceftazidime
C) Metronidazole
D) Imipenem
E) Vancomycin

Answer and Discussion

The answer is E. MRSA is a major problem for elderly patients, especially those in institutional settings. People colonized with MRSA are at increased risk of MRSA infection. They also have a higher risk of death as a result of resistance to typical antibiotics. Poor functional status is associated with being an MRSA carrier. Therefore, nursing homes and other institutional settings must be especially careful to prevent the spread of infection caused by this organism. Hand washing, isolation of infected patients, and proper handling of body secretions are essential to prevent the spread of MRSA. The most common reservoirs for MRSA colonization are the nasal mucosa and oropharynx. Skin contamination from persons already colonized in these areas may also be a source for MRSA infection. Although colonization by MRSA does not require systemic treatment, an active serious infection with MRSA is treated with vancomycin as the preferred antibiotic. Older adults may require dosage adjustment based on renal function. Other regimens include vancomycin plus gentamicin (Garamycin) or rifampin (Rifadin), sulfamethoxazole–trimethoprim (Sulfa), doxycycline, minocycline, and clindamycin. Attempts to identify the original infected person (source case) should be made by swabbing the nasopharynx of patients and staff near to the outbreak and treating those found to have MRSA infection. Staff and patients who are MRSA carriers should be isolated, and some authorities recommend treatment with topical mupirocin (Bactroban), which is applied twice daily for 2 weeks to the nares or other areas of skin carriage (e.g., wounds) to reduce the shedding of MRSA. Colonization recurs in approximately one-half of treated subjects.

> **Additional Reading:** IDSA guidelines on the treatment of MRSA infections in adults and children. *Am Fam Physician.* 2011;84(4):455–463.

Category: Nonspecific system

92. The most common reason for discontinuing acetylcholinesterase inhibitors is
A) Headache
B) Hepatotoxicity
C) Rash
D) Cataracts
E) Gastrointestinal side effects

Answer and Discussion

The answer is E. Gastrointestinal side effects, including nausea, vomiting, and diarrhea, are a class effect and are the most common reason for discontinuation of acetylcholinesterase inhibitors (tacrine, donepezil, rivastigmine, and galantamine). These can usually be minimized by slow titration over an 8- to 12-week period. Reversible hepatotoxicity is seen with tacrine—therefore, this drug is not generally recommended as first-line therapy.

> **Additional Reading:** Alzheimer disease. In: Domino F, ed. *The 5-Minute Clinical Consult.* Philadelphia, PA: Lippincott Williams and Wilkins; 2014.

Category: Neurologic

> Gastrointestinal side effects, including nausea, vomiting, and diarrhea, are a class effect and are the most common reason for discontinuation of acetylcholinesterase inhibitors (i.e., tacrine, donepezil, rivastigmine, and galantamine).

93. Which of the following is considered a risk factor for falls?
A) Hypothyroidism
B) Anemia
C) Addison's disease
D) Vitamin D deficiency
E) All are risk factors for falls.

Answer and Discussion

The answer is E. Many conditions that affect the elderly can increase the risk for falls. Hypothyroidism, anemia, Addison's disease, vitamin B_{12} deficiency, and vitamin D deficiency are some notable causes that should be ruled out when assessing an elderly patient after a fall.

> **Additional Reading:** Management of falls in older persons: a prescription for prevention. *Am Fam Physician.* 2011;84(11): 1267–1276.

Category: Nonspecific system

94. An 87-year-old man is seen by you for a general examination. He has no history of coronary artery disease and remains active, playing golf three times per week. His only other medical problem is mild hypertension for which he takes hydrochlorothiazide. Which of the following statements is true regarding treatment of his elevated cholesterol, which was discovered on a recent blood test?
A) Based on his advanced age, he does not qualify for treatment of his hyperlipidemia.
B) Only lifestyle measures should be used to treat his cholesterol because of the risk of medication use.
C) The decision to treat this man should be based on national guidelines regardless of his underlying medical condition.
D) Treatment of hyperlipidemia should be individualized on the basis of the patient's chronological and physiologic age and life expectancy.
E) The decision to treat hyperlipidemia in the elderly should not be influenced by a patient's terminal diagnosis.

Answer and Discussion

The answer is D. The decision whether to treat high or high-normal serum cholesterol in an elderly individual must be individualized and based on both chronological and physiologic age of the patient. As an example, a patient with a limited life span from a concomitant illness (e.g., metastatic cancer, dementia) is probably not a candidate for drug therapy. However, an otherwise healthy elderly individual should not be denied drug therapy simply on the basis of age alone.

Additional Reading: Treatment of dyslipidemia in the elderly. In: Basow DS, ed. *UpToDate*. Waltham, MA: UpToDate; 2013.

Category: Cardiovascular system

95. Your 50-year-old patient, Roger, chooses to have a colonoscopy, and asks whether his 78-year-old mother, who is also your patient, should be screened. Which one of the following responses is consistent with the recommendations of the USPSTF?
A) She should be screened using high-sensitivity fecal occult blood testing (FOBT).
B) Because of her age, she should be screened at more frequent intervals than persons 75 years and younger.
C) She should not be screened routinely for colorectal cancer.
D) Regardless of whether she has been screened before, Roger's mother should be screened at the recommended intervals throughout her life.
E) She should not be screened using colonoscopy because the harms of the test outweigh the benefits in persons her age.

Answer and Discussion

The correct answer is C. Although considerations may warrant screening in particular patients, the USPSTF recommends against routine screening in adults 76 to 85 years of age. For adults in this age group who have not been screened before, the decision whether to screen should be based on health status, competing risks, and patient preference. Although the direct harms of fecal occult blood testing are minimal, the USPSTF does not endorse a particular screening test in this age group. The USPSTF recommends against colorectal cancer screening in patients 85 years and older because the harms of screening outweigh the benefits.

Additional Reading: Screening for colorectal cancer. *Am Fam Physician*. 2010;81(8):1017–1018.

Category: Gastroenterology system

96. Which of the following medications would be the best selection to treat chronic neuropathic pain in a frail elderly man with a history of cardiac conduction abnormalities?
A) Fluoxitene (Prozac)
B) Amitryptiline (Elavil)
C) Gabapentin (Neurontin)
D) Phenytoin (Dilantin)
E) Cyclobenzaprine (Flexaril)

Answer and Discussion

The answer is C. Gabapentin binds to the voltage-gated calcium channels at the alpha 2-delta subunit and inhibits neurotransmitter release. It has proven efficacy versus placebo in several neuropathic pain conditions. Of the second-generation antiepileptic drugs, gabapentin has the best-documented efficacy in the treatment of neuropathic pain. An antiepileptic drug (e.g., gabapentin) is preferred if the patient cannot tolerate the side effects of tricyclic antidepressants, has cardiac contraindications to the use of tricyclic antidepressants (e.g., conduction abnormalities, recent cardiac event), or is a "frail elder." Treatment with gabapentin should be initiated at a low dose with gradual increases until pain relief, dose limiting adverse effects, or 3,600 mg per day in three divided doses is achieved. An adequate trial of treatment with gabapentin can require 2 months or more.

Additional Reading: Drugs for Pain. *Treatment Guidelines from The Medical Letter.* April 1, 2013

Category: Neurologic

Pictorial Atlas

QUESTIONS

Each of the following questions or incomplete statements is followed by suggested answers or completions. Select the ONE BEST ANSWER in each case.

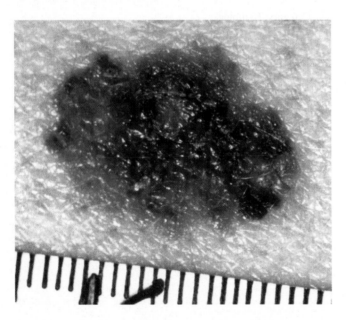

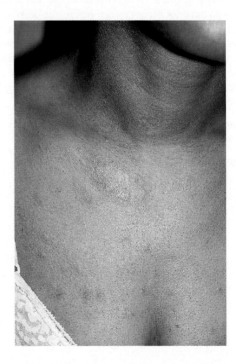

1. A 42-year-old woman presents with the lesion (shown at left) on the back of her calf. She has no significant medical problems and otherwise feels well. The lesion has not bled, but seems to have grown over the last few months. Appropriate initial management of this skin lesion should be

A) Observation and removal if bleeding or further change occurs
B) Complete excision with normal margins
C) Complete excision with wide margins
D) Shave biopsy
E) Electrodesiccation and curettage

2. A 26-year-old woman presents with the above rash. She states the rash is minimally pruritic and developed over the last week. She has had some virus-like symptoms and reports the rash began as a large salmon-colored patch on her chest area. The most likely diagnosis is

A) Tinea versicolor
B) Pityriasis rosea
C) Varicella
D) Psoriasis
E) Coccidioidomycosis

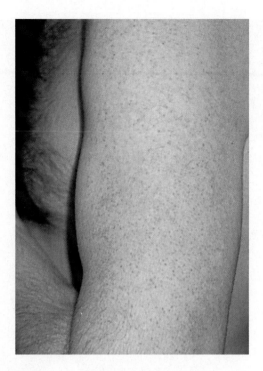

3. An 18-year-old man presents to your office complaining of a sandpaper-like rash that affects his upper outer arms. He is otherwise healthy and has no other symptoms. The most likely diagnosis is
A) Scarlet fever
B) Infectious mononucleosis
C) Keratosis pilaris
D) Seborrheic dermatitis
E) Psoriasis

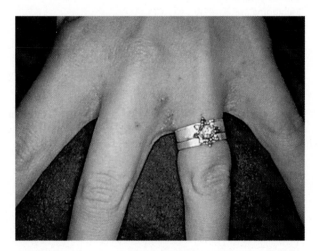

4. A 35-year-old woman presents with a pruritic rash that has been present over the last few weeks. The area affected is in the webs of the fingers, and symptoms are reported to be worse at night. Topical over-the-counter steroids have not been beneficial. The likely diagnosis is
A) Poison ivy
B) Dyshidrotic eczema
C) Scabies
D) Tinea corporis
E) Psoriasis

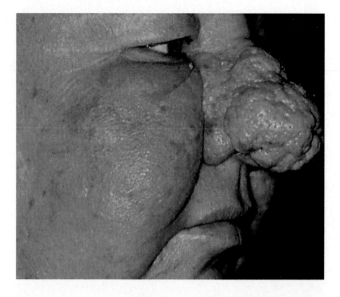

5. A 72-year-old man presents to your office complaining of an area of redness associated with the perinasal region. He states that the rash is often worse in the summer, and he has noticed that sunlight exposure makes it worse. Appropriate treatment of this condition consists of
A) Hydrocortisone cream
B) Tretinoin gel
C) Metronidazole cream
D) Mupirocin ointment
E) Acyclovir ointment

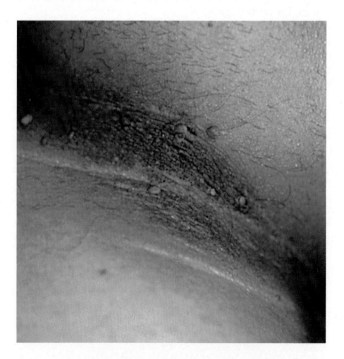

6. Which of the following malignancies is associated with the skin condition shown here?
A) Ovarian carcinoma
B) Gastric carcinoma
C) Malignant melanoma
D) Multiple myeloma
E) Hodgkin's lymphoma

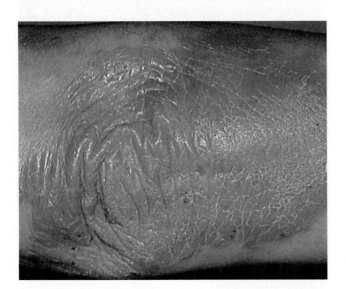

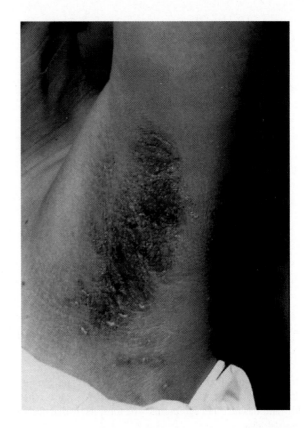

7. A 45-year-old woman presents with a localized area of erythematous scaly patches that comes and goes and typically affects the elbows. The likely diagnosis is

A) Pityriasis rosacea
B) Mycosis fungoides
C) Tinea corpora
D) Nummular eczema
E) Psoriasis

9. You note the above skin disorder during a general medical evaluation. You explain to the patient they are at risk for the development of

A) Alzheimer's disease
B) Tuberculosis
C) Diabetes mellitus
D) Graves' disease
E) Melanoma

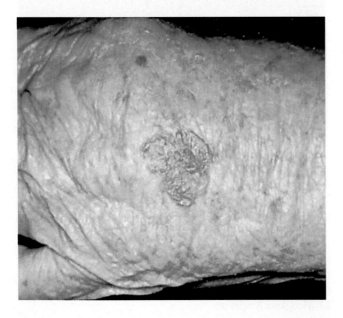

8. A 60-year-old retired construction worker presents with a non-healing skin lesion on the back of his hand that occasionally bleeds when he gets out of the shower. The most likely diagnosis is

A) Basal cell carcinoma
B) Squamous cell carcinoma
C) Superficial spreading malignant melanoma
D) Actinic keratosis
E) Keratoacanthoma

10. A 42-year-old woman presents to the emergency room complaining of shortness of breath and palpitations. An electrocardiogram shows the above tracing. Appropriate management at this time includes
A) Epinephrine
B) Metoprolol
C) Nitroglycerin
D) Adenosine
E) Lidocaine

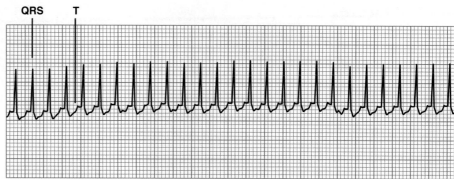

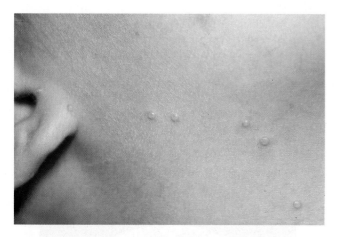

11. A 4-year-old preschooler presents with the skin lesions shown here. The area affected is just below the chin on the child's right side. The lesions have been present over the last month, and the child has reported no symptoms associated with them. The most likely diagnosis is
A) Varicella
B) Herpes zoster
C) *Rhus* dermatitis
D) Molluscum contagiosum
E) Scabies

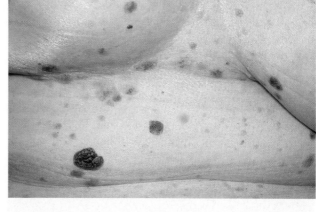

13. An 82-year-old nursing home resident is seen on monthly rounds. The floor nurse points out the skin lesions shown here. The patient is asymptomatic. Appropriate management includes
A) Punch biopsy
B) Topical 5-fluorouracil cream
C) Cryotherapy
D) Hydrocortisone cream
E) Observation

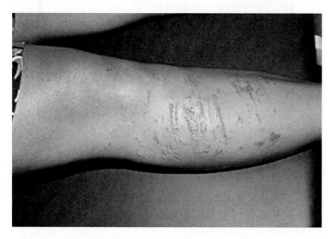
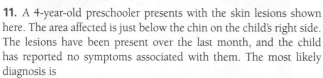

12. A 16-year-old girl who just returned from a camping trip reports an intensely pruritic vesicular rash associated with the lower extremities. The most likely diagnosis is
A) *Rhus* dermatitis
B) Lyme disease
C) Chigger bite
D) Brown recluse spider bite
E) Black widow spider bite

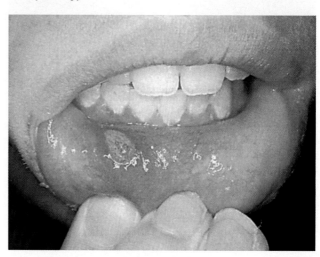

14. An 18-year-old sexually active woman presents with a single ulcer that is located on the lower lip and is painful. She is a smoker and has noticed that the ulcers have been recurrent and correlate with the onset of menses. The most likely diagnosis is
A) Kawasaki disease
B) Aphthous stomatitis
C) Squamous cell carcinoma of the lip
D) Syphilis
E) Koplik's spot

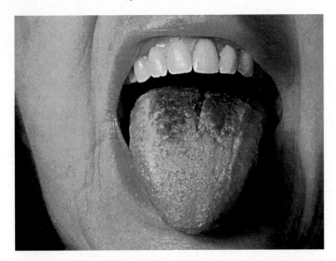

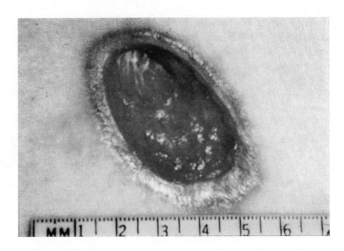

15. Which of the following conditions is the skin finding shown here associated with?
A) Prolonged antibiotic use
B) Sjogren's syndrome
C) Addison's disease
D) Chronic gastroesophageal reflux
E) Malignant melanoma

17. The condition shown here was noted associated with an 88-year-old debilitated nursing home resident. He has no evidence of bacteremia or osteomyelitis. Which of the following is an acceptable treatment?
A) Application of povidone-iodine gauze two times per day
B) Application of hydrogen peroxide 3 times per day
C) Systemic antibiotics for 7 to 10 days
D) Keeping the area clean and dry until granulation tissue forms
E) Surgical debridement

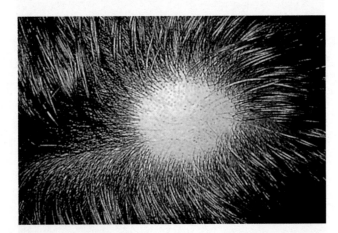

16. A 38-year-old man presents with rapid hair loss that has occurred over the last few weeks. He reports that his father had a similar condition. The most likely diagnosis is
A) Alopecia areata
B) Androgenic alopecia
C) Tinea capitis
D) Trichotillomania
E) Secondary syphilis

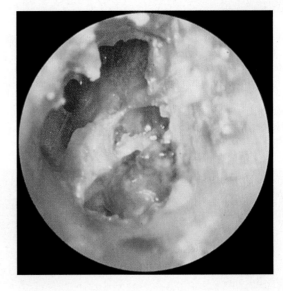

18. A 35-year-old presents with unilateral hearing loss that has been gradual but progressive over the last 6 months. Appropriate treatment of the above condition consists of
A) Prolonged antibiotics for up to 4 weeks
B) Decongestant and antihistamine administration
C) Corticosteroid treatment for 2 weeks
D) Hearing aid amplification
E) Tympanomastoidectomy

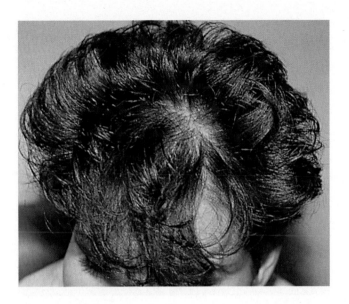

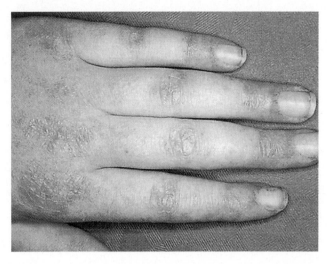

19. A 27-year-old gravida 2, para 2 woman is now 6 months post-partum and complains of excessive hair loss. The most likely diagnosis is

A) Alopecia areata
B) Telogen effluvium
C) Trichotillomania
D) Tinea capitis
E) Hypothyroidism

21. A 55-year-old woman complains of generalized fatigue, weakness, inability to climb stairs, arthralgias, and dysphagia. Physical examination reveals definite proximal muscle weakness, a periorbital heliotrope rash, and skin findings associated with the hands (shown here). The most likely diagnosis is

A) Lupus erythematosus
B) Sarcoidosis
C) Sjögren's disease
D) Dermatomyositis
E) Polymyalgia rheumatica

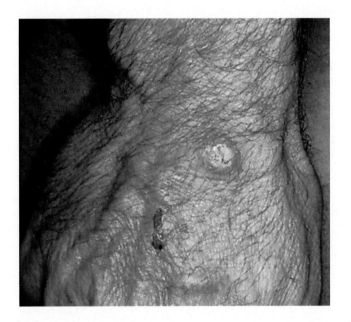

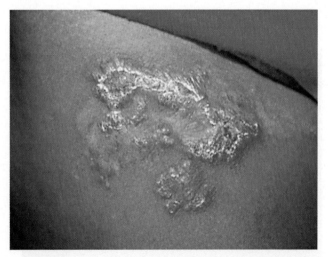

20. A 68-year-old man is seen for a general examination and reports a dome-shaped lesion on the back of the hand that has developed over the last few weeks. The lesion is rapidly becoming larger. The most likely diagnosis is

A) Basal cell carcinoma
B) Squamous cell carcinoma
C) Seborrheic keratosis
D) Actinic keratosis
E) Keratoacanthoma

22. A 50-year-old housewife who enjoys growing roses presents to your office complaining of the lesion shown here. She reports removing a thorn from the area several weeks before. After that, a small painless lump developed that now has crusted over. The most likely diagnosis is

A) Sporotrichosis
B) Blastomycosis
C) Lyme disease
D) Coccidioidomycosis
E) Histoplasmosis

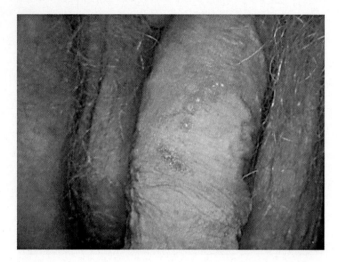

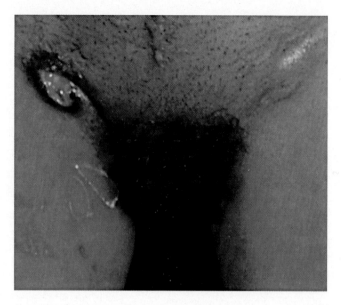

23. A 23-year-old Navy enlisted man is seen in sick bay with the recurrent lesion shown here. The patient reports pain and discomfort associated with the lesion but no dysuria. The likely diagnosis is
A) Molluscum contagiosum
B) Gonorrhea
C) Syphilis
D) Chancroid
E) Herpes infection

24. A 23-year-old black woman presents with a lesion affecting her groin that has developed over the last few days. Dark-field microscopic examination is negative. The etiologic agent that is responsible for the lesion is
A) *Neisseria gonorrhoeae*
B) Herpes zoster
C) *Treponema pallidum*
D) Molluscum contagiosum
E) *Haemophilus ducreyi*

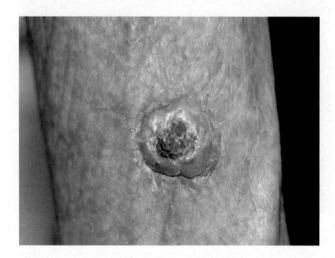

25. The pictured skin lesion developed over a 4-week period. The most likely diagnosis is
A) Melanoma
B) Basal cell carcinoma
C) Keratoacanthoma
D) Dermatofibroma
E) Molluscum contagiosum

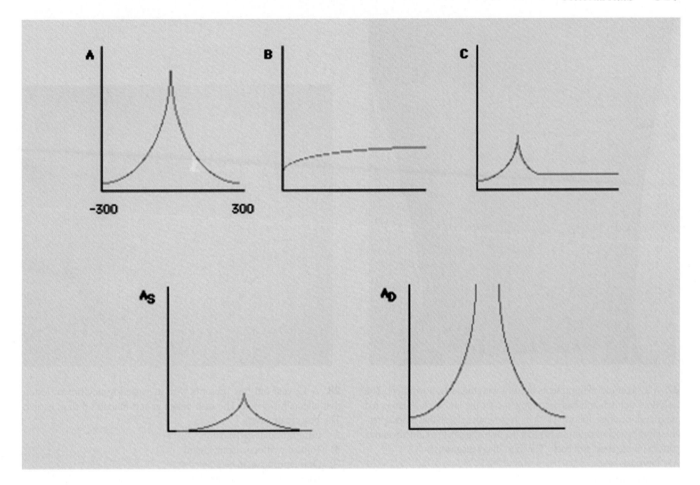

26. Which of the above audiograms represents a likely effusion behind the tympanic membrane?

A) Type A
B) Type B
C) Type C
D) Type As
E) Type Ad

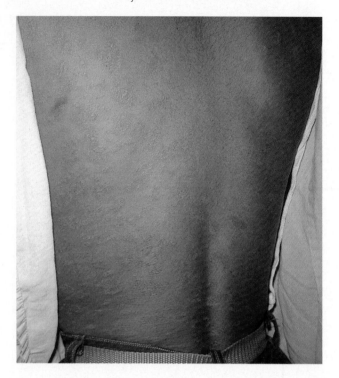

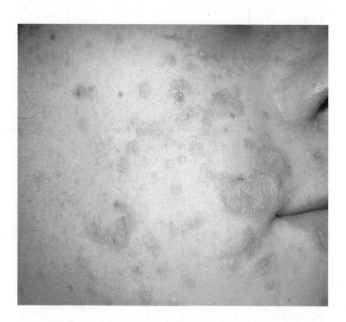

27. A 29-year-old man presents in April with the rash shown here. The rash does not itch and has been present over the last week. A large, red area developed first, followed by a more generalized rash that is now present. Physical examination shows that the rash appears in a Christmas-tree pattern on his chest and back. The most likely diagnosis is

A) Pityriasis rosea
B) Tinea versicolor
C) Herpes zoster
D) Varicella
E) Lyme disease

28. A 12-year-old boy presents with a crusted honey-brown lesion that affects his cheek. The rash began as red macules 3 days earlier. The best treatment is

A) Intramuscular ceftriaxone
B) Topical hydrocortisone cream
C) Oral ciprofloxacin
D) Topical mupirocin ointment
E) Oral acyclovir

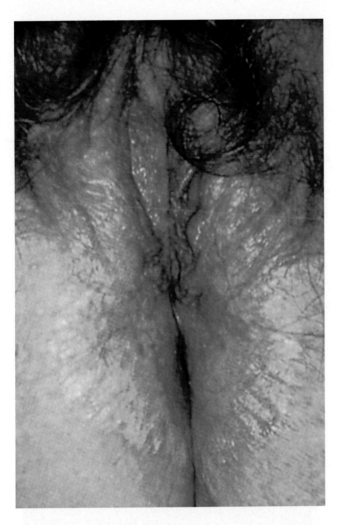

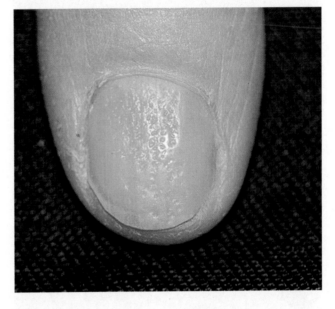

29. A 65-year-old woman presents to your office complaining of gradually increasing dyspareunia. Findings from the physical examination are pictured here. The most likely diagnosis is

A) Yeast vaginitis

B) Herpes genitalis

C) Lichen sclerosis

D) Vitiligo

E) Contact dermatitis

30. A 45-year-old woman presents with pitting of the nails that has developed slowly over the last few months. The most likely diagnosis is

A) Psoriasis

B) Onychomycosis

C) Hyperthyroidism

D) Chronic obstructive pulmonary disease

E) Scleroderma

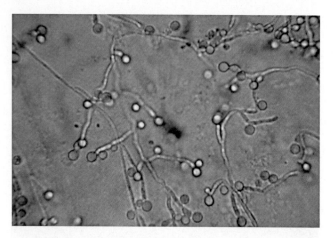

31. A sexually active 24-year-old woman presents to your office complaining of vaginal discharge. Findings from a wet prep are pictured here. The most likely diagnosis is
A) Yeast vaginitis
B) *Gardnerella* infection
C) *Trichomonas* infection
D) Gonorrhea
E) Chlamydia

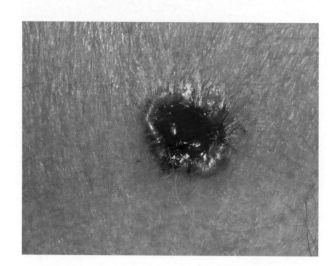

33. An 18-year-old surfer presents with the above skin condition. The most likely diagnosis is
A) Pityriasis rosea
B) Secondary syphilis
C) Seborrheic dermatitis
D) Eczema
E) Tinea versicolor

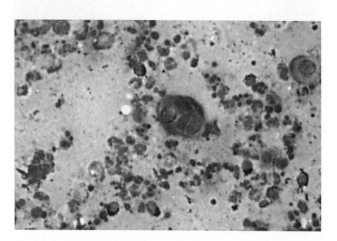

32. The sample shown here was obtained from a penile lesion of a 24-year-old sexually active man. A Tzanck smear was performed. The confirmed diagnosis is
A) Gonorrhea
B) Chancroid
C) Herpes genitalis
D) Syphilis
E) Chlamydia

34. The most likely diagnosis is
A) Pearly papule
B) Basal cell carcinoma
C) Molluscum contagiosum
D) Squamous cell carcinoma
E) Keratoacanthoma

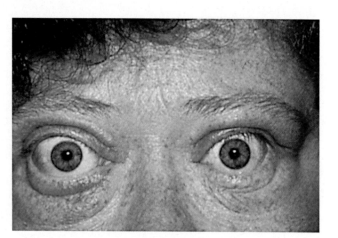

35. The eye findings pictured (at left) were seen in a 40-year-old woman who presented to the emergency room complaining of palpitations. The most likely diagnosis is
A) Scleroderma
B) Graves' disease
C) Amyloidosis
D) Cushing's disease
E) Lupus erythematosus

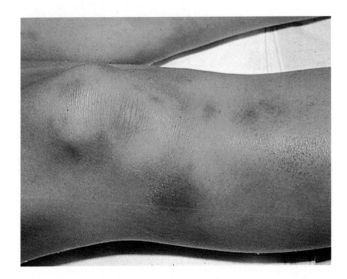

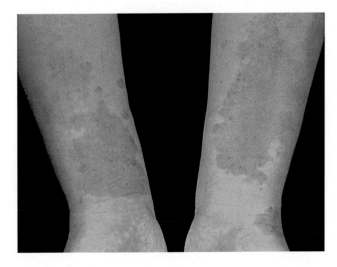

36. An 18-year-old woman presents to your office complaining of tender nodules that have developed on the lower extremities. She has no other symptoms. She continues with her oral contraceptives but has not started any new medications. She denies any fevers and has no history of recent trauma. The likely diagnosis is

A) Erythema multiforme
B) Erythema nodosum
C) Lyme disease
D) Pyoderma gangrenosum
E) Rheumatoid arthritis

38. A 2-year-old girl is brought in by her mother. The child has an erythematous rash that is recurrent and affects the backs of the legs. The most likely diagnosis is

A) Ichthyosis vulgaris
B) Scabies
C) Atopic dermatitis
D) Dyshidrotic eczema
E) Tinea corpora

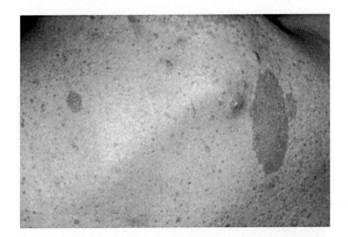

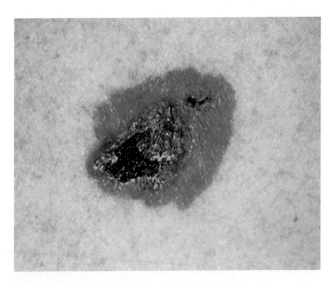

37. A 26-year-old man is seen for an upper respiratory infection. After removing his shirt, you notice the lesions shown here. He reports that his father has similar lesions. The differential diagnosis should include

A) Hypothyroidism
B) Addison's disease
C) Multiple sclerosis
D) Neurofibromatosis
E) Gardner's syndrome

39. Appropriate management of the lesion shown here includes

A) Cryotherapy
B) Electrodesiccation and curettage
C) Shave biopsy
D) Excisional biopsy
E) Laser ablation

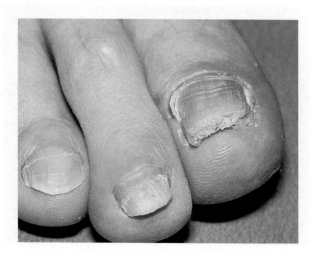

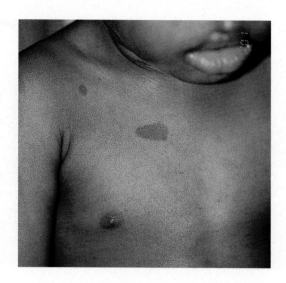

40. The most common etiologic agent that gives rise to the condition shown here is
A) *Trichophyton rubrum*
B) *Candida albicans*
C) *Epidermophytin floccosum*
D) *Aspergillus flavus*
E) *Candida glabrata*

42. A 4-year-old boy is brought to your office by his parents. They are concerned about the multiple skin lesions that have been present since infancy. You explain that the lesions can be a sign for
A) Dysplastic nevi syndrome
B) Diabetes
C) Gastrointestinal cancer
D) Neurofibromatosis
E) Lymphoma

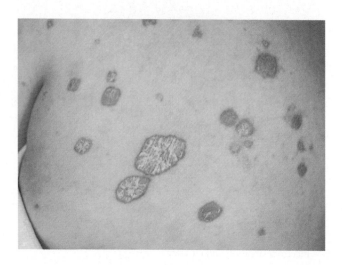

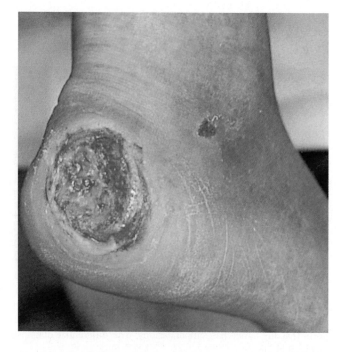

41. A 45-year-old man presents with a chronic, mildly pruritic, and scaly erythematous rash. The most likely diagnosis is
A) Cutaneous T-cell lymphoma
B) Psoriasis
C) Eczema
D) Tinea versicolor
E) Lichen planus

43. A 68-year-old man with a history of a previous myocardial infarction presents complaining of a painful lesion noted on his foot. He has been experiencing pain in his lower legs with ambulation over the last year. The most likely diagnosis is
A) Venous stasis ulcer
B) Arterial ulcer
C) Basal cell carcinoma
D) Livedo reticularis
E) Diabetic foot ulcer

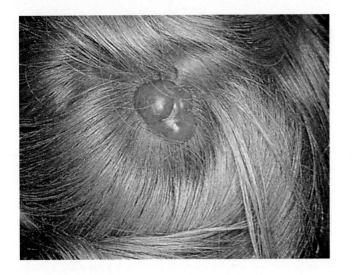

44. A 42-year-old man presents with a small lump that has formed on his scalp. The most likely diagnosis is
A) Syringoma
B) Cylindroma
C) Trichoepithelioma
D) Histiocytoma
E) Dermatofibroma

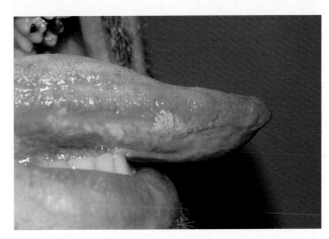

46. Which of the following conditions is associated with the skin finding shown here?
A) Vitamin B$_{12}$ deficiency
B) Hypothyroidism
C) Human immunodeficiency syndrome
D) Periodontitis
E) Gastroesophageal reflux

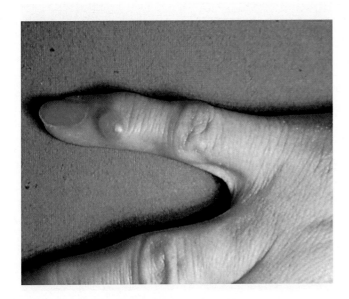

45. A 58-year-old woman presents to your office complaining of a clear fluid-filled cyst that has formed over the distal knuckle of the fifth finger of the right hand. The most likely diagnosis is
A) Epidermoid cyst
B) Sebaceous cyst
C) Mucous cyst
D) Lipoma
E) Synovial cyst

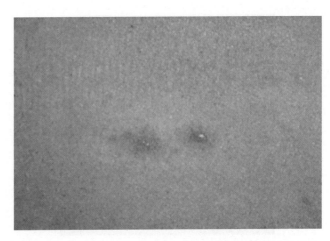

47. A 3-year-old child who attends daycare is brought in by her mother with the lesions shown here noted on the abdomen. The mother reports some low-grade fevers, and the child has not been as active as usual. The most likely diagnosis is
A) Impetigo
B) Coxsackievirus
C) Adenovirus
D) Varicella
E) Scarlatina

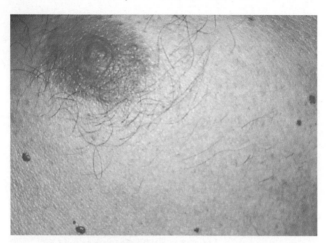

48. A 42-year-old man complains of multiple red lesions that have formed on his chest and abdomen. The most likely diagnosis is
A) Scabies
B) Chigger bites
C) Granuloma annulare
D) Cherry angiomas
E) Erythroderma

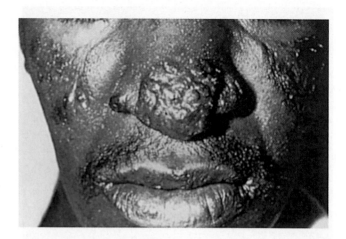

50. A 42-year-old African American presents to your office with the above skin condition. She has a history of chronic sarcoidosis and has experienced multiple exacerbations. The most likely diagnosis is
A) Lupus pernio
B) Erythema nodosum
C) Erythema marginatum
D) Erythema multiforme
E) Psoriasis

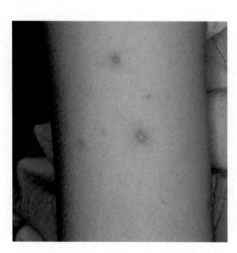

49. A 36-month-old immigrant child is brought in by his mother with a sore throat and an erythematous, pruritic rash that has developed over the last 24 hours. The most likely diagnosis is
A) Varicella
B) Scarlatina
C) Fifth disease
D) Rocky Mountain spotted fever
E) Measles

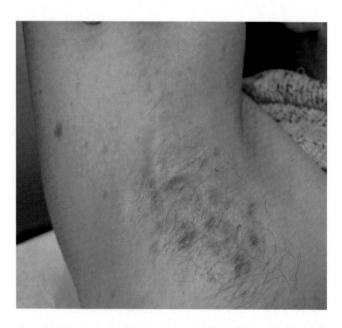

51. A 33-year-old woman presents with complaints of recurrent rashes under the arm that come and go and the development of painful cysts with scar tissue formation. The most likely diagnosis is
A) Hidradenitis suppurativa
B) Reaction to antiperspirant
C) Impetigo
D) Tinea corpora
E) Scrofuloderma

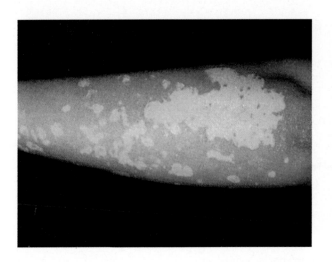

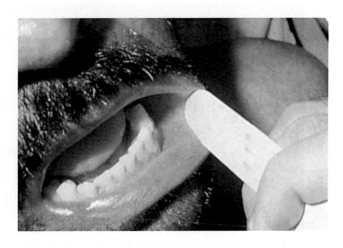

52. A 38-year-old African American presents with the lesion shown here. The lesion shows a "milk-white" fluorescence with a Wood's light examination. The most likely diagnosis is
A) Tinea versicolor
B) Tinea corpora
C) Amelanotic melanoma
D) Vitiligo
E) Leprosy

54. A 36-year-old indigent man from Mexico presents with 1-mm bluish-white macules with an erythematous oral mucosa. Two days later, an erythematous, generalized papular rash develops. The rash began on his forehead and progressed to involve his entire body. He has also had upper respiratory symptoms and a fever. The most likely diagnosis is
A) Human immunodeficiency virus   D) Rubeola
B) Coxsackievirus   E) Scarlet fever
C) Rubella

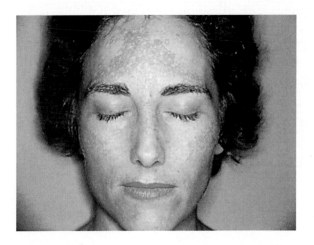

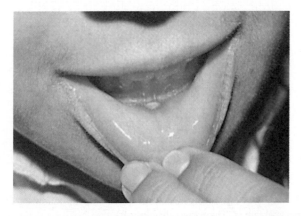

53. A 42-year-old Native American woman presents to your office complaining of dark spots on her face. Her medical history is unremarkable except for two previous uncomplicated pregnancies. She is now taking oral contraceptives. The most likely diagnosis is
A) Solar lentigo
B) Melasma
C) Sunburn
D) Lupus erythematosus
E) Scleroderma

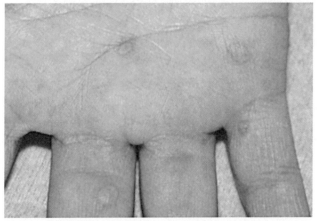

55. The most likely cause for the condition shown here is
A) Herpes virus   D) Lyme disease
B) Coxsackievirus   E) Syphilis
C) Adenovirus

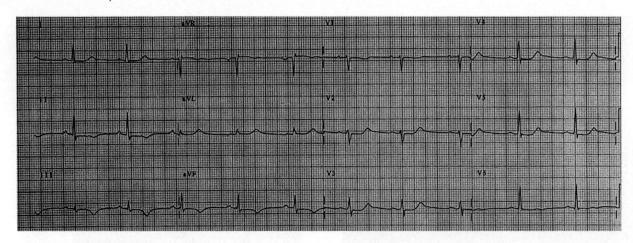

56. Based on the electrocardiographic (ECG) tracing shown here, the most likely diagnosis is
A) Atrial fibrillation
B) Left bundle branch block
C) Third-degree heart block
D) Inferior ischemia
E) Left ventricular hypertrophy

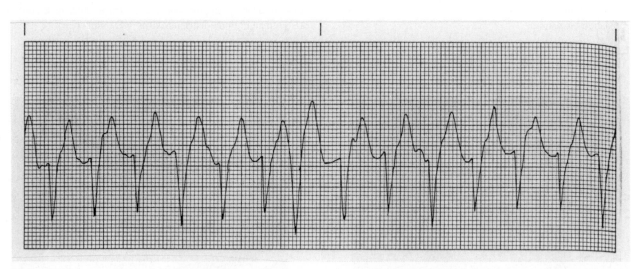

57. A 67-year-old collapses in your office and the following ECG strip is obtained. The correct diagnosis is
A) Atrial fibrillation
B) Ventricular fibrillation
C) Supraventricular tachycardia
D) Ventricular tachycardia
E) Atrioventricular dissociation

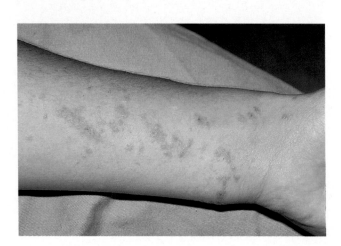

58. A 9-year-old boy is brought in to your office after a weekend camping trip. He complains of a pruritic rash that has developed over the last 24 hours. The most likely diagnosis is
A) Poison ivy
B) Erythema multiforme
C) Lichen sclerosis
D) Varicella
E) Herpes zoster

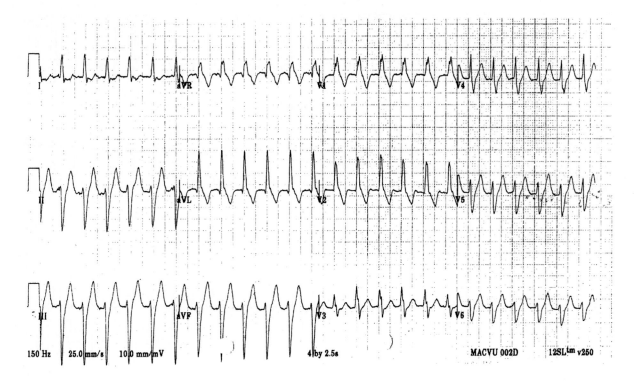

59. Please identify the rhythm shown here.

A) Atrial fibrillation

B) Atrial flutter

C) Supraventricular tachycardia

D) Ventricular fibrillation

E) Ventricular tachycardia

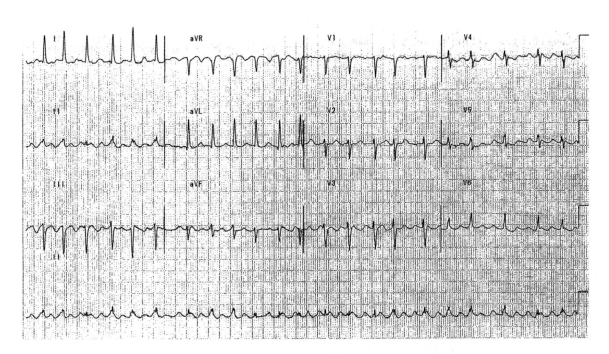

60. A 65-year-old presents to the emergency room complaining of palpitations. Findings from an ECG are shown here. The most likely diagnosis is

A) Acute myocardial infarction

B) Atrial fibrillation

C) Supraventricular tachycardia

D) Ventricular fibrillation

E) Ventricular tachycardia

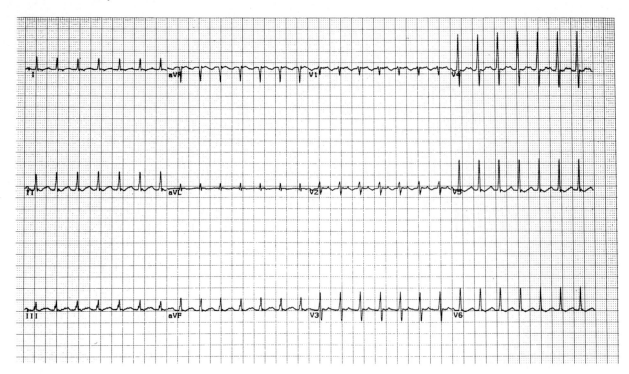

61. A 38-year-old presents to the emergency room complaining of palpitations and shortness of breath. The most likely diagnosis based on the ECG findings shown here is

A) Atrial fibrillation

B) Supraventricular tachycardia

C) Ventricular fibrillation

D) Ventricular tachycardia

E) Wolff–Parkinson–White syndrome

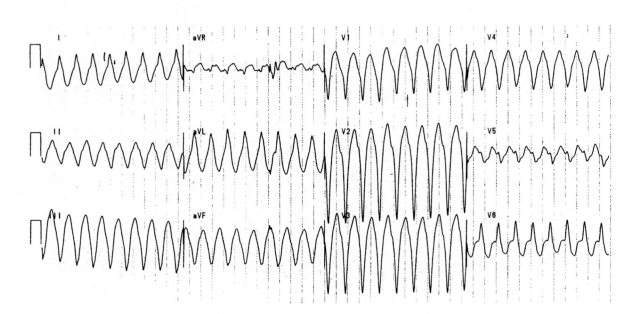

62. A 68-year-old man is found unresponsive. An initial ECG tracing is shown here. Which of the following conditions is present?

A) Atrial ventricular dissociation

B) Ventricular tachycardia

C) Ventricular fibrillation

D) Sinus tachycardia

E) Asystole

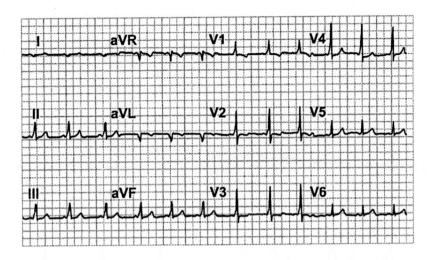

63. Please identify the condition shown here.

A) Hypothermia
B) Wolff–Parkinson–White syndrome
C) Inferior myocardial infarction
D) Atrial fibrillation with 3:1 block
E) Normal sinus rhythm

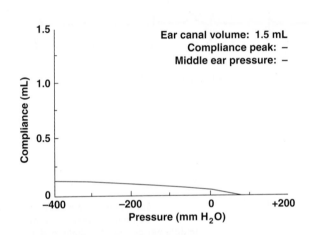

Ear canal volume: 1.5 mL
Compliance peak: –
Middle ear pressure: –

64. The tympanogram shown here would support the diagnosis of
A) Normal tympanic membrane
B) Fluid in the middle ear
C) Negative middle ear pressure
D) Hypermobile tympanic membrane
E) None of the above

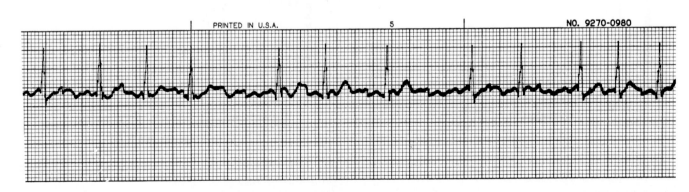

65. A 65-year-old alcoholic presents to your office with shortness of breath and generalized fatigue. An ECG is obtained. The most likely diagnosis is
A) Multifocal atrial tachycardia
B) Supraventricular tachycardia
C) Atrial fibrillation
D) Sinus tachycardia
E) Pulmonary embolism

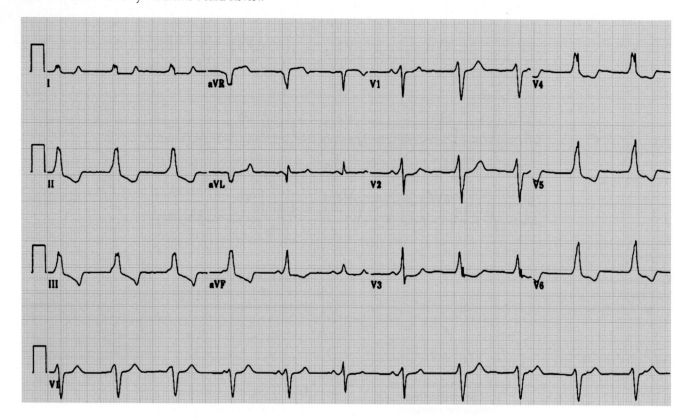

66. Based on the above ECG, the most likely diagnosis is

A) Supraventricular tachycardia with 3:1 block

B) Early myocardial infarction

C) Incomplete right bundle branch block

D) Pericarditis

E) Wolff–Parkinson–White syndrome

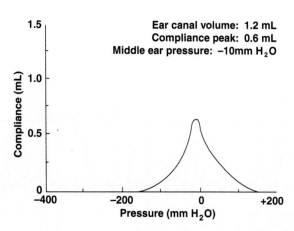

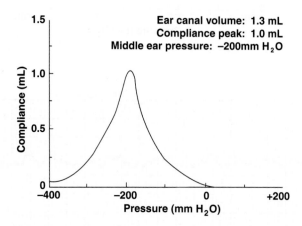

67. A 4-year-old is suspected of having a middle ear effusion. A tympanogram is obtained and reveals the pattern shown here. The most appropriate management is

A) Tympanocentesis

B) Placement of tympanostomy tubes

C) Prophylactic antibiotics for 1 year

D) Decongestant use for 4 to 6 weeks

E) Reassurance

68. The tympanogram shown here was obtained on a 3-year-old girl. The likely diagnosis is

A) Eustachian tube dysfunction

B) Acoustic neuroma

C) Middle ear effusion

D) Sensorineural hearing loss

E) Normal tympanogram

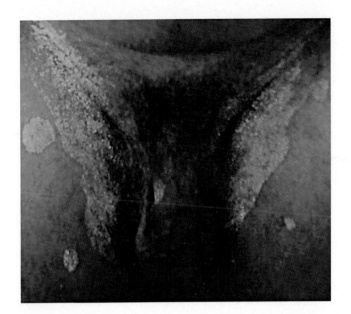

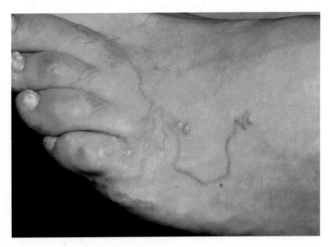

69. A 51-year-old man presents to your office complaining of a rash that affects the groin. Faint redness is noted, with fine scaling and no elevated border. Further examination under a Wood's lamp reveals a bright orange-coral fluorescence. The most likely diagnosis is
A) Tinea cruris
B) Mycoses fungoides
C) Erythrasma
D) Hidradenitis suppurativa
E) Erysipelas

70. An 18-year-old surfer presents to your office with a rash that he noted on his foot. The vesicular rash has been present over the last week and has been enlarging. The most likely diagnosis is
A) Sea lice
B) Cutaneous larva migrans
C) Swimming pool granuloma
D) Jellyfish sting
E) Bathing suit dermatitis

ANSWER AND EXPLANATIONS

1. The answer is B. (*Complete excision with normal margins*) Even in the hands of experienced dermatologists, there is an approximately 15% false-negative rate in determining the presence of melanoma on the basis of examination alone; therefore, histologic confirmation is essential for both tumor diagnosis and staging. A complete excision with normal skin margins is preferable when possible as the first diagnostic step (e.g., excisional biopsy). An incisional biopsy can be performed for larger lesions when complete excision is not practical and when the suspicion of melanoma is low; incisional biopsy does not adversely affect survival. Shave biopsies should be avoided because they may not provide enough tissue for diagnosis and do not allow for accurate depth measurement. All biopsies of lesions suspected of being melanomas should provide a piece of full-thickness skin extending to the subcutaneous fat.

Additional Reading: Cutaneous melanoma: update on prevention, screening, diagnosis, and treatment. *Am Fam Physician.* 2005;72(2):269–276.

Category: Integumentary

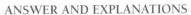 When considering the diagnosis of melanoma, shave biopsies should be avoided because they may not provide enough tissue for diagnosis and do not allow for accurate depth measurement. All biopsies of lesions suspected of being melanomas should provide a piece of full-thickness skin extending to the subcutaneous fat.

2. The answer is B. (*Pityriasis rosea*) Pityriasis rosea is a self-limited, exanthematous skin disease that develops acutely and is characterized by the appearance of slightly inflammatory, oval, papulosquamous lesions on the trunk and proximal areas of the extremities. Pityriasis rosea is largely a disease of older children and young adults. It is more common in women than in men. A prodrome of headache, malaise, and pharyngitis may occur in a small number of cases, but except for itching, the condition is usually asymptomatic. The eruption commonly begins with a "herald patch": a single round or oval, sharply demarcated pink or salmon-colored lesion on the chest, neck, or back, 2 to 5 cm in diameter. The lesion soon becomes scaly and begins to clear centrally, leaving the free edge of the scaly lesion directed inward toward the center. A few days or a week or two later, oval lesions similar in appearance to the herald patch, but smaller, appear in crops on the trunk and proximal areas of the extremities. The long axes of these oval lesions tend to be oriented along the lines of cleavage of the skin. This characteristic Christmas-tree pattern is most evident on the back, where it is emphasized by the oblique direction of the cleavage lines in that location. Most cases of pityriasis rosea need no treatment other than reassurance and proper patient education. Topical steroids with moderate potency are helpful in the control of itching. They can be applied to the pruritic areas two or three times daily. Topical antipruritic lotions such as prax, pramagel, or sarna may also be helpful.

Additional Reading: Pityriasis rosea. *Am Fam Physician.* 2004;69(1):87–91.

Category: Integumentary

3. The answer is C. (*Keratosis pilaris*) *Keratosis pilaris* is defined as hyperkeratotic follicular papules on the extensor surface of the upper arms or upper anterior thighs and occasionally on the malar area of the face. It may be associated with atopy and dry skin. A sandpaper-like feel is noted in these isolated areas. The condition is considered benign and is treated with topical lactic acid cream or lotion. Lesions that are associated with the face typically resolve at puberty.

Additional Reading: The generalized rash: Part II. Diagnostic approach. *Am Fam Physician.* 2010;81(6):735–739.

Category: Integumentary

4. The answer is C. (*Scabies*) The condition of scabies is associated with intense pruritus that is noted predominantly at night. The lesions are brownish in color and often form irregular burrow lines that may be marked with scaling at one end and a vesicle at the other end. The lesions are typically found in intertriginous areas and warm, protected areas such as the finger webs, inframammary areas, and axilla. The mite *Sarcoptes scabei* is responsible. Scrapings of the lesion are treated with 10% potassium hydroxide solution and studied under light microscopy. The mite is often identified. Treatment consists of permethrin cream 5% applied from head to toes and left in place for 12 hours before being washed off. Lindane can also be used as an alternative, but not in infants or in pregnant women.

Additional Reading: *Sauer's Manual of Skin Diseases,* 10th ed. Philadelphia, PA: Lippincott Williams & Wilkins; 2010:178–180.

Category: Integumentary

5. The answer is C. (*Metronidazole cream*) Rosacea is a common problem encountered by family physicians. The condition is associated with areas of erythema and telangiectasia on the face. It is exacerbated by sunlight, hot or spicy foods, and alcohol. Pronounced rosacea may appear as acneiform papules, pustules, or ruddiness. Northern Europeans and those of Celtic descent are most commonly affected. Treatment involves oral tetracycline or doxycycline. Topical metronidazole is also effective for milder cases.

Additional Reading: *Sauer's Manual of Skin Diseases,* 10th ed. Philadelphia, PA: Lippincott Williams & Wilkins; 2010:158–159.

Category: Integumentary

6. The answer is B. (*Gastric carcinoma*) Acanthosis nigricans is associated with hyperpigmented areas that typically affect flexural folds (axilla). The two basic types of acanthosis nigricans are benign and malignant. The benign form is associated with obesity, diabetes, Stein–Leventhal syndrome, Cushing's disease, Addison's disease, pituitary disorders, and hyperandrogenic syndromes. Drugs, including glucocorticoids, nicotinic acid, diethylstilbestrol, and growth hormone therapy, have also caused acanthosis nigricans. Many cases are idiopathic. Malignant acanthosis nigricans is associated with an intestinal cancer such as gastric carcinoma.

Additional Reading: *Sauer's Manual of Skin Diseases,* 10th ed. Philadelphia, PA: Lippincott Williams & Wilkins; 2010: 395–396.

Category: Gastroenterology System

7. The answer is E. (*Psoriasis*) Psoriasis usually manifests itself as erythematous scaly patches that affect the knees or elbows. More severe cases can involve multiple areas over the entire body.

Extensor surfaces are predominantly affected. Nail pitting may be present. The condition appears to be hereditary. Diagnosis is usually based on clinical findings. Skin biopsy may be helpful for definitive diagnosis. Treatment consists of topical steroids, intralesional steroids, tar preparations, anthralin, tazarotene, and calcipotriene.

Additional Reading: *Sauer's Manual of Skin Diseases,* 10th ed. Philadelphia, PA: Lippincott Williams & Wilkins; 2010:160–163.

Category: Integumentary

> Psoriasis usually manifests itself as erythematous scaly patches that affect the knees or elbows. More severe cases can involve multiple areas over the entire body. Extensor surfaces are predominantly affected. Nail pitting may be present.

8. The answer is A. (*Basal cell carcinoma*) Basal cell carcinoma is the most common form of skin cancer. The lesions are induced by ultraviolet radiation in susceptible individuals. Risk factors include age older than 40, light complexion, positive family history, and male sex. The lesion has pearly, raised borders with telangiectasia and a central ulcer that may crust. Sun-exposed areas are most commonly affected. Diagnosis is achieved with shave or excisional biopsy. Treatment is accomplished with excision, electrodesiccation and curettage, liquid nitrogen application, Moh's surgery, radiation treatment, and topical 5-fluorouracil cream. Almost 50% of patients with basal cell carcinoma will have another within 5 years.

Additional Reading: *Sauer's Manual of Skin Diseases,* 10th ed. Philadelphia, PA: Lippincott Williams & Wilkins; 2010:305–308.

Category: Integumentary

9. The answer is C. (*Diabetes mellitus*) Although the majority of cases of acanthosis nigricans are benign and associated with obesity, the disease can represent the onset of malignancy as well as a variety of conditions related to insulin resistance. Acanthosis nigricans has been reported in association with a number of malignancies, particular gastrointestinal cancers (e.g., gastric, hepatocellular), and lung cancer. The suspicion for malignancy increases in patients with extensive or rapidly progressive lesions, when there is mucous membrane involvement, or when there is prominent sole and palm disease. The common finding in all nonmalignancy-associated cases of acanthosis nigricans is insulin resistance. This explains the relationship between this skin disorder and diseases such as diabetes mellitus, Cushing's syndrome, and hypothyroidism (most likely due to weight gain and subsequent insulin resistance), and with obesity.

Additional Reading: Velvety axillary lesions. *Am Fam Physician.* 2004;69(2):373–374.

Category: Endocrine system

10. The answer is D. (*Adenosine*) The most important step to make when a narrow QRS tachycardia is noted is whether the patient is experiencing signs and symptoms related to the rapid heart rate. These symptoms include hypotension, shortness of breath, shock, decreased level of consciousness, or chest pain suggestive of coronary ischemia. Determining whether a patient's symptoms are related to the tachycardia depends on several factors, including age and the presence of underlying cardiac disease. Paroxysmal supraventricular tachycardia (PSVT) with a heart rate of 200 bpm may be tolerated by a healthy young adult with no or few symptoms (e.g., palpitations). However, a heart rate of 120 bpm may precipitate angina in an elderly patient with significant coronary heart disease. Adenosine is approved by the Food and Drug Administration (FDA) in the United States only for the intravenous management of PSVT in which the atrioventricular (AV) node is involved. For intravenous adenosine administration, the patient should be supine and should have electrocardiographic and blood pressure monitoring. The drug is administered by rapid intravenous injection over 1 to 2 seconds at a peripheral site, followed by a normal saline flush. The usual initial dose is 6 mg, with a maximal single dose of 12 mg. The most common side effects of adenosine are facial flushing (18%), palpitations, chest pain, and hypotension. Transient asystole is a rare complication. Another important side effect of adenosine is that it may precipitate atrial fibrillation (AF). In patients with Wolff–Parkinson–White syndrome (WPW), AF can progress into ventricular fibrillation. As a result, caution should be used when giving adenosine if WPW is a possible mechanism, and emergency resuscitation equipment should be available.

Additional Reading: Approach to the diagnosis and treatment of wide QRS complex tachycardias. In: Basow DS, ed. *UpToDate.* Waltham, MA: UpToDate; 2013.

Category: Cardiovascular system

11. The answer is D. (*Molluscum contagiosum*) Molluscum contagiosum is a common, superficial viral infection of the skin that typically occurs in infants and preschoolers. The incidence decreases after the age of 6 to 7 years. The condition can be spread via sexual contact in young adults. The lesions are dome-shaped, waxy, or pearly-white papules with a central white core and are 1 to 3 mm in diameter. Frequently, groups of lesions are found. The lesions may resolve spontaneously. Treatment involves removal with a sharp needle or curette, application of liquid nitrogen, antiwart preparations, electrodesiccation and curettage, or trichloroacetic peels for extensive areas. Typically, infants or young preschool-age children should not be treated aggressively.

Additional Reading: *Sauer's Manual of Skin Diseases,* 10th ed. Philadelphia, PA: Lippincott Williams & Wilkins; 2010:235–236.

Category: Integumentary

12. The answer is A. (*Rhus dermatitis*) Poison ivy or poison oak is also referred to as *Rhus dermatitis.* The condition is associated with intensely pruritic linear streaks of vesicles, papules, and blisters. The plants contain a resinous oil that gives rise to an allergic response approximately 2 days after exposure. Contrary to common belief, the fluid in the blisters can neither transfer the rash to others nor cause it to spread. Treatment involves topical steroid creams, Burow's solution, calamine lotion, antihistamines, cool baths with colloidal oatmeal, and oral steroids (for 2 to 3 weeks to prevent rebound dermatitis) for more widespread cases.

Additional Reading: *Goodheart's Photoguide to Common Skin Disorders: Diagnosis and Management,* 3rd ed. Philadelphia, PA: Wolters/Kluwer Lippincott Williams & Wilkins; 2009:63–65.

Category: Integumentary

13. The answer is E. (*Observation*) Seborrheic keratoses are common skin lesions that affect the elderly. They tend to run in families. The average diameter is 1 cm, but they can grow to 3 cm in diameter. The lesions are brown or black, oval in shape, raised, and have a "stuck

on" appearance. They most commonly occur on the face, back, neck, and scalp. They may appear suddenly and become pruritic and crusted. Numerous lesions that appear rapidly may signal the development of an underlying malignancy. Treatment is cosmetic and usually reserved for those that are inflamed or causing symptoms.

Additional Reading: *Sauer's Manual of Skin Diseases,* 10th ed. Philadelphia, PA: Lippincott Williams & Wilkins; 2010:280–283.

Category: Integumentary

14. The answer is B. (*Aphthous stomatitis*) Aphthous stomatitis, also known as *canker sores*, are painful eruptions that affect the mucosal surface of the mouth. The cause is unknown. Lesions typically develop at the same time and resolve in 5 to 10 days. A viral cause has not been proved. A streptococcal bacterium has been implicated. The lesions recur at regular intervals and may correlate with the onset of menses in some women. Treatment consists of toothpaste swish therapy, triamcinolone acetonide (Kenalog in Orabase), or tetracycline solution swish and swallow. Severe cases may respond to systemic corticosteroids.

Additional Reading: *Sauer's Manual of Skin Diseases,* 10th ed. Philadelphia, PA: Lippincott Williams & Wilkins; 2010:361–362.

Category: Integumentary

15. The answer is A. (*Prolonged antibiotic use*) Black hairy tongue results from hyperplasia of the filiform papillae with deposition of keratin on the surface. The condition causes the tongue to have a dark, velvety, hairlike appearance. Associated conditions include smoking, consumption of coffee, prolonged use of antibiotics, and possibly acquired immunodeficiency syndrome. Treatment involves using a toothbrush to scrape off the excess keratin that forms on the tongue's surface.

Additional Reading: *Sauer's Manual of Skin Diseases,* 10th ed. Philadelphia, PA: Lippincott Williams & Wilkins; 2010:363–364.

Category: Integumentary

16. The answer is A. (*Alopecia areata*) Alopecia areata is associated with sudden hair loss that occurs in round patches. The patches are well circumscribed and are not associated with scarring or inflammation. Patients have no other symptoms. The most common area affected is the scalp; however, the condition may also affect the eyebrows or beard. Alopecia areata usually affects children and young adults and is recurrent. A pathognomonic sign for alopecia areata is the "exclamation point" hair, which is wide distally and narrower at the base. These hairs are often found at the periphery of a patch of hair loss. Hair that regrows in the area of alopecia areata is in many cases white. Nail pitting may also be present. The treatment consists of injection of intralesional steroids and topical steroids. Most experience complete regrowth of hair.

Additional Reading: *Sauer's Manual of Skin Diseases,* 10th ed. Philadelphia, PA: Lippincott Williams & Wilkins; 2010:337–343.

Category: Integumentary

Alopecia areata is associated with sudden hair loss that occurs in round patches. The patches are well circumscribed and are not associated with scarring or inflammation.

17. The answer is E. (*Surgical debridement*) When treating pressure ulcers, it is important to maintain a moist environment while keeping the surrounding skin dry. This can be accomplished by loosely packing the ulcer with saline-moistened gauze. Topical antimicrobials such as silver sulfadiazine cream may be helpful in ulcers that appear infected. Topical antiseptics such as povidone-iodine or hydrogen peroxide should not be used in the treatment of pressure ulcers. Systemic antibiotics should be reserved for serious infections (e.g., bacteremia, osteomyelitis). A 2-week trial of topical antimicrobials may be considered for ulcers that do not appear infected but are not improving. Although most patients are successfully managed without surgery, procedures may be appropriate in patients whose quality of life would be markedly improved by rapid wound closure. Stage 3 and 4 ulcers with necrotic tissue should be debrided. Ulcers with minimal exudate that are not infected can be covered with an occlusive dressing to promote autolytic debridement. Ulcers with thick exudate, slough, or loose necrotic tissue should undergo mechanical debridement. Options include wet-to-dry dressings, hydrotherapy, wound irrigation, and scrubbing the wound with gauze. Ulcers with evidence of cellulitis or deep infection should undergo sharp debridement with a scalpel or scissors. Ulcers with a thick eschar or extensive necrotic tissue should undergo sharp debridement as well. However, a thick, dry eschar covering a heel ulcer should generally be left intact. Patients without access to surgical interventions (such as in a long-term care setting) or those who may not be acceptable surgery candidates can be treated with enzymatic debriding agents. Wound debridement should stop once necrotic tissue has been removed and granulation tissue is present.

Additional Reading: Treatment of pressure ulcers. In: Basow DS, ed. *UpToDate*. Waltham, MA: UpToDate; 2013.

Category: Integumentary

18. The answer is E. (*Tympanomastoidectomy*) Cholesteatoma is a growth of desquamated, stratified, squamous epithelium within the middle ear space. The condition occurs when keratin desquamates from the epithelial lining of the sac and gradually enlarges with eventual erosion of the ossicular chain, mastoid bowl, and external auditory canal. The development of a cholesteatoma typically occurs after a retraction pocket has formed in the posterior/superior quadrant of the ear, often as a result of chronic eustachian tube dysfunction. It may also occur after tympanic membrane (TM) trauma, such as a traumatic, inflammatory, or iatrogenic perforation. Without treatment, cholesteatomas may erode the tegmen tympani (the bony covering of the middle fossa), the sigmoid sinus, or even the inner ear. As a result, untreated cholesteatomas can result in lateral sinus thrombosis, sepsis, brain abscess, sensorineural hearing loss, vertigo, disequilibrium, facial paralysis, and even death. Treatment is surgical, usually involving a tympanomastoidectomy.

Additional Reading: Etiology of hearing loss in adults. In Basow DS, ed. *UpToDate*. Waltham, MA: UpToDate; 2013.

Category: Special sensory

19. The answer is B. (*Telogen effluvium*) Telogen effluvium is sudden, diffuse hair loss that occurs 3 to 6 months after a stressful event. The causes include medications (heparin, coumarin, propranolol, haloperidol, and lithium), neoplasms, infection, and crash diets. The stressful event triggers the hair follicles to go into a rest phase, and once the cycle returns a larger amount of hair is lost at one time. Typically, 30% to 50% of the scalp hair is affected. No treatment is needed. Patients should be reassured that normal hair growth should resume.

Additional Reading: Diagnosing and treating hair loss. *Am Fam Physician*. 200980(4):356–362.

Category: Integumentary

20. The answer is E. (*Keratoacanthomas*) Keratoacanthomas usually develop rapidly over a 2- to 6-week time frame. The lesions are dome-shaped with a central keratin-filled plug. They occur most commonly on sun-exposed areas. Many resolve spontaneously; however, because of their similarity to squamous cell carcinomas and their ability to metastasize, they should be removed by excision. Other treatment options include intralesional methotrexate, 5-fluorouracil, interferon, systemic retinoids, or radiation therapy. Complete excision is usually curative; however, recurrences can develop at the site of treated lesions.

Additional Reading: *Sauer's Manual of Skin Diseases*, 10th ed. Philadelphia, PA: Lippincott Williams & Wilkins; 2010:298.

Category: Integumentary

21. The answer is D. (*Dermatomyositis*) Dermatomyositis presents with a heliotrope rash and the presence of Gottron's papules. The rash is violaceous in color and involves the periorbital areas. Gottron's papules are erythematous or violaceous papules or plaques that form over the bony prominences, particularly the metacarpophalangeal joints, the proximal and distal interphalangeal joints. The condition is also associated with a myopathy that involves the proximal muscles. The shoulders and pelvic girdle are mainly affected in a symmetric pattern. Symptoms include fatigue, weakness, inability to climb stairs, or weakness in rising from a squatting or sitting position. Dysphagia is also seen. Approximately 20% of patients have an associated malignancy. Laboratory tests include elevated serum creatine kinase or aldolase, or both. Electromyographic studies and a muscle biopsy can also provide additional diagnostic information. The mainstays of treatment are systemic steroids. Other options include immunosuppressant agents and hydroxychloroquine. Those who are older and have severe myositis, dysphagia, associated malignancy, and a poor response to corticosteroids have a poorer prognosis.

Additional Reading: *Sauer's Manual of Skin Diseases*, 10th ed. Philadelphia, PA: Lippincott Williams & Wilkins; 2010: 386–389.

Category: Musculoskeletal system

22. The answer is A. (*Sporotrichosis*) Sporotrichosis is a granulomatous fungal infection that affects the skin. The lesion is caused by *Sporothrix schenckii*, a fungus that grows on wood and in the soil. The lesions typically affect farmers, gardeners (especially those who grow roses), laborers, and miners. A primary chancre occurs at the site of inoculation. The primary lesion is painless and forms a subcutaneous nodule that breaks down to form an ulcer. Within a few weeks, multiple nodules form along the areas of draining lymphatics and break down to form streaks of ulcers, often affecting the arms or legs. The fluid from unopened ulcers can be cultured and can aid in diagnosis. Treatment consists of saturated solution of potassium iodide, ketoconazole, or itraconazole. Systemic invasion is rare.

Additional Reading: *Sauer's Manual of Skin Diseases*, 10th ed. Philadelphia, PA: Lippincott Williams & Wilkins; 2010:264–265.

Category: Nonspecific system

23. The answer is E. (*Herpes infection*) Genital herpes is primarily associated with herpes simplex virus type 2. The symptoms include painful vesicles that occur in clusters, often on the shaft of the penis in men or vulvar areas in women. Patients often report fever, regional lymphadenopathy, and generalized fatigue in association with an outbreak. The lesions last for 2 to 3 days before the tops of the vesicles rupture. The remaining ulcers crust over and last an additional 5 to 7 days. Recurrences are common in the same area. Asymptomatic shedding of the virus can occur once the outbreak has resolved and can infect others. Diagnosis *can* be achieved with the use of Tzanck smears (which detect large bizarre mononucleate and multinucleate giant cells and nuclear changes of ballooning degeneration). Treatment is accomplished with the use of antiviral medications (acyclovir, valacyclovir, famciclovir, and topical penciclovir). Prophylactic therapy may be indicated in recurrent infections.

Additional Reading: *Sauer's Manual of Skin Diseases,* 10th ed. Philadelphia, PA: Lippincott Williams & Wilkins; 2010:230–232.

Category: Integumentary

24. The answer is E. (*Haemophilus ducreyi*) Chancroid is a sexually transmitted disease that is caused by *Haemophilus ducreyi*. It has a very short (1- to 5-day) incubation period. The primary lesion occurs on the genitalia and forms superficial or deep erosion with surrounding erythema and edema. Marked unilateral and regional lymphadenopathy are present and eventually suppurate, causing buboes in untreated cases. The organisms are arranged like "schools of fish" and are found on smears from active lesions. Treatment consists of a sulfonamide such as sulfisoxazole or third-generation cephalosporin.

Additional Reading: *Sauer's Manual of Skin Diseases,* 10th ed. Philadelphia, PA: Lippincott Williams & Wilkins; 2010:214–215.

Category: Reproductive system

25. The answer is C. (*Keratoacanthoma*) Keratoacanthoma (KA) is a rapidly growing hyperkeratotic nodule with a central keratin plug. A KA typically develops over 3 to 6 weeks, in contrast to the slow growth of typical squamous cell carcinomas (SCCs) over months to years. KAs occur most commonly in areas of sun-damaged skin. KAs are clinically and histologically indistinguishable from well-differentiated SCC. The etiology of KA is not certain, however; human papillomavirus DNA has been found in some cases. KAs have also occurred in skin soon after radiation therapy. Additionally, there are syndromes of multiple KAs developing over years. There is controversy regarding whether KAs are malignant or benign. Although they resemble SCCs histologically, most spontaneously regress with scar formation. There have been reported cases of invasive KAs, some with metastases, leading many experts to consider all KAs a form of SCC and treat them as such. Because of the uncertain malignant potential of KAs, most are treated as well-differentiated SCC.

Additional Reading: *Sauer's Manual of Skin Diseases,* 10th ed. Philadelphia, PA: Lippincott Williams & Wilkins; 2010:298.

Category: Integumentary

Keratoacanthoma (KA) is a rapidly growing hyperkeratotic nodule with a central keratin plug. A KA typically develops over 3 to 6 weeks, in contrast to the slow growth of typical squamous cell carcinomas over months to years.

26. The answer is B. (*Type B*) A flattened tympanogram is represented by choices B and is associated with fluid behind the TM or perforation of the TM.

Additional Reading: Etiology of hearing loss in adults. In: Basow DS, ed. *UpToDate.* Waltham, MA: UpToDate; 2013.

Category: Special sensory

27. The answer is A. (*Pityriasis rosea*) Pityriasis rosea is a common papulosquamous rash that occurs mainly on the trunks of young adults during the spring and fall. The condition begins with the onset of a "herald patch" that is oval and erythematous. Usually within 2 to 10 days, a generalized rash follows. The individual lesions have fine scaling noted around their edges. In many cases, a Christmas-tree pattern is seen over the back. The lesions may continue to appear for 2 to 3 weeks. Most cases resolve by 6 to 8 weeks. Pruritus is often present. The disease is not contagious. Treatment consists of oatmeal colloidal baths, calamine lotion, antihistamines, topical steroids, and ultraviolet-B treatments. Systemic steroids may be necessary for severe cases.

Additional Reading: *Sauer's Manual of Skin Diseases,* 10th ed. Philadelphia, PA: Lippincott Williams & Wilkins; 2010:164–168.

Category: Integumentary

28. The answer is D. (*Topical mupirocin ointment*) Impetigo is caused by group A β-hemolytic streptococci or *Staphylococcus aureus* and typically affects young children. The lesions begin as erythematous papules that expand to form crusted patches with a honey-brown appearance. More severe cases may cause bullae to form. The infection occurs more commonly around the nose and mouth and in the intertriginous areas; there are no constitutional symptoms. Examination is usually made on clinical presentation. Treatment for mild infections includes 2% topical mupirocin ointment. More severe cases respond to dicloxacillin, cephalexin, or erythromycin. Impetigo is highly contagious. Glomerulonephritis is a rare complication of impetigo that is caused by certain strains of *Streptococcus.*

Additional Reading: *Sauer's Manual of Skin Diseases,* 10th ed. Philadelphia, PA: Lippincott Williams & Wilkins; 2010:203–204.

Category: Integumentary

29. The answer is C. (*Lichen sclerosis*) Lichen sclerosis is caused by thinning of the vulvar skin and gives rise to itching and dyspareunia. Atrophy of the skin occurs and gives rise to a shiny whitish appearance. Diagnosis is accomplished with punch biopsy. A slight increase in squamous cell carcinoma has been found in areas that are affected with lichen sclerosis. Treatment consists of potent topical corticosteroids. In addition, a topical antifungal preparation should be used to prevent secondary yeast infections.

Additional Reading: *Sauer's Manual of Skin Diseases,* 10th ed. Philadelphia, PA: Lippincott Williams & Wilkins; 2010:365.

Category: Integumentary

30. The answer is A. (*Psoriasis*) Pitting of the nails is commonly associated with psoriasis. Erythematous scaly plaques are usually noted on other parts of the body. Thirty percent of patients with psoriasis have a positive family history for the condition. Men and women are affected equally. Other conditions that are related to nail pitting include alopecia areata and eczematous dermatitis. Chronic obstructive pulmonary disease is related to clubbing. Subungual hyperkeratosis is associated with onychomycosis.

Additional Reading: *Sauer's Manual of Skin Diseases,* 10th ed. Philadelphia, PA: Lippincott Williams & Wilkins; 2010:160–163.

Category: Integumentary

31. The answer is A. (*Yeast vaginitis*) Yeast vaginitis causes approximately one-third of all vaginal infections. Risk factors include pregnancy, diabetes, use of intrauterine devices, recent antibiotic use, immune deficiency, or corticosteroid use. Diagnosis is made by examination of a vaginal smear under high-power microscopy after potassium hydroxide has been added. Budding yeast and pseudohyphae are noted. Topical antifungals are effective, as are single-dose oral antifungals.

Additional Reading: Vaginitis: Diagnosis and Treatment. *Am Fam Physician.* 2011;83:807–815.

Category: Reproductive system

32. The answer is C. (*Herpes genitalis*) Tzanck smears are used in the diagnosis of herpes infections. The preparation detects multinucleated giant cells. A sample obtained from unroofed vesicles that have appeared within 24 hours provides the best specimen for diagnosis. A #15 blade is used to scrape the base of the vesicle, and the material is spread onto a slide and allowed to dry. Giemsa's, Wright's, or methylene blue is used to stain the cells. After staining, the sample is gently flooded with tap water to remove excess stain. Oil immersion is used for viewing with the microscope.

Additional Reading: *Goodheart's Photoguide to Common Skin Disorders: Diagnosis and Management,* 3rd ed. Philadelphia, PA: Wolters/Kluwer Lippincott Williams & Wilkins; 2009:328–331.

Category: Reproductive system

33. The answer is E. (*Tinea versicolor*) Tinea versicolor is a common skin infection caused by the organism *Pityrosporum orbiculare* (also known as *Malassezia furfur, Pityrosporum ovale,* or *Malassezia ovalis*). The condition usually affects adolescents and young adults in tropical environments. The organism is a yeast that is a constituent of the normal skin flora. A number of factors may trigger conversion to the mycelial or hyphal form that is associated with clinical disease, including hot and humid weather, use of topical oils, hyperhidrosis, and immunosuppression. Tinea versicolor usually responds to medical therapy, but recurrence is common, and long-term preventative treatment may be necessary. Versicolor refers to the variety and changing shades of colors present in this condition. Lesions can be hypopigmented, light brown, or salmon-colored macules. A fine scale is often noted, especially after scraping. Individual lesions are typically small, but frequently coalesce to form larger lesions. Typically the lesions are limited to the outer skin, most commonly on the upper trunk and extremities, and are less common on the face and intertriginous areas. Most patients are asymptomatic; however, some may complain of mild pruritus. The condition may occur in patients who are immunocompromised. It is most evident in the summer because the organism produces a substance that inhibits pigment transfer to keratinocytes, thus making infected skin more demarcated from uninfected, evenly pigmented skin. The diagnosis of tinea versicolor is made by microscopic examination of skin samples with 10% potassium hydroxide (KOH). Both hyphae and spores are evident in a pattern that is often described as "spaghetti and meatballs." The differential diagnosis includes seborrhea, eczema, pityriasis rosea, and secondary syphilis. Seborrheic lesions are more frequently located on the central trunk, are more erythematous, and have thicker scales. With eczema, patients usually have more scaling, pruritus, and involvement of the extremities. Patients with pityriasis usually have a herald patch, more peripheral scale around border lesions, and confinement of lesions to the central trunk, and the lesions do not show hyphae on KOH prep. Secondary syphilis usually involves the hands and feet, and the lesions do not show hyphae on KOH prep. Topical antifungal therapy given for 2 weeks is the treatment of choice for patients with mild and limited disease. Virtually any topical antiyeast preparation can be used with cure rates exceeding 70% to 80%. Patients should be informed that the healing process continues after the treatment is complete. A return to normal pigmentation may take months after the completion of successful treatment. Oral medications are more convenient for patients with extensive disease and may also be more effective in patients with recalcitrant infection. Most oral antifungal agents, with the exception of griseofulvin or terbinafine, may be used. Additionally, ketoconazole 2% shampoo in a single application or daily for 3 days may be considered as an option for treatment, especially with mild infections.

Additional Reading: Tinea versicolor. In: Basow DS, ed. *UpToDate.* Waltham, MA: UpToDate; 2013.

Category: Integumentary

34. The answer is B. (*Basal cell carcinoma*) The clinical presentation of basal cell carcinoma (BCC) can be divided into the following three groups:

1. *Nodular:* The most common form of BCC. It typically presents on the face as a pink or flesh-colored papule. The lesion usually has a pearly or translucent quality, and a telangiectatic vessel is frequently seen within the papule. Ulceration is frequent, and the term *rodent ulcer* refers to these ulcerated nodular BCCs.
2. *Superficial:* The second most common subtype. Superficial BCC is most likely to occur on the trunk of the affected patient. The lesion typically presents as a slightly scaly papule or plaque that is most often pale red in color; the lesion may be atrophic in the center and is usually surrounded with fine translucent micropapules. Men are more likely to be affected.
3. *Morpheaform:* Also known as sclerosing BCC, this is the least common subtype. These lesions are typically smooth, flesh-colored, or very lightly erythematous papules or plaques that are frequently atrophic; they usually have a firm or indurated quality with ill-defined borders. Some experts categorize morpheaform, infiltrative, and micronodular as "aggressive-growth" BCC because they behave similarly. Infiltrative and micronodular BCCs are less common than the morpheaform BCC.

Additional Reading: Epidemiology and clinical features of basal cell carcinoma. In: Basow DS, ed. *UpToDate.* Waltham, MA: UpToDate; 2013.

Category: Integumentary

35. The answer is B. (*Graves' disease*) Exophthalmos can be related to hyperthyroidism (i.e., Graves' disease). Patients with hyperthyroidism may report nervousness, tremor, weight loss, hair loss, palpitations, tachycardia, and muscle weakness. Pretibial myxedema is also seen in those with Graves' disease. The eye findings are related to edema and lymphoid infiltration of the orbital tissue. Unfortunately, exophthalmos usually does not resolve after treatment.

Additional Reading: Overview of the clinical manifestations of hyperthyroidism in adults. In: Basow DS, ed. *UpToDate*. Waltham, MA: UpToDate; 2013.

Category: Endocrine system

36. The answer is B. (*Erythema nodosum*) Erythema nodosum is an acute inflammatory reaction of the subcutaneous fat. Women between the ages of 20 and 30 years are most likely to be affected. Causes include use of oral contraceptives or sulfonamides, pregnancy, sarcoidosis, histoplasmosis, tuberculosis, inflammatory bowel disease, lymphoma, leukemia, Behçet's disease, and streptococcal infections. Up to 40% of cases may be idiopathic. Typically, the lesions begin as bright red, tender nodules. The lesions tend to occur bilaterally on the lower extremities and occasionally on the arms. Constitutional symptoms (fever, arthralgias, and malaise) may also be present. The lesions become dark brown or violaceous during the resolution phase. Spontaneous resolution occurs in 3 to 6 weeks after onset regardless of the cause. Treatment consists of symptomatic treatment, nonsteroidal anti-inflammatory drugs, and systemic corticosteroids once an infectious cause is ruled out.

Additional Reading: *Sauer's Manual of Skin Diseases*, 10th ed. Philadelphia, PA: Lippincott Williams & Wilkins; 2010: 134–135.

Category: Integumentary

> Erythema nodosum is an acute inflammatory reaction of the subcutaneous fat. Women between the ages of 20 and 30 years are most likely to be affected. Causes include use of oral contraceptives or sulfonamides, pregnancy, sarcoidosis, histoplasmosis, tuberculosis, inflammatory bowel disease, lymphoma, leukemia, Behçet's disease, and streptococcal infections. Up to 40% of cases may be idiopathic.

37. The answer is D. (*Neurofibromatosis*) Neurofibromatosis is also referred to as *von Recklinghausen's disease*. It is associated with autosomal-dominant inheritance and is characterized by multiple, macular, pigmented skin lesions called *café au lait spots* and skin tumors called *neurofibromas*. Axillary or inguinal freckling (Crowe's sign) is considered to be pathognomonic for neurofibromatosis. Ocular lesions (Lisch nodules) are asymptomatic, pigmented iris hamartomas that are seen in 80% of cases. The disease has been associated with defects on chromosomes 17 and 22. Neurofibromas may cause neurologic symptoms. Seizures, paraplegia, and mental retardation may occur secondary to the condition. Treatment consists of surgical removal of symptomatic or disfiguring lesions. Patients should be monitored for the development of neurofibrosarcomas, optic gliomas, acoustic neuromas, and pheochromocytomas. Those who are affected should also receive genetic counseling.

Additional Reading: *Goodheart's Photoguide to Common Skin Disorders: Diagnosis and Management*, 3rd ed. Philadelphia, PA: Wolters/Kluwer Lippincott Williams & Wilkins; 2009:491–492.

Category: Nonspecific system

38. The answer is C. (*Atopic dermatitis*) Atopic dermatitis is also referred to as *atopic eczema*. The condition is associated with erythematous pruritic areas that occur in association with hay fever, asthma, allergic rhinitis, or allergic sinusitis. The flexor surfaces are commonly involved. The course is variable with flares and remissions. The condition affects children and adults. The diagnosis is made based on history and clinical presentation. Treatment consists of topical steroids, antihistamines, tar baths and ointments, and Burrow's solution. Severe cases may require systemic steroids, cyclosporine, or phototherapy.

Additional Reading: *Sauer's Manual of Skin Diseases*, 10th ed. Philadelphia, PA: Lippincott Williams & Wilkins; 2010:117–123.

Category: Integumentary

39. The answer is D. (*Excisional biopsy*) Malignant melanoma lesions are treated with surgical excision. Biopsies must include epidermis, dermis, and subcutaneous fat. Shave biopsy should not be done. Knowledge of depth of invasion is essential for proper staging and treatment. Melanoma in situ (epidermal only) should be removed with margins of 0.5 cm. Melanoma that is <1.5 mm deep should be removed with a margin of 1 cm. Lesions that are 1.51 to 4 mm deep should have 1- to 2-cm margins. Lesions deeper than 4 mm should have a margin of 2 to 3 cm. Lymph node dissection is indicated if metastasis is suspected or if the lesion is of intermediate depth. Sentinel node biopsy is increasingly used in patients with proven melanoma that is >1 mm deep.

Additional Reading: *Sauer's Manual of Skin Diseases*, 10th ed. Philadelphia, PA: Lippincott Williams & Wilkins; 2010: 313–315.

Category: Integumentary

40. The answer is A. (*Trichophyton rubrum*) Onychomycosis is usually caused by *Trichophyton rubrum*. Diagnosis is generally made by clinical presentation; however, fungal elements can be confirmed with observation under a microscope using potassium hydroxide 10% preparation of nail plate scales. Nail clippings can also be used for culture.

Additional Reading: *Sauer's Manual of Skin Diseases*, 10th ed. Philadelphia, PA: Lippincott Williams & Wilkins; 2010:347–350.

Category: Integumentary

41. The answer is B. (*Psoriasis*) Psoriasis typically involves the scalp (including the postauricular regions), the extensor surface of the extremities (particularly elbows and knees), the sacral area, buttocks, and penis. The nails, eyebrows, axillae, umbilicus, or anogenital region may also be affected. Occasionally, the disease is generalized. Typical lesions are well demarcated, variously pruritic, ovoid or circular, erythematous papules or plaques covered with overlapping thick silver appearing, slightly opalescent shiny scales. Papules sometimes extend and coalesce to produce large plaques in annular patterns. The lesions heal without scarring, and hair growth is usually unaltered. Nail involvement occurs in 30% to 50% of patients and may clinically resemble a fungal infection, with stippling, pitting, fraying, discoloration or separation of the distal and lateral margins of the nail plate (onycholysis), and thickening, with hyperkeratotic material under the nail plate.

Additional Reading: Psoriasis. *Am Fam Physician*. 2013;87(9): 626–633.

Category: Integumentary

42. The answer is D. (*Neurofibromatosis*) Café au lait skin lesions are seen in neurofibromatosis. The lesions are medium-brown freckle-like macules distributed most commonly over the trunk, pelvis, and flexor creases of elbows and knees; they are present at birth or develop in infancy in >90% of all patients.

> **Additional Reading:** Neurofibromatosis Type 1. In: Domino F, ed. *The 5-Minute Clinical Consult.* Philadelphia, PA: Lippincott Williams and Wilkins; 2014.

> Category: Nonspecific system

43. The answer is B. (*Arterial ulcer*) Arterial ulcers are usually caused by atherosclerosis in the elderly. Men are more commonly affected. Pain is common, as is claudication. Distinguishing features of arterial ulcers are their sharply defined borders and round, punched-out appearance. They tend to be smaller than venous ulcers and are usually deep enough to expose muscle or tendons. Commonly affected sites include the toes, pretibial areas, and dorsum of the feet. Patients may have signs of livedo reticularis, pallor, and cyanosis. The legs may feel cold and clammy. Decreased peripheral pulses are commonly noted. Treatment consists of alleviating underlying risk factors. Pentoxifylline can be used in some cases. Surgical evaluation should be considered.

> **Additional Reading:** Arterial Ulcer Checklist. *Advances in Skin & Wound Care:* 2010;23(9):432.

> Category: Cardiovascular system

44. The answer is B. (*Cylindromas*) Cylindromas appear as numerous smooth, rounded tumors that occur in various sizes on the scalp. They have the appearance of a group of grapes. Rarely, the tumors cover the entire scalp and are referred to as *turban tumors.* Cylindromas are considered benign and can be observed.

> **Additional Reading:** *Sauer's Manual of Skin Diseases,* 10th ed. Philadelphia, PA: Lippincott Williams & Wilkins; 2010:300.

> Category: Integumentary

45. The answer is E. (*Synovial cyst*) A synovial cyst appears as a translucent, pea-sized cyst that commonly forms adjacent to the joints of the fingers. The cysts form as a result of small tracts that lead from the synovial space of joints to the surface of the skin. The fluid contained is synovial fluid. Occasionally, the cysts resolve spontaneously. Aspiration can be attempted, but care must be taken not to introduce infection into the joint. Compression of the area after aspiration may help to prevent recurrence.

> **Additional Reading:** *Sauer's Manual of Skin Diseases,* 10th ed. Philadelphia, PA: Lippincott Williams & Wilkins; 2010:288.

> Category: Musculoskeletal system

46. The answer is C. (*Human immunodeficiency syndrome*) Oral hairy leukoplakia is a marker for human immunodeficiency syndrome and is thought to be caused by the Epstein–Barr virus. The condition appears as white plaques that have the look of corrugated cardboard. The lesions are fixed and not friable and appear on the lateral surface of the tongue. Although the condition rarely causes symptoms, burning of the tongue can occur. Treatment consists of acyclovir, topical tretinoin, and podophyllin. Oral hairy leukoplakia can be distinguished from oral candidiasis by the fact that the latter scrapes off easily with a tongue blade. Oral candidiasis typically affects the dorsal aspect of the tongue and buccal mucosa.

> **Additional Reading:** *Sauer's Manual of Skin Diseases,* 10th ed. Philadelphia, PA: Lippincott Williams & Wilkins; 2010:240–245.

> Category: Nonspecific system

47. The answer is D. (*Varicella*) Varicella (chickenpox) is described as "dew drops on rose petals" in its appearance. The lesions are red macules that progress rapidly from papules to vesicles, pustules, and then crusted lesions. The lesions are intensely pruritic. Lesions affect the entire body and oral mucosa, especially the palate. A characteristic feature is multiple lesions in varying stages of development and healing. A Tzanck smear can be helpful in confirming the diagnosis. Treatment is usually supportive, but can include the use of acyclovir. Aspirin should be avoided because of the risk of developing Reye's syndrome. Varicella vaccine is recommended for all children at 12 to 18 months of age.

> **Additional Reading:** *Goodheart's Photoguide to Common Skin Disorders: Diagnosis and Management,* 3rd ed. Philadelphia, PA: Wolters/Kluwer Lippincott Williams & Wilkins; 2009:194–196.

> Category: Nonspecific system

> Varicella (chickenpox) is described as "dew drops on rose petals" in its appearance. The lesions are red macules that progress rapidly from papules to vesicles, pustules, and then crusted lesions.

48. The answer is D. (*Cherry angiomas*) Cherry angiomas are common asymptomatic lesions that appear red in color and blanch with pressure. The diagnosis is clinical. They are more common in elderly patients. They occur more commonly on the trunk and are benign.

> **Additional Reading:** *Field Guide to Clinical Dermatology.* Philadelphia, PA: Lippincott Williams & Wilkins; 1999:120–121.

> Category: Integumentary

49. The answer is A. (*Varicella*) The manifestations of varicella in most children generally develop within 15 days after the exposure, and typically include a prodrome of fever, malaise, or pharyngitis, followed by the development of a generalized vesicular rash, usually within 24 hours. The lesions are commonly pruritic and appear as groups of vesicles over a 3- to 4-day period. The patient with varicella typically has lesions in different stages of development on the face, trunk, and extremities. New lesion formation generally stops within 4 days, and most lesions have fully crusted by day 6 in normal hosts.

> **Additional Reading:** Clinical features of varicella-zoster virus infection: chickenpox. *Up to Date, April 2013.*

> Category: Nonspecific system

50. The answer is A. (*Lupus pernio*) Lupus pernio is associated with chronic sarcoidosis and consists of indurated plaques associated with discoloration of the nose, cheeks, lips, and ears. The lesion is more common in African American women. The nasal mucosa is frequently involved. Lupus pernio is often associated with bone cysts and pulmonary fibrosis. The course of the disease with lupus pernio is prolonged; spontaneous remissions are rare.

> **Additional Reading:** Sarcoid: Muscle, bone, and vascular disease manifestations. *Up to Date, August 2010.*

> Category: Nonspecific system

51. The answer is A. (*Hidradenitis suppurativa*) Hidradenitis suppurativa is a painful, erythematous, and nodular condition that affects the axilla, genitalia, and perianal areas. Hallmarks for the disease include open comedones, enlarged follicular orifices, and scarring. Nodules become inflamed and pus filled, rupture, drain pus and blood, and then cause scarring. Sinus tracts can form. The disease often waxes and wanes. *Staphylococcus* bacteria are frequently the causative agent. Treatment consists of appropriate antibacterial agents based on culture and sensitivities. Intralesional corticosteroids can also be used to reduce the inflammatory response. For severe cases, excision and skin grafting may be necessary. The condition may regress as the patient approaches middle age.

Additional Reading: Hidradenitis suppurativa. In: Domino F, ed. *The 5-Minute Clinical Consult.* Philadelphia, PA: Lippincott Williams and Wilkins; 2014.

Category: Integumentary

52. The answer is D. (*Vitiligo*) Vitiligo is a disorder associated with depigmentation of the skin that is thought to be related to an autoimmune-mediated loss of melanocytes. Fifty percent of those who are affected have a family history of vitiligo. The lesions appear as hypopigmented chalk-white lesions and are more obvious on people who have dark complexions. The condition is bilateral and symmetric in appearance and typically forms around orifices (i.e., mouth, eyes, nose, and anus). Vitiligo is often cyclical. Some may experience partial repigmentation. Diagnosis is made clinically. A Wood's light examination reveals a "milk-white" fluorescence over the lesion. Treatment is limited, but includes potent topical steroids, psoralen plus ultraviolet A photochemotherapy, minigrafting, and cosmetics to hide areas.

Additional Reading: *Sauer's Manual of Skin Diseases,* 10th ed. Philadelphia, PA: Lippincott Williams & Wilkins; 2010:381–382.

Category: Integumentary

53. The answer is B. (*Melasma*) Melasma, also referred to as *chloasma,* is described as the "mask of pregnancy." The condition typically affects women with dark complexions and appears as hyperpigmentation of the skin, usually associated with the face. It is caused by long-term sun exposure, pregnancy, and oral contraceptives. In many cases, the condition is idiopathic. Diagnosis is made clinically. Treatment involves the use of bleaching creams, hydroquinone, and chemical peels for more resistant cases. In some instances, the condition disappears after pregnancy or the discontinuation of oral contraceptives.

Additional Reading: *Sauer's Manual of Skin Diseases,* 10th ed. Philadelphia, PA: Lippincott Williams & Wilkins; 2010:380–381.

Category: Integumentary

54. The answer is D. (*Rubeola*) Rubeola, or measles, is caused by a ribonucleic acid virus that invades the respiratory epithelium of the oropharynx. Transmission occurs via a respiratory aerosol route. The condition begins with a respiratory illness prodrome (cough, coryza, and conjunctivitis—the "3 Cs") followed by discrete erythematous macules and papules that coalesce. Pruritus is usually absent. The rash lasts for up to a week and resolves with desquamation. Koplik's spots are described as 1-mm bluish-white macules that form on the oral mucosa (especially the buccal mucosa opposite the molars) 2 days before the onset of the generalized rash. The rash typically begins on the forehead or behind the ears and then spreads centrally to involve the face, trunk, arms, and legs. Pneumonia is the most common complication. No specific therapy is indicated for measles.

Most cases resolve within 2 weeks. Vitamin A may decrease morbidity and mortality in severe cases. Immunization is recommended for all children who are 15 months or older.

Additional Reading: Clinical presentation and diagnosis of measles. In: Basow DS, ed. *UpToDate.* Waltham, MA: UpToDate; 2013.

Category: Nonspecific system

55. The answer is B. (*Coxsackievirus*) Hand-foot-and-mouth disease is caused by coxsackievirus A16. Outbreaks commonly affect children 1 to 5 years of age during the summer or early fall. Transmission occurs via a fecal–oral route. The rash appears as shallow erosions that affect the oral mucosa. The lesions are painful and can interfere with eating. The oral lesions are followed by an exanthem that consists of oval or angulated fluid-filled vesicles that form on the palms and soles. In contrast to most viral illnesses, lymphadenopathy is minimal or absent. The diagnosis is made clinically. Cultures to confirm the infection can be obtained from the throat or stool. Treatment is supportive.

Additional Reading: Clinical manifestations and diagnosis of enterovirus and parechovirus infections. In: Basow DS, ed. *UpToDate.* Waltham, MA: UpToDate; 2013.

Category: Nonspecific system

56. The answer is D. (*Inferior ischemia*) The inferior surface of the heart is usually supplied by the right coronary artery (right dominant coronary circulation). Occasionally, the inferior aspect is supplied by the circumflex artery, which branches to form the posterior descending artery (left dominant coronary circulation). Arterial occlusion related to the right coronary artery gives rise to inferior ischemic changes noted on ECG. These findings include ST-segment depression in leads II, III, and aVF.

Additional Reading: Electrocardiogram in the diagnosis of myocardial ischemia and infarction. In: Basow DS, ed. *UpToDate.* Waltham, MA: UpToDate; 2013.

Category: Cardiovascular system

> Arterial occlusion related to the right coronary artery gives rise to inferior ischemic changes noted on ECG. These findings include ST-segment depression in leads II, III, and aVF.

57. The answer is D. (*Ventricular tachycardia*) Ventricular tachycardia (VT) is defined as three or more successive ventricular complexes. Nonsustained VT is a series of repetitive ventricular beats that have a duration of <30 seconds, whereas sustained VT lasts >30 seconds. Typically, the rate of VT is >100 beats per minute, but may vary significantly. The rhythm is usually regular, although there may be slight irregularity of the R–R intervals. The morphology of the QRS complex during VT is usually different when compared with the sinus beat. The QRS axis is typically shifted, often to the left but occasionally to the right. The width of the QRS complex is generally >0.16 seconds. The VT is monomorphic when all of the QRS complexes of an episode are identical. When the QRS complexes show markedly different morphologies, the VT is said to be polymorphic and the R–R intervals may be grossly irregular.

Additional Reading: ECG tutorial: ventricular arrhythmias. In: Basow DS, ed. *UpToDate.* Waltham, MA: UpToDate; 2013.

Category: Cardiovascular system

58. The answer is A. (*Poison ivy*) Intense pruritus and erythema are the most common presenting signs of poison ivy dermatitis. Patients develop papules, vesicles, and/or bullae, often arranged in characteristic linear or streak-like patterns where the plant has made contact with the skin. Symptoms of poison ivy in sensitized individuals generally develop within 4 to 96 hours after exposure and peak between 1 and 14 days after exposure. New lesions can present up to 21 days after exposure in previously unexposed individuals. Lesions may occur at different points in time depending on the degree of exposure to different points on the skin and the thickness of the exposed skin. This may give the impression that the poison ivy is spreading from one region to another. Blister fluid is not antigenic and is not responsible for spreading the rash. Patients may, occasionally, carry the dried antigenic resin on clothing or under fingernails, thus spreading their own dermatitis or exposing household or other contacts. Without treatment, poison ivy dermatitis usually resolves in 1 to 3 weeks. The most common complication of poison ivy dermatitis is secondary bacterial infection of the skin with *Staphylococcus aureus* or β-hemolytic group A *Streptococcus*. Bacterial infections can be polymicrobial.

> **Additional Reading:** Diagnosis and management of contact dermatitis. *Am Fam Physician.* 2010;82(3):249–255.

> **Category:** Integumentary

59. The answer is E. (*Ventricular tachycardia*) Ventricular tachycardia (VT) is a potentially life-threatening event. ECG changes show wide QRS complexes with no discernible P waves. The rate is >120 bpm. The patient may report palpitations, dizziness, or syncope, or circulatory collapse may occur. Asymptomatic (isolated) VT is usually not treated. Sustained VT can degenerate to ventricular fibrillation. Hypotensive VT requires immediate treatment with synchronized direct current (DC) shock. Lidocaine is used for drug treatment. Antiarrhythmics may be needed to prevent recurrent VT.

> **Additional Reading:** Monomorphic ventricular tachycardia in the absence of apparent structural heart disease. In: Basow DS, ed. *UpToDate.* Waltham, MA: UpToDate; 2013.

> **Category:** Cardiovascular system

60. The answer is B. (*Atrial fibrillation*) Atrial fibrillation (AF) is frequently seen in the offices of family physicians. ECG findings include the absence of obvious P waves and the irregularly irregular response of QRS complexes. Intra-atrial contractions may show rates of >350 bpm. The ventricular rate may vary depending on the atrioventricular nodal conduction, but typically is elevated. Treatment involves the management of underlying causative disorders, control of ventricular rate, restoration of sinus rhythm if possible, and prevention of systemic emboli.

> **Additional Reading:** Overview of atrial fibrillation. In: Basow DS, ed. *UpToDate.* Waltham, MA: UpToDate; 2013.

> **Category:** Cardiovascular system

61. The answer is B. (*Supraventricular tachycardia*) Supraventricular tachycardia is often referred to as *narrow complex tachycardia*. The condition is characterized by sustained tachyarrhythmia with a QRS complex that appears normal and has a duration > 120 msec. Patients whose condition is unstable should receive immediate synchronized cardioversion. Those who are hemodynamically stable can be treated with vagal maneuvers (Valsalva, cough, carotid massage), adenosine, verapamil, or diltiazem. One should make sure that the patient does not have ventricular tachycardia because calcium channel blockers are contraindicated.

> **Additional Reading:** Clinical manifestations, diagnosis, and evaluation of narrow QRS complex tachycardias. In: Basow DS, ed. *UpToDate.* Waltham, MA: UpToDate; 2013.

> **Category:** Cardiovascular system

62. The answer is B. (*Ventricular tachycardia*) Ventricular tachycardia (VT) is a potentially life-threatening event. ECG changes show wide QRS complexes with no discernible P waves. Hypotensive VT requires immediate treatment with synchronized DC shock. Lidocaine is used for drug treatment. Antiarrhythmics may be needed to prevent recurrent VT.

> **Additional Reading:** ECG tutorial: ventricular arrhythmias. In: Basow DS, ed. *UpToDate.* Waltham, MA: UpToDate; 2013.

> **Category:** Cardiovascular system

63. The answer is B. (*Wolff–Parkinson–White syndrome*) Wolff–Parkinson–White (WPW) syndrome is caused by an accessory pathway that links the atria and ventricles, bypassing the atrioventricular node. The ECG shows a short PR interval and slurred upstroke at the beginning of the QRS complex known as a *delta wave* (best seen in V_2, V_3, and V_4). Antegrade and retrograde conduction both occur, causing a reciprocating tachycardia. AF in the setting of WPW can be a medical emergency. Ventricular rates can be excessive and lead to ventricular fibrillation. DC cardioversion should be considered when AF is present in the setting of WPW.

> **Additional Reading:** Epidemiology, clinical manifestations, and diagnosis of the Wolff–Parkinson–White syndrome. In: Basow DS, ed. *UpToDate.* Waltham, MA: UpToDate; 2013.

> **Category:** Cardiovascular system

64. The answer is B. (*Fluid in the middle ear*) Tympanograms can help assist in the diagnosis of middle ear–related problems. A flat tympanometric pattern is typical of fluid within the middle ear. The ear volume is normal, but the mobility is greatly reduced.

> **Additional Reading:** Tympanometry. *Am Fam Physician.* 2004;70(9):1713–1720.

> **Category:** Special sensory

65. The answer is C. (*Atrial fibrillation*) Atrial fibrillation (AF) is characterized by rapid and irregular atrial fibrillatory waves at a rate of 350 to 600 impulses/min. This is accompanied by the presence of normal atrioventricular (AV) nodal conduction, with an irregularly irregular ventricular response of 90 up to 140 to 170 bpm; however, the rate may be higher in some patients. AF in patients with intact AV nodal conduction is associated with the following characteristics on ECG tracings: P waves are absent; fibrillatory or f waves are present at a rate that is generally between 350 and 600 bpm; the f waves typically vary in amplitude, morphology, and intervals; the R–R intervals are irregularly irregular; the ventricular rate usually ranges from 90 to 170 bpm. Ventricular rates <60 bpm are seen with AV nodal disease, drugs that affect conduction, and high vagal tone as can occur in a well-conditioned athlete. Ventricular rates >200 bpm suggest catecholamine excess, parasympathetic withdrawal, or the existence of an accessory bypass tract as occurs in the preexcitation syndrome. The QRS complexes are narrow unless AV conduction is abnormal due to functional (rate-related) aberration, preexisting bundle branch or fascicular block, or preexcitation with ventricular activation via an accessory pathway.

Additional Reading: Overview of atrial fibrillation. In: Basow DS, ed. *UpToDate*. Waltham, MA: UpToDate; 2013.

Category: Cardiovascular system

> ⟳ Atrial fibrillation in patients with intact AV nodal conduction is associated with the following characteristics on ECG tracings: P waves are absent; fibrillatory or f waves are present at a rate that is generally between 350 and 600 bpm; the f waves typically vary in amplitude, morphology, and intervals; the R–R intervals are irregularly irregular; the ventricular rate usually ranges from 90 to 170 bpm.

66. The answer is E. (*Wolff–Parkinson–White syndrome*) The two major features of Wolff–Parkinson–White (WPW) syndrome include a short PR interval (<0.12 second) and a delta wave. The QRS is wide (>0.12 second) and is considered a fusion beat. The initial part of the delta wave results from rapid depolarization of the accessory pathway. Termination of ventricular depolarization is through the normal activation pathway and gives rise to a normal-appearing terminal portion of the QRS complex.

Additional Reading: Epidemiology, clinical manifestations, and diagnosis of the Wolff–Parkinson–White syndrome. In: Basow DS, ed. *UpToDate*. Waltham, MA: UpToDate; 2013.

Category: Cardiovascular system

67. The answer is E. (*Reasurrance*) A normal tympanogram curve is peaked, indicating normal mobility of the TM. The peak compliance occurs at a pressure of −10 mm H_2O (normal = +100 mm H_2O to −150 mm H_2O).

Additional Reading: Tympanometry. *Am Fam Physician*. 2004;70(9):1713–1720.

Category: Special sensory

68. The answer is A. (*Eustachian tube dysfunction*) Eustachian tube dysfunction gives rise to a tympanogram that has a normal compliance curve, but the curve is shifted to the left, indicating a negative pressure in the middle ear. The peak occurs at −200 mm H_2O.

Additional Reading: Tympanometry. *Am Fam Physician*. 2004;70(9):1713–1720.

Category: Special sensory

69. The answer is C. (*Erythrasma*) Erythrasma looks very much like tinea cruris. It can affect the groin, axilla, and webs of the toes. The condition is caused by *Corynebacterium minutissimum*. The area affected fluoresces a bright reddish orange under a Wood's light. The treatment is oral or topical erythromycin.

Additional Reading: *Sauer's Manual of Skin Diseases*, 10th ed. Philadelphia, PA: Lippincott Williams & Wilkins; 2010: 209–210.

Category: Integumentary

70. The answer is B. (*Cutaneous larva migrans*) Cutaneous larva migrans is also called the *creeping eruption*. The causative agent is a hookworm (*Ancylostoma duodenale* and *Necator americanus*). The organisms are found in the feces of dogs, cats, cattle, and monkeys. The larvae penetrate human skin (usually the feet after walking barefoot). The condition is more common in gardeners, sea bathers, plumbers, and farmers. The lesion presents as a thin erythematous, serpiginous, raised tunnellike lesion. The larva die in 4 to 6 weeks; thus, the eruption is typically benign and self-limited. Treatment consists of topical steroids, topical or oral thiabendazole, albendazole, or liquid nitrogen.

Additional Reading: Acute Pruritic Rash on the Foot. *Am Fam Physician*. 2010;81(2):203–204.

Category: Integumentary

Study Grid

Category (approximate % of the general examination questions)	Wrong answer	Type of test-taking "error"			
		Did not read all of the question/ or choices	Didn't use keywords	Lured by a distractor	Guessed w/o using partial knowledge
Nonspecific system (10%)					
Nephrologic system (2%)					
Respiratory system (10%)					
Cardiovascular system (10%)					
Endocrine system (7%)					
Neurologic (2%)					
Integumentary (5%)					
Gastroenterology system (5%)					
Musculoskeletal system (10%)					
Psychogenic (5%)					
Hematologic system (2%)					
Special sensory (2%)					
Patient/population-based care (7%)					
Reproductive system (5%)					

Index